1 MONTH OF
FREE
READING

at

www.ForgottenBooks.com

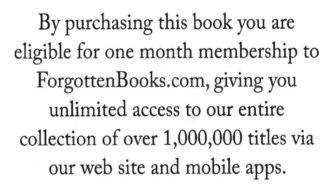

By purchasing this book you are
eligible for one month membership to
ForgottenBooks.com, giving you
unlimited access to our entire
collection of over 1,000,000 titles via
our web site and mobile apps.

To claim your free month visit:

www.forgottenbooks.com/free974258

ISBN 978-0-260-82901-6
PIBN 10974258

For support please visit www.forgottenbooks.com

SURGICAL DISEASES AND INJURIES OF THE GENITO-URINARY ORGANS

Surgical Diseases and Injuries of the Genito-Urinary Organs

By

J. W. Thomson Walker

M.B., C.M.Ed., F.R.C.S.Eng.

Hunterian Professor of Surgery and Pathology, Royal College of Surgeons
of England (1907); Surgeon to the Hampstead General and North-West
London Hospital; Assistant-Surgeon to St. Peter's Hospital for Stone;
Urinary Surgeon to the Radium Institute.

With 24 Colour and 21 Black-and-White
Plates, and 279 Illustrations in the Text

Cassell and Company, Ltd

London, New York, Toronto and Melbourne

1914

PREFACE

In the following pages I have given an account of the diseases and injuries of the urinary system, and of the male genital system, which I hope will prove of value to members of the profession engaged in general practice, and may also assist those on the threshold of a surgical career.

A textbook should reflect the current opinion of the day, and should at the same time bear the impress of the experience and individual views of the author. I have endeavoured to give each its proper place in this volume.

For the benefit of those anxious to obtain a more extensive knowledge of any subject, a few references to recent articles from the literature of different countries have been provided. Many valuable articles have of necessity been omitted from these lists, but references to these may be obtained through the channels I have quoted.

In writing these pages I have drawn largely on my own experience and have referred to many personal cases. Many procedures which are of merely historical interest have been omitted, and space has thus been found for a more adequate discussion of modern methods.

The claims of a pathological as opposed to an anatomical classification of diseases have received full consideration.

I decided to retain the anatomical classification for the reason that this work lays no claim to be a purely scientific treatise on the diseases of the genito-urinary organs, but is intended to serve as an aid to clinical work; and my personal experience of using textbooks arranged in the anatomical and in the pathological classification is that it is easier to refer to the former in an obscure case than to the latter.

In recent works there is observable a tendency to slur over the science and to make prominent the art of urinary surgery. With this I am not in sympathy. It is, I believe, impossible to carry out good work on a superficial knowledge of the pathological conditions with which the surgeon has to deal.

The pathology given in the following pages is not the pathology of the post-mortem room. It is the living pathology met with by the surgeon in the operating theatre, and, as such, is of vital importance to proper treatment.

Special attention has been paid to both the immediate and the late results of operation, and, whenever possible, reliable statistics in regard to these have been given. This will, I hope, prove of value to the practitioner in considering the question of prognosis.

The illustrations, with very few exceptions, are from cases that have been under my care, or from specimens that have been removed by operation.

Professor A. R. Ferguson, of Cairo, generously provided a series of beautiful microscopical sections illustrating bilharziosis, from which Figs. 121, 122, and 123 were drawn. To him and to Professor F. C. Madden, who also helped me in this section, I wish to express my warmest thanks.

The cystoscopic drawings are, I believe, of exceptional value. They were obtained direct from the patient, and are chosen from a large collection made during a number of years. For these and for many other illustrations I have to thank the patience and skill of Mr. Thornton Shiells. To Dr. G. Dupuy my thanks are due for his skilful realism in drawing the illustrations of operations.

I have to express my gratitude to my friend Sydney G. MacDonald, F.R.C.S., who undertook the arduous task of reading proofs, and to whom I am indebted for many valuable suggestions.

To my publishers I offer my especial thanks for the generous enthusiasm with which my suggestions in regard to the illustrations of the volume were adopted, and for their forbearance in many delays.

J. W. THOMSON WALKER.

January, 1914.

CONTENTS

Part I.—The Kidney

CONTENTS

Part II.—The Ureter

Part III.—The Bladder

Part IV.—The Urethra

Part V.—The Prostate

Part VI.—The Seminal Vesicles and Cowper's Glands

CONTENTS

Part VII.—The Testicle

LIST OF PLATES

xiii

LIST OF PLATES

LIST OF PLATES

SURGICAL DISEASES AND INJURIES OF THE GENITO-URINARY ORGANS

PART I.—THE KIDNEY

CHAPTER I

SURGICAL ANATOMY

Situation of the kidney.—The kidneys lie obliquely on the posterior wall of the abdomen, the upper end of each being 2½ cm., the hilum 3½ cm., and the lower pole 4 cm. from the middle-line. The anterior surface has an antero-external aspect.

The upper border of the kidney corresponds to the middle of the 11th dorsal vertebra, and the lower border to the lower border of the transverse process of the 3rd lumbar vertebra about 5 cm. above the iliac crest. The left kidney reaches to the upper border of the same process. The hilum of the kidney corresponds to the 2nd lumbar vertebra. The upper two-thirds of the kidney lies under cover of the 11th and 12th ribs, the lower one-third descends below them. The 12th rib may, rarely, be absent; it may be short and only come into relation with a small part of the posterior surface of the kidney, or it may be long and project beyond it. A short 12th rib, less than 7 cm. long, is always horizontal; a longer rib is oblique.

Relations of the kidney (Figs. 1, 2).—The posterior relations are the diaphragm, and the anterior layer of the transversalis aponeurosis which separates it from the quadratus lumborum muscle. A strong process of this aponeurosis, the costo-vertebral ligament, reaches from the tips of the transverse processes of the 1st and 2nd lumbar vertebræ to the 12th rib. Between the fibres of origin of the diaphragm from the external arcuate ligament and the 12th rib the pleura is uncovered and comes into relation with the kidney. The psoas muscle is also

B

related to a small part of the kidney at its lower pole. The more important structures met with in exposing the kidney from the lumbar aspect are as follows : the skin, subcutaneous fascia and fat, the latissimus dorsi muscle and the external oblique, the serratus posticus inferior, internal oblique, the lumbar fascia, the 12th intercostal nerve and vessels, the perirenal fascia and perirenal fat.

The anterior surface of the right kidney is covered by peritoneum along the outer border and upper part of its surface. At the upper part it is in relation to the under surface of the right

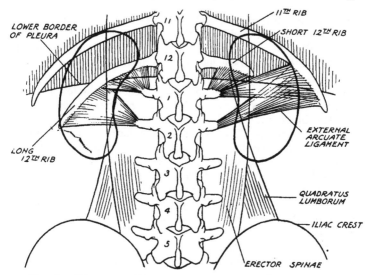

Fig. 1.—Diagram of the general relations of the kidneys.

lobe of the liver and internally to the vena cava. The hepatic flexure of the colon crosses the lower one-third and is adherent to it. In this situation a nephro-colic ligament has been described. The descending part of the duodenum is in direct contact with an area along the inner border, and the common bile-duct is in close relation to the inner border of the organ. In relation to the anterior surface of the left kidney, and separated from it by peritoneum, are the stomach and spleen, the former lying in contact with the upper pole and the latter with an area along the outer border. Below the stomach area the tail of the pancreas and the splenic artery are in contact with the kidney. The duodeno-jejunal junction is related to the inner border at the region of the hilum. Below this the splenic flexure of the colon crosses the kidney and passes down its outer border, and the left colic artery lies upon its anterior surface. It is attached to the diaphragm above and outside the kidney by the phreno-colic ligament. At the lower pole, in the angle formed by the flexure of the colon, the coils of small intestine are separated from the kidney by peritoneum.

The suprarenal capsules are in contact with the upper pole of each kidney and attached to it by areolar tissue. The connection is not very firm in normal kidneys, and diminishes with age ; in disease of the kidney it may be densely adherent.

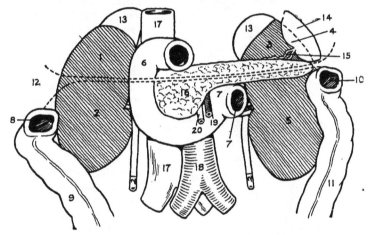

Fig. 2.—Diagram of the anterior relations of the kidneys.

1 and 2, Peritoneum-covered surface of right kidney in apposition with liver and with small intestine ; 3 and 5, peritoneum-covered surface of left kidney in apposition with stomach, with spleen, and with small intestine ; 6, duodenum ; 7, duodeno-jejunal junction ; 8, hepatic flexure of colon ; 9, ascending colon ; 10, splenic flexure ; 11, descending colon ; 12, attachment of transverse mesocolon ; 13, suprarenals ; 14, gastric surface of spleen ; 15, splenic vessels ; 16, pancreas ; 17, inferior vena cava ; 18, aorta ; 19, superior mesenteric artery ; 20, superior mesenteric vein ; 21, ureters.

Investment of the kidney.—The kidney lies embedded in a layer of fine fat, the fatty capsule, contained in a fascial envelope, the fascia propria or perirenal fascia. (Figs. 3, 4.) The perirenal fascia appears between the transversalis fascia and peritoneum, and divides into an anterior and a posterior layer at the border of the kidney. · The anterior layer covers the front of the kidney and crosses the middle line to join the corresponding layer of the opposite side, passing in front of the abdominal aorta and inferior vena cava. A thin layer splits off at the hilum and covers the renal blood-vessels. The posterior layer, or fascia of Zucker-kandl, lies behind the kidney, and, after sending a layer to the renal vessels, passes on to be attached to the sides of the bodies of the vertebræ. At the upper pole of the kidney the layers unite after having enclosed the suprarenal capsule, and are attached to the under surface of the diaphragm, forming a suspensory ligament. At the lower pole the anterior layer is continued onwards, lining the peritoneum, and the posterior layer is gradually lost in the extraperitoneal fat without uniting with the anterior layer.

The perirenal fascia thus forms an envelope which is open on its internal and inferior aspects. It is strengthened by an additional covering of fascia, the fascia of Toldt, which is distributed between the fascia propria and the hepatic flexure of the colon and the descending part of the duodenum on the right side, and the splenic flexure of the colon on the left side.

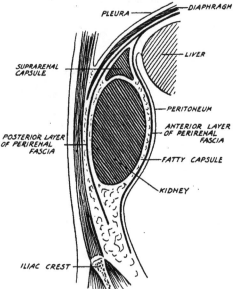

Fig. 3.—Diagram of the arrangement of the perirenal fascia in vertical section.

The kidney is immediately surrounded by a fine layer of fibrous tissue in which are some non-striped muscle fibres. This capsule passes in at the hilum to become continuous with the outer layer of the pelvis of the kidney, and also invests the renal vessels. The capsule is easily stripped from the kidney as far as the hilum.

From the outer surface of this capsule a network of fine fibres passes out in all directions to the perirenal fascia. In the meshes of this is deposited a layer of fine yellow fat—the fatty capsule—forming a bed in which the kidney lies. This layer is thicker over the posterior and outer aspects of the kidney. It does not exist before the tenth year.

Structures at the hilum. The renal pelvis (Fig. 5).—At the level of the lower end of the kidney the ureter begins to expand into a trumpet-shaped extremity which passes the hilum

and enters the sinus of the kidney. This is the renal pelvis. At
the junction with the ureter a narrow part may frequently be

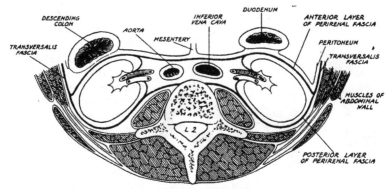

Fig. 4.—Diagram of the arrangement of the perirenal fascia in
transverse section at the level of the 2nd lumbar vertebra.

seen. As it passes upwards the pelvis usually separates into
two primary divisions—a smaller upper and a larger lower branch
—and each of these separates into three or more subdivisions,

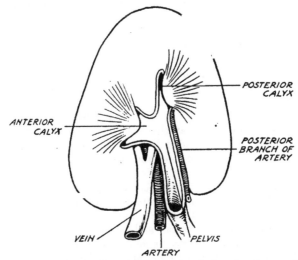

Fig. 5.—Diagram of the arrangement of the structures at the
hilum in transverse section of the kidney.

called calyces (average number, nine), which receive the apices
of the pyramids of the kidney on which open the large collecting

tubes. Each calyx surrounds two or sometimes three papillæ. The calyces are arranged in an anterior and a posterior series. Modifications of the primary division are not uncommon. (Fig. 6.)

The average capacity of the renal pelvis is about 3½ drachms. Distension of 2 drachms or less in the living subject causes pain (*see* p. 176).

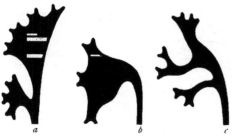

Fig. 6.—Tracings from collargol shadow-graphs showing different types of renal pelvis and variation in calyces. (*See* Plate 2, Fig. 1, and Plate 4, Figs. 2, 3.)

a, Dichotomous pelvis ; *b*, simple pelvis ; *c*, compound branching pelvis.

The renal artery (Fig. 7). — The left artery is 1 cm. shorter than the right. Small branches are given off from the main trunk or the primary divisions, which pass to the fatty capsule and form a network round the kidney. At the hilum the renal artery divides into three or four branches. Two or three of these pass into the sinus in front of the pelvis, and one passes behind it: one of the anterior branches passes to the upper pole and may reach it directly without entering the hilum. The retropelvic branch passes over the upper border of the pelvis and runs downwards under the edge of the posterior lip of the hilum.

The branches further subdivide and enter the kidney at the columns of Bertini between the pyramids, each pyramid being surrounded by four or five arteries. These run alongside the pyramids and curve towards the base of the pyramid. The arteries do not anastomose either at the base or around the pyramids. The arterial supply is divided into an anterior and a posterior system, which are independent, and each branch of which is a terminal artery. The anterior system is larger than the posterior, which is formed by the single posterior primary branch. The arteries of the kidney communicate on the surface of the organ with those of the adipose capsule, and through these with the diaphragmatic, lower intercostal, and lumbar arteries. This anastomosis with parietal arteries is not sufficient to carry on an adequate blood supply if the renal artery is blocked.

An additional renal artery is present in about 20 per cent. of bodies. The accessory artery may arise from the trunk of the renal artery, from the aorta, or from one of the parietal arteries, such as the inferior phrenic. The vessel may pass into the kidney at the hilum, or it may enter the surface of the kidney at the upper or lower pole on either the anterior or posterior surface. Such a vessel is more frequent on the left side and above the normal renal artery. An abnormal renal artery may pass in front of or behind the ureter. When the kidneys are abnormal in shape and position an abnormal blood supply is very common. Irregularities in the .veins are also common. The surgical importance of these abnormalities lies in the facts that in nephrectomy an abnormal vessel may escape ligature and cause serious hæmor-

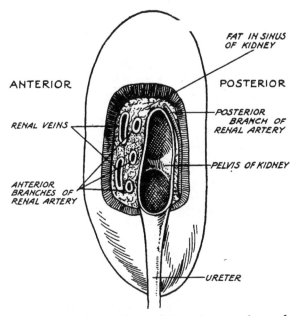

Fig. 7.—Diagram of the relations of the veins, arteries, and pelvis at the hilum of the kidney. A cornice of kidney tissue has been cut away to display these structures.

rhage, and that hydronephrosis may result from pressure of the vessel on the ureter. In my experience, an aberrant artery, the size of a crow-quill, passing to the upper pole, is very commonly met with in performing nephrectomy. The artery is derived from the suprarenal or phrenic artery.

On the surface of the kidney the area corresponding to each pyramid is usually marked out by lines of paler colour, and a depressed line can be seen running parallel to the convex border a little in front of its most prominent part. This is Brödel's line, and, with the other pale areas, it indicates the lines along which the arteries course. Brödel's line is the most vascular part of the kidney, and should for this reason be avoided in incising the organ. The least vascular line is that which separates the anterior and posterior arterial systems and runs parallel to and a little behind the curved border. This is the exsanguine line of Hyrtl, and is the best line for nephrotomy incision.

The renal veins (Fig. 7).—The small renal veins are collected by large anastomosing venous arches running parallel with the surface of the kidney. The veins emerge from the kidney

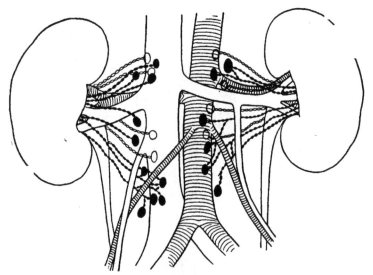

Fig. 8.—Diagram of the lymphatic vessels and glands of the kidneys, showing their relations to the blood-vessels.

substance between the papillæ of the pyramids and anastomose between the calyces. Numerous branches then combine to form two large trunks in front of the pelvis. These and a smaller posterior branch unite to form the renal vein. The left renal vein receives the spermatic or ovarian vein.

Lymphatics of the kidney (Fig. 8).—The lymphatics are collected into four to seven large trunks, which emerge at the hilum. They pass partly in front of the vein and partly behind it, to glands lying in front of and behind the vena cava on the right side, and alongside the aorta on the left side. In their course they run in a sort of mesentery between the layers of the fascia to the glands. This extends from the inner border of the kidney and the ureter on the outer side to the aorta on the left and the inferior vena cava on the right (Grégoire). They do not anastomose with neighbouring lymphatic plexuses.

The glands earliest affected in malignant disease of the kidney are found at the hilum and lying along the side of the aorta between it and the spermatic vein, and along the vena cava. These glands lie in small numbers above the renal vessels and in larger numbers below them. The mediastinal glands are then the seat of deposit.

The renal pedicle.—The pedicle of the kidney consists of the renal vein, the renal artery, the lymphatic vessels, and the nerves, together with a varying amount of fat. The pedicle is about 4 cm. long. It is shorter on the right side than on the left. It is longer in kidneys which lie low down and in those which show fœtal lobulation. When the kidney is abnormally movable the pedicle becomes elongated, and the organ in its excursion swings downwards and towards the median line round the attachment of the artery and the vein. When the kidney is raised into a lumbar wound the artery and vein are increased in length by stretching. On the right side the wall of the inferior vena cava is dragged outwards, but on the left side the aorta is more resistant. The pedicle is seldom transverse. Usually it passes obliquely upwards towards the middle line. When the kidney is brought into a lumbar wound this obliquity is increased. The circumference of the pedicle varies greatly. It is increased by an early branching of the renal artery, and in diseased kidneys may be greatly thickened by masses of fibrous fatty tissue.

Attachments of the kidney.—The following structures combine to support the kidney. They prevent the organ from being displaced, but allow it to move freely (3 to 5 cm.) with respiration.

1. The renal vessels.
2. The peritoneum.
3. The attachment of retroperitoneal surfaces of the duodenum, colon, pancreas.
. The adhesion to the suprarenal capsule.
5. The perirenal fascia and the supporting network of fibres that pass to it from the renal capsule.
6. The perirenal fat.
7. The fascia of Toldt.
8. The intra-abdominal pressure.

CHAPTER II

PHYSIOLOGY AND PATHOLOGY OF THE RENAL FUNCTION

THE following functions are combined in the kidney :—

1. The kidneys separate from the blood a fluid of different molecular composition, namely the urine.
2. They exercise a selective power by which certain substances are removed from the blood. These substances, if allowed to accumulate in the blood, produce uræmia.
3. They have a synthetic action which places them in a line with other glandular organs. Hippuric acid is built up and secreted by the kidneys.
4. An internal secretion which affects nitrogenous metabolism is suggested by certain experiments.

The urine differs from the blood in reaction, in the absence of the proteins of the blood, in the presence of hippuric acid in the urine, and in the different percentage of its constituents.

The most important factor in producing variations in the renal secretion is the velocity of the blood flow through the organ. This is affected by variations in the general blood pressure. When the aortic blood pressure falls below 40 cm. of mercury the flow of urine stops. Constriction of the renal arteries by stimulation of the renal nerves, or pressure upon the renal artery so as to obstruct its flow, and obstruction to the renal vein, diminish the blood flow and reduce the secretion of urine.

EXAMINATION OF THE RENAL FUNCTION

An estimate of the function of the kidneys in disease of these organs may be formed (1) by the discovery of symptoms of renal failure, (2) by an examination of the urine, or (3) by certain tests of the renal function.

1. SIGNS AND SYMPTOMS OF RENAL FAILURE

Pain is a sign that the kidneys are diseased, but it is not a reliable indication of interference with the renal function. The kidneys may be the seat of advanced disease and their function seriously impaired, and the patient be entirely free from pain.

Thirst, worst at night, is the most frequent symptom of interference with the renal function. It is marked in 26·7 per cent. of cases of urinary obstruction. The tongue early becomes˙ dry (12·9 per cent.), at first along the centre and later over the whole surface. It has a glazed, cracked appearance that is distinctive. In the later stages of urinary septicæmia the tongue is dry and covered with a brownish fur (*parrot tongue*). Loss of appetite is constantly present, and in severe cases a buccal dysphagia becomes established from the dryness of the mouth. Nausea and vomiting are late symptoms. Frontal headache is present in 22 per cent. of cases of urinary obstruction. The skin is dry and harsh, and these patients seldom sweat.

The complexion is sallow and muddy. Emaciation is often present, and is very marked if there be septic inflammation of the kidneys. Hiccough is a sign of grave import; it may be slight and gradually increase, exhausting the patient's strength. Drowsiness is a constant and grave symptom of renal failure. In obstructive anuria, however, the mind remains clear for days. Restless delirium is a frequent symptom, and is most marked at night.

The temperature is not raised unless septic complications are present. In cases where the kidney is being slowly destroyed by obstruction the temperature is slightly subnormal, and in obstructive anuria it is continuously subnormal. In chronic septic pyelonephritis a subnormal temperature is present, and may be interrupted from time to time by rises of temperature from exacerbations of the disease. In acute septic pyelonephritis and during the development of a pyonephrosis the temperature is high and swinging. In suppression of urine following urethral operations the temperature rises rapidly after a rigor, and remains high during the course of the disease. There is no œdema, nor are there changes in the heart and vessels. If the renal failure is due to septic infection there may be rigidity and tenderness over one or both kidneys. In acute septic pyelonephritis and in some cases of pyonephrosis one kidney is frequently enlarged.

2. Examination of the Urine

The average **specific gravity** of the urine varies from 1018 to 1020. It is temporarily decreased by copious draughts. of fluid, and increased by any condition which tends to reduce the watery contents of the urine, such as profuse sweating or diarrhœa. A continuously low specific gravity when associated with other signs of disease is a grave symptom. In all forms of polyuria except diabetes mellitus the specific gravity is lowered. Thus, in hysterical polyuria it may be 1005 or less. The specific gravity is estimated with sufficient accuracy by means of a urinometer, which should float free in the urine. The figure is obtained by reading off the lowest mark that can be seen with the eye at the level of the fluid.

The average quantity of **urea** excreted in twenty-four hours in a healthy individual is about 33 grammes (500 grains), or 2 per cent. The excretion of urea is diminished in disease of the kidneys, but there are many extrarenal causes for variation in the quantity of urea contained in the urine, such as diet, absorption, tissue metabolism, and hepatic action.

Urea forms only about 80 per cent. of the total nitrogen compounds in the urine, and if accurate observations are to be made the total nitrogen excretion should be estimated.

Temporary variations in the urea output are valueless in estimating the renal function unless the diet and other factors which influence the production of urea are carefully controlled. Continuous reduction in the urea is of greater value, and shows that the function of the kidneys is seriously impaired. The elimination of chlorides in the urine does not furnish any precise information in regard to the activity of the renal function.

Quantity of Urine

Polyuria.—The quantity of urine passed in twenty-four hours amounts to 40 to 50 oz. (1,200 to 1,500 c.c.). Considerable variation may be observed, depending upon the removal of water from the body by the skin, lungs, intestines, etc., the amount of fluid ingested, and other physiological factors.

Transient polyuria occurs after an attack of fever or an epileptic attack. There is continuous polyuria in the different forms of diabetes, in chronic interstitial nephritis, whether in the form of chronic Bright's disease or the result of back-pressure in urinary obstruction.

Frequent contraction of the bladder is said to increase the quantity of urine secreted, and in all forms of disease where there is increased frequency of micturition there is, as a rule, an increased quantity of urine.

Polyuria is a constant symptom in the chronic interstitial nephritis that results from urinary obstruction (stricture, enlarged prostate). (Chart 1.) The polyuria in such cases is a grave symptom of permanent reduction of the renal efficiency. The quantity excreted varies from 80 to 100 oz. in twenty-four hours. It is liable to sudden falls, each of which marks a temporary reduction in the already enfeebled renal function. The percentage of urea and other urinary constituents is much reduced. The total quantity of these bodies passed in twenty-four hours may be only slightly below the normal standard, but may be much smaller.

Polyuria is observed in cases of advanced calculous disease, where the kidney tissue has been reduced to a mere shell and is the seat of chronic interstitial nephritis and chronic septic nephritis. There is polyuria in the early stage of tuberculous disease of the kidney, due to congestion of the organ. Temporary polyuria usually follows the removal of a diseased kidney, and at the same time the specific gravity is raised and the quantity of urea increased. (Chart 2.) This polyuria is due to the relief of a reno-renal depressant reflex which a diseased kidney exerts upon its healthy or less diseased neighbour.

Polyuria may alternate with oliguria in cases of chronic septic pyelonephritis. In this disease there is polyuria with a subnormal temperature alternating with attacks of oliguria with a rise of temperature. (Charts 3, 4.)

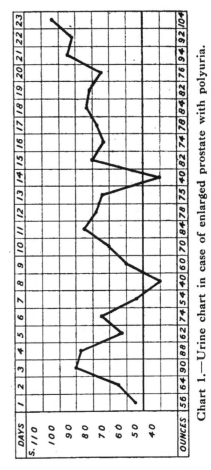

Chart 1.—Urine chart in case of enlarged prostate with polyuria.

Nervous or hysterical polyuria.—This form of polyuria occurs in young adults, in nervous, excitable individuals, both male and female. It may commence suddenly and continue for a few hours or for several weeks.

The patient may be subject to attacks of this nature from time to time. The urine is pale, clear, and of low specific gravity, and the percentage of the urinary constituents is reduced. No albumin or other abnormal constituent is present. The patient complains of frequent micturition and scalding as the urine passes.

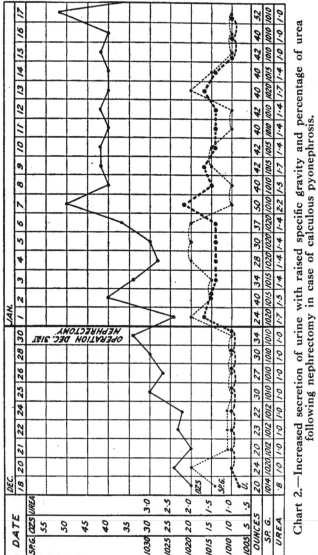

Chart 2.—Increased secretion of urine with raised specific gravity and percentage of urea following nephrectomy in case of calculous pyonephrosis.

In a prolonged attack the urine is increased by one or two pints in the twenty-four hours. Thirst is not a marked feature of the malady. There are usually obscure abdominal pains which are never severe or definitely localized.

Oliguria and anuria.
—Oliguria is a diminished secretion of urine; anuria is a total cessation of the secretion. The agencies which bring about oliguria and anuria may be classified in the following manner :—

(1) Hysterical anuria.
(2) Anuria due to changes in the general circulation of the body.
(3) Reflex anuria :
   (*a*) Urethra.
   (*b*) Bladder.
   (*c*) Ureter.
   (*d*) Kidney.
(4) Infective anuria :
   (*a*) Hæmatogenous
     (i) Toxic.
     (ii) Bacterial.
   (*b*) Ascending urinary.
(5) Urinary-tension anuria :
   1. Obstruction—
     (*a*) Gradual.
     (*b*) Sudden.
   2. Sudden relief of tension.
(6) Anuria from destruction or removal of renal tissue :
   (*a*) Gradual destruction.
   (*b*) Sudden complete destruction or removal.

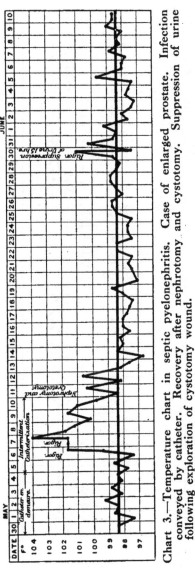

Chart 3.—Temperature chart in septic pyelonephritis. Case of enlarged prostate. Infection conveyed by catheter. Recovery after nephrotomy and cystotomy. Suppression of urine following exploration of cystotomy wound.

(1) **Hysterical anuria.**—There may be diminution or complete suppression in cases of severe hysteria. Anuria has lasted for several hours, or even for some days. Apart from continuous vomiting, no symptoms of uræmia have been observed in such cases. A copious polyuria immediately follows the anuria.

(2) **Circulatory anuria.**—After severe and prolonged operations the secretion of urine is temporarily reduced or suspended. This may last for several hours, and is due to the low blood pressure of shock and collapse. The effect of the anæsthetic, and perhaps the absorption of antiseptics, may play a subordinate part. Where the kidneys are diseased and the active renal tissue much reduced this may be the exciting cause of continuous and fatal anuria. Usually the function is restored when the blood pressure again rises. In shock following grave injuries to the body, in the collapse of cholera, and in other conditions of extreme lowering of the blood pressure, anuria is present.

(3) **Reflex anuria.** —The passage of an instrument along the

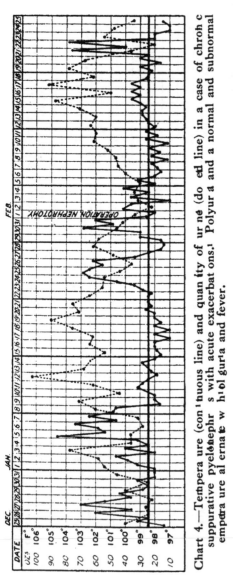

Chart 4.—Temperature (continuous line) and quantity of urine (dotted line) in a case of chronic suppurative pyelonephritis with acute exacerbations. Polyuria and a normal and subnormal temperature alternate with high oliguria and fever.

urethra may be followed by suppression of urine. In such a case the urethra may be healthy, or it may be the seat of stricture or other disease. In some cases no blood follows the passage of the instrument, and post-mortem examination of the urethra fails to reveal the slightest abrasion. The kidneys are sometimes the seat of chronic interstitial nephritis or chronic septic nephritis, and they have been found deeply congested; but in some cases nothing abnormal has been discovered.

Suppression of urine is more likely to occur when an instrument has been roughly passed, and where the disease for which it is used is in the deeper part of the urethra. In the majority of cases there has been difficulty in passing an instrument, and this has been followed by some bleeding. Some hours later, usually immediately after the first passage of urine, the patient has a rigor, and the temperature rises to 103° or 104° F., after which no urine is secreted.

The majority of these cases are due to septic absorption. Some are apparently due to a combination of septic absorption and a reflex effect on the circulation of the kidneys, while a few are purely reflex in nature.

Surgical interference with the bladder may be followed by suppression of urine, especially if the kidneys are already diseased.

Reflex impulses from a ureter, started by a stone or the catheter, may inhibit the secretion of the corresponding kidney. The function of the second kidney may be inhibited, and complete anuria result, by reflex impulses from a stone in the ureter. The corresponding kidney is affected partly by blocking of its ureter and partly by reflex impulses from the ureter. The second kidney may be healthy in such a case, but almost invariably it is impaired by disease.

Sudden kinking of the ureter by torsion of the pedicle in a case of movable kidney may bring about a temporary diminution in the secretion, or a complete suppression. The function is re-established when the torsion is relieved.

There is a reflex depressant effect exerted by one diseased kidney on its healthy or less diseased neighbour. In cases of pyonephrosis, unilateral suppurative pyelonephritis, and other irritative conditions, the total quantity of urine is usually much reduced. On removal of the diseased kidney the activity of the remaining kidney, relieved of the depressant reflex, is greatly increased.

Surgical interference with one kidney is said to produce a reflex inhibition of the activity of its neighbour. Although it appears probable that some such effect may be temporarily

c

produced, it can only last during the time of the operation, and if the second kidney is adequate before the operation this cause will not induce postoperative anuria. Other factors which are much more potent in producing anuria after a kidney operation are the effect of the anæsthetic and of absorbed antiseptics on the remaining kidney and the low blood pressure of shock. Further, the remaining kidney may have been inadequate before the operation, and the removal of its neighbour only makes this evident. Irritation of the kidney pedicle by a drainage tube after nephrectomy has been found to produce reflex anuria (Israel).

(4) **Infective anuria.** (a) *Hæmatogenous.*—In acute nephritis caused by a hæmatogenous infection in septicæmia, influenza, pneumonia, typhoid fever, and in auto-intoxication from gastrointestinal infections, suppression of urine is frequently present and may be fatal. Anuria following urethral operations where the kidneys are healthy and no ascending infection has occurred is probably toxic in nature in many cases.

(b) *Ascending.*—An acute ascending affection of the kidneys from the bladder, arising from an old-standing cystitis or induced by means of septic instruments, may cause complete and rapidly fatal anuria. Chronic septic pyelonephritis secondary to disease of the lower urinary organs is accompanied by oliguria, which becomes more pronounced with acute exacerbations of the disease, and complete anuria may supervene.

(5) **Urinary-tension anuria.**—(a) Gradually increasing obstruction to the outflow of urine, such as is met with in enlarged prostate, produces a slight dilatation of the kidney and chronic interstitial nephritis, and in this way the secreting tissue of the kidney is slowly destroyed. The onset of anuria in these cases is referred to under the heading of Anuria from Destruction of Renal Tissue (*see* below).

(b) Rapid occlusion of both ureters is met with in malignant growths of the bladder involving both ureteric orifices, and in other pelvic growths such as carcinoma of the uterus. Where a calculus suddenly blocks the lumen of the ureter of a solitary kidney, or where both ureters become simultaneously blocked, obstructive anuria results. The calculous anuria is partly obstructive and partly reflex.

(c) Anuria may follow the sudden relief of urinary hypertension. When the urine has been secreted under increased tension for some time, as in enlarged prostate, and the kidneys are the seat of interstitial changes, the sudden emptying of an over-distended bladder is frequently followed by suppression of urine. This suppression is probably due to sudden engorgement of the renal vessels. It is more likely to occur in old than in young men.

(6) Anuria from destruction or removal of renal tissue. —The removal of a solitary kidney, or a working kidney whose neighbour is destroyed by disease, is followed by anuria and death in a few days. When nephrectomy has been performed, and the second kidney is active, but incompetent from disease to perform the total renal function, the patient may survive the operation and gradually sink with symptoms of increasing renal failure, and die some months after the operation. Where disease, such as stricture, enlarged prostate, or calculus or tuberculosis of the kidney, has gradually destroyed the tissue of the kidney, there is usually polyuria. This is interrupted from time to time by attacks of oliguria or anuria brought on by slight causes. (Chart 5.) Finally an attack of anuria proves fatal.

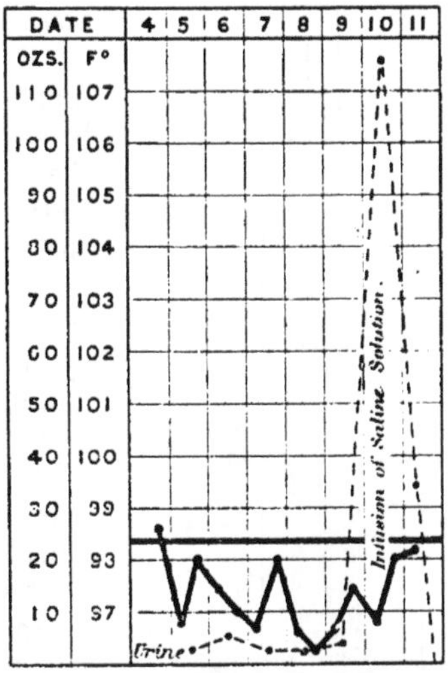

Treatment of anuria.—The following measures should be adopted in cases of anuria: Diuretics are administered, such as caffeine (5 gr.), diuretin (10 gr.), theocin sodium acetate (5 gr.), hot Contrexéville water, and citrate of potash (25 gr.).

Hot fomentations and poultices are applied over the loins.

The patient is placed in a hot pack or a vapour bath.

Chart 5.—Urine and temperature in obstructive anuria, showing subnormal temperature and practically complete anuria, interrupted by a copious polyuria.

A saline infusion of several pints (sodium chloride, 1 dr. to the pint) is slowly introduced into the rectum.

In severe cases the introduction of one to two pints or more of saline solution into a vein has a powerful diuretic effect. It has recently been pointed out that the kidneys are embarrassed by the introduction of chlorides, and these should be replaced by sugar solutions, which are powerfully diuretic.

In urgent cases a pint of glucose solution (25 per cent.) is infused into a vein. This solution is hypertonic, and increases the molecular content of the blood.

In less urgent cases the injection may be given subcutaneously or intramuscularly. Jeanbrau recommends an isotonic solution of glucose (47 grm. per 1,000), or of saccharose or lactose (90 grm. per 1,000).

A solution of 5 per cent. of glucose is isotonic, and I use this in preference to saline solution in anuria.

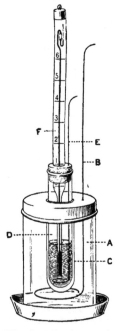

Fig. 9.—Beckmann's apparatus for estimating the freezing-point of the urine.

A, Glass jar; B, stirring rod; C, outer glass tube; D, inner glass tube for urine; E, platinum stirring rod; F, Beckmann's thermometer.

Nephrotomy is followed by re-establishment of the secretion in some apparently desperate cases. This will be discussed in connection with the diseases causing anuria.

Hysterical anuria is treated by bromides, valerian, etc. Diuretics should be administered, and care exercised that the patient has no opportunity of fraudulently disposing of urine that may be passed.

In circulatory anuria the treatment is directed to raising the blood pressure by means of strychnine, ergot, adrenalin, and pituitary extract, and by saline infusion.

In reflex anuria the cause of the reflex inhibition should be removed (see Calculous Anuria, p. 279, and Pyelonephritis, p. 127).

In infective anuria it may be necessary to incise one or even both kidneys (see Pyelonephritis, p. 135).

Sudden relief of long-established severe obstruction—as, for example, the complete emptying of a chronically overdistended bladder in a case of enlarged prostate—should be avoided.

3. Tests of the Renal Function

(1) Cryoscopy.—For details of the method of cryoscopy of the urine and blood the reader is referred to special works dealing with this subject.[1]

By estimating the freezing-point (Fig. 9) the molecular concentration of a fluid is ascertained, and as the molecular concentration is proportional to the osmotic pressure the latter may thus

[1] Thomson Walker, "The Estimation of the Renal Function in Urinary Surgery." 1908.

be measured. The osmotic pressure of the urine is constantly higher than that of the blood, and the work of extracting this fluid of greater osmotic pressure from one of lower osmotic pressure is performed by the kidney. If these organs are diseased their power of bringing about a change in the osmotic pressure of the fluid passing through is reduced. The osmotic pressure therefore falls, and approaches more nearly that of the blood.

When the kidneys are diseased the molecular content of the urine is reduced, and the freezing-point of the urine is raised. The freezing-point of the urine is indicated by the sign $\triangle$, or, to avoid confusion with other fluids, $\triangle U$ may be used. In the healthy state this is liable to considerable variations. It is usually between $-1\cdot30°$ and $-2\cdot20°$ C., but after copious libations it may rise to $-1°$ C., and when the urine is concentrated by profuse sweating the figure may be $-2\cdot30°$ C., or lower. In nervous polyuria the point may be reduced to $-0\cdot46°$ or $-0\cdot17°$ C.

A fallacy is introduced by the precipitation of urates in many urines when the temperature is lowered.

The variations in the point $\mathbf{A} U$ are so considerable in healthy individuals that cryoscopy of the urine alone has little value as an indication of the renal function.

Cryoscopy of the blood.—The freezing-point of the blood is remarkably constant at $-0\cdot56°$ C., and the point $\mathbf{A}$ of the serum is practically the same as that of the blood. Where one kidney is inefficient no change is found in the point $\triangle$, but when the function of both kidneys is reduced the point $\mathbf{A}$ is lowered. A point $\mathbf{A}$ of $-0\cdot57°$ or $-0\cdot58°$ C. indicates a reduction in the total renal function, and a point $\triangle$ of $-0\cdot60°$ C. is a contra-indication to nephrectomy. Lowering of the point $\mathbf{A}$ to $-0\cdot60°$ C. or under may be observed apart from disease of the kidney in cardiac and respiratory affections, and in diabetes, epilepsy, and other conditions. Further, the normal point $\mathbf{A}$ of the blood does not prove that the kidneys are efficient, for the blood may have been hydræmic and the point $\mathbf{A}$ raised, and the renal lesion only succeeds in reducing the point $\triangle$ to normal. This method is not always trustworthy, although it may give useful information when it is impossible to separate the urines of the two kidneys for examination.

Comparative cryoscopy of the urine and the blood.—The freezing-point of the normal urine is $-1\cdot5°$ to $-2°$ C., and that of the blood serum $-0\cdot56°$ C. The quotient of these will be $2\cdot3°$ to $3\cdot5°$ C., and when this figure diminishes we may conclude that there is a diminution in the permeability of the kidney. There is, however, too wide a range of variation in the freezing-point of the urine in the normal individual for reliable information to be obtained by this means. If the volume of the urine be taken into account, this fallacy will be corrected. Thus the quotient is multiplied by the number of c.c. of urine secreted in twenty-four hours. The figures thus obtained vary in healthy individuals from 3,000 to 5,000. The remarkable tendency of the blood to remain at a constant molecular concentration under any condition reduces the value of this test.

Cryoscopy of the urine and estimation of the chlorides. —Koranyi believes that the glomeruli of the kidney filter through a solution of sodium chloride from the blood, and as this passes down the tubules water is absorbed and molecules of sodium chloride are removed, and replaced by molecules of urea, uric acid, etc., from the blood. He therefore proposes to estimate the renal

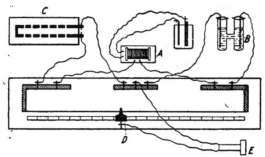

Fig. 10.—Apparatus for measuring the electrical
conductivity of urine.

A, Induction coil ; B, Vessel containing fluid ; C, rheostat ; D, movable contact ; E, telephone.

function by noting the relation between the point $\triangle$ U (the total molecular content) and the sodium chloride content in 100 c.c. of urine. This is expressed by the formula $\frac{\triangle}{NaCl}$. In the normal state this does not exceed 1·7. The result depends, however, not upon the permeability of the kidney, but upon the rapidity of secretion, which affects the time allowed for interchange of the sodium chloride molecules. This again depends upon the rate of circulation through the kidney. In order to overcome such fallacies the formula has been corrected by adding to it the volume of urine in cubic centimetres for twenty-four hours and the total body-weight in kilogrammes. The formula becomes so complicated that the figures obtained are of very doubtful value.

Wright and Kilner have suggested a method by which the molecular content of the blood is measured by means of dilution with a standard solution of sodium chloride. At a certain point of dilution destruction of the red blood-corpuscles (hæmolysis) takes place, and the amount of dilution required to produce this is an index of the molecular concentration of the blood.

Estimation of the electrical conductivity of the urine has been used to estimate the molecular content, and the figure compared with that of salt solution. (Fig. 10.) Further, the electrical resistance of the urine has been compared with that of the blood and a hæmo-renal index obtained; but neither this method nor the estimation of the surface tension of the urine, which has also been used, has been widely adopted.

It may be said of all these methods of estimation of the molecular content of the urine, that the delicacy of the instruments required and the skill necessary for their observation preclude them from general clinical use, and that the results they have given could equally well and much more easily be obtained by testing the specific gravity by means of the ureometer.

(2) **Methylene-blue test.**—The methylene blue should be pure and free from arsenic, and must dissolve completely in · water. Methylene blue is absorbed from the intestine or from an intramuscular injection into the blood, and excreted by the kidney, and to a less extent by the liver. Some of the latter is reabsorbed from the intestine. The blue cannot be recognized in the blood. It appears in the urine partly as blue and partly in the form of a chromogen or colourless body which is transformed into blue by boiling with acetic acid.

After cleansing the skin, 15 minims of a 5 per cent. aqueous solution are slowly injected into the muscles of the buttock. Chromogen appears in the urine in from fifteen to twenty minutes, and a trace of blue is detected half an hour after the injection. The urine rapidly becomes olive green and then emerald green bluish green, prussian blue, and finally a deep blue colour. The colour may not, however, pass beyond emerald green. During the first four or five hours of the elimination chromogen is present in greater quantity than blue, and may be detected by extracting the blue with chloroform and then boiling the cleared urine with acetic acid. (Chart 6.) The excretion of blue is at its height in four or five hours, remains stationary for several hours, and then gradually declines. In from forty to sixty hours it has usually disappeared. The chromogen disappears from the urine some hours before the methylene blue. In pathological conditions of the kidney, such as chronic interstitial nephritis, tuberculous kidney, or hydronephrosis (Charts 7, 8), the appearance of methylene blue is delayed for one, two, or more hours. An early onset and rapid

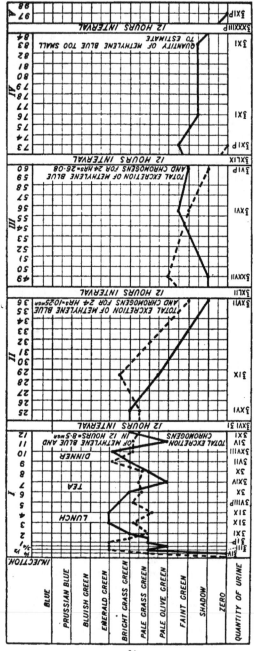

Chart 6.—Elimination of methylene blue (continuous line) and chromogen (dotted line) in a healthy individual. The total quantity of methylene blue and chromogen passed in each twenty-four hours is given in milligrammes, and the quantity of urine in ounces.

24

elimination have been observed in parenchymatous nephritis. In surgical disease of the kidneys elimination of blue may be prolonged for several days. I have observed the excretion during a period of eight days and seventeen hours in a man of 67 years who suffered from enlarged prostate and interstitial changes in the kidneys. After the first twenty-four hours only traces of blue are passed in such cases, and the total quantity of blue eliminated is usually much reduced. The quantity of blue may be estimated by a colorimetric method, but it is usually sufficient

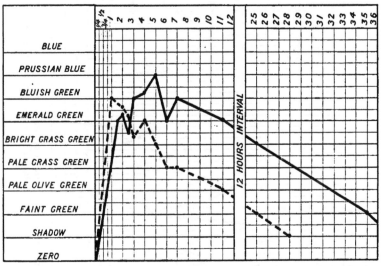

Chart 7.—Elimination of methylene blue (continuous line) in tuberculous kidney. Delayed commencement and rapid short elimination.

to note the varying depth of colour, and from this to judge of the quantity eliminated.

Intermittent elimination may occur, and is said to result from an inhibitory action on the kidney of bodies produced in the liver in hepatic disease, but I have observed it in the healthy.

(3) **Indigo-carmine test.**—An injection of 20 c.c. of 0·4 per cent. solution of indigo carmine is made into the muscles of the buttock. The urine becomes tinged in five minutes, the excretion reaches its highest point in half to three-quarters of an hour, and then falls gradually and disappears in about twelve hours. Delay in the commencement and a diminution in the quantity of dye eliminated are indications of a reduced renal

function. · The quantity of fluid which must be injected is a drawback to this method. The solubility of indigo carmine does not permit of more concentrated solution being used.

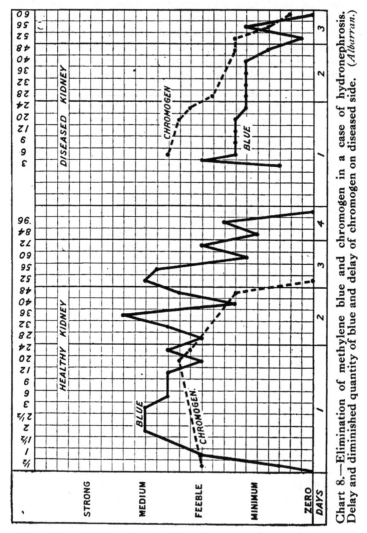

Chart 8.—Elimination of methylene blue and chromogen in a case of hydronephrosis. Delay and diminished quantity of blue and delay of chromogen on diseased side. (*Albarran.*)

Rosaniline, iodide of potassium, and salicylic acid have been tried as tests of the renal function, but have not been found satisfactory.

(4) **Phenol-sulphone-phthalein test.**[1]—A cubic centimetre of a solution containing 6 mg. of phenol-sulphone-phthalein is injected subcutaneously in the upper arm, and the urine is collected. The urine is rendered alkaline by the addition of sodium hydrate (25 per cent.), and assumes a brilliant purple-red colour. The sample of urine is diluted to 1 litre with distilled water and compared in a Duboscq's calorimeter with a standard solution ($\frac{1}{2}$ c.c. of the injection fluid in a litre of water rendered alkaline by the addition of NaOH). In normal cases the colouring material appears in from five to ten minutes; 40 to 60 per cent. of the drug is excreted in the first hour, 20 to 25 per cent. in the second hour, and 60 to 85 per cent. in two hours. The presence of blood in the urine introduces a fallacy, and renders the test more difficult even after filtering the urine.

This test is at present under trial.

(5) **Toxicity-of-urine test.**—The normal urine is highly poisonous, but the exact nature of the poison is unknown. The injection of a certain quantity of urine into a rabbit causes symptoms of poisoning, and after a varying interval the animal dies. For rabbits the lethal dose is stated at 40 to 50 grm. per kilo of body weight. Variations in this dose are stated to be due to the accumulation of poisons in the body from which the urine was derived, or, on the other hand, increased elimination of poisons in the urine. The urine has been injected into the veins, the serous cavities, the cellular tissues, and intracerebral injections have been used. Most observers who have used the method are agreed that so long as the figures are not considered to be mathematically exact the estimation of the toxicity of the urine will afford useful information. By a comparison of the toxic properties of the urine and the blood in renal disease more exact data may be obtained, but even here there is some degree of fallacy, for the toxicity of the blood tends to remain constant, accumulated poisons being stored in the tissues.

(6) **Phloridzin test.**—When phloridzin is administered by the mouth or subcutaneously a temporary glycosuria follows. The production of sugar has been shown to take place in the kidney. The quantity of sugar excreted does not depend upon the dose of phloridzin, provided sufficient is given to produce the maximal effect. A second injection of phloridzin given shortly after the first will produce a greater quantity of sugar proportionally than the first injection.

The source of the sugar is apparently the tissue protein, and

[1] Geraghty, *Trans. Amer. Assoc. Genito-Urinary Surgeons*, vol. v., 1910

the phloridzin influences the kidney so that it manufactures sugar from this body.

A subcutaneous injection of 10 mg. of phloridzin is given. Sugar can usually be detected in the urine in a healthy individual in fifteen minutes, occasionally after thirty minutes. The glycosuria is at its height from three-quarters to one hour after the injection, and has usually ceased in two to two and a half hours. An injection of 10 mg. of phloridzin will normally produce from 1 to 2 grm. of glucose. Certain drugs reduce the secretion of sugar; among these are glycerine, salicylate of soda, antipyrin, and piperazin.

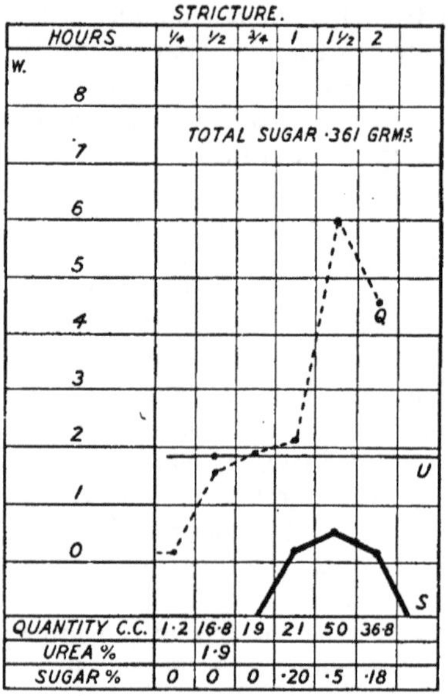

Delay in the appearance of sugar in the urine indicates an interference with the renal function. A prolonged duration of glycosuria, especially if it coincides with a total reduction in quantity, points to a lowered renal activity. The lowest limit of normal glycosuria lies between 50 cg. and 1 grm., and the highest between 2 and 2·50 grm. Occasionally a diminished production of sugar (*hypoglycosuria*) or an increased production (*hyperglycosuria*) may be observed in diseases which do not directly affect the kidneys, and even in normal individuals, but this is exceptional. In almost all cases of renal disease, when the lesion is bilateral there is some variation in the phloridzin glycosuria. Usually this takes the form of diminution of the quantity eliminated. Sometimes there is complete absence of sugar.

Chart 9.—Stricture of the urethra. Delayed, shortened, reduced elimination of sugar.

In urinary obstruction (stricture, enlarged prostate) there is diminished elimination of sugar. (Charts 9, 10.) When the kidneys are damaged, and when pronounced renal complications are present, sugar may be absent. In primary surgical diseases of the kidneys the sugar may be diminished or absent. (Charts 11, 12.)

A diminished phloridzin glycosuria indicates a depressed renal

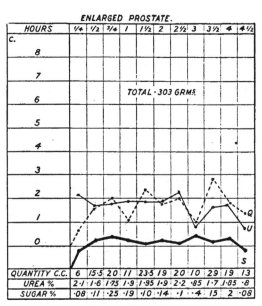

ENLARGED PROSTATE.

HOURS	1/4	1/2	3/4	1	1 1/2	2	2 1/2	3	3 1/2	4	4 1/2

TOTAL ·303 GRMS.

QUANTITY C.C.	6	15·5	20	11	23·5	19	20	10	29	19	13
UREA %	2·1	1·6	1·75	1·9	1·95	1·9	2·2	·85	1·7	1·85	·8
SUGAR %	·08	·11	·25	·19	·10	·14	·1	·4	15	2	·08

Chart 10.—Prolonged diminished phloridzin glycosuria (S) in enlarged prostate.

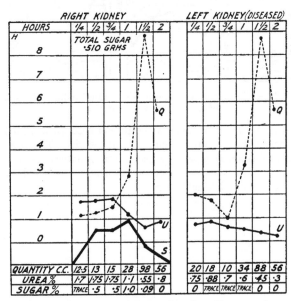

	RIGHT KIDNEY						LEFT KIDNEY (DISEASED)					
HOURS	1/4	1/2	3/4	1	1 1/2	2	1/4	1/2	3/4	1	1 1/2	2

TOTAL SUGAR ·510 GRMS

QUANTITY C.C.	12·5	13	15	28	98	56	20	18	10	34	88	56
UREA %	1·7	1·75	1·75	1·1	·55	·8	·75	·88	·7	·6	·45	·3
SUGAR %	TRACE	·5	·5	1·0	·09	0	0	TRACE	TRACE	TRACE	0	0

Chart 11.—Calculous hydronephrosis. Traces of sugar on diseased side.

29

function which is usually due to disease of the kidney, and complete absence of sugar should be regarded as a sign of advanced renal disease.

Compared with the urea output and the general symptoms of renal inadequacy, the phloridzin test is more delicate. The fallacy

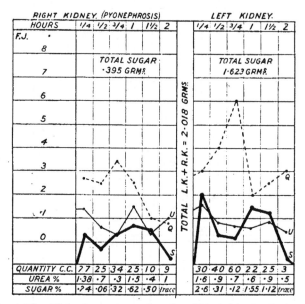

Chart 12.—Calculous pyonephrosis. Diminished elimination of sugar on diseased side.

to which it is especially liable is the pronounced effect which minor renal changes may produce upon the glycosuria. The test, which we owe to Casper, is especially useful for unilateral renal disease, and is used with catheterization of the ureters, each kidney being drained for two and a half hours.

CHAPTER III

EXAMINATION OF THE KIDNEYS

I. INSPECTION AND PALPATION

Inspection.—A kidney which has attained a large size becomes prominent on the surface of the abdomen. The prominence is more readily seen in the recumbent than in the erect posture. There is usually well-marked fullness in the flank on the affected

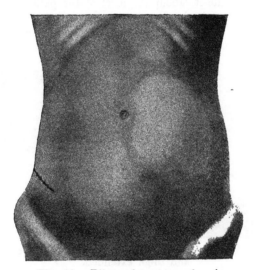

Fig. 11.—Bilateral hydronephrosis.

The left kidney is distended ; the right has been the subject of a plastic operation.

side, but the greatest prominence is on the anterior surface of the abdomen (Fig. 11).

With the patient lying on the back, a large, rounded swelling will be seen to one side, or a little above the level, of the umbilicus. If the abdominal wall is thick and the tumour very large, only a general fullness of one side of the abdomen is apparent. In some

31

cases of hydronephrosis the pelvis of the kidney is greatly distended
with fluid, while the kidney itself is less prominent. A vertical
groove will frequently be observed on the swelling, and indicates
the division between pelvis and kidney.

Palpation.—The patient lies on his back on a high couch,
the abdomen fully exposed, the shoulders raised on a pillow, and
the knees flexed, with the feet planted on the table. I usually
dispense with the flexion of the knees, or, at most, place a pillow
beneath them. The surgeon either sits on the edge of the couch,
or stands alongside it, about the level of the patient's pelvis on
the side to be examined. To examine the right kidney, he places
the finger-tips of the left hand beneath the patient's loin and presses
gently upwards in the angle formed by the last rib with the erector

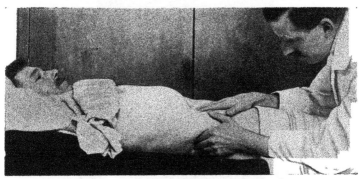

Fig. 12.—Palpation of right kidney, with patient recumbent
and thigh extended.

spinæ mass of muscles. The right hand, well warmed, is placed
flat upon the surface of the abdomen, with the tips of the fingers
a little above the level of the umbilicus and about midway between
this and the margin of the ribs (Fig. 12). With the knees fully
flexed the axis of the surgeon's hand lies almost transverse (Fig. 13).
With the knees slightly flexed or fully extended the hand can be
placed with its long axis in the long axis of the patient's body—a
position more favourable for palpation of the kidney. The patient
is directed to take deep inspirations, but not to force expiration.
As the abdomen recedes at each expiration the fingers sink in,
and the deeper position is maintained during the next inspiration,
and at each succeeding expiration the fingers sink deeper. There
should be no plunging with the tips of the fingers. When the fingers
have sunk deeply, the posterior hand should try to raise the kidney
at each inspiration. To examine the left kidney, the position of

the surgeon and his hands are changed to the other side of the patient, the left hand being used for the front of the abdomen and the right hand being behind.

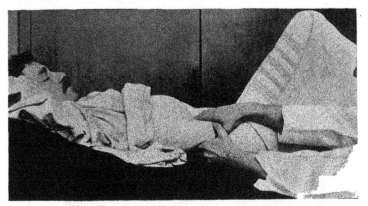

Fig. 13.—Palpation of right kidney: dorsal position with knee flexed. Note interlocking of thumbs.

The patient may also be examined lying upon the side with the knees flexed. The uppermost loin is palpated, the surgeon standing behind the patient (Fig. 14).

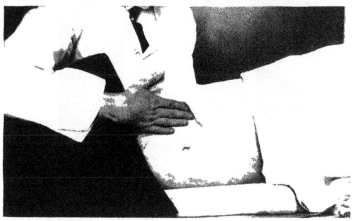

Fig. 14.—Palpation of kidney with patient lying on sound side.

In thin patients and in children the whole loin may be grasped just below the last rib by placing the hand behind and the thumb

D

in front.   Additional pressure may be applied to assist the sinking-in of the thumb by pressing upon it with the fingers of the other hand.

The same method may be practised with the patient standing

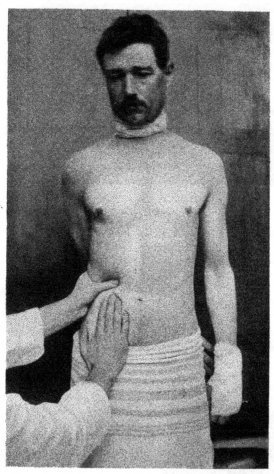

Fig. 15.—Palpation of kidney in erect posture.

(Fig. 15), but it is more difficult to get relaxation of the abdominal muscles in this position.

By palpation the size, outline, shape, and movements of an enlarged or otherwise abnormal kidney will be ascertained.   The difficulties in examining a renal tumour are stoutness of the patient and rigidity due to contraction of the abdominal muscles. Contraction of the muscles may be caused by pain and tenderness of the kidney, or by rough handling or the application of a cold hand, or by nervousness on the part of the patient. A general anæsthetic may be necessary to overcome this.

Signs of renal tumour.—The following are the characteristic signs of an abdominal tumour formed by the kidney (tumours caused by movable kidneys will be specially described under that heading) : The borders of the kidney are all rounded; there are no sharp edges. The reniform shape can frequently be distinguished. Kidney tumours project forwards into the abdomen, and although the depression of the loin may be obliterated, there is no projection of a definite tumour laterally or backwards. The tumour passes backwards into the kidney area at the angle formed by the ribs with the spinal muscles, and the fingers pressed in here do not sink in behind the tumour. With the fingers in this position and the other hand on the front of the abdomen, the kidney tumour, if a small one, can be projected against the anterior hand by a sudden push, and gives a characteristic sensation, called by French surgeons " ballottement." When the tumour is a large one, and already in contact with the abdominal wall in front, the hands in these positions can so grasp the tumour as to move it backwards and forwards between them. Renal tumours descend with inspiration unless they are fixed by adhesions. They move rather less freely with respiration than tumours of the spleen, liver, or suprarenal body. Unless the renal tumour is very large it does not reach the middle line, but it may, when of exceptional size, cross the middle line, and even fill the whole abdominal area. When of moderate dimensions it can usually be separated from the liver. The edge of the liver may sometimes be felt on the surface of the enlarged kidney. Renal tumours rarely extend into the iliac fossa. A renal tumour due to a large growth is usually tense and elastic to the touch. Sometimes the tumour is hard and nodular, or the consistence may vary in different parts, being soft and fluctuating at one part and hard at another. Kidneys distended with fluid are tense and elastic. It is seldom possible to detect fluctuation in these tumours. Occasionally large masses of calculi may be felt in the kidney as very hard, irregular nodules. The colon can often be felt crossing the tumour vertically. On percussion the tumour is dull, and the dull note merges into that of the spinal muscles behind. Anteriorly there is a zone of comparative resonance when the colon is pressed forwards in front of the tumour ; or if the colon is collapsed, and dull on percussion, it can be rolled beneath the fingers. An enlarged right kidney may push the ascending colon downwards and inwards. On the right side percussion will usually show an area of resonance between the renal dullness and that of the liver, which can be demonstrated when the patient is standing.

Differential diagnosis of renal tumour.—Tumours of the kidney may be confused with enlargements of the liver or spleen, ovarian tumours, suprarenal tumours, malignant growths of the large-intestine, and perinephritic tumours and inflammations. (1) An *enlarged liver* has no intestine in front of it, and does not give the sensation of ballottement. The outline of the dullness may be characteristic, and the sharp lower edge may be felt, or there is an absence of roundness at the edge. Jaundice and biliary colic, when present, point to disease of the liver and gall-bladder, while urinary symptoms may give the clue to urinary disease. A floating lobe of the liver may be confused with a movable kidney. In all cases where there is difficulty in diagnosis, pyelography gives invaluable information in regard to the position of the kidney and the presence of dilatation of the organ (p. 42). (2) The *spleen* has no bowel in front, and is therefore absolutely dull on percussion. It has a sharp, well-defined edge, and a notch in this which may be distinguished. There is usually resonance between the posterior edge and the spinal muscles, and there is frequently hollowing in this position if the tumour is large. Ballottement cannot be obtained. The enlargement of a splenic tumour takes a downward and inward direction ; that of a renal tumour extends downwards, not inwards. The lower end of a large splenic tumour crosses the middle line ; that of a renal tumour does not, although a very large renal growth may cross the middle line at its point of greatest circumference. The history of the case and examination of the blood may help. Urinary symptoms, such as hæmaturia, are very important when present. (3) *Ovarian tumours* are dull in front, and there is resonance in the flanks. The enlargement has taken place from below upwards. The tumour can be felt in the pelvis from the vagina or rectum, and there are changes in the position of the uterus. A small ovarian tumour with a long pedicle has been mistaken for a renal tumour. (4) *Suprarenal tumours* are seldom distinguished from those of the kidney. The kidney may be recognized as a reniform swelling on the surface of the mass, but if felt at all will probably be indistinguishable from a round nodule of growth. (5) *Malignant growths of the large intestine* may simulate renal growths. In position and in distribution of the dullness they may be similar, and the outline of the intestinal tumour may be rounded on palpation. Mobility may be a feature of intestinal growths, and it may be possible to reduce such a growth into the loin in a manner similar to a renal tumour. The presence of changes in the urine or of intestinal symptoms will influence diagnosis in one or other direction. Intestinal growths are not reniform in outline. (6) *Perinephritic growths* may closely simulate renal tumours in all respects, and the diagnosis may only be made by exploration. *Perinephritic inflammation and suppuration* may originate above a malignant growth of the intestine, or may result from appendicitis or other causes. The diagnosis of the cause of the inflammation will be made by the history of the case.

II. RADIOGRAPHY OF THE KIDNEY AND RENAL PELVIS

The Röntgen rays were first used in the diagnosis of renal calculus by Macintyre in 1896, and have proved of immense value in urinary surgery.

In examining a kidney by this means the plate should show both kidney areas, the last two ribs on each side, the transverse processes of the vertebræ, and each iliac crest, and it should be possible to trace clearly the shadow of the psoas muscle. If these landmarks are not seen the plate must be classed as of poor quality, and the value to be placed upon the reading of it is reduced.

In a plate of good quality the shadow of a normal kidney can be distinguished. The outline of the lower pole and the outer border are most definite; the inner border can sometimes be seen, but the upper pole can seldom be distinguished unless the organ is displaced downwards clear of the ribs. The left kidney throws a more definite shadow than the right, which is frequently obscured by the liver.

Stoutness of the patient and a loaded bowel give rise to difficulty in obtaining a good radiogram. It is possible to obtain a negative of first quality even in very stout subjects. Careful preparation of the bowel is of the utmost importance. A loaded bowel will produce a cloudy opacity which obscures the kidney. It is equally important to avoid over-purgation, as the large intestine becomes distended with air and reduces the value of the plate. A mild aperient, such as a dose of liquorice powder, should be given on two successive nights previous to the examination. The patient should eat very sparingly on the day before, and should fast on the day of the examination.

It is important for purposes of localization and comparison that the radiographer should be able to reproduce with mathematical exactness the position and the relation to each other of the patient, the tube, and the plate at any subsequent time, and in order to do this a fixed position must be used. The radiographer must clearly indicate on the plate which is the right and which the left side of the patient.

At the first examination both kidney areas should be examined, and the light should be centrally placed in relation to the patient. Should more detailed information be required to elucidate some point, oblique rays may be used, or one spot may be examined by means of a diaphragm. Inspection with the fluorescent screen may be used as a preliminary to the production of a radiogram, but it is an unreliable method of examination and cannot replace radiography. The photographic negatives should be examined in preference to prints in doubtful cases.

It cannot be too strongly insisted that every radiographic examination in urinary disease must include the whole urinary tract. Both kidneys, both ureters, the bladder, and the urethra must be examined.

RADIOGRAPHY IN RENAL CALCULUS

Radiography is used for the following purposes in renal calculus :—

1. Diagnosis of the calculus.
2. Examination of the condition of the calculous kidney.
3. Localization of the calculus.
4. Examination of the second kidney.

1. Diagnosis of renal calculus. (*a*) **Position of the shadow.**— In the radiogram the bodies of the vertebræ and transverse processes, the last two ribs, and the iliac crests will be visible, and these act as landmarks. The following points in regard to the normal relations of the kidney to the bony skeleton are therefore extremely important. The upper part of the kidney lies under cover of the last two ribs, the upper border corresponding to the middle of the 11th dorsal vertebra and being covered by the shadow of the 11th rib. This rib may therefore be taken as representing the upper limit of the renal area. The lower border reaches the level of the lower border of the transverse process of the 3rd lumbar vertebra. The right kidney lies a little lower than the left. In radiograms the lower border of the kidney usually comes a little lower than this, and the upper border scarcely so high. The outer border usually lies well beyond the tip of the 12th rib, but the varying length and obliquity of this rib make it an unreliable guide.

I have adopted the following method of measurement by which the outer border of the normal kidney can be indicated and any increase in size demonstrated. If the narrowest transverse measurement of the 1st lumbar vertebra be taken, and this measurement

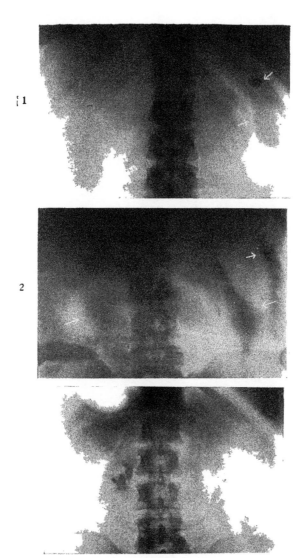

Fig. 1.—Shadow thrown by gall-stone in renal area (upper arrow);
shadow of right lobe of liver (lower arrow). (P. 39.)

Fig. 2.—Shadows thrown by bismuth-covered fæces during administration of bismuth. (P. 41.)

Fig. 3.—Shadow thrown by intra-abdominal calcareous glands.
The shadow lies on the psoas-muscle shadow at the level
of pelvis of kidney, but just internal to it. (P. 39.)

PLATE 1.

doubled and projected transversely from the middle of the outer edge of the vertebral body, a point will be found.

If the same measurements be made in regard to the 2nd and 3rd lumbar vertebræ, two other points are found. By joining these three points the outer border of the kidney is roughly indicated. The kidney does not, however, lie flat on an even bed of muscle. The inner border is tilted so that the hilum and pelvis face forwards and inwards. As a result, shadows of calculi lying in the pelvis of the kidney may appear in the kidney area as if embedded in the substance of the organ.

The inner border of the kidney corresponds with fair accuracy to the outer border of the psoas shadow, and the hilum lies in this line at the level of the 2nd lumbar vertebra. The pelvis of the kidney lies at this area and overlaps the psoas shadow. In full expiration and in full inspiration, in the supine and in the erect posture, the kidney shadow lies higher or lower respectively, and in some cases the excursion is considerable.

Shadows in the renal area are, so far as position is concerned, most probably calculi embedded in the kidney (Plate 20, Figs. 1, 2) ; those in the pelvic area are stones in the renal pelvis. Lying outside and below the kidney is the colon, and this also passes in front of the kidney, so that opaque bodies in the colon may give shadows in the renal area. This difficulty

Fig. 16.—Gall-stone which threw a radiographic shadow in renal area.

more frequently arises on the left side, where the colon covers a larger area of the kidney, than on the right. This does not affect the pelvic area, but in this area calcified glands in the lumbar chain or in the mesentery may throw shadows (Plate 1, Fig. 3). Immediately outside the renal area on the right side at the level of the 1st lumbar vertebra are the gall-bladder and ducts. Rarely, a shadow may be thrown by a gall-stone and appear in this area. Plate 1, Fig. 1, shows the shadow of a gall-stone which I removed from the cystic duct ; Fig. 16 shows the gall-stone itself. The patient had been unsuccessfully explored for renal calculus in South Africa.

The kidney which contains a calculus may be movable or displaced. When the outline of the kidney is seen in the negative the relations of the suspected stone shadow to it will be evident.

The displacement is usually vertical; seldom, if ever, outward. A stone in the pelvis of a horseshoe kidney is much nearer the middle line than the normal pelvis, and is usually at a lower level. After an operation upon the kidney the organ is usually found displaced downwards, and may be partly hidden behind the shadow of the iliac crest.

Distension of the renal pelvis with collargol solution (Pyelography, p. 42) may give valuable assistance in localizing a doubtful shadow.

(*b*) **Size, shape, and number.**—Small stones usually throw a round or oval shadow. Stones the size of a split pea may be recognized unless composed of pure uric acid. The size of the shadow is several times greater than that of the stone, if the stone be opaque throughout. Movement of the stone due to deep breathing will cause a round stone to throw an elongated shadow. When a prolonged exposure has been given, some very small stones, which are eventually passed through the ureter, do not cast a shadow on even a good plate.

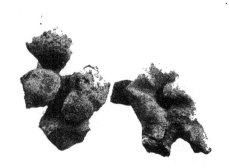

Fig. 17.—Branched calculi removed from kidney.

Large stones are usually branched, and the main mass throws an extensive, heavy shadow (Plate 20, Fig. 1, and Fig. 17). The branches which are connected by a narrow neck may appear isolated. In the larger masses of stone the shadows extend downwards beyond the kidney area, and may be partly hidden by the iliac crest. A collection of stones may throw a single shadow.

(*c*) **Density of the shadow.**—The density of the shadow depends upon the size and composition of the calculus. A large mass of calculus will throw a heavy, uniform shadow, whatever its composition may be ; a small calculus will throw a shadow whose definition and opacity depend upon its composition. Oxalate-of-lime stones are the least permeable to the rays and throw the densest shadow, the rare cystin and xanthin calculi throw a shadow slightly less dense, calcium phosphate is next, and triple phosphate is much less opaque. Pure uric-acid stones throw little, if any, shadow, and are not recognizable in the body. Calculi are seldom composed of a single ingredient, and a coating of phosphates will occasionally render a uric-acid calculus opaque.

Fallacies.—Fallacies due to the size and composition of a calculus have already been noted. Opaque substances in the bowel may closely simulate renal calculi. A shadow of very irregular shape is unlikely to be caused by a calculus. Sometimes the shape is that of some recognizable object, such as a coin. A long, opaque body lying transversely is not renal, and is usually in the bowel.

In a patient who has been taking bismuth, shadows which are indistinguishable in size, shape, position,. and density from those of renal or pelvic calculi may be thrown by bismuth-covered fæces. The bismuth shadows shown in Plate 1, Fig. 1, remained for several months, in spite of repeated purgation.

Calcified glands belonging to the lumbar group or lying in the mesentery, or the deposit of phosphates upon silk ligatures used in a previous operation, may simulate renal or pelvic calculi. Indefinite shadows are sometimes found in the kidney or pelvic area, which have proved to be due to thickened scars in the kidney or to phosphatic deposit in an inflamed or tuberculous renal pelvis.

Fallacy due to gall-stones has already been mentioned.

In an aseptic case the absence of a stone shadow after two or more examinations, when a plate of first quality has been obtained, excludes all but a pure uric-acid calculus.

When the urine is alkaline the absence of a stone shadow excludes calculi of any composition, for it is certain that phosphates will have been deposited upon a uric-acid calculus and render it opaque.

2. **Condition of the kidney.**—In slight dilatation of the kidney the measurement given above will serve roughly to demonstrate the change. I have introduced a more accurate method of measurement of the kidney shadow. A ureteric catheter, alternately opaque and translucent in segments of half an inch, is passed up the ureter of the diseased kidney ; on the plate the shadow value of half an inch is obtained, and by using this the shadow of the kidney can be measured in half-inches.

In a greatly enlarged calculous kidney the shadows extend downwards and outwards beyond the normal limits.

The stone shadows may merge with, and be partly hidden by, the iliac shadow. The upper limit does not, however, extend higher than the normal kidney at the level of the 11th rib.

Where a very large branched shadow or many stone shadows are observed, the kidney will be found practically destroyed.

Isolated stone shadows widely separated indicate that the kidney is dilated with pus or urine, and a large kidney outline will confirm this.

The use of collargol in the diagnosis of hydronephrosis will be described later (p. 176).

3. Position of the calculus.—Several cases are recorded in which symptoms of stone were present in one kidney, and radiography showed that this kidney was free from calculus, but that the second kidney was the seat of calculi.

Shadows lying far out in the kidney area are cast by calculi embedded in the calyces, and the position of the shadow will indicate whether the stone lies at the upper or the lower pole of the kidney. A stone shadow lying over or above the 12th rib shadow and far out, in a short, stout patient, is likely to give rise to difficulty in its removal.

Pyelography is valuable in accurately localizing the position of the calculus.

4. Examination of the second kidney.—When a stone shadow has been found in one kidney, information in regard to the second kidney may be obtained by examination of the plate. If the outline of this kidney is seen and is normal, this will demonstrate the presence of a second kidney, although it will not indicate functional power. The most frequent disease of the second kidney, when one organ is the seat of calculus, is the formation of calculi, and the absence of stone shadows in the kidney will exclude this.

RADIOGRAPHY IN HYDRONEPHROSIS AND PYONEPHROSIS

A large, dense shadow is thrown by a distended kidney. The upper and inner parts are difficult to define, but there is a sharp and easily distinguishable outer and lower border. It is impossible to distinguish, in a radiograph, between a hydro- and a pyonephrosis.

Pyelography (Plates 2, 3, 4).—Voelcker and Lichtenberg introduced a method by which the early stages of dilatation of the renal pelvis can be recognized. These observers inject a warm solution (2 to 5 per cent.) of collargol, an innocuous preparation of silver, through a ureteric catheter into the renal pelvis. A radiogram is now made, and the size and shape of the renal pelvis can be seen. Lime-water, argyrol, and other solutions have also been used, but are less opaque. I have used this method in a large number of cases, and have obtained striking pictures of the renal pelvis which clearly demonstrate the position of the pelvis and the presence or absence of dilatation.

A catheter is passed up the ureter so that the eye enters the renal pelvis, and the contents are allowed to run off. The bladder is emptied and the cystoscope removed, leaving the ureteric catheter in position. The collargol solution is heated and slowly introduced. I use a 10 or a 20 per cent. solution, and introduce it by means

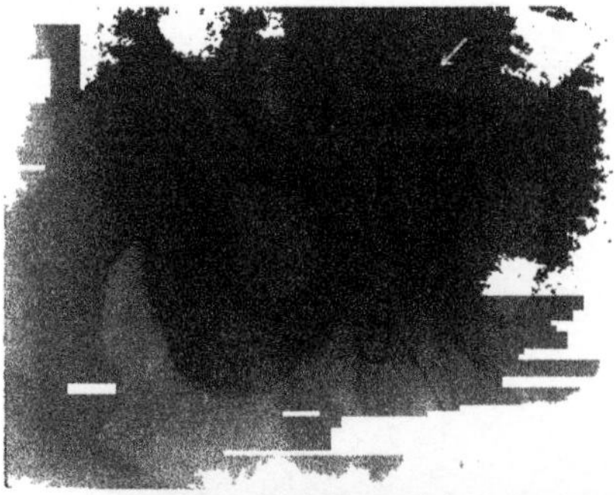

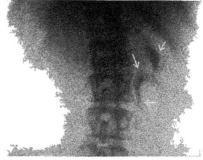

Fig. 1.—Pyelography : Injected pelvis showing dichotomous outline and calyces. Note axis of upper end of ureter and
of pelvis are in line. (P. 42.)

Fig. 2.—Pyelography : Collargol which has regurgitated into bladder
(arrow). Opaque catheter in ureter. (P. 42.)

Fig. 3.—Pyelography in movable kidney : Kinking of ureter and
dilatation of upper calyx. The lowermost arrow points to
the upper end of ureter, the middle one to the kinked
pelvo-ureteral junction, and the uppermost one to the
dilated calyx. (Pp. 79, 176.)

PLATE 2.

of an all-glass syringe of 20 c.c. capacity. The barrel of the syringe, filled with solution and with the piston in place, is attached to the catheter by means of the needle, and held 6 in. to 1 ft. above the level of the body. The fluid passes slowly in, and is assisted by an occasional touch on the piston. No force is used, and the injection is stopped whenever the patient feels the pain of distension of the pelvis; the syringe is removed, the catheter plugged, and the radiograph is taken. The ureteral catheter should be opaque to the X-rays. The fluid is now allowed to flow off. The catheter is removed in ten minutes. Pain is usually only present when the pelvis is fully distended, but occasionally there is an attack of renal colic. In the radiographic plate the uretero-pelvic junction should be examined for kinking, and the pelvis and calyces for dilatation. The earliest stage of dilatation is shown by clubbing of the calyces. Later, the calyces become much enlarged and approach the surface of the kidney, and the kidney tissue between them is reduced (Plate 3, Fig. 1). The angle formed between the lowest calyx and the ureter and pelvis becomes more and more acute as dilatation proceeds, and eventually there is only a narrow slit remaining (Plate 3, Figs. 1, 3). A hydronephrosis shows as a mass of opaque nodules separated by thin, clear lines—renal type (Plate 4, Fig. 1); or as a large opaque mass with small bosses projecting from its surface—pelvic type (Plate 3, Figs. 2, 3). In the normal kidney the point of the ureteric catheter enters the upper calyx of the renal pelvis, and can be seen here in a collargol plate (Plate 4, Fig. 3). In hydronephrosis the catheter impinges on the upper wall of the dilated pelvis (Plate 3, Fig. 3).

Braasch has recorded cases of renal tumour, tuberculosis, and other renal diseases in which he has used the method.

RADIOGRAPHY IN RENAL TUBERCULOSIS

Clark, Brown, and others have shown that radiographic shadows are thrown by chronic tuberculous "abscesses" of the kidney. The opacity depends in part upon the presence of phosphatic salts in the milky or putty-like substance found in these "abscesses," but also upon the greater bulk of the kidney which contains these collections. In Plate 5, facing p. 58, are shown the outline and details of structure of a tuberculous kidney converted into a multilocular sac filled with putty-like material.

RADIOGRAPHY IN NEW GROWTHS OF THE KIDNEY

Large growths of the kidney cast a dense, ill-defined shadow which extends beyond the normal limits of the kidney.

DANGERS OF RADIOGRAPHY

All possible care must be exercised by the radiographer in avoiding undue exposure of the patient, rough handling, or too severe pressure upon the kidney. I have seen a severe attack of hæmaturia with an increase in all the symptoms follow a radiographic examination of a tuberculous kidney, and a serious crisis of fever and reduced renal function supervene in bilateral calculous disease.

The collargol method must be used with the greatest possible care and gentleness, and is only safe and reliable in the hands of an expert.

LITERATURE

Blum, *Amer. Journ. Derm. and Gen.-Urin. Dis.*, March, 1912, p. 136.
Braasch, *Ann. Surg.*, Nov., 1910, p. 645.
Brown, *New York Med. Journ.*, March 31, 1906, p. 683.
Clark, *Med. News,* Dec. 9, 1905.
Keyes, *Trans. Amer. Urol. Assoc.*, 1909, p. 351.
Macintyre, *Lancet*, July 11, 1896.
Voelcker und **Lichtenberg,** *Münch. med. Woch.*, Jan. 16, 1906 ; *Beitr. klin. Chir.*, 1907, lii. 1.
Walker, Thomson, *Lancet,* June 17, 1911 ;· *Trans. Med. Soc. Lond.*, 1912.

III. EXAMINATION OF THE BLADDER IN SURGICAL DISEASES OF THE KIDNEY

The examination of most surgical diseases of the kidney is incomplete without examination of the bladder with the cystoscope. The method of performing cystoscopy will be described in the section dealing with diseases of the bladder.

The cystoscope may be required to localize the disease.

There may be disease of the bladder which has caused no vesical symptoms but has given rise to symptoms pointing to disease of the kidney. When a papilloma of the bladder is seated at one ureteric orifice there is often pain in the kidney on that side, and this, combined with hæmaturia from the papilloma, may cause a diagnosis of renal hæmaturia to be made if the cystoscope is not used. This is especially the case when the ureter and kidney are dilated from obstruction by a growth in the bladder. In such a case there is a painful enlarged kidney with hæmaturia, and without cystoscopy the kidney may be regarded as the source of the hæmaturia.

In tuberculosis and other diseases of the kidney there may be signs of cystitis with no symptoms of disease of the kidney. The secondary nature of the vesical disease will be demonstrated by the condition of the ureteric orifice and area surrounding it and the efflux.

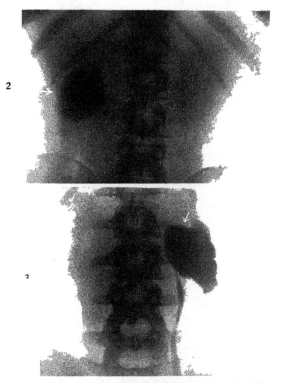

Fig. 1.—Dilated calyces in ureteral calculus. (Pp. 43, 176.)

Fig. 2.—Hydronephrosis caused by aberrant renal vessels. Dilated
renal pelvis shown by oval collargol shadow. (Pp. 43, 176.)

Fig. 3.—Hydronephrosis (pelvic type) in movable kidney. Three
arrows point to ureter; the upper and lower to segments
filled with collargol, the middle to an empty segment,
probably a descending wave of contraction. The outer
arrow points to the dilated kidney, the uppermost one
to the greatly dilated pelvis. (Pp. 43, 176.)

PLATE 3.

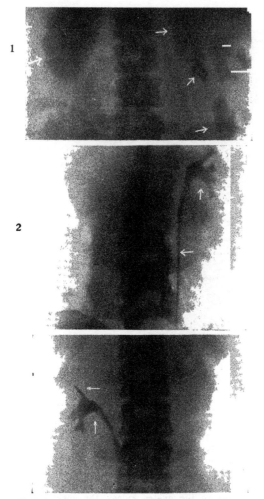

Fig. 1.—Double hydronephrosis. On the left is a hydronephrotic
kidney filled with collargol. The clear bands (lower arrow)
indicate the fibrous septa. On the right is a very large
hydronephrosis, the arrows pointing to shadows of widely
separated calculi in the kidney. (Pp. 43, 176.)

Fig. 2.—Pyelography : Normal trumpet-shaped pelvis and calyces.
Arrows point to catheter in ureter, open angle between this
and lower calyx, upper and lower calyces. (Pp. 43·6.)

Fig. 3.—Pyelography : Normal trumpet-shaped pelvis with calyces.
The point of the opaque catheter (arrow) is lying in the
upper calyx. An arrow points to the lower calyx, and
another to the open angle between this and the ureter
and pelvis. (P. 176.)

PLATE 4.

In many cases of pyuria and hæmaturia there are no definitely localizing symptoms, and cystoscopy is necessary to exclude disease of the bladder. In these cases a blood-stained or purulent efflux will indicate the kidney as the source of the hæmaturia or pyuria, and show which side is diseased.

Information may be obtained as to the state of the diseased kidney by observing the ureteric orifice. An open, rigid ureteric orifice denotes dilatation of the ureter and renal pelvis. A "dragged-out" ureteric orifice (Fenwick) is present in cases of advanced tuberculosis of the kidney or ureter. Here the orifice is displaced outwards and upwards, and resembles a tunnel. In cases where the efflux is a semi-solid pipe of pus the kidney is functionally destroyed and is converted into a thin-walled sac. Large quantities of purulent urine are poured out of the ureteric orifice in cases of acute and subacute pyelonephritis. A cloudy efflux is present in the minor grades of pyelitis. Where no efflux is present on one side, and the cause is not some temporary cessation of the renal function, the kidney may be absent on that side, or the ureter may be blocked by kinking or some other cause, or there may be a fistula of the ureter.

When the kidney is absent or totally destroyed, there will be no movement at the ureteric orifice. When the kidney is present and secreting, and the ureter blocked, there will be an occasional sluggish movement at the orifice, although there is no efflux. In the case of a fistula of the ureter the rhythm and force of the movements at the ureteric orifice may be normal, although there is no discharge of urine into the bladder. Lastly, information may be gained in regard to the presence and condition of a second kidney when one is diseased. The absence of a ureteric orifice on one side will usually denote the absence of the kidney on that side. The muscle of the trigone on the side corresponding to the congenitally absent ureter is often absent. Rarely, the ureter may open in some abnormal situation, such as the prostatic urethra.

The presence of a normally placed ureter and the observation of an efflux from it will in all but the rarest cases demonstrate the presence of a kidney on that side.

In very rare cases two normally placed ureteric orifices lead to the ureters of a solitary kidney, one of the ducts crossing the middle line. In such a case the condition may be demonstrated by passing an opaque bougie into the ureter and obtaining a radiogram, or by pyelography.

When there is disease, such as tuberculosis of one kidney and the bladder, the area of bladder mucous membrane around the ureteric orifice of the second kidney, and the orifice itself, may be free from disease. This is strong evidence but not absolute proof that the second kidney is not tuberculous. If the efflux is clear on this side, this is further evidence, but it is necessary to examine the urine of this kidney separately in order to make certain of the health of the organ.

Examination of the urine of each kidney.—In rare cases when there is known to be complete blocking of one kidney, or when a fistula drains away the urine from one kidney, it may be assumed that the urine passed through the bladder is derived from the other kidney, and examination of this urine will demonstrate the condition of the kidney. In all other cases the urine which is passed is a blend of that secreted by the two kidneys.

In order to examine the functional activity of one kidney, and frequently to localize disease to one kidney, it is necessary to examine the secretion of each organ separately. The urine of each kidney is obtained by means of separators or ureteric catheters (p. 367).

Exploration of the kidney.—Exploration of the kidney by operation may be necessary in the following cases :—

1. To make a diagnosis in an abdominal tumour of doubtful nature. Laparotomy will be the best method.

2. To ascertain the nature of disease already localized to the kidney. An oblique lumbar incision and extraperitoneal examination of the kidney is the method best suited to this purpose.

3. To ascertain the extent and connections and the condition of the lymphatics in a malignant growth of the kidney which has reached a considerable size. Either a combined lumbar extraperitoneal examination of the kidney with an extraperitoneal exploration through an opening in the peritoneum in front of the colon, or a laparatomy alone, may be used.

4. To ascertain the presence and condition of the second kidney when one is diseased and nephrectomy is proposed. Exploration of the kidney for this purpose can only be necessary in the rarest cases. Cystoscopy and catheterization of the ureters have taken the place of this operation, and it is only when these methods are rendered impossible by inflammation of the bladder that this operation is required. In some cases of tuberculosis of the kidney and bladder, when the bladder has been too irritable to permit of catheterization of the ureters, a course of tuberculin injections lasting three months has caused sufficient improvement to allow of ureteral catheterization. Exploration of the kidney in such cases is carried out through a lumbar incision, and the kidney is examined by inspection, palpation, and incision, and a slip of the kidney substance is examined microscopically. The abdominal route only permits of palpation, and has been proved to be worthless.

CHAPTER IV

ABNORMAL CONDITIONS OF THE URINE

OXALURIA

ABOUT 0·0172 grm. of oxalic acid is passed daily in the urine as calcium oxalate. This is derived from the food, and partly also from the tissues. It is held in solution by the acid phosphate of sodium of the urine. Calcium oxalate is deposited in the form of octahedra or dumb-bell crystals, which are visible to the naked eye as sparkling particles in clear urine. The urine is usually pale and faintly acid. When calcium oxalate appears in a high-coloured urine it is said to result from the decomposition of urea, and is of no clinical importance. Crystals of calcium oxalate are sometimes passed persistently for years with occasional attacks of severe oxaluria. Small masses of crystals clinging loosely together may be passed, and larger masses bound together with a colloid substance form calculi.

Increased excretion of oxalic acid has been observed in jaundice, diabetes, gastritis, enteritis, and pancreatitis, but is not constant in any disease. A deposit of these crystals may take place after eating certain vegetables, such as rhubarb, spinach, tomatoes, sorrel, and gooseberries.

In many cases persistent oxaluria is accompanied by symptoms of dyspepsia and mental depression, or even neurasthenia. The exact relationship of these symptoms to the oxaluria, whether they are the cause or the effect, is not decided.

The symptoms which are directly caused by the presence of large quantities of oxalate-of-lime crystals in the urine are due to irritation of the kidneys and urinary tract. Renal aching is frequently present, and is usually bilateral. It may, however, be more marked on or even confined to one side. Aching along the line of the ureter may also be felt. Unilateral renal coho may result from the passage of large quantities of oxalate crystals. The colic may be severe, and is indistinguishable from that caused by the passage of a calculus down the ureter. Hæmaturia may accompany the colic, and the blood is present in considerable quantities.

In less pronounced cases of oxaluria, blood discs are frequently found microscopically, when no staining of the urine is perceptible to the naked eye.

Some vesical irritation is usually present in oxaluria, and frequenoy of micturition may be the prominent symptom.

When an oxalate-of-lime stone is present, oxaluria may be pronounced; but, on the other hand, there may be only a few crystals or none at all.

All the symptoms of a calculus of the kidney, ureter, or bladder may be simulated by oxaluria. Exercise does not, however, affect the symptoms in the latter condition. Cystoscopy will show that no calculus is present in the bladder, and the X-rays fail to demonstrate a stone in the kidney or ureter.

Treatment.—The diet should contain little oxalic acid and lime, and plenty of magnesia, for the latter favours solution of calcium oxalate. The bowels should be regulated, and all causes of intestinal fermentation removed. Articles of diet that are rich in oxalic acid, and therefore contra-indicated, are rhubarb, spinach, tomatoes, sorrel, gooseberries, strawberries, tea, coffee, pepper, haricots, beetroot, and dried figs, much milk, quantities of carbohydrates in the form of sugar and sweets. Calcium is in excess in the following foods, which should therefore be avoided, viz. veal, milk, eggs, fresh vegetables such as radishes, asparagus, spinach, cereals (especially rice), and hard water.

Foods poor in lime, and therefore suitable, are meat (except veal), fish, bread, fruit, potatoes. Magnesium is abundant in meat, bread, potatoes, peas, apples, and beer, and these articles may be taken.

Mineral acids, such as dilute nitro-hydrochloric, should be given, combined with strychnine. The acidity of the urine should be increased by the administration of acid phosphate of sodium, which is the natural solvent of the oxalate of lime in the urine. It should be dissolved in a large quantity of water and taken between meals in a dose of ½ oz. to 1 oz. daily. It occasionally causes troublesome diarrhœa, and the quantity may have to be reduced on this account. When much irritation is present, sandal-wood oil in capsules (10 minims thrice daily) and a diluent water such as barley water may be given for a week at first, and the acid treatment commenced after the most acute symptoms have subsided.

Mineral waters which contain little lime, or such as are rich in magnesium and sodium phosphates, should be given. To the former belong Contrexéville and Vittel, and to the latter Kissingen. Hard water should be avoided, and also such mineral waters as contain lime (Rosbach, Apollinaris, Kronthal).

PHOSPHATURIA

This term is applied to the presence of undissolved earthy phosphates in the urine. The phosphates form a flocculent deposit, or the urine may be milky and deposit a thick white layer. Occasionally in a clear, well-coloured urine numerous sparkling crystals of triple phosphate are seen.

Phosphoric acid to the extent of 2–6 grm. is excreted daily in the urine in the form of phosphates of potassium, sodium, calcium, and magnesium. It is derived largely from the food, but partly from the tissues.

The acidity of the urine is due to acid phosphate of sodium. The phosphates of lime and magnesium are only soluble in acid urine, and when the urine is faintly acid, neutral, or alkaline these salts are precipitated. When the alkalinity is due to ammonia from decomposition of the urine, ammonio-magnesium phosphate is formed and is deposited. The phosphatic salts of sodium and potassium, which form about two-thirds of the total phosphates, remain in solution, whether they are acid, neutral, or basic.

A temporary phosphaturia occurs after a meal from the digestion of food rich in salts of vegetable acids or alkaline carbonates, and partly from the withdrawal of hydrochloric acid for the gastric secretion.

Phosphaturia is sometimes observed in children, and is here due to an increase of the calcium in the urine and deposit of calcium phosphate, without actual increase in the total phosphatic excretion. This increased calcium output in the urine coincides with a diminution in the calcium in the fæces, and is supposed to be due to an inflammation of the intestinal mucosa. This phosphaturia may be the cause of scalding during micturition, and increased frequency of the act.

In certain individuals of a nervous type, and in others during a period of nervous strain, a copious precipitate of earthy phosphates may be present, so that the urine is milky when passed. Nervons dyspepsia is frequently present, and is said to cause the phosphaturia. The total daily excretion of phosphates is not increased in these cases. The phosphaturia is often intermittent in character, and occurs after a period of unusual anxiety. I have known patients, whose urine was continuously phosphatic at first, improve under treatment, so that the phosphaturia appeared only on the day on which their attendance was expected at hospital or in the consulting-room. These patients not infrequently suffer from intermittent attacks of polyuria, or more strictly " hydruria." I have met with a patient whose urine varied in the course of one day from a milky phosphaturia to a highly acid urine which deposited urates on cooling.

Pronounced phosphaturia accompanied by dyspepsia and prolonged intestinal derangement has been the prelude to bacteriuria in several patients under my observation.

Patients affected with this type of phosphaturia usually complain of symptoms of dyspepsia, and frequently suffer from constipation. There is constant, dull aching over the kidneys, most marked in the morning on rising. The urine scalds when passed, and there is a feeling of dissatisfaction after micturition, and often some increased frequency of the act. The urethral mucosa is reddened, and the trigone red and congested, while the rest of the bladder is healthy in appearance. Such cases usually respond readily to treatment.

A more serious form of phosphaturia has been called "*phosphatic diabetes.*" In this there is an actual increase in the quantity of earthy phosphates, their proportion to the alkaline phosphates being as much as 5 to 2, or even more, instead of the normal 1 to 2. The quantity of urea may be normal, or may be increased, though, in a less proportion than the earthy phosphates. The symptoms consist in extreme nervous irritability, dyspepsia, and aching pain in the back and suprapubic area. There are increased frequency of micturition and scalding, and these symptoms may be very distressing. Cystitis is caused by the presence of masses of phosphates loosely held together in the bladder. There is no decomposition of the urine, which is neutral or faintly alkaline and non-bacterial. Some of my patients have dated the onset of their symptoms from the day on which they entered the cold atmosphere of the temperate zone on returning from the tropics. There may be extreme emaciation.

With a tuberculous heredity such cases as these may eventually develop phthisis, in others diabetes mellitus or insipidus has followed. A proportion of these cases recover and the symptoms disappear. In many patients suffering from chronic posterior urethritis a slight degree of phosphaturia is present, and varies with the changes in the inflammation. In moderate cystitis without decomposition of the urine, phosphates may be present and powder the surface of the bladder mucous membrane. In these cases the phosphaturia is probably due to the local inflammation further reducing the acidity of a faintly acid urine. Decomposition of the urine with liberation of ammonia causes a deposit of ammonio-magnesium phosphate in cases of severe and old-standing cystitis, ulcers, malignant growths, and papilloma, and foreign bodies become encrusted with phosphatic deposit.

Treatment.—Children suffering from phosphaturia should subsist on a diet poor in calcium salts, and a milk diet should be replaced by one consisting partly of meat. In adults the slighter cases are treated by the administration of tonics and mineral acids, such as nitro-hydrochloric acid and strychnine, quinine, phosphorus, and cod-liver oil. Acid phosphate of sodium in doses of 10–20 gr. thrice daily speedily cures some cases, but in others is less efficacious than mineral acids. The two may be combined. Where the phosphaturia is the cause of severe irritation and cystitis, belladonna and hyoscyamus, and occasionally sandal-wood oil, are useful. Opium may be given in full doses in the same forms of phosphaturia, but should not be long continued. Alcohol, coffee, and tea should be avoided. Moderate exercise and relief from worry and anxiety should be recommended. Where the urine is decomposing the treatment is that of chronic cystitis. Sodium acid phosphate is especially valuable in these cases. Its use for increasing the acidity of a faintly acid urine, or for rendering an alkaline urine acid, was first advocated by Dr. Robert Hutchison.

BACTERIURIA—BACILLURIA

Bacteriuria or bacilluria is a condition of the urine in which bacteria are present in such abundance that they render the fluid cloudy to the naked eye. In bacteriuria inflammatory products cannot be detected by the naked eye, or at most are seen in very small quantity. It is also a characteristic of bacteriuria that symptoms of inflammation of the urinary organs are either absent or very slight.

It is difficult to separate some cases of bacteriuria from cases of infection of the urinary tract where there is excessive bacterial growth combined with definite inflammatory reaction.

The phenomenon of bacteriuria represents, however, a special type of urinary infection in which there is excessive bacterial growth and minimal reaction.

Etiology.—Bacteriuria is found in infants and children, as well as in adults. Women are more frequently affected than men.

Pathology.—The bacterium coli is present in pure culture in over 80 per cent. of cases. It is frequently atypical in its cultural characters. The bacillus of typhoid is next most frequent. The staphylococcus albus is sometimes present, and more rarely the proteus vulgaris, a streptococcus, or the bacillus subtilis. These bacteria are usually present in pure culture. Bacteriuria may arise spontaneously, or it may supervene in the course, or follow in the wake, of some urinary disease. In the cases which are spontaneous a history of constipation, diarrhœa, or indigestion can usually be obtained, and in several cases I have observed pronounced phosphaturia immediately preceding the bacteriuria. Other predisposing causes are chronic septic conditions of the mouth and throat, operations upon the rectum and anus, and boils and carbuncles. Typhoid fever precedes the form known as typhoid bacilluria, and other fevers such as smallpox, diphtheria, scarlet fever, and measles may be accompanied by bacteriuria. The bacillus coli is frequently the bacterium present in the urine in these cases of bacteriuria associated with the acute fevers.

Bacteriuria may supervene during the course of a subacute or chronic urethritis of the prostatic urethra, or a chronic prostatitis, or chronic seminal vesiculitis. It may immediately follow the passage of a sound or catheter. It may follow an acute attack of pyelitis, and I have observed a case in which it complicated a movable kidney with intermittent hydronephrosis. In such cases the growth of bacteria is strictly localized to the diseased area. In a prostatic case clear sterile urine may be drawn from the bladder, and in a pyelitic case the ureteric catheter demonstrates that the culture ground is confined to the renal pelvis. In a boy with stone in the ureter whose urine was previously clear and sterile, I have seen a bacteriuria suddenly appear, last for three days, and then as suddenly disappear. The bacteria gain admission to the urinary tract through the kidneys (hæmatogenous infection), or are introduced into the urethra or bladder by the passage of instruments, or may be deposited at the urethral opening in women and female children and ascend to the bladder (urinary or ascending infection).

It has been stated that the bacteria may pass directly from the rectum through the rectal and bladder walls, but of this there is no reliable evidence.

In most cases of hæmatogenous infection the bacteria become implanted in some part of the urinary tract, and continue to proliferate there ; but there are other cases, I believe, where repeated infections from the bowel take place, the bacteria rapidly disappearing after each infection.

In cases of uncomplicated bacteriuria post-mortem examination has failed to discover any lesion of the mucous membrane of the urinary tract. The nidus of bacterial growth in women is the renal pelvis in the great majority of cases ; in males it may be either the renal pelvis or the prostate. When the renal pelvis is affected the condition is frequently unilateral.

The urine is hazy when passed, from the suspension of myriads of bacteria. Frequently an opalescent appearance is observed. On rotating a glass beaker containing the urine, so as to circulate the urine, and holding it to the light, a peculiar appearance is seen, like drifting mist or smoke, that is characteristic of the condition. This phenomenon is due to the suspension of fine particles (the bacteria) in fluid. It is to be seen also in the fluid obtained from a spermatocele, where the spermatozoa form the suspended particles. The reaction is usually acid, occasionally neutral, and rarely alkaline. On centrifuging it, no deposit, or only a very small quantity of deposit, is obtained, and the fluid remains cloudy. In most cases the urine has a peculiar strong fishy odour. It is never ammoniacal. There is usually a trace of albumin, and protein can be detected in most cases.

Under the microscope the field is crowded with bacteria, usually the motile bacterium coli. A few leucocytes may be found, and epithelial cells from the renal pelvis, ureter, and bladder or prostatic urethra. The only constant sign is the bacterial emulsion in the urine. The urine may be constantly cloudy for months or years, or it may clear and the bacteria disappear with almost startling suddenness. Just as suddenly the bacteria may reappear in as great quantity as before. I have seen the urine milky with bacterium coli in the morning, and clear in the afternoon of the same day.

There may be no symptoms at all, but signs of localized inflammation are seldom entirely absent.

In cases of chronic prostatitis or posterior urethritis the symptoms of these diseases are already present, and the bacterial condition of the urine is superadded. In bacteriuria arising without previous urinary disease there may be slight increase in the frequency of micturition, and some urgency or heat and burning on passing water. These symptoms are aggravated by cold and by dietary indiscretions. In children, nocturnal enuresis may result from bacteriuria. Here there is urgency and sometimes frequent micturition during the day; in severe cases there may be diurnal incontinence. In cases where the prostatic urethra or prostate is the seat of the bacterial growth the last few drops of urine are often milky with bacterial emulsion, while the rest of the urine is merely hazy.

In other cases the focus of bacterial growth is confined to the renal pelvis. If the bacteriuria be superadded to some disease the symptoms of that disease will be present. In cases arising spontaneously there may be some aching in the kidney and along the course of the ureter, and the kidney and ureter may be slightly tender. There are, however, cases where there is pronounced bacilluria with recurrent attacks of high fever, but no symptom referable to the urinary organs is present.

Prognosis.—In some cases bacteriuria is transient and appears for a few days only, disappearing under treatment. It may, however, be more persistent, and frequently it continues with exacerbations and remissions for months and sometimes for years. During this time the condition may have no influence on the health of the patient. In all cases there is the danger that a period of lowered resistance from some other cause may be the signal for a virulent bacterial inflammation of some part of the urinary tract.

Where bacteriuria is superadded to some disease already present, such as stone in the ureter or movable kidney, it is the precursor of inflammatory complications.

Diagnosis.—The diagnosis is made by the observation of the characteristic appearance of the urine and bacteriological examination. It is imperative to ascertain whether the bacilluria is the sole condition present, or whether it is superadded on stone, growth, chronic inflammation, or other pre-existing disease. Where bacilluria is an independent condition it is necessary to find out where the focus of infection has commenced (e.g. appendix, bowel), and what part of the urinary tract is affected (e.g. prostate, renal pelvis). The latter can only be ascertained by examination of the prostate, by cystoscopy, and by examination of the urine obtained from each kidney by the ureteric catheter.

Treatment.—The treatment consists in the administration of urinary antiseptics and diluents, local treatment of the focus of inflammation, and removal of the source of bacterial infection.

Of urinary antiseptics the best are urotropine (15–30 gr. daily), oil of turpentine (15–30 minims daily) in capsules, hetralin or helmitol (30 gr. daily), and salol (30 gr. daily). The administration of diuretics and alkaline waters with these antiseptics appears to render the urine less suitable for bacterial growth. Contrexéville, Vichy, or Evian water may be given, or the patient directed to drink large quantities of distilled or barley water.

Rovsing advises that in bacterial infection of the urinary tract a catheter should be retained in the urethra for a week or more while salol is administered by the mouth and large quantities of distilled water are drunk.

An alternative treatment to urinary antiseptics is the administration of large doses of alkalis together with diuretics. Citrate or acetate of potash (60–90 gr. daily) is given with the diuretic waters already mentioned.

Where the focus of bacterial growth is confined to the prostatic urethra and bladder, washing the bladder and urethra by Janet's irrigation method may quickly relieve the symptoms and suppress the bacterial growth. The solutions suitable for this irrigation are permanganate of potash (1 in 10,000 to 1 in 5,000), oxycyanide of mercury (1 in 10,000), or nitrate of silver (1 in 10,000).

When the bacterial nidus is situated in the renal pelvis, this may in some cases be washed with weak nitrate of silver solution (1 in 10,000) through a ureteric catheter.

It is of the utmost importance to empty the bowel and prevent further absorption. A mercurial pill followed by a saline purge should be given, and attention paid to obtaining a regular and free action of the bowel. Small doses of calomel ($\frac{1}{10}$-$\frac{1}{4}$ gr.) may be given regularly after meals, or a larger dose (1–2 gr.) may be given once a week.

In order to reduce the growth of the bacterium coli in the intestine a course of milk soured with the Bulgarian bacillus (B. Caucasicum) may be advised, and continued for several months.

Anti-coli horse serum has been administered with some success in acute cases of bacterium coli infection of the urinary tract, and may be tried. A dose of 25 c.c. of the serum should be injected subcutaneously on three successive days. If improvement has not taken place at the end of that time the treatment should be abandoned. Calcium lactate (20 gr. thrice daily) should be administered by the mouth to prevent the unpleasant effects of the serum.

Treatment by vaccines gives varying results. In some cases the bacteria in the urine rapidly diminish in quantity, and in a few cases disappear, when the bacteriuria has been uninfluenced by other methods of treatment. In cases apparently cured by vaccines recurrence may suddenly take place. In cases treated by vaccines, and also in those treated by serum, the opsonic index of the blood may rise while the state of the urine remains unchanged.

Vaccines should be prepared from cultures taken from the patient's urine. In bacterium coli infections small doses of vaccine up to 10 or 15 millions are less efficacious than higher doses from 30 millions and upwards. These should be given in graduated series up to 100 millions, or even higher, at intervals of a week.

Where the bacteriuria is superimposed on some pre-existing disease of the urinary tract, the latter must be suitably dealt with as a preliminary to treatment of the bacilluria. The onset of bacteriuria in a case of movable kidney or ureteric calculus should be the signal for operative measures.

HÆMATURIA

In hæmaturia the amount of blood in the urine may be so small that the microscope is required for its detection, or there may be so great a quantity that the fluid appears to consist wholly of blood.

An appearance resembling blood is given to the urine in bæmoglobinuria, and after the ingestion of some drugs, such as senna, rhubarb, sulphonal, etc. The final test for hæmaturia is the discovery of red blood-corpuscles by the microscope. The urine in hæmoglobinuria has a peculiar purple colour; it contains no clots, and there are no blood corpuscles even after centrifugalizing.

Hæmaturia may take origin in any part of the urinary tract, and may be caused by a large number of surgical diseases. In examining a case of hæmaturia it is necessary first to localize the bleeding to one part of the urinary tract, and then to diagnose the disease which causes it.

1. **Localization of hæmaturia.**—The discharge of blood from the meatus, apart from micturition, will indicate that the source of hæmorrhage is anterior to the compressor urethræ muscle. At any part of the urinary tract behind the compressor urethræ blood will mix with the urine and will only be discharged with it.

Hæmaturia with other symptoms.—Hæmaturia may be the solitary symptom, or it may be accompanied by other symptoms which indicate the source of the hæmorrhage.

Hæmaturia with pain.—Severe pain in one kidney and ureteric colic will localize the hæmorrhage to this kidney, the renal pelvis, or the ureter. Dull aching in one kidney is not so reliable a symptom. A papilloma or malignant growth of the bladder at one ureteric orifice may give rise to hæmaturia with unilateral renal aching.

Pain at the end of the penis on micturition points to the base of the bladder or the prostatic urethra as the source of the blood; while pain at the base of the sacrum, in the rectum or perineum, will point to the prostate.

Hæmaturia with frequent micturition.—Frequent micturition suggests the localization of the point of hæmorrhage to the prostatic urethra or bladder. Copious bleeding which has come from the kidney may, however, cause irritation of the bladder, and this is more likely when clots are present in the urine.

In some diseases of the kidney, such as tuberculosis, reflex irritation of the bladder is a prominent feature. It follows that hæmaturia with frequent micturition may be caused by disease of the kidney when the bladder is healthy.

Hæmaturia with obstruction.—Urethral obstruction may be temporarily produced by the impaction of a clot in the urethra, but the combination of obstruction and hæmaturia is most frequently due to prostatic or urethral disease.

A papilloma of the bladder situated near the internal meatus, or one provided with a long pedicle, may cause hæmaturia with attacks of obstruction.

Examination of the urine.—The colour of the urine may be of some assistance. The longer the blood remains in contact with the urine the more likely is it to be discoloured. The higher the source of blood in the urinary tract the more likely is it to be well mixed with the urine. Blood in a highly acid urine is brownish in colour, and in an alkaline urine bright red. When much pus is mixed with the blood, and the urine is decomposing, a dirty-brownish, muddy appearance is given to the urine.

The urine may have a brownish or smoky appearance. This indicates that the blood is small in quantity, well mixed with the urine, and the reaction acid. Such bleeding is usually renal in origin. In renal hæmaturia the blood precipitates very slowly, so that a sediment forms only after several hours. In coffee-coloured urine the source of bleeding is frequently the kidney or kidney pelvis, but the blood may come from the bladder or prostate, especially if there be urethral obstruction. Purple urine denotes venous bleeding, which may be derived from any part of the urinary tract.

If the urine has a delicate pink colour the blood usually comes from the bladder or the prostatic urethra. Bright-red blood indicates copious bleeding from an arterial source, and may be discharged from any part of the urinary tract. Disease of the bladder or prostate is the most frequent cause of such bleeding.

Type of hæmaturia.—The blood may be present at the beginning or at the end of micturition, or thoroughly mixed with the urine. Blood appearing at the beginning of micturition (initial hæmaturia) has a urethral origin, and usually comes from the prostatic urethra. Terminal hæmaturia may mean that the first urine is clear and' blood appears at the end of micturition, or that the earlier part of the stream is blood-stained and the last part pure blood. The blood in this type is derived from the prostatic urethra or the bladder. No inference can be drawn as to the source of blood which is mixed with the whole of the urine (total hæmaturia).

Presence of clots.—The formation of clots depends largely upon the proportion of blood in the urine. Blood poured out in large quantities from the kidney or renal pelvis may clot in the ureter. Slender worm-like clots, 10 or 12 in. in length, are sometimes passed in such cases, and are diagnostic of the source of the bleeding. More frequently, however, the clots passed from the ureter are small plugs, ½ in. in length. The blood may be rapidly passed into the bladder and clot, there forming irregular masses or flat clots which indicate the position of the clotting but not the source of the hæmorrhage. Vesical hæmorrhage will produce these flat or irregular clots. Urethral bleeding may form a clot which lies in the urethra and is discharged with the urine. This will form a long worm-like clot, not unlike that derived from the ureter, but it is thicker and shorter, and frequently shows enlargements and contractions corresponding to the varying calibre of the urethra.

Albumin can be demonstrated in the urine in hæmaturia, even where the amount of blood is very small. In cases of renal hæmaturia, however, the quantity of albumin is in excess of what might be expected to be present from the admixture of blood. If on estimation the proportion of albumin to hæmoglobin prove to be more than 1·6 to 1, this points to a renal affection as the cause of the hæmaturia (Newman).

In renal hæmaturia the corpuscles often appear as pale discs, almost devoid of colouring matter, while the corpuscles that are added to the urine in the lower urinary tract are less changed.

Epithelial and other elements may be found in the urine, and give an indication of the source of the bleeding.

Casts of the renal tubules, if present, indicate a renal source of the hæmaturia. Epithelial cells from the kidney, pelvis and ureter, bladder or urethra, may be discovered and help to localize the source of the hæmorrhage.

Examination of the patient.—This may reveal signs of disease which point to the source of bleeding. The kidneys, ureters, and bladder should be examined by abdominal palpation, and the prostatic and membranous urethra, the prostate, seminal vesicles, bladder base, and lower ureters examined from the rectum.

Cystoscopic examination.—The cystoscope is the means by which the source of the hæmaturia can be localized with certainty. On cystoscopy, some disease of the bladder, such as papilloma, may be discovered; or the bladder may be found healthy, and the hæmaturia will be known to originate in the kidney, or kidney pelvis. On examining the ureteric orifices, changes may be observed, such as ulceration or tuberculous deposit, which will assist in the localization of the hæmaturia. Where no gross changes are present at the ureteric orifices there is sometimes a slight staining of the lips of the orifice on the side whence the hæmaturia is proceeding. Examination of the efflux from the ureters may show blood-stained urine issuing from one or both sides. (Plate 5, Fig. 1.) When the quantity of blood is small it may be extremely difficult to detect any change in the efflux. The hæmaturia may sometimes cease suddenly before the cystoscopy, so that the examination must be repeated. Finally, the ureters should be catheterized and a sample of urine obtained from each kidney for microscopical examination. This examination should only be carried out by an expert, for the

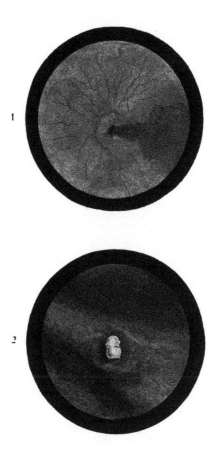

Fig. 1.—Hæmaturia. Blood-stained efflux
from left ureter. (P. 58.)

Fig. 2.—Semi-solid pus issuing from
ureter in case of chronic suppurative pyelonephritis. Acute
cystitis. (Pp. 65, 125.)

PLATE 5.

technique is difficult, and bleeding is easily produced in passing the ureteric catheter, and thus the object of the examination is likely to be defeated.

2. **Diagnosis of the cause of hæmaturia.**—Hæmaturia may appear in almost any disease of the urinary organs. The character of the hæmaturia and the position it occupies in the symptomatology of each disease will be fittingly described under the various diseases. There is, however, one form of hæmaturia which cannot be referred to any single disease, and it must therefore be dealt with in this place.

Essential renal hæmaturia.—This name has been given to a group of cases in which hæmaturia has been localized to one kidney, and nephrotomy, with, in some cases, an examination of the kidney after removal, has failed to reveal the cause of the hæmorrhage. More careful examination of these kidneys, however, shows that in most of them a partial chronic nephritis exists, and in a few there is a varicose condition of one or more of the renal papillæ. The partial chronic nephritis which is present in these cases gives rise to no changes visible to the naked eye, so that the condition is readily overlooked when the kidney is examined by nephrotomy. Further, it is not found in every microscopic section of the kidney substance, so that it may be overlooked unless careful search be made in a number of such sections.

In a section of the renal cortex the tubules and glomeruli are normal in appearance, except at one part where there is a patch of fibrous tissue separating the renal tubules. The fibrous tissue may be poor in nuclei, or there may be an abundant infiltration of small round cells. Frequently the fibrous tissue forms a streak radiating towards the capsule; occasionally it is subcapsular. The capsule is frequently thickened, and there may be a patch of thickening at the spot where an intertubular streak of fibrous tissue reaches the surface of the kidney. One or several completely sclerosed and atrophied glomeruli may be seen; sometimes there is only a thickening of the capsule of Bowman. The walls of the vessels do not appear changed, but occasionally I have found the veins dilated, and there may be some perivascular infiltration of round cells. The tubules are frequently found filled with blood. The epithelium of the kidney is unchanged. A few cases have been recorded in which hæmaturia without other symptoms and without albuminuria has been caused by a more extensive unilateral chronic nephritis (Poirier, Loumeau).

The characters of essential renal hæmaturia are as follows: It is spontaneous, and no cause can be assigned for the onset; it is not affected by rest or movement. The blood is abundant and well mixed, and the urine has a dark port-wine colour. Clots are very rarely formed. The hæmaturia is strictly unilateral ; it may suddenly cease after some weeks or months, and may as suddenly reappear and become persistent. In the intervals of clear urine no albumin can be detected and no tube casts found. No bacteria are found in the urine. There is occasionally a dull aching pain on the side from which the hæmaturia proceeds : this is unaffected by movement. The kidney is not tender or enlarged.

In thirteen cases of unilateral symptomless hæmaturia in which I explored the kidney and removed a portion for examination the microscope showed patches of fibrosis of varying size in the cortex in all. The capsule was frequently thickened, solitary sclerosed glomeruli were sometimes found, and there was blood in the convoluted tubules in seven cases. It is possible that the cause of these changes may be the excretion of bacteria by the kidneys in constipation and other conditions (*see* p. 120).

A varicose condition of one or more of the renal papillæ has been described by Fenwick and by Whitney and Pilcher. The origin of this varicose condition appears to be doubtful, and it may possibly result from a patch of interstitial nephritis similar to the condition described above. The type of hæmaturia and absence of other symptoms are similar.

Profuse unilateral renal hæmaturia which is unaccompanied by other symptoms is sometimes met with as a premonitory or early symptom of chronic Bright's disease. Roy, Harmonic, and Israel have described cases in which the symptoms of chronic Bright's disease developed several years after a spontaneous, symptomless hæmaturia. Newman has recorded a case of severe renal hæmaturia which preceded other symptoms of tubercular disease by two years. " Symptomless " hæmaturia is a symptom of some growths of the kidney from a very early stage of their development.

Treatment of essential hæmaturia.—Exploration of the kidney by operation is necessary in such cases of unilateral hæmaturia. If a papilla of the kidney shows congestion it may be cut away with a sharp spoon. Where no such appearance is observed and nephrotomy fails to discover any lesion in the substance of the kidney, the wounds in the kidney and renal pelvis should be closed with catgut sutures. The hæmaturia in the majority of cases ceases after the exploration, apparently as a result of pressure upon the bleeding vessel by the sutures. For this reason, and also because bilateral nephritis may give rise to unilateral hæmaturia, nephrectomy should not be performed. Very rarely hæmorrhage commences again and necessitates a second operation.

Hale White describes five cases of renal hæmaturia in which the kidney was explored by nephrotomy and no lesion found. Two of these cases had a recurrence of hæmorrhage, in three there was none. Decapsulation may be combined with nephrotomy, but the results are similar to those of nephrotomy alone, the hæmaturia recurring in rare cases.

Treatment of hæmaturia.—It is only in exceptional cases that treatment of hæmaturia apart from operative measures is required. The following drugs may be used, viz. morphia, ergot, ergotine, tincture of hamamelis, and calcium chloride or lactate. Of these, morphia and calcium lactate are the best. A hypodermic injection of morphia is given, and the patient placed on calcium lactate, 10 gr. in cachets being given every four hours for forty-eight hours. After this period the calcium lactate should be omitted.

Local treatment.—In renal hæmaturia, dry cupping over the loin, and icebags over the kidney, may be employed. Adrenalin has been injected into the renal pelvis through a ureteric catheter, 1 drachm of a 1-in-5,000 solution being used.

Vesical hæmaturia.—A catheter should be passed and the bladder washed out with hot boric solution, or with a hot, very weak solution (1 in 15,000) of silver nitrate. Large quantities of these solutions must be used, the stream being supplied from an irrigator or a large glass hand-syringe. A double-way catheter with continuous irrigation is often useful.

After washing the bladder, 10–12 oz. of a solution of antipyrin (10 per cent.) are introduced and left in for a few minutes, or 1 or 2 drachms of adrenalin solution (1 in 2,000) are injected into the bladder, left for a few minutes, and then run out. If clots are present in the bladder they may be washed out through a large catheter, or, better, through a large evacuating catheter such as is used in lithotrity. The rubber lithotrity bulb may be attached and the clots sucked out.

These methods should not be persisted in for long, and, if the clots are of large size and the bladder has become distended with them, suprapubic cystotomy should be performed, the clots cleared out, and a stream of hot boric solution (115° to 120° F.) passed through a catheter in the urethra, and allowed to well out of the suprapubic opening. A large drainage tube (1 in. diameter) should then be placed in the bladder, and the foot of the bed raised on blocks.

LITERATURE

Albarran, *Presse Méd.*, 1904, p. 657.
Fenwick, *Clinical Cystoscopy.* London, 1904.
Graff, *Folia Urol.*, 1908, p. 274.

LITERATURE—*continued*

Israel, *Deuts. med. Woch.*, Feb. 27, 1902 ;
    Mittheil. aus d. Grenzgeb. d. Med. u. Chir., 1899, p. 471.
Klotzenberg, *Zeits. f. Urol.*, 1908, p. 125.
Kretschner, *Zeits. f. Urol.*, 1907, S. 490.
Legueu, *Ann. d. Mal. d. Org. Gén.-Urin.*, 1891, p. 564.
Pilcher, *Ann. Surg.*, 1909, p. 652.
Rovsing, *Brit. Med. Journ.*, 1898, ii. 1547.
White, Hale, *Quart. Journ. Med.*, 1911, p. 509.
Whitney, *Boston Med. Surg. Journ.*, 1908, p. 797.

PYURIA

The presence of pus in the urine is, except in a few rare cases, a sign of inflammation of some part of the urinary tract. The inflammation may be confined to one segment of the urinary tract, such as the urethra, the bladder, or the renal pelvis, or it may be more widely spread, and affect the bladder and pelvis of the kidney. While pyuria is always due to inflammation, the ultimate cause of the inflammation varies. There may be a bacterial infection of an otherwise healthy urinary tract, or there may be bacterial infection superadded to stone, stricture, growths, or other gross lesions. Further, one bacterial inflammation may be superimposed or follow upon another of a different character : thus, a staphylococcal or streptococcal inflammation may be added to a tuberculous inflammation. It is necessary to localize the origin of the pus as a preliminary to making a diagnosis of the cause.

1. **Examination of the urine.** (*a*) **Quantity.**—Apart from acute inflammation of the urethra, the distribution of which will be evident from the discharge of pus at the meatus, the largest quantities of pus are derived from purulent collections in the kidney. In cases of long-standing bladder inflammation the quantity of deposit may be large, but the proportion of pus is not so great.

(*b*) **Character of the pus.**—Pus in small quantities makes the urine cloudy and opaque, and in large quantities milky. This may be equally produced by a copious urethral discharge and a pyelonephritis, but the clinical features of the cases are so obviously different that no question of differential diagnosis need arise. Pus from the urethra is mixed with a certain amount of mucus, so that the deposit, which settles quickly to the bottom of the glass, has a fluffy, feathery appearance. The urine in inflammation of the bladder gives a deposit which is billowy and fluffy, and occupies a large part of the glass without sinking heavily to the bottom. The urine is generally high-coloured and has a high specific gravity. In severe grades of old-standing cystitis the urine may be like coffee to which a large proportion of milk has been added. The sediment, after standing for an hour or two, is thickly viscous, and clings like slime to the bottom of the vessel.

Renal pus—that is, pus which is produced in the renal pelvis or in a dilated kidney—gives a milky urine when passed, and a characteristic deposit on standing. A heavy solid layer of yellow or yellowish-green pus with a flat, even surface lies at the bottom of the vessel and rolls heavily to the lowest part when the vessel is canted. The supernatant fluid is cloudy with suspended pus or bacteria. The urine is usually pale in colour and of low specific gravity. When a suppurative renal disease is combined with cystitis, there is the solid layer of pus at the bottom of the glass, and above this is a layer of billowy, fluffy muco-pus.

(c) **Odour and reaction of the urine.**—There is no unusual odour in the pyuria of a purulent urethritis. In bacteriuria, when the bacterial growth is excessive and the pyuria in minimal amount, the odour of the urine is "fishy."

In chronic cystitis the urine becomes decomposed and has a pungent, ammoniacal odour. As a rule, purulent urine from the kidney has no strong or characteristic odour, but a purulent collection in a dilated kidney may be offensive, and a pyelitis with excessive bacterial growth may possess a very strong, penetrating smell.

That " acid pyuria is from the kidney and alkaline pyuria from the bladder " is no longer accepted as accurate. The following bacteria produce acute cystitis in which the purulent urine remains acid, viz. the bacillus coli, gonococcus, and bacillus typhosus; while the tubercle bacillus produces a subacute or chronic cystitis with an acid urine. The bacillus coli is the most frequent cause of cystitis. The staphylococcus, streptococcus, and proteus are the bacteria of alkaline cystitis. These bacteria cause the ammoniacal decomposition of the urine found in chronic non-tuberculous cystitis.

The pyuria of pyelitis is usually acid, but not invariably so. Ammoniacal decomposition may take place from the same causes as in the bladder. A slightly alkaline urine from the kidney is mixed with the acid urine from the second kidney, and the blended urine is acid. Catheterization of the ureters separates the alkaline and acid urines in these cases.

(d) **Type of pyuria.**—The urine should be passed into two glasses. Pus appearing at the beginning of micturition has a urethral origin. When the urine is clear at the beginning of micturition and purulent at the finish, the pus comes from the prostate or bladder.

Intermittent pyuria is the special characteristic of the discharge from an inflamed dilated renal pelvis. The urine is clear, or almost clear, for days or weeks, and during this time renal symptoms are present and increase in severity. Then the urine suddenly becomes thick with pus and the renal symptoms disappear. This is repeated at varying intervals. Intermittent pyuria may also be observed when an abscess sac repeatedly discharges into the bladder or urethra, or there is a diverticulum of the bladder which has become infected.

(e) **Chemical and microscopical character of the urine.**— Albumin is present in pyuria in a small amount, which is proportional to the quantity of pus present. When nephritis is present, as in pyelonephritis, the quantity of albumin is greater. In catarrhal pyelonephritis the albumin will only give a cloud, while in suppurative pyelonephritis it may be present in large quantity.

If the albumin appears to be present in excessive quantities, renal complication may be suspected. The proportion of albumin to the number of pus corpuscles per cubic millimetre may assist the diagnosis. The albumin should bear the relation of 1 in 1,000 when the pus corpuscles number 100,000 per c.mm. In a urine which contains 40,000 per c.mm. and shows 2 per 1,000 of albumin, the albumin must be derived from another source than the pus. Epithelial elements may be present in the urine, but have rather less significance in regard to localization here than in hæmaturia. Tube casts are found in the slighter forms of pyelonephritis, and are of importance in localizing the process where symptoms are absent or slight.

2. **Presence of localizing symptoms.**—The symptoms of prostatic disease and disease of the seminal vesicles, and rectal examination, will clearly distinguish pyuria which proceeds from these organs from that derived from the bladder and kidneys. In these cases clear urine may be drawn by catheter from the bladder, while the urine which is passed is purulent. The symptoms of inflammation of the bladder will demonstrate that that organ is diseased, but the cystitis may be produced by secondary infection of the bladder from the kidney by way of the ureter, or there may be reflex bladder symptoms from the kidney without actual vesical disease. The renal symptoms in these cases are frequently minimal, while the bladder symptoms are prominent.

3. **Other methods of examination.** (a) **Cystoscopy.**—The cystoscope is a means of localizing disease causing pyuria in a large number of cases which would otherwise remain obscure. When the cause of the pyuria lies in the bladder the disease will be diagnosed at the same time. When the kidney is at fault the source of the pyuria will be localized to one or both organs.

The examination of the ureteric orifices should not be neglected, even when all the symptoms point to cystitis and the cystoscope lends support to the view.

Disease of the bladder exclusively surrounding one ureteric orifice, changes at the orifice itself, and the observation of murky or purulent urine coming from one ureter will show that there is disease of the kidney, whether renal symptoms are present or not. When the quantity of pus in the urine is small and the bladder inflamed, it may be very difficult to distinguish the pyuria by examining the ureteric efflux. In such cases catheterization of the ureters will become necessary. A urine with a moderate quantity of pus and shreds is readily distinguished as purulent at the ureteric orifice; when the pus is present in quantity the appearance of the efflux is unmistakable. Pipes of semi-solid pus are observed issuing from the ureteric orifice in some cases of advanced suppurative disease of the kidney. (Plate 5, Fig. 2.)

(b) **Catheterization of the ureters.**—When cystitis is present, catheterization of the ureters may be difficult. A general anæsthetic will be required, and a good deal of patience must be exercised. The various forms of separator are quite unsuitable for use in such cases. The urine collected from each ureter is compared, each urine is examined microscopically and chemically, and cultures are made. Very important information may thus be gained which cannot be obtained by other methods. In a case of chronic cystitis it may be possible to show by this means that purulent urine comes from one kidney and contains tubercle or colon bacilli, while the urine collected from the other ureter is healthy.

(c) **Radiography.**—In cases of long-standing pyuria radiography may show the presence of stones in one or both kidneys when no symptom of their presence has been observed.

CHYLURIA

In chyluria there is fat in emulsion in the urine so finely divided that no globules of fat are found with the microscope. The urine is milky, and on standing a layer like cream separates and rises to the surface. Shaking with ether extracts the fat and clears the urine. The condition is found in filariasis, in which the lymphatics are blocked with the filaria worms above the entrance of the lacteals. The obstruction causes dilatation of the lymphatics of the renal pelvis, ureter, and bladder, and eventually rupture of these vessels and mixture of chyle with the urine. The urine is clear in the morning after fasting.

F

PNEUMATURIA

Gas is discharged with the urine and appears usually at the end of micturition, producing a gurgling, bubbling, or whistling noise and a peculiar sensation.

Pneumaturia may result from the introduction of air into the bladder by means of a catheter or during evacuation after lithotrity. The gas may come from the intestine, escaping into the bladder by a vesico-intestinal fistula. There may rarely be spontaneous development of gas in the urinary tract. In some of these cases sugar is present in the urine, and the pneumaturia results from fermentation of the sugar and the formation of alcohol, setting free carbonic acid gas. This results from the action of organisms, usually the Bacillus coli communis, but occasionally the Proteus vulgaris. Where sugar is not present in the urine the spontaneous formation of gas has been said to be derived from the blood or to be due to the action on the urine of gas-producing bacteria, such as the B. coli and the B. lactis aerogenes.

Treatment.—When no fistula exists, treatment consists in removing the cause of the fermentation by washing the bladder and administering urinary antiseptics. Glycosuria should be treated.

The treatment of fistula of the bladder will be discussed later (Chap. XXXIX).

LITERATURE

Luetscher, *Johns Hopkins Hosp. Bull.*, Oct., 1911, p. 261.
Schnitzler, *Internat. klin. Rundschau*, 1894, pp. 265, 306.
Wildbolz, *Correspond. Bl. f. Schweiz. Aerzte*, 1901 p. 683.

CHAPTER V

CONGENITAL ABNORMALITIES OF THE KIDNEY AND URETER

FŒTAL lobulation of the kidneys occasionally persists throughout life. The only clinical importance of this fœtal form is that these kidneys, according to the view of some authorities, are specially vulnerable to disease. Küster and Wagner state that they frequently become tuberculous.

Complete absence of both kidneys is most frequently found in acephalic fœtuses and other monsters. The condition has no clinical importance.

Supernumerary kidneys are rare. A third kidney has occasionally been found post mortem, and very rarely on operation.

CONGENITAL ABSENCE OR ATROPHY OF ONE KIDNEY —FUSED KIDNEYS

These conditions are of extreme practical importance. I collected 93 cases of death from uræmia or anuria commencing within the first few days after an operation on one kidney, and found that there was no second kidney in 10 of the cases, and that the second kidney was " completely atrophied " in 8. In over 19 per cent. of these cases, therefore, the fatal result was due to the absence or atrophy of one kidney.

CONGENITAL ABSENCE OF ONE KIDNEY—UNSYMMETRICAL KIDNEY

The frequency with which unsymmetrical kidney or extreme congenital atrophy of the kidney occurs is about 1 in 2,400 bodies (Morris). The left kidney is more frequently absent than the right, and male subjects are more frequently affected in the proportion of two to one (left 127, right 97—Mankiewicz).

The renal vessels of the side on which the kidney is wanting are usually absent, or are quite rudimentary, being represented by a few small twigs which ramify in the retroperitoneal fat. The ureter is usually absent (93 per cent.). When present, it is represented by a solid fibrous cord of varying length which finds attachment to the bladder at its lower end and disappears in the retroperitoneal fat at its upper end. There may be no trace of the ureteric opening, and this half of the trigone of the bladder may be atrophied. A small dimple may sometimes mark the situation which the ureteric orifice would occupy, and sometimes an orifice is actually present opening into a lumen which extends for 1 to 2 cm. along the fibrous cord. The suprarenal gland is absent on the same side in 27·7 per cent. of cases.

Associated with congenital absence of one kidney there is some congenital malformation in the genital system in 70·8 per cent. of cases, almost without exception found on the same side as the renal defect. Thus, in the female subject there has been uterus bicornis with imperfect development of the horn of the uterus on the side of the absent kidney, absence of the uterus, ovary, and Fallopian tube, formation of a septum in the vagina, and absence of the vagina; in the male, absence or atrophy of the testis, vas deferens, and seminal vesicle have been observed.

Other congenital malformations have also been noted, such as hare-lip and cleft palate, accessory auricles, double thumbs, web fingers and toes.

The single kidney is usually larger than the natural size, but there are cases in which it is not increased in size. Sometimes the organ may be as much as twice the size of a normal kidney, or even larger. Such excessive growth cannot be regarded as due to compensatory hypertrophy. It may occupy the natural position in the loin, or it may sometimes be misplaced and lie in the iliac fossa or over the lumbar vertebræ or the sacrum. The kidney is sometimes lobulated, and may have lost its reniform outline and become rounded or globular or even irregular, but more frequently it retains its natural shape. The ureter is single and enters the bladder in the usual position. Occasionally the ureteric orifice in the bladder may be misplaced towards the middle line, or it may open in some abnormal position such as the urethra or vas deferens.

Congenital Atrophy of One Kidney

Congenital atrophy to the extent that the affected kidney is almost obliterated is very rare. Morris found only 3 such cases in 15,904 post-mortem examinations. Less complete atrophy of the kidney is more frequently observed. The atrophy may be due to chronic Bright's disease, to blocking of the ureter, or to embolism.

The chief difference between cases of extreme congenital atrophy and congenital absence is that in the former some rudiment of the kidney is always found and the ureter is present, though sometimes merely in the form of a fibrous cord.

The rudimentary kidney may be a fibro-fatty nodule, or it may be a fibrous nodule with cysts and traces of renal tissue. The shape and appearance may be that of a fœtal kidney with the well-marked lobulation.

Clinical facts relating to congenital absence or atrophy of one kidney.—To the surgeon, complete atrophy and total absence are synonymous terms.

A single kidney is prone to be attacked by disease. Calculus is especially frequent in these kidneys. Newman collected 8 cases of single kidney affected with calculus; Mosler found that 9 out of 12 cases of single kidney had calculi. Malignant growths have also been observed, while cases of tuberculous disease, hydro- and pyonephrosis, and chronic nephritis are recorded.

Such diseases are rendered more serious by the fact that they develop in a single kidney. Apart from this, however, the absence of one kidney does not of itself shorten life. This condition is found in bodies from infancy to old age. Newman collected 17 cases aged over 60 years.

In the great majority of cases of single kidney the condition has been found accidentally post mortem. A few cases of nephrectomy of a single kidney are recorded. I have collected 18 such cases. It is imperative, therefore, that proof of the presence of a second kidney should be obtained whenever nephrectomy is proposed.

The presence of some congenital abnormality of the genital organs, or even some congenital malformation elsewhere, should put the surgeon on his guard when dealing with a case of kidney disease. In 103 cases of congenital absence of the kidneys collected by Ballowitz, where the state of the genital organs was mentioned, there were 73 (70·8 per cent.) in which some malformation was present, and the majority of these were females (28 male and 41 female).

The following means may be used to obtain proof of the presence of a second kidney, viz. (1) cystoscopy, (2) catheterization of the ureters, (3) lumbar exploration.

1. *Cystoscopy.*—In those cases where a kidney is congenitally absent the ureter is also absent, and there is, in many cases, no ureteric opening in the bladder.

The ureteric orifice is absent in 33·3 per cent. of such cases (73 in 234 cases—Mankiewicz). It will therefore be possible to make a diagnosis of congenital absence of a kidney by cystoscopy in one-third of the cases. Rarely the half of the trigone is absent or rudimentary on the side of the absent kidney (Fig. 18). This has been observed on the left side (4 cases) but not on the right. In some cases a dimple may be seen in the position of the ureteric orifice. In a small number of cases there is a normal ureteric orifice which leads into a short tunnel in a rudimentary ureter extending upwards for a few centimetres. In such a ureter the normal rhythmic contractions of the functioning ureter are absent, and there is no efflux. It does not follow, however, that every ureter that is motionless under observation lacks a functional kidney. It frequently happens that while the surgeon is examining the ureteric orifice the ureter ceases to contract, and there may be a pause of several minutes' duration.

2. *Catheterization of the ureters.*—By this method there is provided a means of proving that a patent ureter exists, and that a

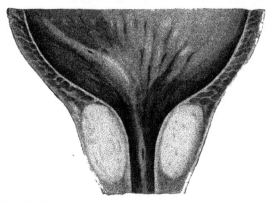

Fig. 18.—Bladder and prostatic urethra in a case of solitary kidney, showing absence of left half of trigone and of left ureteric orifice.

functionally active kidney is present, and the functional value of the kidney may be tested by the various methods which have already been described (p. 20).

If the catheter passes 12 or 13 in. along the ureter without hindrance, the patency of the duct is demonstrated ; but if the catheter is arrested at some point near the bladder orifice, it does not follow that the lumen ends here. The point of the catheter may be arrested by catching in a fold of mucous membrane, especially where there is over- or under-distension of the bladder, or a loaded rectum. A catheter with a smooth, rounded end is the best for use where such a fold is encountered, and various degrees of distension of the bladder and elevation of the pelvis should be tried, and, if necessary, the rectum should be unloaded with an enema. A general anæsthetic may give assistance.

There are also pathological causes for the catheter being arrested at some point in the ureter, but these need not be discussed here, for their presence will already have led to the conclusion that a kidney exists on this side. The withdrawal of urine from a catheter lodged in a ureter is an almost certain proof that a kidney exists on this side. There are, however, rare cases in which two ureters arise from one kidney, and open into the bladder in the normal position (*see* p. 75). Pyelography (p. 42) will give valuable information in such cases.

3. *Lumbar exploration of the kidney.*—A preliminary operation may be performed to demonstrate the presence of the second kidney. The organ is exposed by a lumbar incision, and, if a kidney be found, the size, appearance, consistence, and the microscopical character of a slip cut from its substance are examined.

Unless there is some suspicion as to the absence or atrophy or disease of a second kidney, this method is not likely to be used, but should the other methods already described fail, and a suspicion of such a condition be raised, the use of lumbar exploration is fully justified.

Operative interference in a single kidney has been frequently undertaken, in most cases without previous knowledge that the kidney attacked was a single organ. Winter records 4 cases of nephrolithotomy for calculous anuria in a single kidney where the patients recovered. In 18 cases of death from anuria after operation upon a kidney, where the other kidney was completely atrophied or absent, I found that nephrotomy had been performed for tuberculosis once and for stone once. In the remaining 16 cases nephrectomy of the single kidney was performed for the following conditions : Tuberculosis 3, calculus 3, hydronephrosis 4, displaced and floating kidney 3, cystic and hydatid cyst 2, carcinoma 1.

Solitary or Fused Kidney

Fusion of the kidneys into one mass gives rise to an organ presenting great variety in shape and size. The lowest degree of fusion is found where two kidneys are united by a fibrous band, and the highest where the two kidneys are indistinguishably fused in a single mass. Different names have been conferred upon some of the varieties. There are the horseshoe kidney, the S-shaped kidney, the long kidney, the shield-like kidney, etc. Some of these merit further notice.

The horseshoe kidney.—This represents the most common and the smallest degree of fusion. Morris found the frequency of horseshoe kidney to be 1 in 1,000.

The horseshoe is formed by a union of the lower ends of the

kidneys by means of a band passing across the aorta and vena cava. More rarely the upper ends of the kidneys are united so that the concavity is downwards. The fused kidneys lie nearer the middle line than normal, and they are usually misplaced downwards. The misplacement is never so great as in the more complete forms of fusion, but the uniting band frequently lies as low as the bifurcation of the aorta. The bond of union may be merely a flat band of fibrous tissue, or it may be composed of renal tissue, which is spread out into a thin layer, or forms a bulky mass uniting the lateral organs. The traces of a median division have sometimes been observed on the anterior surface of the isthmus. The uniting mass

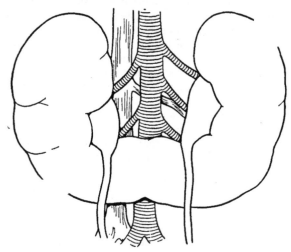

Fig. 19.—Horseshoe kidney and abnormal renal vessels. The ureters pass in front of the uniting band.

has taken the form of a third kidney, to each pole of which the lower pole of an abnormally placed kidney was welded (Rayer) ; or the kidneys may be united by a large quadrilateral mass. One kidney may be much smaller than the other.

The blood-vessels of each kidney may be normal in number, but abnormalities of character and distribution have frequently been recorded (Fig. 19), and are found in the more complete degrees of fusion rather than in the more perfectly formed kidneys. They may be asymmetrical. An increase in the number of arteries is frequent, and the isthmus may receive a special artery. The principal artery of each kidney arises from the aorta above the level of the renal pelvis and passes downwards in front of the pelvis. A smaller artery arises at each side from the aorta or iliac artery below the kidney and ascends to the lower pole of each kidney. Considerable variation is observed in the renal pelvis and ureter. Each kidney has usually a single pelvis and ureter, the ureter passing over the front of, very rarely behind, the uniting band (Fig. 19). The pelves may be increased in number and irregular in form, and are turned more to the front than normal. Very rarely the isthmus possesses a special ureter, which opens into the bladder in the position normally occupied by one ureter, while the ureter belonging to one of the kidneys is misplaced and opens into the bladder in some unusual position.

Diagnosis.—The clinical diagnosis before operation of a diseased horseshoe kidney has only once been made, and that by Israel, in a student of medicine aged 23 years. The patient had suffered for four years from attacks of pain in the back and right side, recurring every fourteen days and accompanied by diminution of the urine. During an attack there was an ill-defined swelling in the gall-bladder region, which reached as low down as the umbilicus. It was tender, and did not move with respiration or in varying positions of the body. The kidneys could not be felt in the normal position. The diagnosis of a horseshoe kidney depended upon the median position of the swelling and the impossibility of feeling the kidneys in the normal position, and this was confirmed by operation.

Suggestions have been made by different authors for the diagnosis of disease in horseshoe kidneys. According to König, one may suspect a horseshoe kidney if one feels a horseshoe-like swelling in front of the lumbar vertebræ. In a case in which Kümmel operated for stone and hydronephrosis in one half of a horseshoe kidney, the shadows in the radiograph were situated immediately adjacent to the bones of the 2nd and 3rd lumbar vertebræ, obscuring the transverse processes; and he suggests that the median position of the shadows should raise the suspicion of a horseshoe kidney. Burghart regards as supremely important the detection of a large, pulsating, somewhat elastic tumour with irregular contour in front of and below the abdominal aorta, and over which a systolic bruit is audible, while there is no delay in the pulse in the peripheral arteries. Davidsohn found hypertrophy of the heart from compression of the aorta by the transverse band.

This malformation of the kidney and also the fixed misplaced kidney have been mistaken for a malignant growth. Oliver relates such a case.

Pyelography with an opaque catheter in the ureter should enable a diagnosis to be made in such cases (p. 42).

The long simple kidney and the S-shaped kidney.—In both these varieties there is an end-to-end fusion of the kidneys, and the combined organ is situated on one side of the vertebral column. In the simple long kidney the hilus of both the component kidneys is turned in the same direction. The ureter of the upper kidney passes to the opposite side of the bladder and opens in the normal position, and there is thus no crossing of the ureters. Both ureters have been known to open on the same side of the bladder. In the S-shaped kidney, or sigmoid kidney, the pelves of the component kidneys face in opposite directions (Fig. 20). The ureters may run parallel, or they may cross and open into opposite sides of the bladder.

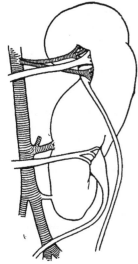

The shield-like or discoid kidney. —The kidneys are completely fused, and form a large, flat, lobulated mass, which usually lies in the middle line of the body, low down about the bifurcation of the aorta. There are usually two ureters, very rarely one. Another form of fused kidney is quite irregular in shape and in the number and distribution of the vessels. I have recorded an example of this form of kidney, for which I am indebted to Prof. Johnston Symington of Belfast. (Fig. 21.) This occurred in a female subject aged 19. There was no kidney on the left side. On the right side a kidney was situated in the right iliac fossa, and extended upwards to the level of the intervertebral disc between the 3rd and 4th lumbar vertebræ. The lower portion was bent nearly to a right angle with the upper part, and dipped into the pelvis, extending as low as the 3rd sacral vertebra. The kidney mass was supplied by three renal arteries, one from the right side of the aorta, one from the right common iliac, and a third from the bifurcation of the aorta. There were two ureters, which passed down and opened into the bladder in the usual situations.

Fig. 20.—Sigmoid kidney. (*After Brösike.*)

MISPLACED KIDNEYS

Fixed misplacements are almost invariably congenital, movable displacements are usually acquired. Fixed misplacements only will be discussed in this place. The movable displaced kidney will be considered later.

In the malformation of the kidney described above it was noted that in the slighter degrees of fusion of the organs the kidneys were either normally placed or were misplaced downwards to a slight degree, whereas in the more severe degrees of malformation the misplacement was considerable. It follows, therefore, that when

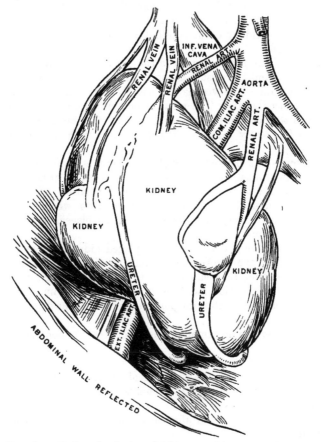

Fig. 21.—Solitary misplaced kidney with two ureters, each of which opened in the natural position in the bladder.

we consider fixed misplacements of the organs, many of the kidneys are malformed. A few fixed misplaced kidneys are normal in size and contour, but there is considerable malformation of the misplaced organ in the great majority of cases. The remaining kidney, if not fused, may be normal in structure and position; but occasionally there is no second kidney, or it is atrophied. The position of the misplaced kidney is at the bifurcation of the aorta, on the promontory of the sacrum, over the sacro-iliac synchondrosis, in the iliac fossa, or in the hollow of the sacrum. The suprarenal capsule is misplaced with the kidney in 9 out of 24 cases (Newman). Both kidneys may be misplaced. If only one kidney is misplaced, it is more frequently the left. The frequency with which fixed misplacements of the kidney occur is about 1 in 1,000 bodies (Morris found 13 in 12,768).

Where the left kidney is misplaced the descending colon crosses the middle line, and the first part of the rectum is on the right side of the sacrum. The vessels are usually abnormal in origin, number, and distribution. The renal artery may spring from the bifurcation of the aorta or from the iliac artery. Genital malformations are as frequently found with malplaced as with malformed kidneys.

Symptoms.—The pelvic kidney (Beckenniere) is more frequent in men than in women, but it is more likely to cause trouble in women. It gives rise to disturbances of menstruation, of pregnancy, and of parturition. Apart from disease, to which these kidneys are unduly liable, most cases of renal misplacement cause no clinical symptoms.

As Israel points out, disease of a misplaced kidney frequently gives rise to pain in the corresponding lumbar region, and is apt to distract attention from the real cause of the symptom. Persistent interference with defæcation has been noted as a symptom.

Wehmer considers the following points important in the diagnosis of a misplaced kidney :—

1. The discovery of a tumour lying upon the promontory or sacrum.

2. The absence of the kidney from the same side.

3. Together with these, the presence of pyuria or hæmaturia, and of spasm of the bladder, especially connected with menstruation in women.

4. The demonstration of an abnormal course of the rectum by means of air inflation.

5. Exclusion of origin of the tumour from the pelvic organs. Ovarian cysts and hydatid cysts are most difficult to distinguish. Hochenegg felt the pulsation of several arteries on the anterior surface of the tumour, which corresponds to the hilum, and found a very short ureter on catheterization. Psychic disturbances are noted by Hochenegg and Israel as accompanying congenital misplacement of the kidney.

The only published clinical preoperative diagnosis of a pelvic kidney has been made by Müllerheim. Israel suggested such a condition as extremely probable in a patient sent to him as a case of malignant growth of the rectum, and his suggestion proved correct. When a doubtful tumour is found in this situation, an exploratory laparotomy has been necessary to make a diagnosis. Catheterization of the ureter with an opaque bougie and pyelography would make the renal nature of such a tumour clear.

Treatment.—When the nature of the tumour has been recognized it will be necessary to have certain proof of the presence and activity of a second organ before removing the misplaced kidney. When this is obtained, Wagner recommends the removal of the misplaced organ, even if it is normal, where profound psychic disturbances are present, or where interference with the bowel causes general symptoms.

Frank found a pelvic left kidney and a malformed uterus on laparotomy, and displaced the kidney upwards above the brim of the pelvis, and fixed it there.

Nephrectomy has frequently been performed.

Israel removed the kidney extraperitoneally by a lateral incision, after allowing an exploratory laparotomy wound to heal. Cragin removed a misplaced kidney through the vagina, and Hochenegg another by a sacral route. Two cases are on record in which a solitary misplaced kidney was removed from the pelvis (Buss and Polk). In both cases there was maldevelopment of the genital organs. The patients died, on the seventh and eleventh days respectively, of uræmia.

LITERATURE

Ballowitz, *Virchows Arch.*, 1895, clxi. 309.
Buss, *Zeits. f. klin. Med.*, xxxviii. 4, 5, 6.
Heiner, *Folia Urol.*, Oct., 1908.
Israel, *Nierenkrankheiten*, 1901 : *Berl. klin. Woch.*, 1889, xxvi. 715.
Kümmel, *Arch. f. klin. Chir.*, 1901, vol. lxiv.
Manby, *Lancet*, 1885, i. 161.
Mankiewicz, *Centralbl. f. d. Krankh. d. Harn- u. Sex.-Org.*, 1900, v. 513.
Morris, *Surgical Diseases of the Kidney and Ureter*, vol. i. 1901.
Müllerheim, *Deuts. med. Woch.*, 1902, xxviii. 46.
Newman, *Scot. Med. Surg. Journ.*, vol. i., No. 1, p. 53 ; *Movable Kidney*,
Oliver, *Brit. Med. Journ.*, Feb. 26, 1898.   [1907.
Owen, *Med. Press and Circ.*, May 10, 1899.
Polk, *New York Med. Journ.*, Feb. 17, 1883.
Preindlsberger, *Wien. klin. Rundschau*, 1901, p. 197.
Walker, Thomson, *Renal Function in Urinary Surgery*, p. 155. 1908.
Ward, *Brit. Med. Journ.*, 1908, i. 978.
Winter, *Arch. f. klin. Chir.*, 1903, vol. lxix.

CHAPTER VI

MOVABLE AND FLOATING KIDNEY

THE normal kidney descends with inspiration and ascends with expiration, the excursion varying from $\frac{1}{2}$ to $1\frac{1}{2}$ in. In many normal individuals where the abdominal wall is not thick or resistant, the lower pole of the right and sometimes of the left kidney can be felt.

Where one-half or more of the kidney can be felt and grasped between the fingers on inspiration the organ is unduly movable.

Anatomy of movable and of floating kidney.—A *floating* kidney is entirely surrounded by peritoneum, which also clothes its pedicle and forms a mesonephros. A floating kidney is a congenital malformation, and is very rare. It cannot be diagnosed from a movable kidney without operation, and an intraperitoneal operation is required for its relief.

A *movable* kidney moves behind the peritoneum and remains an extraperitoneal organ.

The movable kidney moves within the perirenal fascia. The perirenal fascia is often greatly thickened, and the perirenal space enclosed within its layers is elongated. The delicate perirenal fat immediately surrounding the organ is usually diminished in amount, and sometimes is entirely absent; it is occasionally present in considerable quantity. The fine fibrous threads which normally connect the fibrous capsule of the kidney with the perirenal fascia and cross the fatty envelope are thicker, tougher, and longer than in the normal state. The fibrous capsule may present no change, but milky patches of thickening are frequently observed and often the whole capsule is thicker and tougher. It strips easily from the cortex of the kidney. The renal vessels are elongated, the artery more so than the vein, as a result of the rigidity of the aorta compared with the vena cava. The walls of the renal vessels are usually thickened. There is no inflammatory matting of the vascular pedicle. Except in the rarest cases, the suprarenal capsule retains its normal position.

The attachments of the kidney to the duodenum and ascending colon on the right side and the pancreas and descending colon on

78

the left are usually separated. Thick bands of adhesions between the kidney and the colon may, however, be found, and adhesions may form between the right kidney and the duodenum. The kidney may become adherent to the structures surrounding it in an abnormal position, such as the iliac fossa.

The kidney has been found in a congenital lumbar hernia and in a diaphragmatic hernia. I have met with a case in which a kidney could be completely projected by straining or coughing into a thin-walled lumbar hernia which had resulted from a badly repaired lumbar incision. The kidney could be grasped in the fingers and its outline and pedicle traced.

Changes in the kidney substance may be referred either to interference with the blood supply or to obstruction of the outflow of urine, and they may be acute or chronic.

Torsion of the pedicle may occur even when a movable kidney has but a moderate range of mobility. The renal vein obstructed, the organ becomes engorged with blood. The kidney is enlarged and dark purple in appearance, and the fibrous capsule may be raised up by subcapsular hæmorrhages. The urine is partly, and may be completely, suppressed. It contains blood and blood casts. After a time the torsion is relieved and the kidney returns to its normal condition.

Kinking or twisting of the ureter may be caused by rotation of the kidney on its transverse axis and twisting of the ureter over the renal vessels, or by the kidney swinging at the end of its vascular pedicle and causing the ureter to become folded so that its lumen is occluded. The normal ureter is extremely mobile, and some degree of fixation by adhesions is necessary before kinking or twisting of the tube can produce obstruction. (Plate 2, Fig. 3, facing p. 42.) The urine is pent up, and the pelvis distended. By pressure the pyramids of the kidney become flattened and the kidney is hollowed out, until eventually only a thin layer of kidney substance remains. This condition is brought about by repeated attacks of obstruction of the ureter, which give rise to intermittent hydronephrosis. The upper end of the ureter is frequently found adherent for an inch or more to the surface of the dilated pelvis.

Chronic interstitial nephritis may be present in a movable kidney, and is due either to interference with the circulation or to pressure from obstruction of the ureter.

Occasionally the undue mobility of the kidney is accompanied by enteroptosis. The stomach is frequently dilated.

The movable kidney may be the seat of stone, tuberculosis, or new growth, or there may be hydronephrosis, caused by folding of the ureter over an abnormal blood-vessel.

Statistics of frequency, sex, age, and side affected.— The frequency of movable kidney is variously stated as from 44 per cent. to 56 per cent. in women, and 0·48 per cent. to 6 per cent. in men. At most, from 5 to·10 per cent. of women and from ½ to 1 per cent. of men have an abnormally movable kidney. A smaller number suffer from symptoms caused by the undue mobility. The average age is 33½ years (McWilliams). The right kidney is affected in 8 of every 10 cases, and both kidneys in 5 per cent. of cases.

Etiology.—No one cause will satisfactorily explain the occurrence of abnormal mobility of the kidneys in all cases.

Three facts must be explained by any fundamental cause of movable kidney : (1) the preponderance of the condition in women (8 in 9 cases) ; (2) the frequency with which the right side is affected (8 in 10 cases); (3) the prevalence of the condition between the ages of 20 and 50.

The following factors are of importance :—

1. **Congenital mobility.**—Congenital nephroptosis has been observed by Dr. W. R. Stewart and others, but the cases were examples of floating kidney. It is exceptional to meet with movable kidneys in children, and the condition develops at some period after puberty.

2. **Anatomical factors.**—The kidneys lie in a shallow recess on each side of the vertebral bodies, the paravertebral fossa. Wolkow and Delitzen state that in those persons with abnormally movable kidneys the paravertebral fossæ are shallow and more widely open at their lower ends than in normal individuals. In women they are shallower and more open than in men, and on the right side more than on the left.

According to Mansell Moullin there is a slight rotation of the vertebræ to the right in a large number of right-sided people, and this makes the right lumbar recess shallower.

The liver does not cause downward displacement of the right kidney.

Becker and Lennhof look upon the build of the trunk as an important predisposing factor. Women with a long trunk and narrow waist more frequently have movable kidney than those with a short trunk and broad waist. These authors constructed a body index as follows : The distance in centimetres from the suprasternal notch to the upper margin of the symphysis pubis is divided by the narrowest circumference of the abdomen and multiplied by 100.· The normal quotient is 75. Where the quotient is above 75 one kidney will be movable; where it is below this figure there is no movable kidney. This method has been elaborated by Harris, who used the level of the tip of the 10th costal cartilage as a more exact transverse measurement. He also used a series of lateral and antero-posterior measurements made with callipers to show that there was a diminution in the size of the zone at the level of the 10th rib in cases of movable kidney.

3. Atrophy of the perirenal adipose capsule.—In rapid emaciation the perirenal fat frequently disappears, and the kidney becomes unduly movable. This can only be a factor in the causation of a few cases of movable kidney.

4. Weakness of the abdominal walls.—Glénard states that general enteroptosis always accompanies movable kidney, and results from weakness of the abdominal walls. This has been disproved by several observers. Godard-Danhieux examined 131 cases of movable kidney without finding enteroptosis. Einhorn observed 27 cases of enteroptosis in which the kidneys were not movable. Where enteroptosis and nephroptosis coexist, they do not bear the relation of cause and effect.

The relaxation of the abdominal wall after repeated pregnancies probably explains some cases, but movable kidney is frequently found in young nulliparæ with strong abdominal muscles.

In 61 cases of movable kidney, 38 of the patients were married, and of these only 22 had borne children (McWilliams).

5. Injury and pressure.—In 11·4 per cent. of cases there is a distinct history of a blow, severe muscular strain, or other injury in the region of the kidney, which preceded the discovery of the movable kidney.

The wearing of corsets has been stated to cause movable kidney. The waist line is, however, below the lower pole of the kidney, and, unless undue pressure is exerted at the upper part of the abdomen, the corset gives support to the kidney rather than causes its displacement. In races in which the corset is not worn movable kidney is observed.

6. Drag of adhesions between the kidney and bowel.—Bands of adhesions, probably secondary to chronic constipation, pass between the cæcum and ascending colon and the right kidney, and the drag of these is a cause of movable kidney (Arbuthnot Lane). Adhesions may also be observed between the descending colon and the left kidney.

7. Pathological conditions of the kidney.—Tumours of the kidney, hydronephrosis, renal calculus, or other disease may coexist with movable kidney, and in some cases may appear to be a contributory factor in the causation of the mobility.

Symptoms.—A movable kidney may have a wide range of movement and be unaccompanied by symptoms. When a patient.

G

with a movable kidney discovers the abnormality subjective symptoms frequently develop, and it is generally accepted as unwise to inform a patient of the presence of undue mobility of the kidney if no symptoms exist. The symptoms which accompany movable kidney may be directly connected with the kidney, or they may be referred to other organs.

1. **Symptoms referred to the kidney.**—These are (*a*) pain and discomfort, (*b*) undue mobility, (*c*) enlargement of the kidney, and (*d*) changes in the urine.

(*a*) *Pain and discomfort.*—The patient is often conscious of the movement of the kidney within the abdomen. Renal pain is felt in two positions—posteriorly, at the angle formed by the last rib with the erector spinæ mass of muscle; and anteriorly, at a point about 2 in. below and internal to the tip of the 9th costal cartilage. This corresponds to the position of the pelvis and vascular pedicle. The anterior area is that most frequently affected, and the pain is usually of a heavy aching character. There may also be attacks of severe pain on the side of the abdomen on which the kidney is movable, and this pain is most severe at the point indicated above. These attacks are followed by tenderness and sometimes by enlargement of the kidney.

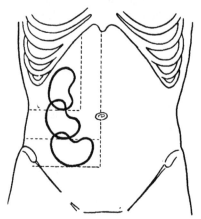

Fig. 22.—Chart of areas of mobility in three cases of movable kidney. The dotted lines show limits of excursion.

The pain of movable kidney is initiated or aggravated by movement and relieved by rest. It is sometimes first experienced on turning in bed, and may be felt on lying in certain positions. The aching is increased during the menstrual period.

(*b*) *Undue mobility of the kidney.*—In examining the kidney the patient should be placed in the recumbent position described on p. 32. The examination should be made with gentle, firm pressure, the fingers of the examining hand sinking into the abdomen at each expiration and holding their position at inspiration. She should also be examined standing up facing the surgeon. If the loin can be grasped with the hand, the thumb should be placed in front above the upper pole of the displaced kidney with the fingers behind the loin. The fingers of the other hand are used to palpate the organ. The kidney can sometimes be made prominent on the surface of the abdomen in this way, and its outline distinguished with the eye.

Three grades of mobility of the kidney are described: (1) where the kidney can be readily grasped below the ribs; (2) where the fingers can be inserted above the upper pole; (3) where the kidney moves freely about the abdominal cavity. (Fig. 22.)

In slight degrees of abnormal mobility the kidney usually moves in a line parallel with the vertebral column, but sometimes it swings

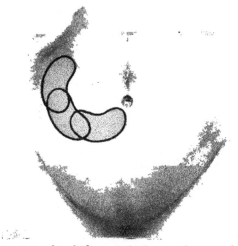

Fig. 23.—Movable kidney swinging on its vascular pedicle.

round so that the lower pole approaches the bodies of the vertebræ. The latter has been called the " cinder sifting " movement (Morris). It is difficult or even impossible to detect this movement without the help of a general anæsthetic. In another form of abnormal movement the upper end of the kidney falls forward while the lower end remains in contact with the posterior abdominal wall. In the wider ranges of movement the kidney descends below the costal margin. At first the direction is vertical, and then the lower pole swings towards the vertebral column at the full length of its vascular pedicle, and the hilum, which at first faces towards the middle line, swings round to face directly upwards. (Fig. 23.) The lower pole passes transversely and may cross the middle line by 1 or 2 in. Finally, there are cases where the vascular pedicle is so long that it exerts no control on the excursions of the kidney, and the organ may be found in almost any part of the abdomen and may descend into the true pelvis.

Where the mobility of the kidney is marked, the organ is un-influenced by the respiratory movements, but many kidneys which are abnormally movable and of which the mobility is causing symptoms move with respiration.

A movable kidney of normal size presents the following char-acters : The organ has a smooth, rounded surface, and the reniform shape can frequently .be detected. The tumour escapes from the grasp of the fingers with a sudden slip that is characteristic. The patient experiences a sickening sensation when the organ is squeezed. The tumour can be reduced into the loin, and in this position may no longer be palpable. The kidney will usually drop again when the patient sits or stands.

A kidney may be found freely movable at one examination while at the next it cannot be felt. It is therefore unwise, where movable kidney is suspected, to base a negative diagnosis on a single examination.

(c) *Enlargement of the kidney.*—Intermittent hydronephrosis is an occasional result of abnormal mobility. The enlargement of the kidney may follow some muscular effort. In two cases under my care an attack of pain and distension of the kidney was in-variably brought on when the patient was confined to bed. There were numerous bands of adhesion between the movable left kidney and the descending colon in .these cases, and the obstruction prob-ably resulted from the drag of a loaded colon. In the earlier attacks the hydronephrosis is small, but after several attacks it becomes large and forms a prominent swelling in the abdomen.

After remaining for a variable time the swelling disappears and there is a marked transient polyuria. The hydronephrosis does not completely disappear between the attacks of acute distension, although it is so soft as to be unrecognizable on abdominal palpa-tion. A loose, partly filled, hydronephrotic sac will be found on operation in the interval between attacks of acute distension.

(d) *Changes in the urine.*—Hæmaturia may occasionally follow muscular effort and be accompanied by attacks of pain. It is not a frequent symptom. Very rarely there is moderate continuous hæmaturia, which ceases when the patient is confined to bed.

Albuminuria is frequently observed, and disappears on resting.

Tube casts may be present in the urine. These are due to venous congestion; they are present in 8 out of 180 cases of movable kidney (Newman). They disappear after the operation of nephropexy.

Transient polyuria coincides with the relief of an attack of hydronephrosis. Anuria may result from torsion of the renal pedicle, and has been known to last nine days without ill after-effects. Frequent micturition may be observed during an attack of pain, and is due to reflex impulses from the kidney, or it may follow the relief of a hydronephrosis, and is due to the increased quantity of urine.

2. Symptoms referred to other organs.—These consist of (a) gastro-intestinal, (b) nervous symptoms.

(a) *Gastro-intestinal symptoms* may be referred to the stomach. There is epigastric pain and burning unconnected with taking food. A sensation of sinking is complained of, and there is loss of appetite and nausea. Eructation, a feeling of distension of the stomach, and vomiting are frequent symptoms. In these cases the stomach is usually distended, and may be displaced. The patient becomes thin and emaciated. The right kidney is the one which is movable in these cases, and the condition is probably due to the drag of adhesions on the second portion of the duodenum (Frank), or of a thickened band of peritoneum upon the pylorus (Bramwell).

Symptoms which are referred to the large intestine are constipation and flatulent distension of the colon. The attacks are recurrent, and so severe as to lead to a suspicion of intestinal obstruction from malignant growth or other cause. The symptoms are probably caused by adhesions between the kidney and large intestine.

Jaundice may be prominent. There are recurrent attacks commencing with severe epigastric pain, and the gall-bladder may be distended. These attacks cease after fixation of the kidney. They have been ascribed to pressure of the kidney on the common bile-duct, but are more probably due to dragging of the kidney upon the second part of the duodenum.

(b) *Nervous symptoms.*—A varying degree of neurasthenia accompanies movable kidney in many cases. There are depression and irritability, giddiness, palpitation, neuralgic pains, loss of appetite, and sometimes loss of weight.

It is held by Suckling that some forms of insanity are due to movable kidney, and are cured by fixation of the organ.

Acute attacks, or Dietl's crises.—The patient suffering from movable kidney is liable to acute attacks or crises which may be due to the kidney dragging on the pylorus or bowel by adhesions, or to torsion of the vascular pedicle, or kinking of the ureter. Such an attack may follow some muscular effort.

If the stomach or bowel is affected there is epigastric or general abdominal pain. The patient lies with the knees drawn up, or sits with the thighs acutely flexed on the abdomen, clasping the knees (Newman). Vomiting and collapse are usual. The abdominal muscles are rigid, and the rigidity may be most marked on the side of the movable kidney. Later the abdomen becomes distended and tympanitic. The stomach may be found distended, or the colon prominent. The bowels are constipated, and the temperature may be raised one or two degrees.

In cases in which the ureter is obstructed there is no distension of the stomach or bowel, but on one side of the abdomen a large tender swelling rapidly develops. The swelling has the characters of a renal tumour. The urine is diminished, and there may be complete anuria. After lasting a few hours or some days, the swelling subsides and the symptoms disappear.

If torsion of the renal vessels is the cause of the crisis the symptoms are again those of an acute abdominal condition. In addition the urine becomes scanty, albuminous, and sometimes bloody, and complete suppression may supervene. The pain is most severe in the region of one kidney, and this organ is found to be enlarged and tender if it can be felt through the rigid abdominal muscles. When the attack passes off the secretion of urine is re-established, and polyuria may follow. The urine contains blood, and hyaline, granular, and blood casts.

Diagnosis.—The great majority of cases of movable kidney occur in patients of moderate or slight build, in whom the abdomen is easily palpable, and the kidney readily felt and the condition diagnosed.

The following conditions may give rise to difficulty in the diagnosis of a movable kidney :—

1. *A distended gall-bladder.*—There may have been an attack of jaundice or of hæmaturia which will point to the swelling being gall-bladder or kidney respectively. A distended gall-bladder is always palpable, whereas a movable kidney sometimes disappears completely. The range of movement of the gall-bladder is more restricted. When a movable kidney is reduced into the loin it only reappears on the patient breathing very deeply or sitting up. A distended gall-bladder reappears whenever the pressure of the examining fingers is removed. The kidney may be felt apart from the enlarged gall-bladder. The area of dullness over a distended gall-bladder is continuous with that of the liver, and there is never bowel in front of it. The two conditions may coexist.

2. *Riedel's lobe of the liver.*—The swelling moves with the liver in respiration, and the movement is greater than that in a

kidney. The dullness is continuous with that of the liver, and the edge of the swelling is sharp. The right lobe of the liver dragged down by an adherent contracted gall-bladder may resemble an enlarged movable kidney. The edge is hidden by adherent bowel, but there is an absence of roundness of the outer border and lower pole.

I have had a case of splenic leukæmia with enlarged spleen and liver referred to me as a case of bilateral movable kidney with anæmia.

3. *A small ovarian tumour with a long pedicle.*—The tumour can be reduced into the pelvis, but not into the loin. Careful examination will usually show that the pedicle of the ovarian cyst is attached below. Vaginal examination may demonstrate the pelvic attachment of the swelling.

4. *A malignant growth of the large intestine* may simulate a movable kidney. It may be possible to reduce the swelling into the loin in a manner similar to a movable kidney. Symptoms of intestinal obstruction are occasionally produced by a movable kidney, and this makes the diagnosis more difficult. A prolonged history of intestinal disturbance and the absence of urinary symptoms will point to a tumour of the bowel.

Where difficulty arises as to the nature of a swelling in the region of the kidney, the introduction of collargol into the renal pelvis through a ureteric catheter, followed by radiography (pyelography), should be used to show the position of the renal pelvis and calyces. By this means the relation of the kidney to the tumour will be demonstrated. (Plate 2, Fig. 3.) Radiography after a bismuth meal will further demonstrate the relation of the intestine to the tumour.

While the recognition of a movable kidney is essential for the diagnosis, and a movable kidney is frequently the cause of symptoms which are referred to other organs, it does not follow that where symptoms such as neurasthenia are present with a movable kidney the nervous symptoms result from the renal mobility. If the neurasthenia is known to have been present before the kidney became movable, and if the replacement of the kidney and its retention by lying in bed or the application of some mechanical support have no effect in allaying the symptoms, it is likely that the two conditions are independent. But if movement aggravates the symptoms and rest or support affords relief, there is a relation of cause and effect between the undue mobility of the kidney and the neurasthenia.

Treatment. Selection of cases.—The careful selection of cases for the different methods of treatment is the only means of obtaining satisfactory results. In cases where no symptoms are present and there does not appear to be any change taking place in the kidney itself, as shown by enlargement or tenderness of the organ or changes in the urine, it will only be necessary to limit violent exercises, such as horse-riding, and to warn against lifting heavy weights. The bowels should be carefully regulated. Should symptoms appear, active treatment of the mobility will become necessary. In such cases a choice will have to be made between palliative and operative treatment.

In certain cases *palliative treatment is contra-indicated* and operative treatment is imperative :

1. Where there are signs that the mobility is causing disease of the kidney. This includes cases in which the kidney is tender or enlarged, cases of intermittent hydronephrosis, cases in which hæmaturia or albuminuria is present, or there are tube casts in the urine, or slight or severe attacks of torsion of the renal pedicle have occurred.

2. Where the kidney is exerting harmful traction upon other organs. This includes cases where there are gastric and intestinal crises and attacks of jaundice.

3. Where the kidney lies below the waist line and is uncontrolled by any mechanical apparatus, and the use of a mechanical apparatus causes pain and aggravates the symptoms.

4. Where the patient is going to reside in tropical or uncivilized countries.

5. Where the patient has to perform manual labour, and the expense of maintaining an apparatus in good order cannot be borne.

In all other cases palliative treatment may be tried before resorting to operation.

In certain cases *operative treatment is contra-indicated*, because doomed to failure :

Where general enteroptosis is present.

Where severe neurasthenia is present and no symptoms can be referred to the kidney.

In a few cases of movable kidney with neurasthenia, control of the renal movements by a mechanical apparatus will alleviate or cure the neurasthenia, and in these cases also fixation of the kidney by operation will be followed by a similar result. This view is generally held, but a few writers go further and advocate operation in all cases of neurasthenia with movable kidney.

Palliative treatment. 1. Treatment by rest and increasing the body fat.—It is claimed by a very few writers that this method can bring about a cure of the renal mobility. They hope by increasing the general fat of the body to produce a simultaneous deposit around the kidney, which will fix it in position. Such a result is not obtained in practice. The method is, however, useful in treating cases of movable kidney in which neurasthenic symptoms are present. In these cases a " rest cure " should be the first resort and an operation the last.

The patient is strictly confined to bed, and in severe cases full Weir-Mitchell isolation should be exacted. The bowels are carefully regulated, and the food is chosen with the view of increasing the body-weight. Milk is given in large quantities, graduated according to the digestive powers. General massage is administered, but the kidney areas are not subjected to manipulation. The treatment extends over a month or six weeks.

This is a useful preliminary to treatment by means of mechanical apparatus.

2. **Treatment by mechanical apparatus.**—Treatment by this means is especially indicated when enteroptosis is present. It is suitable for any case of movable-kidney, with the exceptions already mentioned.

Three forms of apparatus will be described :

(a) *Kidney truss.*—The truss made by Ernst consists of a thin, carefully padded metal plate which exercises pressure upon the abdominal wall by means of two springs. The pressure concerns the lower and inner margins of the plate, so that the kidney is forced upwards and outwards. It must of necessity be applied when the patient is lying down. The truss must be very carefully fitted, and the patient trained and practised in its proper adjustment. She is able to take active exercise.

(b) *Kidney belt.*—A kidney belt is an abdominal belt which is specially adapted for the relief of movable kidney. It consists of a broad band of jean or coutil which surrounds the waist and comes down over the iliac crests and is accurately moulded to the hips. The lower border follows the curve of the groin along Poupart's ligament, and in the middle line in front it slightly overlaps the pubic bones. The upper border is about the level of the umbilicus. The belt is stiffened by whalebone or light steel busks. It is laced in front and behind. At each side there is a broad inset of silk elastic. There are two perineal straps to prevent the belt from riding upwards.

A kidney pad is added with the view of exerting pressure upon the movable kidney and retaining it in place. This may be horseshoe-shaped or oval. The pad may be fixed in the lining of the belt, and consists of a rubber bag with a fine tube which pierces the belt and has a turncock. Or it may be a closed air sac or rubber bag containing glycerine, which fits into a pocket in the lining of the belt. The belt must be put on when the patient is recumbent, and is worn over a silk or fine woollen under-vest.

A belt of similar construction can be fitted to the lower part of a corset, and by this means the perineal straps, which are irksome, become unnecessary.

The pads which are used in these belts do not control the movements of the kidney; were they sufficiently large and firm to do so they would exert injurious pressure upon the bowel. Their use appears, however, to give a feeling of security to the wearer, and for this reason they may be worn.

(c) *Corset for movable kidney* (*Gallant*).—The corset is made from measurements taken from the patient. At the bottom the front steels must overlap the upper half-inch of the symphysis pubis and fit very snugly over the hips, stretching tightly from one to the other to flatten and reduce the hypogastrium. The circumference must be equal to the natural waist, but there should be well-marked incurving of the sides, so that the clothing is supported, the corset prevented from slipping upwards, and a fashionable outline afforded to the figure. At the back and sides the upper portion must accurately fit the thorax, while in front ample room must be provided for the replaced stomach. Below the waist the corset must be inflexible and inelastic, and the portion above the waist must permit free play to the trunk and thoracic walls.

If the hips are poorly developed, pads should be stitched inside the lower part of the corset to give rotundity to the figure and avoid painful pressure on the iliac crests and anterior spines.

One lace begins at the eyelet above the waist line, and is continued down to the bottom of the corset. In the upper part a thin, flat hat-elastic is loosely threaded, so as to keep the corset in contact with the thorax but not to cause pressure.

The following directions must be followed in putting on the corset:

The lower lacing is freely loosened and the corset applied to the body over a fine woollen or silk vest.

The patient lies on her back on a bed, and the legs are flexed to a right angle.

The abdomen is massaged, by stroking upwards, for ten minutes. The corset is then drawn well down over the hips and fastened in front, beginning with the lowest hook. Without lowering the thighs the lace behind is drawn as tight as possible and tied. The corset must not be drawn down after the front has been fastened.

The lower part above the pubes must fit so snugly that the

hugers can barely be inserted between the corset and the pubes when the patient is lying down. On rising, sitting, or walking the corset should not slip upwards.

Gallant holds that from 90 to 95 per cent. of movable kidneys with symptoms are cured of the symptoms by wearing this corset.

Operative treatment.—The preparation of the patient is similar to that in other kidney operations. The position depends upon the incision employed: for the oblique posterior incision the patient lies on the side with a pillow beneath the loin; for the vertical posterior incision she lies prone with an air pillow beneath the abdomen; and for the anterior incision the dorsal position is adopted.

1. **The incision.**—The usual incision is the oblique posterior, passing downwards and forwards from the angle formed by the last rib and the erector spinæ mass of muscle for 4 or 6 in. The advantage of this incision is the good exposure and the possibility of unlimited extension. In it the latissimus dorsi and the three layers of abdominal muscles and the lumbar aponeurosis are cut.

A vertical posterior incision along the outer border of the erector spinæ muscle is used by Edebohls. The latissimus dorsi is pushed aside, and the external oblique pulled forwards. The lumbar aponeurosis is split vertically. The advantage of this incision is the slight disturbance of muscles. A disadvantage is that the exposure is limited.

An anterior incision has been used by some surgeons (Harlan, Stanmore Bishop, Watson Cheyne). It runs from the anterior edge of the latissimus dorsi forwards for 4 in. parallel with the costal margin. Stanmore Bishop opened the peritoneal cavity; Watson Cheyne pushes the peritoneum inwards and exposes the front of the kidney. This incision is less suitable for dealing with disease of the kidney which may accompany the undue mobility. The advantage claimed for it is that it allows of the kidney being replaced and fixed in its normal position, whereas the posterior incision necessitates the fixation in an abnormal position.

2. **Removal of the fatty capsule.**—All authorities are agreed that the adipose tissue immediately surrounding the kidney should be carefully removed. The perirenal fat, the posterior layer of perirenal fascia, and the fat between this and the quadratus lumborum and psoas muscles must be dissected away, and the muscles laid bare. This can only be carried out satisfactorily through a free incision.

3. **Methods of fixation.**—i. By sutures passing through the kidney capsule or kidney substance. The suture material may be

catgut, silk, kangaroo tendon, or a strip of tendon from the erector spinæ muscle of the patient left attached at one end. Strong catgut and kangaroo tendon are the best of these.

If the suture is to be passed through the capsule alone, a small slit is made in it and a director passed along underneath, stripping it up for a varying distance and ending at a second small slit. The suture material is threaded along this tunnel and passed through the muscles of the abdominal wall. Several such sutures may be passed, and they may be placed at the convex border of the kidney or on the posterior surface. The sutures may be passed through the kidney substance about ½ in. from the convex border, and then through the muscles of the abdominal wall at the upper edge of the wound.

ii. By stripping the capsule of the kidney (decortication). An incision through the fibrous capsule of the kidney is made along the convex border, and the capsule seized with dissecting forceps and stripped from both surfaces as far as the hilum, where it is clipped away. This is done with the view to producing adhesions between the stripped surface of the kidney and the surrounding structures.

iii. By stitching the stripped capsule to the parietes. Many variations of this method have been introduced. The stripped capsule may be rolled up on the anterior and posterior surfaces of the kidney without carrying it as far as the hilum, and stitches introduced through the rolled capsule and the muscles of the abdominal wall. The capsule may be stripped in a number of wedges, each of which is stitched to the abdominal wall. The kidney may be slung by passing a strip of capsule through a slit in the ligamentum arcuatum externum (Foulerton).

iv. By partial stripping and suture through the substance of the kidney. It may be necessary to explore the kidney, and the incision is placed along the convex border of the kidney. The nephrotomy wound is closed by four or five thick catgut sutures passed through the kidney substance. These are tied and left long. An elliptical incision through the fibrous capsule leaves an area of unstripped capsule, which contains the nephrotomy incision and the sutures closing it. The capsule is stripped from the anterior and posterior surfaces of the kidney. The ends of the catgut sutures are passed through the upper and lower muscular edges of the wound, and are tied after the wound has been closed. Or the highest suture is passed through the muscles of the last intercostal space and tied.

v. By methods designed to promote granulation. Long strips of gauze are placed below the lower pole of the kidney to promote granulation and the formation of a fibrous sling to support the kidney (Jaboulay).

vi. The formation of a shelf of peritoneum or fibrous capsule. Stanmore Bishop opened the peritoneal cavity by an anterior incision and replaced the kidney in its proper position. The peritoneum covering the lower third of the kidney was divided transversely, and the capsule stripped downwards and inwards from the anterior surface of this portion of the kidney. The divided peritoneum was replaced and sutured. Sutures were passed directly backwards through the peritoneum, detached capsule, and posterior abdominal

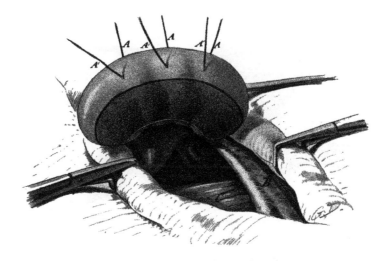

Fig. 24.—Method of fixation of kidney.

The kidney has been delivered from the lumbar wound and its posterior surface decapsulated. Three catgut sutures (A, A') are passed through the substance of the organ. B, Last rib; C, quadratus lumborum muscle.

wall, so as to form a chain of sutures extending from immediately below the renal pelvis along the internal and inferior edge of the kidney and a short distance round the external edge. The sutures were tied behind after division of the skin and subcutaneous fat over the muscular layer.

Watson Cheyne exposes the kidney by an anterior incision and pushes aside the peritoneum. The muscles of the posterior abdominal wall are cleared of fat. The fibrous capsule is stripped from the posterior surface of the lower pole of the kidney, and another flap of capsule from the outer half of the remaining part of the posterior surface, and the capsule is stripped as far as the

convex border. The kidney is replaced, and the flaps of the capsule are stitched down to the muscles of the posterior abdominal
wall, so that the raw surface is kept in contact with the muscles.

I use a free oblique lumbar incision, and prepare the posterior
abdominal wall carefully by dissection of the fascia and fat. Only
the posterior surface of the kidney is stripped of capsule, as it is
undesirable that the anterior surface should become adherent to
the colon. Three catgut stitches are passed through the kidney an
inch from its convex border. The upper suture is passed through
the intercostal muscles of the last space, and the lower two are

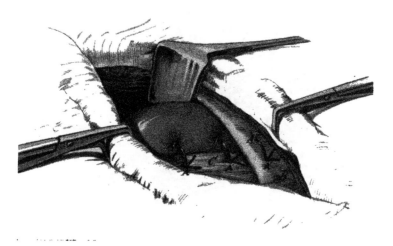

Fig. 25.—Method of fixation of kidney.

The upper suture is passed through the last intercostal space, the other through the quadratus
lumborum muscle. A, A', Catgut sutures ; B, last rib ; C, quadratus lumborum muscle.

passed through the outer edge of the quadratus lumborum.
(Figs. 24, 25.) The patient is confined to bed for four weeks.

Results.—The operative mortality is stated at 1 per cent.,
but it is lower than this in the practice of most surgeons. The
statistics in regard to the success of operation vary. Keen found
that of 116 cases examined not less than three months after
operation 57·8 per cent. were cured, 12·9 per cent. improved,
and in 19·8 per cent. the operation failed. Failure may consist
in recurrence of the mobility or the persistence of pain. Of 42
cases examined by McWilliams, 22 were cured, 8 greatly benefited,
7 somewhat relieved, and 5 unrelieved of symptoms. Improvement
in many cases was only seen some months after the operation.

There were 48 per cent. of cures where parenchymatous sutures were used, and 52 per cent. of cures where no parenchymatous sutures were employed.

Wilson and Howell examined 41 cases after nephropexy had been performed at St. Bartholomew's Hospital, and found 12 cured, 8 greatly improved, 12 improved, and 9 unaffected by the operation.

Failures, are, I believe, due to incomplete removal of fat, want of stripping of the kidney, tearing out of sutures too tightly tied, and too short confinement to bed. It is immaterial whether the kidney is fixed in normal position or lower down, so long as the pedicle and ureter are not twisted.

LITERATURE

Barling, *Brit. Med. Journ.*, 1908, i. 972.
Billington, *Brit. Med. Journ.*, May 1, 1909.
Bishop, Stanmore, *Lancet*, July 6, 1907, voL ii.
Cheyne, Watson, *Lancet*, April 24, 1909.
Gallant, *Journ. Amer. Med. Assoc.*, Nov. 7, 1908.
Glénard, *Les Ptoses Viscérales.* Paris, 1899.
Guiteras, *New York Med. Rec.*, 1903, p. 561.
Keen, *Ann. Surg.*, Aug., 1890.
Lane, Arbuthnot, *Lancet*, Jan. 17, 1903.
Morris, *Surgical Diseases of the Kidney and Ureter.* 1901.
Moullin, Mansell, *Brit Med. Journ.*, March 10, 1900.
Newman, *Movable Kidney.* 1907.
Treves, *Pract.*, Jan., 1905.
Walker, Thomson, *Lancet*, Aug. 11, 1906.
Walkow und **Delitzen**, *Die Wandernicrc.* Berlin, 1899
Wilson and **Howell**, *Movable Kidney.* 1909.

CHAPTER VII

INJURIES TO THE KIDNEY

I. WITHOUT EXTERNAL WOUND

THE kidney is well protected by the lower ribs and the spinal muscles, and injuries of this organ are comparatively rare. In 7,741 injuries found post mortem, 10 (0·12 per cent.) were injuries of the kidney, and in only one of these was there an open wound. The relation of injuries to surgical diseases of the kidney is 7·81 per cent. (Küster).

The right side is more frequently affected than the left, and the injury is rarely bilateral (142 right, 118 left, 12 bilateral). The usual age is from 10 to 30 years. There is a great preponderance of male subjects. Of 299 cases, 281 (93·9 per cent.) were male and 18 (6·1 per cent.) were female.

Etiology.—The form of injury which produces the rupture may be a direct blow on the loin or over the lower ribs, such as a kick or a fall across a beam or cart-wheel, or the passage of a wheel over the loin, or compression between buffers; or the violence may be indirect, such as a fall from a height on the buttocks or forcible acute flexion of the body. In these cases of indirect violence Tuffier holds that the kidney is injured by impact against the 12th rib or the transverse process of the 1st lumbar vertebra.

In cases where the body is acutely flexed from a fall or muscular exertion the laceration of the kidney arises from flexion on its transverse axis.

Küster ascribes an important rôle to hydrostatic pressure within the kidney in the production of laceration. He experimented by distending the veins, arteries, and renal pelvis, and applying violence to the surface of the organ, and produced deep transverse lacerations which extended into the pelvis.

The part of the kidney adjacent to the hilum is that most frequently torn. The most friable part of the kidney substance is at the junction of the cortex and medulla. The mobility of the kidney is some protection against rupture.

Pathology. 1. Lesions of the kidney.—The fatty capsule

alone may be torn, without injury to the renal parenchyma. Around the kidney there is an accumulation of blood, which later becomes organized and eventually constitutes a layer of fibrous tissue. Less frequently a cyst containing blood is formed. From a slight subcapsular rupture of the kidney, blood may be poured out and accumulate beneath the fibrous capsule of the organ.

In a more severe degree the fibrous capsule is ruptured and there is extravasation of blood in the substance of the kidney, especially at the base of the pyramids, and at the same time blood is effused into the renal pelvis. The lacerations are usually transverse or slightly oblique, and radiate from the hilum. There is commonly one large tear with several smaller lacerations, and there is always bruising of the parenchyma in the neighbourhood. Lacerations are more frequent on the anterior than on the posterior surface of the kidney, and at the lower than at the upper pole.

In severe degrees of rupture the rent passes from the surface to the pelvis in a transverse or oblique direction. The whole of one pole of the kidney may be detached. The kidney may be broken up into several fragments and the substance pulped. Sometimes a large branch of the renal artery is ruptured, and the ureter may be torn.

Rarely the organ may be split along its convex border, or it may be torn from its pelvis and vessels.

When the kidney is ruptured, blood is poured out and collects in considerable quantity within the fatty capsule. With extensive laceration and pulping of the kidney there is sometimes comparatively little effusion of blood. The blood may track along the spermatic vein and cause discoloration of the skin at the external abdominal ring, and of the scrotum or labium.

In most cases there is laceration of the renal pelvis or of a calyx, so that urine is mixed with the effused blood. A large collection of urine and blood may be formed which becomes limited by adhesions (pseudo-hydronephrosis).

Blood is also poured into the renal pelvis and passes into the bladder. The ureter may be ruptured or a clot may block its lumen, so that no blood reaches the bladder.

2. **Lesions of other organs.**—Rupture of the kidney is frequently complicated by other lesions. The peritoneum may be torn, when blood and urine are poured into the peritoneal cavity. This happens more frequently in children than in adults, since the perinephritic fat is not developed before the tenth year, and the peritoneum is therefore in more intimate relation with the kidney up to that age. Fracture of one or more ribs occurs in 5 per cent. of cases (Tuffier). The spinal column may be injured,

and the pelvic girdle is occasionally fractured (2 per cent.). There may be injuries to the bowel, liver, spleen, bladder, and lungs.

In 36 post-mortem examinations of subcutaneous renal lesions Güterbock found fracture of the ribs in 21, laceration of the liver in 20, of the spleen in 13, of the suprarenal capsule in 9, and of the bowel and mesentery in 3.

Repair.—In the slighter degrees of rupture the process of repair takes place very rapidly. A clot forms between the edges of the wound, and the surrounding parenchyma is infiltrated with blood lying between and within the tubules. In this zone the epithelium of the tubules degenerates, the area thus affected taking the wedge shape of an infarct with the broadest part at the surface of the kidney. Outside this area there is a zone where the inter-tubular connective tissue proliferates, and the round-cell infiltration thus produced invades the clot and eventually forms fibrous tissue. The tubules nearest the edge of the wound degenerate and are hidden by the round-cell infiltration. In the less damaged tissues regeneration of the damaged epithelium takes place, but there is no new formation of tubules. The glomeruli atrophy slowly, and persist for a long time in the cicatrix.

The wound in the kidney may be firmly healed in three weeks. Occasionally healing may be delayed for many months, and débris and clots are found in the wound with little attempt at cicatrization.

Wounds of the renal pelvis leave a fibrous scar which does not cause narrowing of the receptacle. Occasionally a fistula remains, and if this heals there is pocketing in the interior of the renal pelvis. When the kidney has been extensively lacerated and pulped the whole organ may be converted into a fibrous mass in which little kidney tissue remains. The blood which was effused is either absorbed (rarely it remains as a cyst), or it may become infected and suppuration occur.

Infection and suppuration in the form of perinephritic abscess, suppurative nephritis, pyonephrosis, and peritonitis occur in 11·8 per cent. of cases.

Symptoms.—Shock is present to a varying degree in all the more severe grades of rupture.

The symptoms may not appear immediately on receipt of the injury. I have seen a gamekeeper fall heavily on his shoulder while dragging a shot stag down a steep hillside, pick himself up, resume his part in dragging the animal for another mile, and then take his turn in trundling the 16-stone weight in a wheel-barrow for another mile and a half. There were no signs during that evening or throughout the night, but next morning he noticed blood in his urine and then became faint. When I saw him he was pale and sweating, with a rapid, feeble pulse and a drawn, anxious face, and he had been sick. He passed a large quantity of blood, and the hæmaturia continued for a week. There was tenderness over the left kidney with rigidity of the abdominal muscles on this side. He made a good recovery.

The symptoms which are characteristic of rupture of the kidney are pain, tumour, hæmaturia, and variations in the quantity of urine.

Pain.—Pain after an injury to the loin may result from the bruising of the tissues, or it may be due to fracture of the ribs. The pain which points to an injury of the kidney radiates along the line of the ureter and is accompanied by retraction of the testicle. This pain is severe, and is present especially when the hæmorrhage is copious and clots are passed down the ureter. There is also a dull heavy pain, deeply seated in the loin, which is increased by palpation, by movement, coughing or sneezing.

The abdominal muscles are rigidly contracted, and palpation of the loin is difficult and painful.

The pain may last for a week or more.

Tumour.—Even in slight lacerations of the kidney there may be perirenal swelling. When a large quantity of blood and urine is effused it forms a prominent swelling in the loin, which may be found soon after the injury, or its appearance may be delayed for some days. The swelling is dull on percussion and very tender on palpation, and may be slightly movable. It is usually diffuse and obscured by the rigidity of the abdominal muscles or distension of the bowel (pseudo-hydro-hæmatonephrosis).

If the swelling be smooth and clearly outlined and ballottement can be obtained the renal pelvis has been distended with blood and a hæmatonephrosis formed. The condition is very rare.

Hæmaturia.—There is blood in the urine in nearly all cases of rupture of the kidney (91·5 per cent.). In slight cases it may be the only symptom.

Hæmaturia may be absent in cases of slight cortical rupture when the injury does not affect the renal pelvis, or it may fail to appear when the kidney is completely pulped and the ureter torn across, or when the ureter is blocked with clot. In slight injuries the microscope may be required to detect the blood. In other cases the first urine passed after the accident is blood-stained, and then the bleeding ceases.

In severe cases blood is present in large quantity. It usually appears immediately after the injury, but it has sometimes been delayed for several days.

In about 50 per cent. of cases the hæmaturia has disappeared in a week ; in other cases it persists for several weeks, and may be the cause of death at the end of a fortnight or three weeks. Rarely the hæmaturia is intermittent, the urine remaining clear for ten days at a time.

The blood is bright at first, but later a large quantity of dark disintegrated blood may be discharged from the rupture of a collection of blood into the kidney pelvis (*hæmaturia tardive*— Tuffier and Levi).

Clotting of the blood in the renal pelvis may block the ureter and prevent hæmaturia. Clots may be passed down the ureter and give rise to ureteric colic. If there is clotting of the blood in the bladder, retention of urine may be caused by blocking of the urethra with clot, or the bladder may become distended with masses of clot.

Secondary hæmorrhage may occur on the sixteenth or eighteenth day, the primary hæmaturia having ceased a few days after the injury. This is due to suppuration and sloughing of the injured kidney.

Changes in the quantity of urine.—Oliguria or anuria may follow injury to the kidney, and may be due to injury affecting both kidneys, or to injury to one kidney when the second kidney is diseased or atrophied. More frequently the uninjured kidney is healthy and the suppression of urine is due to a depressant reflex exercised upon it by the injured organ.

Marsius has described fibres in the vagi and splanchnic nerves, stimulation of which contracts the renal vessels and suspends the secretion of urine. Stimulation of either vagus stops the secretion of both kidneys.

The interference with the renal function may be temporary, lasting for twelve or twenty-four hours after the injury, or it may persist and cause death. Polyuria frequently follows upon the oliguria, appearing in twenty-four or thirty-six hours, or later up to the twelfth or fifteenth day, and lasting for several days. Polyuria persisting beyond this time is usually due to traumatic nephritis. Discoloration of the skin in the lumbar region appears four or five days after the injury.

In two or three weeks discoloration may be found at the external abdominal ring, passing down into the scrotum or labium. Blood may pass down behind the peritoneum into the pelvis, and on rectal examination can sometimes be felt behind the bladder. Intraperitoneal effusion of blood may be detected in the pouch of Douglas when the peritoneum has been torn.

Complications and sequelæ.—Anuria, retention of urine, and pseudo-hæmatonephrosis have already been referred to in describing the symptoms.

Intraperitoneal hæmorrhage.—Intraperitoneal hæmorrhage occurs when the peritoneum is lacerated, and is most frequently observed in children under the age of 10 years. It occurs in cases of severe injury, and other organs—such as the liver and spleen —are frequently injured, so that it is impossible to say with certainty that the intraperitoneal hæmorrhage comes from the kidney. Such hæmorrhage is usually rapidly fatal.

Septic complications.—When the peritoneum is lacerated there is the further danger of septic peritonitis from infiltration of urine into the peritoneal cavity.

It is seldom possible to make a diagnosis between peritonitis due to rupture of the kidney and that due to rupture of some other organ, such as the bowel.

Infection of the damaged kidney is usually the result of an ascending infection from the bladder, and in a large number of cases results from septic catheterization. There are cases, however, in which no instrument has been passed and infection of the perirenal hæmatoma must have been due to bacteria carried by the blood stream. This has been reproduced experimentally by Albarran.

The infection usually occurs soon after the accident, but may be delayed for some weeks or months. It has been said to occur some years after the injury.

When the perirenal effusion of blood and urine is infected, suppuration takes place and injured portions of the kidney slough, so that a large collection of blood, urine, pus, and disintegrated kidney tissue is formed. Suppuration may extend beneath the diaphragm and affect the pleura.

Septic inflammation may be confined to the kidney substance and cause pyelonephritis or an abscess of the parenchyma. Symptoms usually develop soon after the use of a catheter, and are ushered in by a rigor. The quantity of urine secreted diminishes, and complete suppression may supervene. There is a high, swinging temperature and an increase in the local tenderness and swelling. The uninjured kidney may also be affected by the ascending infection (pyelonephritis) at the same time as the injured kidney or at a later date.

Traumatic hydronephrosis.—Hydronephrosis sometimes follows upon injury to the kidney. The number of undoubted cases recorded is not great; Wildbolz has collected 17. The obstruction may be due to blocking of the ureter with blood clot, rupture of or injury to the ureter, or to pressure upon it of scar tissue. The true hydronephrosis thus formed is sometimes indistinguishable clinically from traumatic pseudo-hydronephrosis, in which a cyst containing blood and urine limited by adhesions is formed outside the kidney.

A swelling appears in the loin in from two to six weeks after the injury, and may attain a very large size. The parenchyma is destroyed in a comparatively short time. Hydronephrosis may develop some months or years after an injury, and is probably due to undue mobility of the kidney, the result of the injury.

Movable kidney.—To traumatism is ascribed an important rôle in the causation of movable kidney. It has already been stated that 94 per cent. of cases of laceration of the kidney are in the male sex, and the figures relating to sex in movable kidney are reversed, namely, 94 per cent. female. From this Küster has inferred that "the result of a lumbar injury in the male is a subcutaneous contusion of the kidney, in the female a movable kidney."

The number of cases in which a movable kidney follows an injury to the loin cannot, however, be very great, for Tuffier examined a large number of patients who had previously suffered from such an injury without finding a single case of movable kidney.

Traumatic nephritis.—Nephritis is a rare sequela of injury to the kidney. The nephritis is insidious, and usually takes the form of a chronic interstitial nephritis, with secondary vascular changes. Less frequently a parenchymatous nephritis develops.

After the hæmaturia has ceased, albumin continues to be present in the urine and there is continuous polyuria, and epithelial and granular casts are found.

There is sometimes a rapidly appearing œdema of the feet and face, or of the entire body. The œdema is said occasionally to be confined to the side of the body corresponding to the injury (Potain).

In some cases the symptoms disappear, but in others they persist, and in the latter cases there may have been chronic nephritis present before the injury.

It is possible that an injury to the kidney may rarely be the cause of calculus, for a portion of blood clot has been found as the nucleus of a renal calculus. The relation of trauma and calculus is, however, very rare.

Injury is said to have been the cause of cysts in the kidney and of malignant growths, but in support of this there is no clear evidence.

Diagnosis.—The history of the case and the presence of bruising or abrasion in the kidney region will point to an injury of the kidney; and if there is renal and ureteric pain, and especially if there is blood in the urine, rupture of the kidney may be diagnosed. Pain and hæmaturia may be absent, from causes already mentioned, and the diagnosis must depend upon the history, local swelling, and rigidity of the abdominal muscles on the affected side.

It is impossible to judge accurately as to the extent of the injury from the amount of blood or pain. A large, rapidly formed swelling in the region of the kidney is a sign of severe laceration.

It is necessary to inquire very carefully into the previous history of the patient, and to examine doubtful cases with the view of excluding disease antecedent to the injury, such as stone, growth, or chronic nephritis.

· **Course and prognosis.**—In favourable cases the urine clears in three or four days, and the symptoms pass off and disappear in a week or ten days.

In severe cases the immediate dangers are shock and hæmorrhage, and the more remote septic complications and anuria.

During the period of shock the appearance of a large rounded swelling in the region of the kidney, or of free fluid in the peritoneal cavity, denotes progressive perirenal or intraperitoneal hæmorrhage respectively. When shock has passed off, if there be no signs of progressive anæmia and the swelling in the loin be moderate and show no sign of increase, it may be concluded that the hæmorrhage is not immediately progressive. Profound anæmia, an increasing lumbar swelling, and signs of free intraperitoneal fluid denote continued hæmorrhage. The danger from hæmorrhage may continue for fourteen or twenty-one days after the injury.

There is a remote danger of recurrent hæmaturia at intervals of some months, and this may continue for years and eventually necessitate nephrectomy.

Septic complications may supervene a few days after the injury, and may follow catheterization, or occur apart from it. Sepsis may be delayed for some weeks or months, and suppuration has been known to occur in a kidney injured some years previously.

The later the onset and the less acute the progress of the septic process, the better is the prognosis. Prognosis is chiefly affected by hæmorrhage and injury to other organs. Recovery takes place in 70 per cent. of uncomplicated cases.

Grawitz found in 108 cases of injury to the kidney that 58 recovered. Of 50 cases, the fatal result was caused by injury to other vital organs in 18, immediate hæmorrhage in 14, delayed hæmorrhage in 8, suppuration in 7, and failure of the renal function in 3.

The mortality is much higher in children than in adults, owing to the greater frequency with which the peritoneum is ruptured.

Treatment.—In cases of slight and moderately severe uncomplicated rupture of the kidney the treatment is non-operative.

The side is strapped with adhesive plaster reaching to the middle line in front and behind to prevent movement, and a broad bandage may be applied over this to give pressure. Icebags should be placed over and under the loin, and the patient kept absolutely quiet in the recumbent position. The food should be fluid. Hæmostatics are of little value, and those which raise the blood pressure, such as ergot, are harmful. Calcium lactate in doses of 10 to 15 gr. every four hours may be tried; it should not be continued longer than forty-eight hours. Morphia should be given hypodermically, and serves the double purpose of relieving pain and quieting the circulation. Shock, if not profound, should not be too energetically treated lest bleeding be encouraged. Warmth to the extremities and the recumbent position will usually suffice. If the patient cannot pass water the bladder should be emptied by catheter under the most rigid aseptic precautions. Clots, if numerous, may be washed out. If the bladder is distended, and on passing a catheter only a little bloody urine is drawn, there is an accumulation of clot in the bladder, which cannot be removed by catheter. An attempt may be made by means of a large evacuating cannula and bulb, such as is used after the operation of lithotrity, to remove the clots by snotion, but this method should not be persisted in if it be not quickly successful. The bladder should, in case of failure, be opened suprapubically, the clots cleared out, and a large rubber drainage tube introduced. The operation should be rapidly carried out. Should no complications supervene, the patient should be kept in bed for a fortnight after the hæmorrhage has ceased and all local tenderness and swelling have disappeared.

Operative interference may be required for the following conditions :—

1. Immediate severe hæmorrhage.
2. Delayed severe hæmorrhage.
3. Suppuration of the injured kidney.
4. Septic peritonitis.
5. Hydronephrosis, pyonephrosis.

Where there is a rapidly increasing swelling in the region of the kidney, or free fluid in the peritoneum, or severe persistent hæmaturia, and especially where there is progressive anæmia, operation is necessary to control the bleeding. An oblique lumbar incision should be made and the damaged kidney exposed. Clots should be cleared away and a careful search made for the bleeding-point. It may be necessary when the hæmorrhage is free to compress the renal pedicle with the thumb and fingers. A single tear in the kidney substance should be closed by cutgut sutures passed through the substance of the kidney. If one or several portions are partly

detached by a number of lacerations, packing with strips of sterilized gauze should be resorted to, and will successfully control the
bleeding. When a large branch of the renal artery is the source
of hæmorrhage, it should, if possible, be picked up in long artery-
forceps and tied with a silk ligature. It may be necessary to
underrun the vessel with a curved needle and silk in order to
tie it securely.

A distended renal pelvis should be incised and the clots turned
out. If this be followed by considerable hæmorrhage, the pelvis
may be packed with gauze.

Detached portions and shreds of kidney tissue should be removed, and rents repaired as far as possible.

When the kidney is injured so that repair does not appear
possible, primary nephrectomy should be performed.

All operative measures should be carried out with the utmost
dispatch; and when the hæmorrhage has been controlled, rectal
and intravenous infusion of glucose solution (1 per cent.) should
be given.

When there is free fluid in the peritoneum and the diagnosis
of injury to the kidney is clearly established, the kidney should
first be exposed and dealt with, and the peritoneal cavity cleared
of clots and blood by an extension of the lumbar incision. When
the diagnosis of injury to the kidney is uncertain, an exploratory
laparotomy will be necessary, the abdomen being opened in the
middle line.

Nephrectomy is called for when there are recurrent attacks
of hæmorrhage after injury to the kidney.

Suppuration of the damaged kidney necessitates lumbar exploration. Free incision, irrigation, and drainage may be all that
is necessary, but nephrectomy should be performed if there is
extensive destruction of the kidney tissue.

Laparotomy and drainage of the peritoneal cavity will become
necessary if septic peritonitis supervene.

Persistent anuria should be treated by nephrotomy and packing.
The treatment of Hydronephrosis and Pyonephrosis will be discussed under those headings (pp. 177, 150).

Results.—The results of operative treatment in injuries of the
kidney have greatly improved in recent years since the necessity
of early aseptic operation has been recognized.

Hæmorrhage accounted for 80 out of a total 190 deaths, septic
complications for 41, anuria for 34, and shock for 11 (Watson).
Of 13 cases of nephrectomy performed on account of dangerous
hæmorrhage only 4 died, and the 6 patients most recently operated
upon all recovered (Güterbock). Willis collected 14 cases of

nephrectomy for injury to the kidney, with 9 recoveries and 5 deaths. Albarran collected 6 cases of operation in which packing of the injured kidney was resorted to, and all recovered.

The operative interference in septic complications is frequently postponed until too late, and the already exhausted patient succumbs. Of 7 nephrectomies of this nature, 4 resulted fatally,

Nephrotomy also has a high mortality. Of 8 cases, 4 died after the operation, and another after a second nephrotomy (Güterbock).

The following general statistics may be quoted with Riese : Of 490 cases of uncomplicated subcutaneous injuries to the kidney, 93 (18·9 per cent.) died. There were 327 treated by expectant treatment, and of these 69 (21·1 per cent.) died, 40 of the deaths being due to hæmorrhage. In 85 cases a conservative operation was performed (46 times on account of bleeding), and 10 died (11·7 per cent.). In 78 cases nephrectomy was performed (54 on account of bleeding), and 14 died (17·9 per cent.).

II. WITH EXTERNAL WOUND

Etiology.—Wounds of the kidney are much less frequent than subcutaneous injuries. They are produced by stabs with a dagger, sword, bayonet, hayfork, etc., or by bullets.

Pathology.—The external wound may lie in the loin, or on the anterior surface of the abdomen, or over the ribs, and according to the site and direction of the wound the intestine, liver, spleen, or pleura may be wounded.

Any part of the organ may be affected, and portions may be detached by bullet wounds. With the older forms of bullet the ball and portions of clothing might be embedded in the organ and remain for considerable periods. A bullet may have a bursting action on the kidney and cause extensive destruction of its substance.

The blood escapes by the external wound, and, if the calyces or the pelvis of the kidney are wounded, urine escapes along with it. There is no perirenal accumulation of blood, except in rare cases in which the wound is a long, sinuous track. The kidney may partly prolapse from a large wound.

The wound is almost invariably infected, so that primary union is very rare, and prolonged suppuration common.

The organs which may be wounded at the same time as the kidney are seen in the diagram illustrating the anterior relations of the kidneys (Fig. 2, p. 3).

Urinary fistulæ occur, but seldom persist. In the American Civil War there was only one permanent fistula in 74 cases of bullet wounds of the kidney.

When healing has taken place the kidney is usually largely destroyed, and presents irregular depressed scars and extensive adhesions to neighbouring parts.

Symptoms.—The symptoms differ in several particulars from those of subcutaneous lesions of the kidney. There is no perirenal swelling of blood and urine. There are external hæmorrhage and escape of urine by the wound, and occasionally prolapse of the kidney.

The pain is persistent, but does not radiate along the ureter. Hæmorrhage from stab wounds may be severe and rapidly fatal. In bullet wounds the external hæmorrhage is seldom severe, but it may be intermittent, recommencing after an interval of about five days.

The escape of urine seldom takes place at first. It usually occurs when the bleeding is diminishing after a few days. Occasionally flatus from a wound in the intestine is passed with the blood and urine from the external wound.

Septic complications occur on the fourth or fifth day after the injury. Hæmorrhage has usually ceased at this time, but it may continue. With the pus, fragments of slough, portions of clothing, and other materials are discharged. The track of the wound may become blocked by débris, and pus and urine collect around the kidney.

Diagnosis.—The diagnosis is made from the position and direction of the wound, the escape of urine, and the occurrence of hæmaturia.

Prognosis.—In wounds of the kidney the prognosis is comparatively good, and operation is frequently undertaken with success. Wounds of other organs increase the gravity of the prognosis. Tuffier found that in 31 cases 8 died, and in 6 of these the fatal result was due to complicating injuries.

The mortality of incised wounds of the kidney is as low as 15 per cent. (Albarran), but bullet wounds have a high mortality —namely, 53 per cent. (Küster). The mortality of bullet and other wounds of the kidney in the American Civil War was 66·2 per cent.

The statistics are all compiled from cases treated before the development of aseptic wound treatment and abdominal surgery. The duration of healing varies from three weeks to three months; rarely it may be prolonged to two years. After healing of the wound, sequelæ such as inflammation in the urinary tract, fistulæ, etc., may cause chronic invalidism. Of 52 recently healed wounds of the kidney Tuffier found 22 with sequelæ.

Treatment.—If the external hæmorrhage is moderate and

diminishing, it will suffice to clean and dress the wound. A careful watch is kept for recurrent hæmorrhage and septic complications. If there is any reason to suspect that a foreign body is lodged in the wound, the track should be freely opened up and the kidney exposed and examined.

If the hæmorrhage is severe and persistent the kidney should be exposed by an oblique lumbar incision. A single wound in the kidney may be closed with catgut sutures. Detached portions of the kidney may require removal, or, if the kidney is extensively lacerated, nephrectomy may be necessary.

When a large vessel is wounded at the hilum it may be very difficult to control the hæmorrhage, and clamps must be placed upon the pedicle. If the blood supply of the kidney is entirely cut off in this way, it will be necessary to remove the kidney. Küster advises that, when a doubt exists as to the blood supply being sufficient to nourish the kidney, the clamps be left on for a day and then removed on the operating table. If the kidney now bleeds when it is pricked, it may be left and packed with gauze; if it fails to bleed, nephrectomy is performed.

A kidney prolapsed into a large lumbar wound is cleansed, examined, and replaced if necessary, being fixed in position by means of catgut stitches. The wound is then cleansed and partly closed, and a large drainage tube inserted.

In complicated cases in which it is probable that other organs are wounded an exploratory laparotomy will be necessary

LITERATURE

Curschmann, *Münch. med. Woch.*, 1902, xlix. 38.
Delbet, *Ann. d. Mal. d. Org. Gén.-Urin.*, 1901, xix. 669.
Keen-Spencer, *Ann. Surg.*, Aug., 1896, xxiv.
Klippel et Chabrol, *Presse Méd.*, 1900, p. 265.   [vol. ii., pt. ii.
Medical and Surgical History of the War of the American Rebellion,
Riese, *Arch. f. klin. Chir.*, 1903, vol. lxxi.
Tuffier, *Arch. Gén. de Méd.*, 1888, cxxii. 298, cxxiii. 335.
Waldvogel, *Deuts. Zeits. f. Chir.*, 1902, vol. lxiv.
Watson, *Boston Med. Surg. Journ.*, July 9, 1903, p. 16.
Wildbolz, *Zeits. f. Urol.*, 1910, iv. 241.

CHAPTER VIII

ANEURYSM OF THE RENAL ARTERY

THIS is a rare condition. Only 25 cases were found by Skillern in the literature.

Etiology.—The condition is usually due to traumatism, but it is sometimes spontaneous (12 traumatic, 7 spontaneous—Morris). In traumatic cases the majority are men in the most active period of life; in spontaneous cases the sexes are about equally divided, and the majority are over 40 years of age. The form of injury which causes the aneurysm is similar to that which produces rupture of the kidney, such as a fall across a cart-wheel. In spontaneous cases endocarditis or arterial degeneration is usually present.

Pathology.—The aneurysm is formed in relation to the main trunk of the renal artery or one of its large branches. It may be fusiform or sacculated, and it may be associated with a false aneurysm formed either by rupture of a branch of the renal artery at another part or by rupture of the aneurysm itself.

The aneurysm may vary from the size of a hazel-nut to a large swelling occupying the whole of the loin and extending inwards as far as the middle line. A small aneurysm may press upon the kidney and cause atrophy of the parenchyma adjacent to it. When the aneurysm is large, and especially when a false aneurysm has been formed, the kidney tissue is extensively destroyed by pressure. The blood may track along the renal vessels and accumulate within the capsule of the kidney, which is greatly distended. Rupture may take place into the renal pelvis, which becomes distended with blood, and the kidney is dilated to form a hæmatonephrosis. Rupture of the wall of the sac and the overlying peritoneum will be followed by escape of blood into the peritoneal cavity.

When the aneurysmal sac increases in size it displaces the colon forwards and inwards, and the liver or spleen upwards. Adhesions are formed with neighbouring structures, which vary in density and thickness. The sac is lined by, and most of its cavity filled with, laminated clot, so that it contains only a small quantity of fluid blood.

Symptoms.—Some of the smaller aneurysms recorded have been discovered post mortem, and have caused no symptoms during life. With large or with false aneurysms there is a tumour situated in the region of the kidney which has, in most cases, followed upon an injury to the loin. The tumour may appear some days or weeks after the injury, but two years, or even fourteen years, may elapse before a swelling is noticed. It is smooth, slightly movable or fixed, and does not move with respiration. It is not painful or tender, unless in a few exceptional instances. Hæmaturia is an early symptom, and usually precedes the discovery of the swelling. It may immediately follow the injury and be continuous, or there may be an interval of months or years, or the hæmaturia may be recurrent. Profuse and rapidly fatal hæmorrhage may be caused by the rupture of an aneurysm into the renal pelvis. Pulsation has rarely been observed. It was present in one case, and very indistinct in two others. In Morris's case there was a loud systolic bruit, best heard in front, over the tumour.

Diagnosis.—The condition has been diagnosed once, and suspected in two other cases. When pulsation is absent the only means of diagnosis is exploratory operation. The conditions with which aneurysm of the renal artery is most likely to be confused are ruptured kidney with hæmaturia, and hæmatonephrosis.

Prognosis.—Albert, Hahn, and Keen have each operated successfully in one case. All the other patients in whom the aneurysm caused a tumour died. Aneurysms cause no symptoms and are discovered accidentally post mortem.

Treatment.—The condition will usually be discovered in the course of an exploratory operation undertaken for a swelling in the loin which has followed an injury. The sac should not be opened up more than is sufficient to recognize the laminated character of the contents.

In breaking down adhesions severe hæmorrhage has taken place and necessitated plugging with gauze. In such a dilemma, and in a case where diagnosis has previously been made, the peritoneal cavity should be opened in the semilunar line. The peritoneum is divided along the outer side of the colon and reflected inwards. The pedicle of the kidney is exposed and ligatured. The aneurysmal sac and kidney are then removed.

LITERATURE

Barnard, *Trans. Path. Soc.*, 1901, lii. 254.
Hahn, *Deuts. med. Woch.*, 1894, xx. 32.
Keen, *Philad. Med. Journ.*, 1900, p. 1038.
Morris, *Lancet*, 1900, ii. 1902.
Skillern, *Journ. Amer. Med. Assoc.*, 1906, xlvi. 37.
Ziegler, *Centralbl. f. Grenzgeb. d. Med. u. Chir.*, 1903, vi. 2.

CHAPTER IX

PERINEPHRITIS AND PERINEPHRITIC ABSCESS

PERINEPHRITIS

CHRONIC perinephritis leads to the formation of a layer of inflammatory tissue around the kidney.

Two forms are observed : a fibrous or sclerotic and a fibro-lipomatous form. They both result from long-continued inflammation which has not reached the stage of suppuration, and it is seldom that a purely fibrous or a purely lipomatous form can be distinguished.

The kidney is invariably diseased. Any form of chronic inflammatory disease may be present, such as pyelonephritis, pyonephrosis, calculus, tuberculosis.

The change takes place in the fatty capsule of the kidney, and in old-standing cases tough adhesions are formed with the surrounding structures, especially the diaphragm, liver, colon, duodenum, and peritoneum.

In the sclerotic form the fatty capsule of the kidney is replaced by a dense layer of fibrous tissue which binds the organ to the surrounding structures. The kidney is usually small and shrunken, and may sometimes be difficult to find at operation. I operated upon a child of 9 years with subacute pyelonephritis and a renal calculus, and found a mass of perinephritic fibrous tissue, $\frac{1}{2}$ to $\frac{3}{4}$ in. in thickness, that cut like cartilage and was fused with the ribs, diaphragm, and peritoneum. On cutting a window through this the kidney was found and the stones were removed.

In the more common fibro-lipomatous form the delicate perirenal fat is replaced by coarse nodular fat with a tough fibrous stroma, the whole mass being adherent to the neighbouring structures. The fibrous capsule of the kidney is firmly adherent to this fibro-lipomatous envelope, but is easily stripped from the kidney itself, so that a subcapsular nephrectomy may, if required, be quickly and easily performed. The mass is closely adherent around the hilum to the pedicle of the kidney, and there may be difficulty in securing the vessels in such an operation.

When the pelvis of the kidney is the chief seat of disease the fibro-lipomatous mass is developed principally in this situation. When one pole of the kidney contains an abscess, this part only may be surrounded by an adherent fibrous or fibro-lipomatous mass.

Symptoms. — The symptoms of chronic perinephritis are slight, and are merged in those of the underlying renal disease. Some part of the aching and tenderness in the loin and the local rigidity of the abdominal muscles in cases of pyelonephritis and pyonephrosis, etc., may be referred to perirenal inflammation.

At the same time a tuberculous kidney may become surrounded by a thick layer of chronic inflammatory tissue without ever having given rise to pain or discomfort.

The volume of the kidney is increased on palpation, but it is impossible to say what part of the increase is perirenal and what renal. The movements of the kidney are not appreciably limited.

The **treatment** of perinephritis is that of the renal disease which has caused it.

PERINEPHRITIC ABSCESS

A perinephritic abscess may occur at any age, and may be primary or secondary.

In 230 cases collected by Küster the age was from 25 to 40. Recently, Townsend has described cases of 5 and 15 years, and Gibney collected 28 cases of children aged from 1½ to 15 years.

Men are more frequently affected than women (140 men to 68 women—Küster), and the right side more often than the left. The abscess is very rarely bilateral.

Etiology.—The primary form may follow injury to the kidney, suppuration occurring immediately, or sometimes after months or years. More frequently it develops during the course of some fever such as typhoid, scarlatina, measles, or pneumonia ; or it may appear when the patient is suffering from tonsillitis, carbuncle, boils, or even eczema.

The secondary form complicates suppuration in some neighbouring organ, such as the kidney (about 25 per cent.), liver, gallbladder, appendix, pelvic organs, or vertebræ, or duodenal ulcer.

Tuberculous perinephritic abscess is very rarely secondary to tuberculosis of the kidney. It is especially found in tuberculous disease of the vertebræ.

Pus from an empyema or an abscess of the lung may track through the costo-lumbar hiatus of the diaphragm and form a perinephritic abscess.

Bacteriology.—The following bacteria are found, and are

given in their order of frequency, viz. bacterium coli commune, streptococcus, staphylococcus. The gonococcus and pneumococcus are rare.

Pathology.—The abscess is usually unilocular, but occasionally there are multiple abscesses. It is situated outside the fibrous capsule, and may lie inside or outside the perinephritic fascia. In the former case the pus will tend to spread down the ureter into the bony pelvis, while in the latter it will appear on the surface of the body over the iliac crest, or pass into the iliac fossa.

There is a tendency to the formation of fibrous tissue in the early stages of the suppuration, so that the pus becomes shut in and tends rather to rupture in one direction than to spread widely in the retroperitoneal tissue.

Four varieties are distinguished according to situation :—

1. Above the kidney, or subphrenic, which is frequently connected with intrathoracic suppuration. The kidney is pushed downwards, and may be felt below the subphrenic mass.

2. Below the kidney, which tends to pass downwards to the iliac fossa, and may rupture into and pass along the psoas sheath and appear in Scarpa's triangle, or may pass into the pelvis and escape at the sciatic notch.

3. In front of the kidney, limited by peritoneum. This form is very rare; it may rupture into the peritoneal cavity, bowel, bladder, or vagina.

4. Behind the kidney—a much more common variety, which may pass through the muscles of the loin at the triangle of Petit.

Symptoms.—When the perinephritic abscess complicates some other disease the symptoms are superadded to those of the primary disease.

When the perinephritic suppuration is primary the onset is usually insidious and the pain slight and insignificant. The general condition of the patient is bad, and there is fever of the high remittent type. The temperature rises to 102° or 103° F. at night, and falls to normal or a little above it in the morning. In rare cases the temperature is not raised. Occasionally the onset is sudden and is heralded by a rigor. It is often difficult to find the cause of the illness at this stage.

Pain and tenderness over the kidney become marked. The pain may radiate to the shoulder or arm, but more frequently it passes downwards to the scrotum or labium. It is increased by movement and by respiration, coughing and sneezing.

There is increasing tenderness on palpation of the loin, and the abdominal muscles of that side are rigid, so that examination is difficult without an anæsthetic.

The patient complains of stiffness of the corresponding thigh, which becomes flexed and rotated slightly outwards. There is restricted extension, but no limitation of flexion. The position is that of contraction of the psoas. There may be transient paralysis of the lower limb.

A characteristic tumour forms in the loin. The waist line is obliterated, and the whole loin bulges outwards and backwards. The anterior swelling is less than appears in cases of enlarged kidney. The tumour does not move with respiration. It may be moved a little between the hands, but it does not give the sensation of ballottement.

There may be œdema of the overlying skin. Very rarely fluctuation can be detected. Some variation in symptoms may be observed according to whether the abscess is situated mainly above or mainly below the kidney.

In the variety above the kidney, in addition to the symptoms of involvement of the pleura and lung there may be jaundice, ascites, and œdema of the legs, and persistent vomiting when the right side is affected. These symptoms are caused by the relation of the abscess to the gall-bladder, inferior vena cava, and duodenum.

An abscess below the kidney is characterized by constipation from the colon being affected, symptoms of involvement of the psoas muscle (*see* above), neuralgic pain referred to the groin and genital organs, and retraction of the testicle. The swelling invades the iliac fossa and may pass under Poupart's ligament.

Pyuria will be present in the cases where the kidney is the cause of the perinephritic abscess, unless the ureter is blocked. In acute cases pus forms in ten or twelve days, while in less acute cases pus may not be detected for three or four weeks. In tuberculous cases the abscess is usually secondary to disease in the vertebra, acute symptoms are absent, and pain and tenderness are slight.

If no operation is performed the patient either dies of septicæmia or the abscess ruptures into some neighbouring organ or on the surface through the muscular triangle of Petit. Küster gives the following statistics of rupture: Pleura and bronchi, 18 cases; intestine (colon), 11 cases; peritoneum, 2 cases; bladder, or bladder and vagina, 3 cases.

Diagnosis.—The condition has been mistaken for typhoid fever or malaria in the early stage, and disease of the hip-joint or pyonephrosis at a later period.

When only fever and general symptoms are present, leucocytosis suggests that suppuration is taking place in the body; a negative Widal reaction will exclude typhoid fever, and examination of the blood will eliminate malaria. Against hip-joint disease there is the freedom of flexion and rotation of the thigh, and the absence of local tenderness.

A pyonephrosis is regular and well defined. It moves with respiration, projects forwards rather than laterally or backwards, and does not cause œdema of the skin. A pyonephrosis may be present and concealed by a perinephritic abscess.

Prognosis.—Spontaneous cure is very rare and cannot be hoped for. Good results are obtained by prompt operation in primary cases. The longer the operation is delayed the worse is the prognosis. The prognosis in secondary perinephritic abscess depends upon the original cause. Küster collected 230 cases at a period when the importance of early operation was imperfectly understood, and found 151 (65·6 per cent.) recovered. Fistulæ persisted in 6 of these cases.

Treatment.—Early operation is the only successful method of treatment. The kidney is exposed by an oblique incision, and the abscess drained. The lumbar muscles are found œdematous, and the abscess lies immediately under the lumbar fascia. The cavity should be explored in all directions, so that no pockets are left undrained. Subphrenic collections of pus and those in the iliac fossa are searched for and opened up.

Counter-openings may be necessary in the loin or elsewhere to ensure free drainage.

If the kidney is the seat of abscess, pyelonephritis, or pyo-nephrosis, it should be freely incised and drained. If nephrectomy be necessary it should be postponed to a later date.

When the abscess has originated in an empyema, this should also be drained.

In old-standing cases, when sinuses have persisted, a diseased kidney or an imperfectly drained empyema may necessitate nephrec-tomy, resection of portions of ribs, or other secondary operations.

Watson compared two series of cases where perinephritic sup-puration had followed injuries to the kidney. Of 21 cases treated without operation 17 died (80 per cent.), while in 28 cases treated by operation 2 died (7·1 per cent.).

LITERATURE

Albarran, *Soc. de Biol.*, 1889.
Guiteras, *New York Med. Journ.*, 1906, lxxxiii. 169.
Küster, *Chirurgie der Nieren.* 1902.
Maas, *Volkmanns Sammlung klin. Vort.*, 1897, p. 605.
Townsend, *Journ. Amer. Med. Assoc.*, 1904, xliii. 1626.
Watson, *Boston Med. Surg. Journ.*, 1903, cxlix. 29, 64.
Zuckerkandl, *Wien. klin. Woch.*, Oct. 13, 1910.

CHAPTER X

SURGICAL INFLAMMATION OF THE KIDNEY AND PELVIS

Classification and nomenclature.—The inflammations of the kidney and pelvis met with in surgical practice may be either non-bacterial or bacterial. The non-bacterial inflammations are caused by the excretion of irritants or by mechanical means. The bacterial diseases are divided for convenience into those produced by the ordinary pathogenic bacteria and those due to the tubercle bacillus, the fungus of actinomycosis, and the spirochæte of syphilis.

When the kidney is affected alone the term " nephritis " is used, and when the kidney substance contains scattered abscesses the condition is named "suppurative nephritis." When a single abscess or several large abscesses are present, then the disease is termed " abscess of the kidney." When the kidney and pelvis are affected " pyelonephritis " is present, and when the pelvis alone is inflamed " pyelitis " exists. If obstruction to the outflow of urine complicates pyelitis or pyelonephritis the kidney becomes distended with pus and urine, and a " pyonephrosis " is formed.

Bacteriology of renal infections.—The bacillus coli communis is the most common cause of renal infection, occurring in 75 per cent. of cases. The next most frequent are the staphylococcus (especially the aureus), the streptococcus, the proteus of Hauser, and the bacillus pyocyaneus. The pneumococcus and gonococcus are rare. The bacillus coli is usually found in pure culture, but occasionally in a mixed infection with the proteus, staphylococcus, or streptococcus. Anaerobic bacteria are occasionally found, especially in pyonephrosis.

The staphylococcus and proteus vulgaris cause decomposition of urea, and the urine rapidly becomes ammoniacal. In the rare pure streptococcal infections and the common bacillus coli infections the urine remains acid. Where the urine of the infected kidney is alkaline the blended urine of two kidneys may be acid.

116

ASEPTIC PYELONEPHRITIS

1. Due to Acute Retention of Urine

Guyon and Albarran have described a form of pyelonephritis observed experimentally in acute retention of urine. There is acute congestion of both kidneys, which may go on to interstitial and intratubular hæmorrhages with desquamation of the epithelium of the tubules. Clinically there is lessened secretion of urine. The urine contains a reduced quantity of salts, and blood, renal cells, blood casts and epithelial casts are present.

When the retention is relieved there is polyuria, and the urine contains casts for some days. If the obstruction is completely relieved and no sepsis is present, the symptoms entirely disappear.

2. Due to the Excretion of Irritants

A mild catarrhal pyelonephritis may be set up by the elimination of certain balsamics such as sandal-wood, copaiba, turpentine, etc. There is pain in the renal region and often increased frequency of micturition. The urine contains a little albumin, and cells derived from the renal pelvis. The symptoms disappear when the drug is withheld.

The excretion of cantharides produces nephritis, at first catarrhal, then interstitial ; there are also catarrhal pyelitis and cystitis. The urine is scanty, high-coloured, and contains blood, albumin, mucus, and fibrin. Microscopically, the urine contains cells from the urinary tract, and also hyaline and epithelial casts. The oliguria may become anuria. The condition may subside when the elimination of cantharides ceases and the patient is placed upon a milk diet ; but it may pass into chronic interstitial nephritis.

3. In Chronic Urinary Obstruction

In long-standing obstruction to the outflow of urine, such as stricture, enlarged prostate, or the pressure of malignant pelvic growths, the ureters become dilated and thickened and lose their contractile power, and the pelvis of the kidney is dilated. The apices of the pyramids become flattened, the sinus of the kidney is hollowed and more spacious, and the calyces are dilated. The lining membrane of the pelvis becomes opaque and tough and loses its brilliancy. The kidney is enlarged, and when not distended with fluid is flabby.

The kidney substance is narrower, both cortex and medulla being reduced in width. The differentiation between the layers remains distinct, but the fine structure is lost. The substance is tough and leathery. Microscopically there is chronic interstitial nephritis in an advanced degree. The interstitial connective tissue is increased, is moderately cellular, and the tubules and glomeruli are widely separated. The tubules become distorted and broken up, the glomeruli fibrous and their vessels occluded. (Fig. 26.)

Both kidneys are affected, but usually to an unequal degree.

Symptoms.—Those of renal disease are generally slight, and may easily be overlooked.

There is dull aching pain in the posterior renal area on both

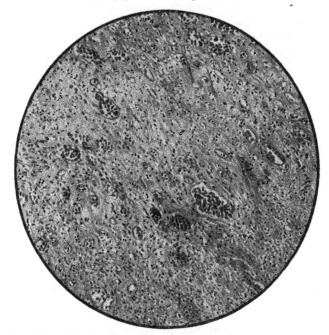

Fig. 26.—Chronic interstitial nephritis due to obstruction from enlarged prostate.

sides, rarely on one side only (25·3 per cent.), with constant thirst, sometimes more marked at night (26·7 per cent.). The tongue is dry (12·9 per cent.), at first along the centre, and later over its whole surface. Loss of appetite is present in 5 per cent., and frontal headache in 22 per cent. There may be appreciable loss of weight. The temperature is slightly subnormal. There are no cardiac or vascular changes. The kidneys cannot be felt on palpation, and are not tender. Polyuria is a constant symptom. The urine is pale and clear. The percentage of urea and other urinary constituents is much reduced, and the specific gravity is low (1005 to 1010). The total quantities of these bodies passed in twenty-four hours may be only slightly below the normal standard, or may be much reduced. The polyuria amounts to 80–100 oz. in twenty-four hours ; it is often more marked at night. No tube casts or other cellular elements are found in the urine.

Treatment.—Operation in advanced cases is fraught with extreme danger. Suppression of urine may immediately follow the operation ; more frequently there is gradual failure of the renal function, with thirst and drowsiness alternating with sleeplessness and restlessness, gradual loss of flesh, and mild delirium at night ; and the patient dies of syncope after gradually increasing cardiac failure, a few days or some weeks after the operation. .

Chronic aseptic pyelonephritis may also be caused by calculus and by new growths of the kidney. If the obstruction to the outflow of urine is complete and intermittent, the kidney becomes distended with urine and a hydronephrosis forms (p. 164). In calculus of the ureter a very pronounced polyuria may be present, which disappears when the calculus is removed, and is apparently due to reflex influences on the kidney of the affected side (*see* Chart, p. 327).

INFECTIVE PYELONEPHRITIS

There are two forms of pyelonephritis, which differ according to whether the infection occurs without previous disease of the urinary tract, or is secondary to some pre-existing urinary disease. The first form, primary pyelonephritis, is believed to be caused by blood-borne bacteria, and is therefore termed " hæmatogenous " ; while the second form is secondary to infection of the lower urinary tract, and is termed " ascending " pyelonephritis. These two forms will be described separately.

1. PRIMARY OR HÆMATOGENOUS PYELONEPHRITIS

Hæmatogenous pyelonephritis is a less common form than ascending pyelonephritis, but it has been shown within recent years to occur with greater frequency than was at one time supposed. The disease is met with in infants, children, and adults. In infants and young children it occurs with comparative frequency. At this age the pelvis is more severely affected than the kidney, and the condition will be more conveniently described under the heading of Pyelitis of Infancy and Childhood (p. 141). Adults are most frequently affected in the most active period of life. The disease also occurs in pregnant women, and presents special features, which will be described under the heading of Pyelitis of Pregnancy (p. 142).

Of my personal cases 56 per cent. were female and 44 per cent. male; while the right kidney was affected in 50 per cent., the left in 42 per cent., and both in 6 per cent. Legueu found the right kidney affected in 93 per cent. of cases.

Etiology.—The large intestine is the chief source of bacteria. A history of chronic constipation can be obtained in a number of cases, and occasionally an attack of diarrhœa has preceded the onset of renal symptoms. Tonsillitis, boils, and carbuncle are sometimes the primary foci. The renal infection may occasionally complicate influenza and typhoid fever.

It is now recognized that bacteria are constantly entering the lymphatics from the intestine and other sources in healthy individuals. The bacteria may be destroyed at the point of entry or at the lymphatic glands, or they may pass through the lymphatic system into the blood stream, in which they circulate. The endothelium and cells of the liver destroy bacteria which are introduced by way of the portal system, and bacteria are excreted in the bile. Similarly a function of the renal parenchyma, especially of the convoluted tubules, is to remove the bacteria present in the systemic circulation.

It has been proved that the virulence of these bacteria is not reduced in their passage through the body. The excretion of bacteria in this way does not give rise to any symptoms which show that the kidneys are damaged. It is stated, however, as the result of experiments on animals, that the secreting membrane is injured by the passage of the bacteria. The damage is probably slight, and is repaired partly or completely by the regenerative powers of the kidney. In some cases long-continued excretion of bacteria or their toxins may be the cause of patches of interstitial nephritis in the kidney.

It is held that the excretion of bacteria does not cause pyelonephritis unless some additional factor is present. Predisposing causes of pyelonephritis are traumatism, excessive functional activity, the elimination of toxic bodies such as cantharides, previons disease of the kidney such as urinary obstruction, calculus, new growth. It is exceptional, however, to find any of these factors present, and it is more likely that chronic toxæmia from constipatiou, an excessive dose and an exceptionally virulent strain of bacteria, are the decisive factors.

Pathology. i. **Hyperacute or fulminating pyelonephritis.** —The kidney is large, plum-coloured, and engorged with blood. The vessels at the base of the pyramids are distended with blood. The cortex is dark, the pyramids are paler. Microscopically, the large vessels and a few glomeruli are engorged with blood, and a few of the pyramids show dilated vessels. The glomeruli and tubules are healthy in appearance, and the nuclei of the renal epithelial cells may be well stained. (Fig. 27.) There may be a few ecchymoses, and sometimes a slight degree of cloudy swelling of the epithelium.

ii. **Acute pyelonephritis.**—The organ is enlarged and con-

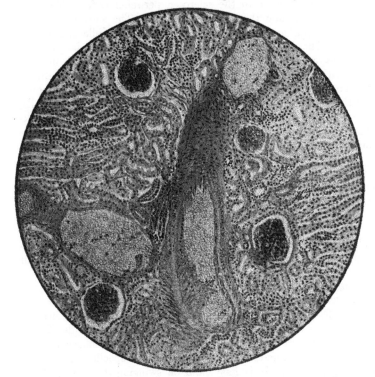

Fig. 27.—Microscopical section of kidney in postoperative suppression of urine.

There is engorgement of blood-vessels. The nuclei of the renal epithelium are well stained.

gested. Scattered over the surface are bosses varying in size from a millet-seed to a large pea. On section the cortex shows congestion, and dots and patches of greyish yellow, some of which are wedge-like in shape and correspond to the bosses on the surface of the organ. Ecchymoses are frequently observed. The epithelium of the convoluted tubules shows cloudy swelling and sometimes desquamation, and there is proliferation of the endothelium of the glomeruli. The greyish patches and wedges are densely infiltrated areas, where the tubules and glomeruli are obscured by round cells. Here and there the centre of these may have broken down so as to form a tiny abscess. The infiltration may surround a glomerulus or a small blood-vessel. The pelvis shows proliferation and desquamation of the epithelium with ecchymoses.

iii. **Subacute and chronic.**—The kidney is small, very tough, and densely adherent to the sclerosed perirenal tissue. The surface is irregular and the capsule adherent. The substance of the organ is tough and fibrous, the cortex and medulla are poorly defined. The colour is either uniformly greyish, or is pale red with grey areas. Sometimes there are small cysts, which may be filled with pus. Microscopically there is advanced chronic interstitial nephritis with sclerosis of glomeruli and destruction of tubules, and the fibrous tissue is infiltrated with densely packed round cells, either uniformly distributed or in patches. The pelvis shows thickening of the mucous membrane and great proliferation of epithelium. There may be phosphatic débris or calculi in the pelvis.

Symptoms. Prodromal symptoms.—The patient frequently has headache, lassitude, and want of appetite for a few days before the onset of the acute symptoms. Habitual constipation may have become more pronounced, or there may have been an attack of diarrhœa.

In 6·25 per cent. of cases (5 out of 80—Lenhartz) there is a sudden desire to pass water, followed by great frequency of micturition and even strangury. These symptoms may last for an hour or two, or for one or two days.

There are several degrees of severity of the symptoms :—

(a) **Mild attack.**—After a rigor the temperature rises to 101° or 102° F. The vesical irritation continues, and there is usually aching across the loins, sometimes more marked on one side. There is tenderness over one kidney, but the organ is not enlarged. The urine is usually abundant and pale, with a low specific gravity and a stale-fish odour. It is hazy, and on swinging the glass a drift-cloud appearance or shimmering is seen, which is characteristic of bacilluria. The bacillus coli communis is present in pure culture.

In a few days the temperature begins to subside, and in ten or fourteen days it is normal. The tenderness of the kidney disappears. The urine may clear and become sterile, or it may remain hazy with bacteria. In rare cases hæmaturia is an early symptom, and persists for many weeks after all other symptoms have subsided.

(b) **Acute attack.**—The initial rigor is severe and the temperature rises to 102° or 103° F. The patient is prostrate, often drowsy, and may be delirious. There is at first general abdominal pain or backache, and then heavy aching pain in one loin; occasionally attacks of severe renal colic. The abdominal muscles are rigid, especially on one side. There is intense tenderness in the region of the kidney in front, and at the angle of the last rib and the erector spinæ muscles behind. The kidney can usually be felt enlarged, unless the abdominal muscles be so rigidly contracted as to prevent examination. The second kidney is not painful or tender.

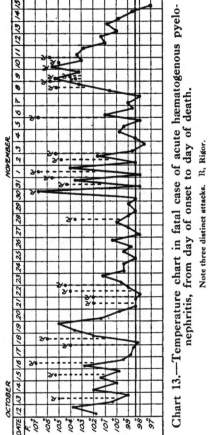

Chart 13.—Temperature chart in fatal case of acute hæmatogenous pyelonephritis, from day of onset to day of death. Note three distinct attacks. R, Rigor.

The urine is scanty, acid, very rarely alkaline in reaction, and contains bacteria, pus cells, and red blood-corpuscles. According to Dudgeon the bacteria lie between the cells, phagocytosis taking place sparingly in urine. This is not, however, invariable, for I have frequently seen evidence of active phagocytosis in all forms of bacteria. There are hyaline, granular, and blood casts, and epithelia from the renal pelvis and bladder may be found. The blood in the urine is usually small in quantity.

When the urine of each kidney has been examined separately, that from the diseased kidney has shown the characters just described, while that from the second kidney has been normal or has shown polyuria. After the first few days the bladder symptoms pass off. On examination of the blood there is a leucocyte count of 18,000 to 20,000. The bacillus coli has been found in the blood, especially in young children.

The temperature may fall slightly and then the rigor is repeated, the temperature shooting up to 105°, 106°, or even 107° F. (Chart 13), and falling to normal or slightly above it. After two or three weeks the acute symptoms may subside; the temperature falls gradually or quickly.

When the patient is allowed to get up the symptoms may all reappear. The recurrent attack is due either to infection of the second kidney or to recrudescence of the disease in the organ first attacked. After the second attack has subsided, convalescence may be established, but sometimes recurrent attacks are brought on each time the patient gets up, for several months.

Instead of taking a benign course after a fortnight or so, the rigors may be frequently repeated, the temperature rising to 105° or 107° F. after each, falling occasionally to normal, but usually keeping above 100° F. There is often a lull, during which the patient appears to improve, and then another series of rigors follows. The kidney remains large and tender, and the urine scanty and bacterial. The tongue becomes dry and brown, the appetite is lost, and the patient rapidly emaciates. Hiccough appears occasionally, and then grows more persistent and distressing. The mind becomes dull and clouded, and the patient gradually sinks, and dies in from three to six weeks after the onset of the illness.

(c) **Fulminating attack.**—The patient, previously in good health, is seized with a severe rigor, and the temperature mounts to 104° or 105° F. He becomes heavy, drowsy, or even comatose. Vomiting occurs, and there is abdominal pain and sometimes backache, and the abdomen is rigid. The urine is scanty and contains bacteria, casts, epithelia, and sometimes blood. There may be complete suppression of urine.

The patient may die comatose without developing any symptoms which point to the kidney, except the condition of the urine.

Chronic pyelonephritis (hæmatogenous).—When the acute stage of pyelonephritis has subsided, chronic pyelonephritis frequently follows, and recurrent subacute or acute attacks occur from time to time. The renal symptoms are very slight. There may be aching in one kidney, but the organ is not tender or enlarged. The urine is abundant, pale, faintly acid, and hazy with pus, and contains small shreds. The pus settles in a flat, creamy, or dead-white layer at the bottom of the glass. Bacilluria is seldom present in the milder forms of chronic pyelonephritis, but bacteria are plentiful.

The chief complaint is of chronic vesical irritation. There is increased frequency of micturition, partly from the polyuria and partly from cystitis. Micturition is either equally frequent night and day, or the nocturnal frequency is the greater. This nocturnal polyuria is very characteristic of chronic pyelonephritis. On cystoscopy the general surface of the bladder is healthy, or there may be a patchy cystitis. The trigone is red and often puffy, and the inflammation is chiefly confined to, or more marked on, one side. On this side, which corresponds to the diseased kidney, the ureteric orifice is surrounded by a zone of inflammation, and not infrequently an irregular greyish patch may be seen below it, representing a delicate film of necrosis of the surface epithelium. In the more chronic conditions these appearances may be absent, there is congestion at the bladder base, and the opening of the ureter appears a little thickened and reddened. The efflux from the ureter of the diseased side is abundant and cloudy with pus. In very chronic cases it is often scanty and thick, and occasionally it is reduced to a putty-like pipe of pus which is squeezed out of the ureter at long intervals. (Plate 5, Fig. 2.)

In other cases the vesical symptoms are prominent, and the case is frequently regarded as one of chronic cystitis. There is frequent and painful micturition. The urine contains mucus and bladder epithelium, bacilluria is usually present, and the urine has a fishy and sometimes an ammoniacal smell. In these cases recurrent attacks of subacute or acute pyelonephritis frequently occur. In some cases there are recurrent attacks of urethritis.

In another class of cases the bladder is healthy, there is a long history of renal aching but no enlargement or tenderness. The urine contains a few bacteria and some pus, and the ureteric catheter shows that these come from one kidney. The quantity of urine is continuously lowered (8 to 10 oz. in twenty-four hours), and there are recurrent attacks of complete anuria lasting for twenty-four to thirty-six hours.

Diagnosis.—In fulminating cases the symptoms are those of a sudden and profound toxæmia. Infective endocarditis, acute influenza, the onset of lobar pneumonia, and malaria have been diagnosed in such cases. Examination of the urine usually makes the diagnosis plain.

In acute cases the abdominal pain and rigidity of the muscles have led to the mistaken diagnosis of cholecystitis, subphrenic abscess, abscess of the liver, appendicitis with retrocolic abscess. The discovery of a large tender kidney, together with changes in the urine, will lead to a correct diagnosis.

Rarely an exploratory laparotomy may be necessary to clear up the diagnosis.

In chronic pyelonephritis the most frequent mistake in diagnosis is to regard the chronic cystitis as primary and to overlook the renal infection. The diagnosis is made by the cystoscope and by examining the urine drawn from each kidney by the ureteric catheter. All subacute and chronic cases of pyelonephritis should be examined with the X-rays for calculus.

Prognosis.—In mild cases of acute pyelonephritis the prognosis is good. Recovery without operation is the rule. Recurrent attacks occur, however, and in a large percentage of cases bacilluria and slight chronic pyelitis or pyelonephritis persists. This may disappear, or it may continue for many years, and may be the cause of an acute attack ten or twelve years after the first.

In acute cases the prognosis is very grave, and operation will frequently be necessary. In fulminating cases the issue is often fatal. If the diagnosis has been made, an early operation gives a more hopeful outlook. Chronic pyelonephritis persists for many years, and eventually destroys the kidney. There is the danger of secondary stone formation in the kidney and bladder, and of ascending pyelonephritis of the second kidney.

Treatment.—The treatment is medicinal, serum, vaccine, or operative.

Medicinal treatment consists in confining the patient to bed and applying hot fomentations to relieve pain, and turpentine stupes or dry cupping over the loins to relieve congestion. Urinary antiseptics should be given, such as urotropine, metramine, hetralin, or helmitol in doses of 5 or 10 gr. every four hours. Alkalis and diuretics should be freely administered, such as potassium citrate in doses of 50 or 60 gr. daily, Contrexéville water and distilled water. The bowels should be freely opened, and calomel given in doses of $\frac{1}{20}$ to $\frac{1}{8}$ gr. thrice daily. This treatment is suitable for mild cases and the early stage of acute cases. If bacteria persist in the urine when the acute symptoms have subsided, urinary antiseptic treatment should be continued and vaccine treatment adopted.

Serum treatment.—This consists in the injection of serum, usually anti-colon-bacillus serum, since in the great majority of cases the infection is due to the bacillus coli. A dose of 25 c.c. is injected hypodermically each day for three days, and at the same time calcium lactate in doses of 20 gr. thrice daily is given by the mouth in order to prevent the joint-pains and rashes which may result from the serum. Should no effect be produced in three days, the treatment should be abandoned. Dudgeon obtained satisfactory results in most instances by this treatment in 12 cases of acute pyelonephritis. In 5 of his cases the effect was rapid and permanent, in 4 there was considerable benefit, in 3 there was no benefit. In chronic cases the treatment has no effect.

Vaccine treatment.—This consists in injecting graduated doses of dead bacteria obtained from cultures of the patient's urine, or of a stock vaccine should there not be time for the preparation of an autovaccine. Small doses of two or three million colon bacilli should be used at first, and repeated in four or five days, rising rapidly to 10, 15, 20, 25, 30 millions, and so on to 100 millions, then to 150 millions for six doses, then 200 millions for six or twelve doses. The injection should be made once a week after the first three doses; and should any reaction, shown by a rise of temperature, malaise, and headache, occur, the dose should be reduced and a longer interval allowed.

In acute cases the results of the vaccine treatment have been unsatisfactory. In 10 cases only one showed a change in temperature (Williamson); in a large number of patients treated by Dudgeon there was "no material improvement except in a very few instances." In chronic cases, with or without acute exacerbations, where no complication, such as growth or stone, is present, the treatment may be of great service and bring about a cure when all other methods have failed. The treatment is a long and tedious one, and may last for six months or a year or even longer. The doses must be carefully graduated and sudden large increases avoided, as an overdose is frequently followed by a recurrence of symptoms, and if this has occurred the vaccine appears to have less effect. In several cases under my care the urine has been rendered sterile after six or twelve months' treatment.

Operative treatment.—The operations that have been performed are nephrotomy, decapsulation and opening of surface abscesses, partial resection, and nephrectomy, but only nephrotomy and nephrectomy need be considered.

I have collected 40 cases of operation in acute hæmatogenous pyelonephritis from the literature, with the following results :—

Unilateral Operations	Cases	Recovered	No change	Died
Nephrotomy	12	3	2	7
Decapsulation and opening of surface abscesses ..	6	6	0	0
Partial resection	2	2	0	0
Nephrectomy	17	17	0	0
Bilateral operations				
Nephrotomy	2	2	0	0
Nephrectomy and nephrotomy	1	1	0	0
	40	31	2	7

The results of nephrotomy are even less satisfactory than this table shows. I have performed the operation twice in the acute stage, and seen three cases in which it had previously been performed. All these patients survived. This makes 20 cases of nephrotomy with 7 deaths. The after-results of nephrotomy are unsatisfactory. Chronic pyelonephritis persists, and nephrectomy may be required at a later date.

The best results in acute cases have been obtained by nephrectomy. This should not be too long delayed. If at the end of five or seven days the acute symptoms persist and the patient is beginning to lose ground, nephrectomy should be performed.

In chronic cases operation will be called for on account of recurrent exacerbations of acute inflammation, or of persistent cystitis, or for secondary calculus, or sometimes for anuria If the second kidney is shown to be healthy by examination of its urine, nephrectomy should be performed. I have found nephrotomy sufficient when reflex oliguria and attacks of anuria were caused by chronic unilateral pyelonephritis.

LITERATURE

Adams, *Journ. Amer. Med. Assoc.*, 1899, xxxiii. 1512.

Barnard, *Lancet,* Oct. 28, 1905.

Brewer, *Ann. Surg.*, Dec., 1904, p. 1010 ; *Surg., Gyn., and Obst.*, June, 1908, p. 699.

Dudgeon, *Lancet,* 1908, i. 616.

Finkelstein, *Jahrb. f. Kind.*, 1896, xliii. 148.

Guyon et **Albarran,** *Arch. de Méd. Expér.*, 1897.

Herringham, *Clin. Journ.*, 1910, xxxv. 241.

Legueu, *Ann. d. Mal. d. Org. Gén.-Urin.*, 1904, xxii. 1441.

Lenhardt, *Münch. med. Woch.*, 1907, Nr. 16.

Pawlowsky, *Zeits. f. Hyg. u. Infect.*, 1900, xxxiii. 261.

Pousson, *Ann. d. Mal. d. Org. Gén.-Urin.*, 1902, p. 514.

Rolleston, *Pract.*, April, 1910, p. 439.

Sampson, *Johns Hopkins Hosp. Bull.*, 1903, No. 153, p. 336.

Walker, Thomson, *Pract.*, May, 1911 ; *Renal Function in Urinary Surgery.* 1908.

2. Secondary or Ascending Pyelonephritis

This disease results from an extension of infection from the lower urinary organs. It is the last phase of many chronic diseases of the bladder and urethra, such as malignant growths, stone, enlarged prostate, stricture. It frequently follows surgical interference in the bladder or urethra, such as the passage of instruments, or operations upon stone, and for this reason has been termed " surgical kidney." Ascending pyelonephritis usually, but not invariably, attacks kidneys which are already the seat of chronic aseptic pyelonephritis due to obstruction in the lower urinary tract. (Plates 6, 7.)

Etiology.—The bacteria already mentioned are the active agents in the production of ascending pyelonephritis. They are introduced into the bladder by a sound or other instrument

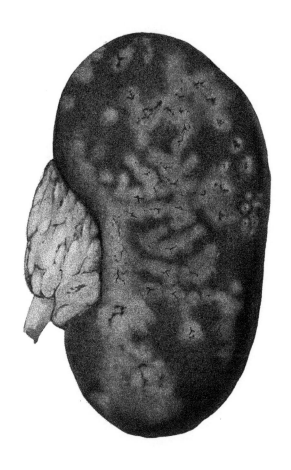

Ascending pyelonephritis in case of enlarged prostate.
(Pp. 128, 130.)

PLATE 6.

which has not been sterilized, or they may be carried from an infected urethra on a sterilized instrument.

Infection from the bladder may reach the kidney by the following paths :—

    1. *Blood-vessels.*

        (*a*) General circulation.

        (*b*) Anastomosis between the vesical, uterine, ovarian, and renal arteries (Sampson).

    · (*c*) Along the blood-vessels of the ureter.

    2. *Lymphatics of the ureter* in the muscular and outer coats.

    3. *Ureter.*

Infection ascending along the ureter is the most frequent method. It spreads either by direct continuity of the inflammatory process or by ascent of motile bacteria against the stream of urine.

The presence of organisms in the bladder, or even in the ureter, is not necessarily followed by an ascending infection of the kidney. Albarran injected cultures of virulent organisms into the bladder and ureter without producing ascending pyelonephritis.

There are natural barriers to the ascent of infection. The lower end of the ureter penetrates the wall of the bladder very obliquely, and its longitudinal layer of muscle passes into the trigone. When the bladder is distended the trigone is pushed down and the bladder wall stretched so that the intramural portion of the ureter becomes more oblique and flattened by stretching, and the intravesical tension further closes the lumen by pressure. When the bladder is contracted the intramural portion becomes shortened and less oblique, but the mucous membrane is thrown into folds,. which prevent a reflux of fluid. The condition under which a reflux is most likely to occur is during a powerful contraction of the bladder when the organ contains a small quantity of fluid. The downward flow of urine is a further protection against the ascent of bacteria. The predisposing causes of ascending infection are urethral obstruction, long-continued cystitis, new growths of the bladder, operations on the bladder involving the ureteric orifice, and stone in the bladder or ureter, all of which destroy the natural barriers.

Pathology.—In the early stage ascending pyelonephritis is frequently unilateral; in the later stages it is invariably bilateral, although one side is more diseased than the other. The disease ˊ is bilateral in 83 per cent. of cases.

Three types of pathological change are found :

    1. **Recent acute pyelonephritis.**—The kidney is enlarged, tense, and deeply congested. Scattered over the surface are small

groups of greyish-yellow spots the size of a pin's head or a split pea, or larger, and slightly raised. The kidney substance is dark and congested, and greyish streaks radiate outwards through the pyramids and cortex. A greyish-yellow patch underlies the raised surface nodule. Ecchymoses are observed here and there.

2. **Old-standing, diffuse, subacute, and chronic pyelo-**

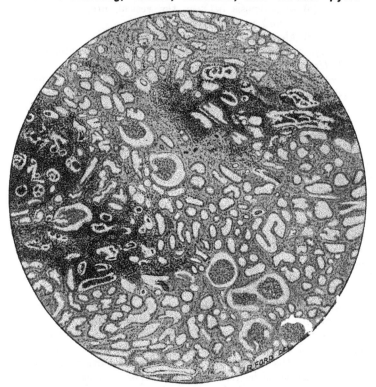

Fig. 28.—Microscopical section of kidney in suppurative pyelonephritis.

The field shows the edge of the affected area and illustrates the spread of inflammation along the line of the tubules.

nephritis.—The kidney is enlarged, and has a mottled dull-red and greyish-yellow surface. Section shows either a uniform dull greyish-yellow appearance or patches of this colour scattered on a dull-red surface. (Plates 6, 7.) Small points of softening may be found in the cortex. The grey streaks and patches consist of dense round-cell infiltration. (Fig. 28.) Bacteria are found in the straight and convoluted tubules and passing through the walls.

3. **Old-standing sclerotic pyelonephritis.**—The kidney is of natural size or smaller than normal. It is surrounded by a dense thick layer of fibro-lipomatous tissue firmly adherent to the capsule. The capsule is usually adherent to the kidney. The surface is irregular and granular. The kidney substance is tough and fibrous. Microscopically there is diffuse chronic interstitial fibrosis. The tubules are widely separated, some forming small cysts and others being broken up and disintegrated. Patches of round-cell infiltration are found here and there. Many sclerosed glomeruli are seen. The ureter may be almost normal, or may be dilated, thickened, and thrown into folds. The pelvis is thickened and may be slightly dilated, and contains purulent urine.

Symptoms.—During the course of chronic cystitis or some obstructive disease, and usually as a direct consequence of surgical intervention, such as the passage of instruments or the removal

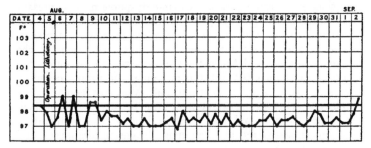

Chart 14.—Continuous subnormal temperature in chronic ascending pyelonephritis in vesical calculus.

of an enlarged prostate, symptoms of acute infective pyelonephritis supervene. The onset of chronic pyelonephritis is insidious, and the symptoms may be insignificant, so that it is usually impossible to say when the disease commenced. Occasionally the onset is marked by an acute attack, which subsides.

1. **Acute ascending pyelonephritis.**—A few hours after surgical interference, or sometimes after exposure to cold, there is a rigor, and the temperature rises to 102° or 104° F. (Chart 3, p. 15). The temperature may, however, be continuously subnormal (Chart 14). The patient is drowsy, and complains of backache, sometimes more marked on one side. The skin is dry and harsh, the face heavy and apathetic. There is burning thirst, the mouth is dry and parched : the tongue is dry, red, and glazed ; later it becomes covered with a brown or black fur (" parrot tongue "). Nausea and vomiting are frequent symptoms, and there is absolute constipation. The abdomen becomes tense

and distended with flatus. Hiccough sets in and becomes increasingly troublesome. Rigidity of the abdominal muscles is usually present, and often more marked on one side. There is tenderness over both kidneys at first, but after twenty-four hours this usually becomes confined to one side. The tender kidney is enlarged, the second kidney is not palpable. There has frequently been polyuria before the attack, and now the urine suddenly becomes scanty, or there is complete suppression. The temperature may remain at 102° F. or over, or it may fall, and rise again after another rigor, and then become high and swinging while the rigors are repeated at irregular intervals. Herpes of the lips is frequently observed.

The patient becomes more and more drowsy, the abdominal distension increases, vomiting grows more frequent, and hiccough is constant. The pupils are small and react sluggishly to light. Convulsions are extremely rare. Uræmic dyspnœa may be present and is occasionally paroxysmal. Cheyne-Stokes breathing may be observed in the last stages. Muttering delirium supervenes, and the patient passes into coma and dies. Occasionally the mind remains clear and the patient is restless and anxious; the temperature is high (105° F.) and swinging, the urine absolutely suppressed. Later there is delirium, and eventually coma.

In less severe cases the excretion of urine becomes re-established. It is scanty at first and may contain blood. The temperature falls, flatus is passed and the abdominal distension disappears, and the symptoms subside.

In other acute cases the urine continues to be secreted in good quantity, but there are recurrent attacks of very severe hæmorrhage.

In mild cases the temperature rises to 102° or 103° F. after a slight chill, the quantity of urine is reduced, and there are slight tenderness over the kidneys, headache, nausea, and sometimes vomiting. The bowels are constipated. The urine becomes purulent. In some cases the urine becomes foul and there are signs of cystitis without any rise of temperature. As the cystitis subsides, blood begins to appear in the urine, and on cystoscopy the hæmorrhage is found to be renal. In this type severe hæmorrhage may continue until relieved by operation.

2. **Chronic suppurative pyelonephritis.**—An acute attack of septic pyelonephritis which subsides is usually followed by chronic septic pyelonephritis. In rare cases, where the obstruction in the lower urinary tract is relieved, the kidneys may return to their normal state.

The onset of chronic suppurative pyelonephritis is frequently

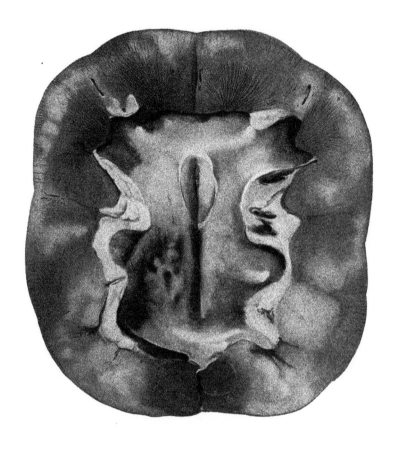

Dilatation of renal pelvis, pyelitis, and suppurative nephritis in enlarged prostate. Same kidney as shown in Plate 6. (Pp. 128, 130.)

PLATE 7.

insidious. It is engrafted on chronic aseptic pyelonephritis (p. 117), and it is often impossible to state when the septic complication ensued. When the syndrome is fully developed, the condition is known as *urinary septicæmia*. The patient has a sallow, earthy appearance, the skin is dry and harsh and seldom sweats. There is gradual, persistent loss of weight. The lips are dry; the tongue is at first dry along the middle, then over the whole surface, and it becomes glazed, red, and cracked; the mouth and throat also become dry. There are loss of appetite, dyspepsia, and occasionally nausea. The bowels are constipated. The patient suffers from frontal headache, and is frequently drowsy. There is polyuria, amounting to 80–100 oz. in twenty-four hours. The urine is pale, neutral or faintly acid, has a specific gravity of 1008–1010, or

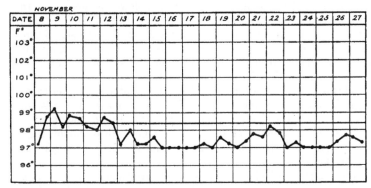

Chart 15.—Continuous subnormal temperature in case of bladder growth with chronic septic pyelonephritis.

even less. It is hazy and contains flakes, and may occasionally give the characteristic drift-cloud appearance of bacilluria. There is a trace of albumin, and a small deposit of pus which settles as a thin creamy layer. The urine contains pus, sometimes a few casts, and bacteria. There may be slight renal aching, but the kidneys are not enlarged or tender.

There is frequent micturition, in increased quantity, more marked at night (nocturnal polyuria), but this symptom may be masked by the symptoms of previously existing prostatic or bladder disease. The temperature varies from 97° to 97·6° or 97·8° F., occasionally rising to 98° or to normal. (Charts 14, 15.)

An injection of methylene blue either fails to colour the urine or the elimination is delayed, reduced, and prolonged.

After the injection of phloridzin, either no sugar is produced by the kidneys, or only a trace.

The course of chronic septic pyelonephritis may be interrupted by acute or subacute attacks at long or short intervals. (Chart 4, p. 16.) These are brought on by the passage of an instrument or by injudicious exposure to cold and fatigue, or may come on apparently without exciting cause. Such an attack resembles the acute attacks already described, but is usually milder in character. During the attacks the quantity of urine diminishes, and there may even be a period of temporary suppression, lasting some hours, and the patient rapidly emaciates. After the attack improvement takes place, the urine is secreted in as great quantity as before, but the patient has lost ground. Sometimes the patient dies during an acute exacerbation.

Chronic septic pyelonephritis may last several years, and its progress apart from acute exacerbations is slowly progressive. In the later stages the quantity of urine diminishes, and the headache, thirst, anorexia, drowsiness, and other symptoms increase. There are seldom, if ever, uræmic convulsions. The patient may die almost suddenly without an increase in the symptoms, or may gradually sink with a failing renal function.

Diagnosis.—The occurrence of acute symptoms such as those detailed above, after the passage of an instrument in a case of obstructive urinary disease, presents no difficulty in diagnosis.

If the urine becomes clear while the temperature remains high and swinging and the kidney large, it is likely that a pyonephrosis has developed.

The diagnosis of chronic suppurative pyelonephritis is of high importance in diseases of the urethra, prostate, and bladder. The symptoms are insidious and slight, and must be carefully investigated. The condition of the urine is very important in diagnosis. The tests for the renal function are also invaluable. Where operative treatment of the renal disease is proposed, it will be necessary to catheterize the ureters and examine each urine separately.

Prognosis.—Many patients die during the acute attack of ascending pyelonephritis, and of those that recover the majority suffer from chronic pyelonephritis. Should the urinary obstruction be removed, the further progress of the disease will probably be arrested, but the kidneys are permanently damaged.

Chronic ascending pyelonephritis is usually slowly progressive, and is eventually fatal after some years.

Treatment. 1. Acute ascending pyelonephritis.—*Prophylactic measures* include the sterilization of all urethral instruments and of all basins, syringes, lotions, etc., and the cleansing of the surgeon's hands and of the patient. They consist also in practising the utmost gentleness in all manipulations. Roughness means bruising and laceration, and this, together with the damage produced by obstruction, paves the way for sepsis.

Non-operative treatment consists in dry cupping, hot fomentations, turpentine stupes, or poultices applied to the loin to relieve the renal congestion. A hot pack or hot vapour bath should be given to induce sweating. Pilocarpine may be injected hypodermically, but should be carefully watched. It is important to get the bowels opened and to relieve the abdominal distension. A large dose of castor oil or a strong saline purge should be given, but it is frequently returned' if the patient has commenced vomiting. Turpentine and soap-and-water enemata, to which 20 minims of oil of rue are added, help to bring away flatus, and a rectal tube should be introduced high up in the rectum.

If the patient is able to keep fluids down, large draughts of warm Contrexéville water should be given, and may be combined with theocin sodium acetate 3-8 gr. every four hours, or theobromine sodiosalicylate (diuretin) 10 or 15 gr. every four hours. Pituitary (infundibular) extract (20 per cent., B., W. & Co.) may be used in a dose of 0·5 c.c. This has the advantage of being given subcutaneously, but its powerful effect in raising the blood pressure necessitates great caution in its use; I combine it with atropine. Glucose solution should be introduced into the subcutaneous tissues in large quantities, several pints being injected slowly. Infusion of glucose solution (2½ per cent.) into a vein (median basilic) is the most rapid and powerful means of re-establishing the renal secretion. Two or three pints are infused.

Operative treatment.—There are two indications for operative treatment :

    i. The relief of urinary obstruction, if present.

    ii. The relief of congestion and drainage of the kidney.

Should the measures detailed above prove ineffectual and no improvement be apparent in two or three days, or if the patient appear to be failing before this, operation will become necessary.

If there is unrelieved urinary obstruction, this should first receive attention. The operation which is performed for the relief of the obstruction is not necessarily that which would have been chosen had no kidney complication developed. The operation should give the freest drainage with the least amount of shock. Suprapubic cystotomy and drainage with a large tube are the best means of carrying this out. It is a temporary measure. Operation for the permanent cure of the obstruction can be performed later if the patient survives.

For relief of the renal congestion and sepsis nephrotomy should be performed. The kidney is freely incised along the convex border, and a large rubber drain introduced into the pelvis. If there is free hæmorrhage a mattress stitch may be inserted to control it, the rest of the kidney wound being left open or packed with antiseptic gauze. Another large drain is placed outside the kidney before uniting the edges of the parietal wound. As a result of this operation the temperature falls to normal, and within a few hours the dressings are flooded with urine. The temperature may remain normal and the progress to complete recovery be uninterrupted, or the temperature may rise again to 100° or 101° F. for a few days and then gradually fall. The secretion of urine, however, is re-established, and the crisis is over.

It is of vital importance that these operations be carried out with the utmost celerity. The operation for obstruction and that for relief of the renal congestion and sepsis are done at one sitting. Saline infusion, rectal and intravenous, should be given on the return from the operation. There is some danger of hæmorrhage from the kidney about the seventh or tenth day after operation. Should this occur, the tube is removed and the kidney rapidly plugged with gauze. I have operated in this manner with successful results on patients who were weakened by over-long delay, on others in the final unconscious stage of the disease, and on a patient with one kidney, anuric for three days and with a temperature of 106° F.

Nephrectomy is not indicated in these cases, since nephrotomy suffices to tide over the crisis; the shock in nephrectomy is greater, the disease is not cured by it, and the second kidney, if it is not acutely septic, is damaged to an unknown degree by back pressure. Nephrectomy may, however, be necessary in the hæmorrhagic type of pyelonephritis on account of the severe and continuous hæmorrhage.

2. **Chronic ascending pyelonephritis.**—In the majority of cases chronic ascending pyelonephritis is bilateral, one kidney, however, being more seriously damaged than the other. The *prophylaxis* of chronic ascending pyelonephritis consists in the early removal of enlarged prostate, the efficient treatment of stricture, the removal of calculi, and other measures directed against the existence of chronic obstruction and chronic sepsis in the lower urinary organs.

When chronic pyelonephritis has become established, operative interference in the bladder and urethra must be undertaken with the utmost caution. When an operation for enlarged prostate is proposed the bladder should be opened suprapubically and drained for a week or more before the prostate is removed. In a case of stricture, external urethrotomy with drainage of the bladder would be preferred to internal urethrotomy or dilatation with instruments. Urinary antiseptics (see under Hæmatogenous Pyelonephritis, p. 126) and diuretics should be freely administered.

If the disease is proved to be unilateral and the second kidney ascertained to be healthy by means of the ureteric catheter and tests for the renal function, the kidney may, after removal of all lower urinary obstruction, be incised or removed. It is seldom, however, that these circumstances combine to make surgical intervention possible.

Vaccine treatment has not given encouraging results. The administration of renal extract has been tried in these cases and in chronic aseptic pyelonephritis. It does not influence the cause, or, in the cases I have seen treated by it, modify the progress of the disease.

LITERATURE

Albarran, *Traité de Chirurgie* (Le Dentu et Delbet), iii. 760.
Israel, *Nierenkrankheiten.* Berlin, 1901.
Legueu, *Bull. de la Soc. de Chir.*, 1901.
Pousson, *Folia Urol.*, Jan., 1909, p. 445.
Sampson, *Johns Hopkins Hosp. Bull.*, Dec., 1903.
Walker, Thomson, *Pract.,* June, 1903.
Weir, *Med. Rec.*, 1894, xl. 325.
Wilms, *Münch. med. Woch,.* 1902, Nr. 12, p. 476.

CHAPTER XI

SURGICAL INFLAMMATION OF THE KIDNEY AND PELVIS (Concluded)

PYELITIS

THE intimate relation between the kidney and its pelvis makes it impossible for severe inflammation to be wholly confined to one or the other. At the same time there are cases where the brunt of the inflammation falls upon the pelvis, and the kidney is but slightly involved, so that clinical evidence of nephritis cannot be obtained. These are cases of mild subacute or chronic inflammation, which may either follow upon an acute attack of pyelonephritis or arise *de novo*.

Etiology.—Mid-adult life is most frequently affected in either sex. The infection may be blood-borne (hæmatogenous), or it may ascend from the lower urinary organs by the ureter or the lymphatics of the ureter.

As in pyelonephritis, diseases of the lower urinary organs which cause obstruction and inflammation are the most frequent causes. Thus, enlarged prostate, stricture, stone in the bladder, gonorrhœa (18 per cent.—Finger), bladder growths, etc., are predisposing causes.

In one class of cases a calculus is present in the pelvis. This may be either the cause or the result of the pyelitis.

Pathology.—The mucous membrane in slight catarrhal forms is hyperæmic, and in more severe forms is thickened and velvety, and sometimes shows petechiæ and superficial ulceration. In old-standing pyelitis, especially where calculi are present, the wall of the pelvis is thick and leathery, the mucous membrane dull and opaque, sometimes there are small colloid-filled cysts (*pyelitis cystica*), or tiny sago-grain lymph follicles (*pyelitis granulosa*). Pyelitis, whether ascending or hæmatogenous, may be unilateral. In the later stages of ascending pyelitis the condition is usually bilateral.

Symptoms.—In cases of non-calculous pyelitis the symptoms are usually insignificant, if the cases of acute pyelonephritis, already described, are excluded. There may be a slight rise of temperature to 100° F. at night, but the temperature is often unaffected.

Slight constant renal aching is complained of, either at the angle formed by the last rib and the erector spinæ mass of muscles, or anteriorly a little below and internal to the tip of the 9th rib. There may be a little tenderness on pressure at this point, but often this is absent. The kidney is not enlarged.

Urine.—Changes in the urine form the most important signs of pyelitis. There is polyuria, most marked at night. The urine is pale and opalescent, the specific gravity low (1008 or 1010). It is acid and usually odourless, but sometimes there is the stale-fish smell of bacilluria.

On standing the urine deposits a flat, creamy layer of pus, which moves heavily when the glass is tilted. The supernatant fluid is pale and cloudy, and there may be the characteristic drift-cloud appearance on making the urine circulate in a glass. There is a slight cloud of albumin. Microscopically, tailed cells and over-lapping epithelial cells (*see* under Pyuria, p. 147) are present, but no tube casts. Bacteria are present and may be abundant.

With the cystoscope the ureteric efflux is copious, frequently repeated, and cloudy to a varying degree. The movements at the ureteric orifice are vigorous. The edges of the orifice may be healthy, but are frequently reddened and sometimes thick. (Plate 16, Fig. 1, facing p. 234.) A halo of congestion or inflammation may surround the orifice in an otherwise healthy bladder. Where cystitis is present these appearances may be obscured, and there may be nothing apart from the efflux to distinguish one orifice from the other when the disease is unilateral. In slight degrees of pyelitis the urine shows only a faint haze and a few flakes, and the cystoscopic changes consist in a faint blush around the orifice, which is open and with slightly thickened lips.

It will sometimes be found on examination of the urine of each kidney, drawn by a ureteric catheter, that the urine of the diseased pelvis is alkaline, while that of the healthy side is acid. The blend of the two urines is acid if alkaline cystitis is not present.

In cases where pyelitis is secondary to cystitis, the symptoms of the latter may obscure those due to the pyelitis. In this case the urine may be alkaline and stinking and ammoniacal. It contains pus and mucus, giving the deposit a billowy appearance.

Diagnosis.—In making a diagnosis the following questions must be answered :—

    1. In a case of cystitis from any cause is pyelitis present ?

    2. Where pyelitis is present is the kidney involved ?

    3. Is there a calculus in the renal pelvis ?

1. Where the signs of pyelitis are obscured by cystitis the diagnosis depends upon the cloudy efflux from the ureteric orifice, the appearance of the orifice, and the examination of the urine of each kidney obtained by the ureteric catheter.

2. It is often extremely difficult to state whether the kidney is involved in a slight chronic pyelitis. The history of a severe acute onset points to renal inflammation, and so do tenderness and enlargement of the organ, an excessive quantity of albumin, the discovery of tube casts, and proofs of an inadequate renal function as shown by symptoms (see under Chronic Pyelonephritis, p. 117) and by the methylene-blue and phloridzin tests.

3. There may be difficulty in the diagnosis of a pelvic calculus when there has been no pain or hæmaturia and no history of stone. The X-rays will settle the diagnosis.

Treatment.—The first indication for treatment is to remove any local irritant or any cause of back pressure or sepsis in the lower urinary organs.

The removal of a calculus from the renal pelvis may suffice to cure the pyelitis.

Enlarged prostate and stricture must be treated. If the pyelitis is of long standing and there is reason to suspect that the kidney is involved, it may be necessary to drain the bladder by suprapubic cystotomy for a fortnight or more before proceeding to the operation for radical cure of the prostatic obstruction.

The treatment of the pyelitis consists in the administration of urinary antiseptics (urotropine, hetralin, helmitol, metramine, etc.) and diuretics (Contrexéville, Evian, Vittel, and other alkaline diuretic waters).

Vaccine treatment should be tried in chronic cases (see under Pyelonephritis, p. 126).

Instillations of argyrol and other silver preparations have been made through a ureteric catheter passed along the ureter into the renal pelvis. The method is not free from the danger of obstruction resulting from swelling of the mucous membrane at the outlet of the pelvis, and should be used with the utmost caution, and not practised if the temperature be elevated. Kelly and Casper have employed this method in cases of chronic gonorrhœal pyelitis, and Stockmann recommends it in all cases of chronic pyelitis. From 10 to 15 c.c. of a 1–2 per cent. solution of nitrate of silver are instilled into the renal pelvis on several successive days or on alternate days, or a solution of 1 in 2,000 to 1 in 1,000 may be used in larger quantities.

My experience of this method has been favourable. I reserve it for cases where medicinal and vaccine treatment have failed.

It should only be used by those who are experienced in ureteral catheterization.

Should these methods fail in chronic cases, and diuretics and urinary antiseptics fail in more severe and acute cases, the kidney should be exposed and opened, and the pelvis washed out and drained through the wound. A small rubber tube may be fixed in the pelvis by a catgut stitch through the renal capsule, and the pelvis washed with silver nitrate solution daily for ten days, when the wound is allowed to close. The cystitis should then be treated by bladder-washing.

PYELITIS OF INFANCY AND CHILDHOOD

A form of acute pyelitis which occurs in infants and children merits separate discussion.

Many of the cases are met with in infants under 2 years, but the disease also occurs in older children. Dr. J. Thomson records 8 cases at the ages of 7½, 10, 10, 12, 14, 14, 18, 20 months.

The majority are girls, but cases in boys have been recorded, and Morse found that 40 per cent. of his 50 cases were boys.

Constipation is very frequently present, and there may have been occasional attacks of diarrhœa. There is frequently a history of soreness around the anus, painful defæcation, or blood in the motions. The symptoms begin suddenly with a rise of temperature and a chill or rigor, which may be severe and repeated. Delirium, squinting, and vomiting follow, and the child is restless and distressed. The temperature is high, 104° or 106° F., and remittent in type. There is pallor and anorexia. Emaciation is slow.

The local symptoms may be slight and insignificant. Attacks of screaming—due to colic—occur, and tenderness on palpation in the region of the kidney has been suspected in some cases. Increased frequency of and pain on micturition is sometimes observed, but this symptom may be wanting, and occasionally the urine is held for an unusually long time to avoid pain on passing it if there is soreness of the vulva.

The first indication that there is any urinary trouble is often given by a yellowish staining of the diapers. The urine is strongly acid. There is a little albumin (usually less than 0·1 per cent.), while pus is present in considerable amount. Hyaline and finely granular tube casts are occasionally found. Red blood-corpuscles may be seen in the early stage. Some epithelial cells from the kidney pelvis or quantities of squamous cells from the bladder are present, and bacteria in large numbers, which are found to be the bacillus coli in the majority of cases, but occasionally the staphylo- or streptococcus.

Diagnosis.—This depends upon the presence of pus and bacteria in the urine. Thomson looks upon pyrexia " and extreme distress without any other symptoms sufficient to produce them," and the occurrence of rigors, in a child under 2 years, when malaria can be excluded, as important points in diagnosis.

The condition has been mistaken for malaria, irregular typhoid, and general tuberculosis.

Prognosis.—There is a tendency to spontaneous recovery, but the condition sometimes ends fatally. The cases improve rapidly under treatment. The temperature falls and the symptoms subside in a week or ten days. The pus may remain for several weeks and the bacteria for longer.

Treatment.—Acidity of the urine is reduced by the administration of alkalis, and the urine is kept neutral. Citrate of potash is given in doses of 24 gr., or in severe cases 36 to 48 gr., per day in infusion of digitalis, and continued till danger of a relapse is past. Urotropine, 5 or 10 gr. daily, and salol may be given in addition to the alkaline treatment.

The nurse should be warned not to wipe soiled diapers against the urethra.

Operative measures are very rarely necessary. If the child is steadily losing ground under medicinal treatment, and the symptoms are unilateral, nephrotomy may be performed.

PYELITIS (PYELONEPHRITIS) OF PREGNANCY

When pyelonephritis is already present the effect of pregnancy is to aggravate the disease. Pyelonephritis not infrequently develops during the early months of pregnancy, and the pregnancy is the predisposing cause of the disease.

Pathology.—The bacteriology is similar to that of other renal infections. Albeck found the bacillus coli in 131 out of 159 cases.

The right kidney is almost always attacked (65 in 70 cases—Leguen), and the condition is unilateral. The disease most frequently appears about the fourth month of pregnancy.

It has been ascribed to compression of the ureter by the gravid uterus, but this is doubtful, since the uterus is not likely at this early stage to cause pressure. Mirabeau holds that it is due to hyperæmia of the vesical mucous membrane and the altered relations of the ureters and bladder to the urethra causing urinary obstruction.

When an instrument has been passed the infection is usually looked upon as ascending. In other cases when no infection of the lower urinary tract has occurred, it is considered to be a hæmatogenous infection.

Symptoms.—Bar describes a latent presuppurative stage during which there is bacilluria with continuous fever, but Leguen found a sudden onset in 12 out of 70 cases. There are a rigor and rise of temperature, together with severe unilateral renal pain in paroxysms and frequent painful micturition. The vesical irritation may be the first and most distressing symptom. The urine contains pus and bacteria. The quantity of pus is not a gauge of the severity of the infection, and Legueu states that the urine may be almost clear even with grave symptoms. The general condition usually remains good, although the temperature is high and swinging. In a few cases the disease is bilateral and there is rapid emaciation, with drowsiness, burning thirst, dry tongue, and other signs of uræmia. In the later stages of pregnancy palpation of the abdomen is difficult owing to the large volume of the uterus. There is some rigidity on one side, and the kidney is tender; it may be felt slightly enlarged.

Diagnosis.—The diagnosis depends upon the examination of the urine and the situation of pain and tenderness. A mistaken diagnosis of appendicitis has been made.

Course and prognosis. Effect on the pregnancy and puerperium.—Of 52 untreated cases, premature labour occurred in 13 (25 per cent.) (Leguen). When the acute attack occurs early in the pregnancy and there is an interval of normal temperature before parturition takes place, the puerperium is usually apyretic. If, however, the acute attack is late in the pregnancy there is usually fever during the puerperium, but puerperal infection does not occur.

Effect on the child.—If the pregnancy be interrupted the child is usually ill-nourished, and dies in one-third of cases (Legueu). If the attack occur late, and the pregnancy go on to full term, the child is usually healthy and well-nourished.

Effect on the kidney.—After parturition the pyelonephritis may subside and the urine clear and become sterile, but more frequently bacilluria and some degree of pyelonephritis persist and exacerbations occur during succeeding pregnancies.

Treatment.—*Prophylaxis* consists in careful asepsis in catheterization and in the treatment of constipation during pregnancy. If bacilluria exists or there is chronic pyelonephritis, this should be energetically treated, and the patient warned of the danger of becoming pregnant. The production of abortion or the induction of premature labour is seldom necessary, but it may be called for in a severe case. Urinary antiseptics and vaccine treatment should be given, and in the great majority of cases these yield satisfactory results. (*See* Pyelonephritis, p. 126.)

Operative treatment.—This is very rarely necessary. Nephrotomy has given good results, and is specially indicated when the pyelo-nephritis is unilateral. In severe bilateral pyelonephritis premature labour should be induced. Nephrectomy is a more severe operation. It may be necessary in unilateral pyelonephritis, and does not affect the course of the pregnancy in most cases.

Cova collected 21 cases of nephrectomy, and found that the pregnancy went on to term in 15 and was 5 times interrupted spontaneously and once artificially. The mortality is 9·5 per cent. According to this observer nephrectomy is well borne in the early months of pregnancy, but less so after the fifth month.

LITERATURE

Albeck, *Zeits. f. Geb. u. Gyn.,* lx. 466.
Ayres, *Amer. Journ. Urol.,* 1906, p. 480.
Bar, Soc. d'Obst. de Paris, June 16, 1904.
Box, *Lancet,* 1908, i. 77.
Casper, *Wien. med. Press,* 1895, p. 1417.
Cova, Soc. d'Obst. e di Gin., 1903, p. 692.
Cumston, *Amer. Journ. Med. Sci.,* 1908, p. 87.
Johnson, *Amer. Journ. Urol.,* 1906, p. 566.
Legueu, *Ann. d. Mal. d. Org. Gén.-Urin.,* 1904, p. 1441.
Morse, *Amer. Journ. Med. Sci.,* 1909, p. 313.
Pousson, *Folia Urol.,* 1909, p. 445.
Sampson, *Johns Hopkins Hosp. Bull.,* 1903, p. 336.
Sellei und **Unterberg,** *Berl. klin. Woch.,* 1907, p. 1113.
Smith, Bellingham, *Guy's Hosp. Repts.,* 1906, p. 227.
Thomson, *Scot. Med. Surg. Journ.,* 1902, p. 7.

PYONEPHROSIS

Pyonephrosis is distension of the kidney and its pelvis with pus or purulent urine. In the description of pyelonephritis it was pointed out that obstruction in the lower urinary organs was a frequent predisposing factor, and that some dilatation of the renal pelvis was almost constant in these cases. The degree of dilatation is, however, very slight, and the destruction of renal tissue by intrapelvic pressure is minimal. In pyonephrosis the kidney tissue is destroyed by intrapelvic pressure, and the presence of sepsis may be accidental.

There are two distinct forms of pyonephrosis :

1. Pyonephrosis secondary to uronephrosis (hydronephrosis), or uro-pyonephrosis.

2. Pyonephrosis developing from acute pyelonephritis.

Etiology.—The etiology of uro-pyonephrosis is that of uro-nephrosis. The condition is unilateral, it occurs more often on the right side, it is more common in women, and it is in most cases related to movable kidney, stone, or pregnancy. The actual obstruction is usually situated high up in the ureter, and is due to a stone, or to stricture or duplication of the ureter. The super-added infection may be ascending, from recent cystitis, or it may be hæmatogenous.

Pyonephrosis developing in acute pyelonephritis occurs especi-ally in cases of old-standing disease of the lower urinary organs, such as enlarged prostate, stricture, and growths of the bladder and prostate, and is therefore more frequent in men. The infee-tion is almost invariably ascending. There is frequently bilateral disease, but the second kidney is not necessarily pyonephrotic. The obstruction which gives rise to the dilatation of the kidney is at any part of the ureter, and is due either to stricture or to swelling of the mucous membrane consequent upon the septic inflammation. The bacteria are those of other renal suppurations. Anaerobic bacteria are sometimes found.

A pyonephrosis is " open " when the obstruction is incomplete and pus escapes, and " closed " when the block is complete.

Pathology.—The dilated kidney forms a globular or elongated mass. It frequently reaches the size of a child's head and fills the flank and one side of the abdomen.

The pelvis may be greatly dilated and form a large globular swelling, which is capped by a slightly enlarged kidney. This form is said to occur especially where the pyonephrosis is of ascending origin. The kidney may be greatly distended, form-ing the pouch, while the pelvis is small and hidden. The surface shows rounded grey or dark bosses corresponding to saccules in the pouch and separated by grooves corresponding to septa between these. The kidney is firmly adherent to its surroundings, and is frequently hidden by a thick fibro-fatty layer. There is a single large cavity in the centre formed by the dilated pelvis or the greatly distended sinus of the organ, and with this numerous pouches com-municate. These pouches are separated by firm fibrous septa of varying thickness, and frequently communicate with each other. Sometimes the communication of a pouch with the main cavity is very small, and occasionally a pouch may become completely shut off from the central cavity. In the walls of the secondary pouches there may be small abscess cavities.

The lining membrane of the primary and secondary pouches is smooth and tough, and is occasionally covered with a rough greyish false membrane, which may be gritty with calcareous deposit. The distension of the kidney is brought about by pressure upon the pyramids, which become flattened and then pouched, while the columns of Bertini form the fibrous septa. These septa may become thinned out so that one pouch communicates with another. Microscopical examination of the wall of the sac shows remains of

K

the renal parenchyma. The glomeruli are fibrous, and the tubules undergoing atrophy. There is widespread fibrosis, and scattered through this are patches and areas of recent leucocytic infiltration. Albarran has described areas of compensatory hypertrophy. Partial pyonephrosis may occur, and is due to the blocking of one section of a dichotomous renal pelvis. A small portion or one pole of the kidney may be converted into a pyonephrosis by the blockage of one or several calyces with a stone. The content of a pure pyonephrosis is pus, and this is sometimes thick and almost cheesy. Traces of urea may be found, but are occasionally absent. In a uro-pyonephrosis the contents are urine with a varying admixture of pus.

Calculi may be present in the sac, and may be primary and cause the obstruction, or secondary. When the pyonephrosis is secondary to disease of the lower urinary organs the ureter is large, elongated, tortuous, greatly dilated and pouched, and usually adherent to the surrounding cellular tissue ; the wall is thick and tough, and there are folds and strictures which may be so narrow as to admit only a fine probe. When the pyonephrosis follows a uronephrosis or a descending infection, only the part of the ureter above the site of obstruction is damaged. The ureter is inserted into the dilated pelvis at a point high above the lowest part of that receptacle, and may be adherent to the surface of the sac.

The functional power of the renal tissue of a pyonephrotic kidney may have been entirely destroyed, and only pus is discharged on nephrotomy. Usually, however, a certain quantity of urea (Albarran states 2 to 4 gr. per litre) is found in the fluid discharged by the fistula, and most pyonephrotic kidneys have some amount of functional power.

The second kidney.—When the pyonephrosis is due to old-standing disease of the lower urinary organs, both kidneys are usually affected, although in different degrees. Gosset has shown that the lesion is occasionally unilateral in these cases. When bilateral disease is present, the second kidney usually suffers from chronic pyelonephritis, and there is seldom any marked development of compensatory hypertrophy.

In uro-pyonephrosis the second kidney is usually healthy, and shows compensatory hypertrophy.

Symptoms.—When the pyonephrosis is secondary to lower urinary disease, the symptoms of cystitis or obstruction may obscure those of the renal complication. Usually, however, there are symptoms of ascending pyelonephritis. It may be difficult or impossible to say when obstruction converts the pyelonephritis into pyonephrosis. When the condition settles down into a less acute state, the diagnosis is more readily made.

The advent of suppuration in a case of hydronephrosis is heralded by a rigor, rise of temperature, and other signs of infection.

The symptoms of pyonephrosis are pain and tenderness of the kidney, tumour, and pyuria.

Pain.—At the outset pain is usually pronounced. It is constant, heavy, and boring, and is occasionally severe. When the pyonephrosis is more fully developed pain may be absent, and may occur only when the outlet of the pyonephrosis becomes blocked and the kidney fills up with pus. It may then be severe and radiate down the ureter, causing renal colic. The thigh is often flexed to relax the psoas muscle.

Tenderness on palpation is pronounced at first, but later it may be absent, and only appear during a crisis of retention. When present the abdominal muscles are contracted. Guyon found tenderness absent in 17 out of 26 cases.

Tumour.—The tumour has the characteristics of a renal tumour. It projects below the costal margin, but, as Albarran points out, it is more likely than a hydronephrosis to form adhesions and remain bound down and concealed beneath the ribs. It forms a large, smooth, regular, non-fluctuating, firm tumour from which ballottement can be obtained. During an attack of retention it becomes tense, larger, and tender.

The ureter may occasionally be felt as it crosses the brim of the pelvis, and it may be detected as a thickened band in the lateral fornix of the vagina in the female, or in the rectum in the male.

Pyuria.—This is the cardinal symptom of pyonephrosis. The pus forms a thick, heavy deposit, and the supernatant urine remains cloudy. The pyuria is abundant, and is subject to slight variations in quantity from day to day, and to intermissions lasting a few days. These variations are dependent upon the ease with which the pus escapes from the pyonephrosis.

There are recurrent attacks of complete retention of pus, during which the urine becomes clear, the tumour increases in size and becomes painful, tender, and more tense, and the temperature rises. The attack lasts two or three days, and then the temperature falls suddenly, the symptoms subside, and a large quantity of pus appears in the urine.

Even in the crises of acute retention the urine may still contain pus derived either from the bladder or from a diseased second kidney.

Cystoscopy.—If the infection has been ascending there will be chronic cystitis and evidence of urethral obstruction or of bladder growth. The orifice of the ureter may be lost among the trabeculæ and pouches of the bladder. It may be discovered on a thick ridge and show nothing abnormal, even when the ureter and renal pelvis are widely dilated and their walls greatly thickened. Œdema and thickening of the lips will denote inflammation of the ureter.

The orifice is occasionally found open, round, and immobile, and surrounded by a rigid, thickened margin, or with a thick, œdematous, sometimes ulcerated edge.

In a closed pyonephrosis there is no efflux, but there may be an occasional feeble gaping movement at the orifice. In an open pyonephrosis the efflux varies according to the contents of the pyonephrosis. It may consist of thick worm-like masses of semi-solid pus slowly expressed from the ureter, or there may be a copious intermittent stream of watery pus or of purulent urine. A forcible jet rapidly repeated denotes that the ureter has retained its muscular power, while a slow, continuous stream or a lazy welling of fluid at long intervals shows that the ureter is dilated and atonic.

Catheterization of the ureters will determine whether an obstruction exists, and at what level, and also give information in regard to the presence, health, and function of a second kidney.

Course and prognosis.—In rare cases the pyonephrosis diminishes in size. It is compressed and invaded by the peri-nephritic inflammatory tissue from between the calyces and from the surface, and gradually shrinks, being eventually replaced by a fibro-fatty mass. The ureter becomes obliterated and atrophies. More frequently there is perinephritic suppuration, and this burrows in various directions (*see* Perinephritic Abscess, p. 112), and may rupture into the lung, stomach, peritoneum, or on the surface. The patient eventually dies of exhaustion from long-continued suppuration.

Diagnosis.—If the pyonephrosis is closed the diagnosis will depend upon the history of pyuria, the presence of cystitis, symptoms of septic absorption, and the presence of a renal tumour. Occasionally cases may be met with in which there has never been renal pain or other urinary symptom.

When there is pyuria alone the characters of the pyuria and cystoscopy will lead to a diagnosis. When cystitis is superadded the large quantity of pus in the urine will suffice to distinguish the renal disease. When the pus reaches one-fifth to one-sixth of the whole urine it must come from the kidney.

In two other conditions there may be very large quantities of pus in the urine at intervals, namely, (1) a suppurating diverticulum of the bladder, and (2) a purulent collection communicating with a ureter. The use of the cystoscope, and if necessary the ureteric catheter, will distinguish a diverticulum of the bladder. The second condition is only diagnosed on operation, unless some point in the history of the case reveals its nature.

The differential diagnosis must be made from—

(1) Pyelonephritis without retention. The large quantity of pus points to pyonephrosis, and catheterization of the ureter will show no obstruction.

(2) Tuberculous pyonephrosis. The presence of tubercle bacilli in the urine and of tuberculous lesions elsewhere in the genital system, and the general tests for the presence of tubercle in the body, will distinguish this from pyonephrosis. In such cases there is usually a thick tuberculous ureter which will be diagnosed by abdominal, vaginal, or rectal palpation and with the cystoscope.

The functional value of the pyonephrotic kidney and the presence of disease in the second kidney and the functional power of this organ are estimated by catheterization of the ureters. The urine of each kidney is examined, the quantity, naked-eye and microscopic characters, and the presence of albumin and the quantity of urea being noted. The tests for the renal function (phloridzin, indigo carmine, etc.) are used (p. 20).

The following table gives the results of the examination of the urines in a case of calculous pyonephrosis :—

	RIGHT KIDNEY (PYONEPHROSIS)	LEFT KIDNEY (HEALTHY)
Quantity	206·5 c.c.	107 c.c.
Specific gravity	1004	1011.
Freezing-point (Δ)	−0·18° C.	−0·76° C.
Colour	Pale, limpid	Fairly coloured.
Urea	0·4 per cent.	1·3 per cent.
Uric acid	0·0067 per cent.	0·0150 per cent.
Chlorides	0·0977 per cent.	0·1112 per cent.
Phosphates	0·08 per cent.	0·03 per cent.
Methylene blue	No change in colour of urine	Delayed 1 hour 50 min., d i m i n i s h e d, pale green, and lasted only 18 hours.
Chromogen	Appeared 25 min., small amount	Appeared 25 min., large amount.
Phloridzin glycosuria	0·395 grm.	1·623 grm.

An X-ray examination for stone should be made of the whole urinary tract, including the bladder, lower ureters, and second kidney.

Treatment.—The following methods of treatment will be discussed :—

1. Drainage by ureteral catheter.
2. Plastic operations.
3. Nephrotomy.
4. Partial nephrectomy.
5. Nephrectomy.

1. Drainage by ureteral catheter.—Pawlik and Albarran have advocated this method in selected cases. The ureter is catheterized daily or less often, according to whether a reaction occurs. The pelvis is washed at the same time. The catheter may be progressively increased in size until No. 13 Fr. is reached. Albarran has left the ureteral catheter in place for several weeks, changing it when it became blocked. He uses boric acid, silver nitrate (1 in 1,000), and permanganate of potash (1 in 4,000 to 1 in 500) for washing the kidney. Pawlik recommends massage of the kidney and the application of a firm bandage afterwards. He claims a cure in a pyonephrosis of 150 grm., and Albarran another in one of 60 grm.

Many circumstances combine to limit the application of this method—an intolerant bladder, febrile reaction, strictures of the ureter, subdivision of the pyonephrotic pouch, the presence of calculi, thick caseous contents, etc.—and there can be very few cases where it will possess an advantage over an open operation.

2. Plastic operations.—In cases of uro-pyonephrosis plastic operations have been undertaken with the object of re-establishing the outlet by the ureter. These operations will be discussed under Uronephrosis (p. 179). It is necessary to ascertain first the nature of the obstruction and the functional power of the kidney, and in order to do this a preliminary nephrotomy is necessary. Usually the functional power is so far destroyed that it is not worth while doing such an operation, and the choice will lie between nephrotomy and nephrectomy.

3. Nephrotomy.—This may consist only in incision of the kidney, or an attempt may be made to re-establish the lumen of the ureter.

The pyonephrotic sac is opened by an oblique lumbar incision. The contents are evacuated, and septa between saccules are broken down. Careful search is made for interstitial abscesses and the main cavity, the upper portion of the ureter and the subsidiary cavities are carefully examined for stone, and the perinephritic tissue around the kidney, and especially at the upper and lower poles, should be explored for possible extrarenal collections of pus. Guyon recommends that the edges of the sac should be stitched to the skin in order to avoid perinephritic suppuration. This is not necessary if free drainage be established by large rubber tubes placed both inside and outside the kidney.

This operation is rapid, causes no shock, and preserves the remains of the secreting tissue. It may therefore be performed in the very worst cases, where the patient is weak from severe or prolonged suppuration, and in cases where it is impossible to estimate the value of the second kidney or where this organ is known to be the seat of advanced disease. The mortality of the operation is from 17 (Küster) to 23·3 per cent. (Tuffier).

After the operation an improvement in the work performed by the second kidney is usually observed, and is due to the relief from the depressant reno-renal reflex, and also to the removal of toxins which were being absorbed from the pyonephrosis and excreted by the second kidney. The general health, for similar reasons, greatly improves. In 27 per cent. (Küster) of cases the wound closes, the sac shrinks, and the patient is cured.

In a certain number of cases septicæmia persists, and the work of the second kidney is still poorly performed. This is due to continued suppuration in the thick, fibrous-walled cavity, to unopened pouches, to abscesses in the walls and partitions, to stones being left in the sac (16 per cent. of cases), or to the persistence of the ureteric block and ureteritis. A fistula remains in from 45·6 per cent. (calculous pyonephrosis 34·2 per cent., non-calculous 57·1 per cent.—Tuffier) to 56 per cent. (Küster).

Various means have been adopted to obviate this or to cure the fistula when it has persisted. At the nephrotomy Bazy introduced a bougie along the ureter, and Doyen used a metal sound to dilate the ureter. There is difficulty, however, in finding the opening of the ureter in a large multilocular sac, and Albarran has used the following method : Before the nephrotomy he passes a catheter up the ureter by means of the cystoscope. At the operation this is easily found, and to the end of it is attached a catheter of No. 10 Fr. size. By withdrawing the first catheter the No. 10 catheter is drawn down to the bladder. This second catheter is fixed to the skin of the loin with a thread, and the nephrotomy is finished in the manner described. The ureteric catheter is left in place for four or five days and then changed. A light pliable stilette is passed along the catheter, and a metal conductor screwed on the end of it. The catheter is now withdrawn, and replaced by another which is threaded over the guide. The ureteral drainage

is continued for a month.   By this means the number of cases
of fistula has decreased.

A fistula may be cured by excision of its fibrous wall, the
opening up of the sac, removal of calculi, and the establishment
of free drainage.   Should these measures fail, the patient has the
choice of retaining the fistula or having the kidney removed.   The
presence of a renal fistula does not of itself necessarily shorten
life.   Watson has described a bilateral renal fistula persisting for
thirteen years, and Leguen has seen women become pregnant and
parturition proceed naturally when such fistulæ were present.
Watson fits a tube and metal reservoir to collect the urine discharged.   A small celluloid box the shape of a straw hat may
be used for this purpose.   It is held in position by a rubber waist-
band, and drains into a receptacle.   (Fig. 32, p. 159.)

Secondary nephrectomy is indicated when septicæmia persists ;
when it is believed, from the inadequate secretion of the diseased
kidney and the absence of disease in the second kidney, that a
depressed renal function in the latter will improve after nephrectomy ; and when the patient is gradually losing ground from
prolonged suppuration.

The mortality of secondary nephrectomy is only 5·9 per cent.
(2 in 25 operations, 8 calculous and 17 non-calculous—Tuffier).   If
this is added to the mortality of nephrotomy (23·3 per cent.) the
total mortality of nephrotomy followed by nephrectomy at a later
date is 29·2 per cent.

Nephrectomy.—This operation may be either partial or
total.   Partial nephrectomy is only possible when there is a partial
pyonephrosis with a separate pelvis.   This condition is rare.

Nephrectomy is performed by the lumbar route.   The abdominal
route has been abandoned owing to its high mortality (57 per
cent.—Küster).

Subcapsular nephrectomy should be performed.   The kidney
will usually shell out of the great perinephritic fibro-fatty mass
with comparative ease, whereas the removal of the thick fibro-
fatty capsule with the kidney is fraught with extreme difficulty
and some danger.   It may be necessary to puncture a very large
pyonephrosis with a trocar and cannula, and to remove a large part
of its contents, so as to deal with the pedicle more easily.   The
wound should be protected with pads, and the patient turned
almost on his back while the purulent fluid is being withdrawn
through a rubber tube attached to the cannula.   The ureter
should be dissected out separately, and as much of it removed as
possible.   The mortality of this operation is 17 per cent. (Küster).

Death may take place from shock in patients exhausted by

severe or prolonged suppuration, but the principal danger is inadequacy of the second kidney from disease (40 per cent.—Legueu). Nephrectomy should not, therefore, be undertaken until the condition of the second kidney has been ascertained by catheterization of the ureters and the use of the phloridzin, indigo-carmine, or methylene-blue test. By this means only those cases are submitted to nephrectomy in which there is a functionally adequate second kidney, and the mortality is thereby greatly reduced. In the remaining cases nephrotomy is performed, and at a later date improvement in the condition of the second kidney may render nephrectomy practicable.

As to the time when operation should be performed in a case of pyonephrosis, Bazy, Pousson, and recently Morris have urged the importance of early nephrotomy in all cases with the view to preventing irreparable damage to the kidney.

LITERATURE

Albarran, *Traité de Chirurgie* (Le Dentu et Delbet), viii. 806.
Bazy, XIIe Congrès franç. de Chir., Paris, 1898, p. 56.
Cahn, *Münch. med. Woch.*, 1902, xlix. 19.
Casper, *Wien. med. Presse*, 1895, xxxvi. 38.
Fouguet, Thèse de Paris.
Gosset, Thèse de Paris, 1900.
Greaves, *Brit. Med. Journ.*, July 13, 1907.
Hallé, Thèse de Paris, 1897.
Meyer, *Med. News*, Sept. 12, 1900.
Morris, *Lancet*, 1910, i. 1597.
Watson, *Ann. Surg.*, 1908, No. 3.

ABSCESS OF THE KIDNEY

Under this term will be described a rare condition in which there is circumscribed suppuration in the renal parenchyma, forming a solitary abscess of considerable size. From this category are excluded an abscess formed in a calyx plugged by a stone or other obstruction (*partial pyonephrosis*), and scattered points of suppuration in the kidney substance (*suppurative nephritis*).

Etiology and pathology.—According to Morris, a renal abscess may be formed by (*a*) the fusing together of a number of miliary abscesses, or (*b*) the plugging of a large artery with a septic embolus. The infection may be hæmatogenous in cases of ulcerative endocarditis or pyæmia, or it may be ascending from the lower urinary tract. Injury by wounds or contusions and lacerations and calculus of the kidney are other causes. The abscess may rupture into the renal pelvis and the pus be discharged from the ureter or on the surface of the kidney and form a perinephritic abscess.

Symptoms.—The abscess may give rise to acute or chronic

symptoms. In acute cases the temperature rises after a rigor, and there are severe renal pain, abdominal rigidity and tenderness.

The kidney is not sufficiently enlarged to form a tumour, and, unless the abscess is secondary to infection of the urinary tract or bursts into the renal pelvis, there is no pus in the urine.

Morris states that hæmaturia often precedes the formation of abscess, and, when it does, partial suppression of urine may be expected.

Symptoms may be entirely absent in chronic abscess of the kidney, or they may resemble those of stone.

Treatment.—The abscess will not infrequently be found during an exploratory operation, but if a diagnosis has been made the kidney should be exposed without delay. The abscess should be freely incised, and the kidney carefully searched for other collections of pus and for calculi. Morris has excised portions of the kidney in such cases. If the kidney is extensively destroyed it must be removed, but nephrectomy should be reserved for cases where the destruction of renal tissue is widespread.

RENAL AND PERIRENAL FISTULÆ

Fistulæ which open on the lumbar region may take origin in the kidney or ureter, or they may be unconnected with the urinary tract. In a small number of cases fistulæ connected with the kidney appear spontaneously or follow an injury. The great majority of renal and perirenal fistulæ follow upon an operation.

1. PERIRENAL FISTULÆ UNCONNECTED WITH THE URINARY ORGANS

Perinephritic abscess, if untreated, ruptures on the skin, having reached the surface by the triangle of Petit ; or it may be incised and a postoperative fistula persist.

The origin of perinephritic abscess, when the kidney is not diseased, has been discussed (p. 112).

The subsequent fistula may be single, and open in the lumbar region, or there may be several openings, which are often connected by subcutaneous tracks. A large inflammatory mass may surround or displace the kidney (Fig. 29). There is frequently a perinephritic cavity. Beyond this the sinus may lead by a tortuous track through the diaphragm into the pleural cavity, into the iliac fossa, or elsewhere, according to the origin of the abscess. The quantity of pus which escapes varies at different times in the same individual. From time to time retention of pus may cause an attack of pain and fever, relieved by the discharge of a large amount of pus from the fistula.

Diagnosis.—The original seat of suppuration may be shown by the history of the case or by the presence of scars (Fig. 30). Much

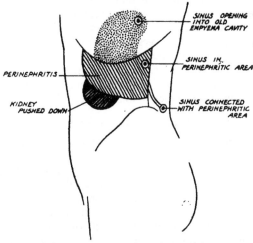

Fig. 29.—Diagram of area of perinephritic suppuration following empyema.

information can be obtained by the injection into the sinus of an emulsion of bismuth and then taking a radiogram. Examination

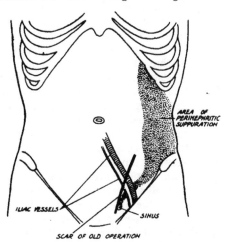

Fig. 30.—Diagram of area of perinephritic suppuration in case of dermoid of kidney.

Note the fistulous track passing beneath the iliac vessels.

of the urine, cystoscopy, and catheterization of the ureter on the fistulous side demonstrate that there is no urinary infection, and that the ureter on this side is patent and the kidney active.

Treatment.—The treatment is surgical, and may require extensive operations, such as the exploration of the perinephritic tissue, the search for a retrocæcal appendix, or the obliteration of a cavity in the pleura by resection of ribs. Before resorting to operation the effect of injections of bismuth paste (vaseline 20, paraffin 10, lanoline 10, subnitrate of bismuth 10) may be tried. The injections are made twice a week with a glass syringe.

2. Spontaneous Renal Fistulæ

In this category are placed a small group of fistulæ which do not follow operation on the kidney.

Wounds of the kidney cause a urinary fistula only when the renal pelvis or calyces are injured. A fistula persists for some months and sometimes for years, but is rarely permanent (*see* under Wounds of the Kidney, p. 107). An untreated pyonephrosis ruptures into the perinephritic tissue, and the pus either finds its way to the surface of the body or opens into the pleural cavity, a bronchus, the stomach, duodenum, or elsewhere, giving rise to a reno-cutaneous, reno-pulmonary, reno-intestinal, or reno-gastric fistula.

The discharge is purulent or uro-purulent. There may be considerable difficulty in diagnosis. To symptoms of pyonephrosis there are superadded those of rupture of a large abscess into a bronchus or elsewhere.

Fig. 31.—Collection of calculi discharged from spontaneous fistula of kidney.

The opening of the fistula is usually small, so that the escape of pus into the bronchus or elsewhere is intermittent. In the intervals there is retention of pus in the kidney or around it, causing fever and recurrent rigors.

A small number of cases have been recorded in which calculi have been discharged from a spontaneous renal fistula. Fig. 31 shows a number of small calculi discharged from a spontaneous sinus in a man aged 78. A small abscess formed on the right side, 1½ in. below the iliac crest and the same distance external to the posterior superior iliac spine; this was incised, and the sinus persisted and discharged small calculi. The radiogram (Plate 8, Fig. 1) shows a large calculous mass in the right kidney with a number of small shadows of calculi lying in the sinus. There was a history of litholapaxy ten years previously,

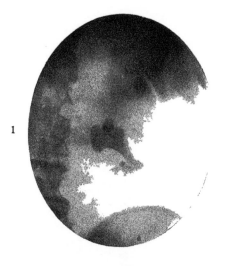

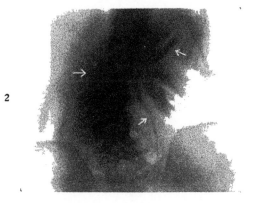

Fig. 1.—Shadows of large calculus in kidney and number of small calculi (arrow) lying in spontaneously formed fistula. A number of calculi were discharged through the fistula. (*See* p. 156 and Fig. 31.)

Fig. 2.—Hydronephrosis due to adhesions round vertebræ in scoliosis. Arrows point to lateral curvature of spine, to opaque catheter in ureter, and to three of the dilated calyces. (P. 168.)

PLATE 8.

and of bladder symptoms, but no renal symptoms, and the general
health was unimpaired.

3. POSTOPERATIVE RENAL FISTULÆ

These fistulæ are cutaneous and open in the lumbar region,
generally at the posterior end of the operation scar. There is
commonly a single fistula; occasionally two or more exist, and
communicate by subcutaneous tracks. The latter are most frequently found in tuberculous disease.

The orifice of the fistula is often retracted and hidden in folds
of skin. If placed far back in the lumbar region it is more likely
to be on the level of the surface. It is narrow and the edges are
smooth. In tuberculous disease and in some septic cases there
may be granulations sprouting from the fistula, and tags of scar
tissue around it. The discharge may be urine, urine mixed with
pus, or pus.

The track of the fistula is narrow, and it usually passes in a
straight course down to the kidney. The walls consist of thick,
dense fibrous tissue.

The state of the kidney and ureter varies according to the
disease for which the operation was performed.

The factors which cause a temporary fistula to persist or
become permanent are various.

The fistula may give exit to pus or urine, which would accumulate under tension if it closed. Disease, such as tuberculosis, may
spread along the track, or concretions form in the lumen and
prevent healing. The wall of the fistula may become so thick,
hard, and callous from prolonged use of drainage tubes, or from
continued discharge of urine and pus, that spontaneous healing
is impossible.

After nephrolithotomy there is seldom a fistula, unless urinary
obstruction is present, or unless there are infected calculi remaining
in the kidney.

Pyelotomy for stone has been followed by a fistula, but this
is rare, unless some collateral condition, such as ureteritis or narrowing of the ureter, exists, or unless the drainage by rubber tubes or
other means is unduly prolonged.

Nephrotomy in hydronephrosis where the obstruction has not
been removed is followed by a fistula which discharges watery urine.
In pyonephrosis a uropurulent fistula persists, which is chiefly due
to the ureteral obstruction, but partly also to the thick fibrous
walls being too rigid to collapse.

After nephrectomy a fistula may persist and may be due to
necrotic portions of the kidney or renal pelvis forming part of

the stump of the pedicle, to an infected ligature of thick silk on the pedicle, to infection of the wound from a septic ureter, or to tuberculous infection of the wound. In these conditions a purulent discharge issues from the fistula.

After nephrectomy considerable quantities of urine may be discharged from the wound, derived from fragments of kidney tissue remaining on the stump of the pedicle. These portions of kidney tissue lie on the distal side of the ligature, and are apparently cut off from their blood supply. In a few days they necrose and the secretion of urine ceases. A permanent fistula discharging urine may be caused by a patent dilated ureter allowing the urine of the remaining kidney to ascend from the bladder.

Finally, there are permanent urinary fistulæ made by nephrostomy to effect drainage in a ureter blocked by irremediable disease.

Diagnosis.—In many cases the cause of the fistula and the condition of the kidney are well known, but in others it is uncertain whether the copious purulent secretion contains urine.

The discharge should be examined for urea, which can be detected if even a small quantity of urine is present. After an intramuscular injection of methylene blue, a urinary discharge will be tinged with blue.

By catheterization of the ureters or separation of the urines in the bladder, it is found either that the fistula drains away all the urine secreted by the kidney, or that it drains away only a part of it, the remaining urine, usually a small quantity, passing down the ureter.

Catheterization of the ureter on this side will also give information in regard to the presence of stricture.

Treatment.—In some cases nephrostomy has been performed with the view of producing a permanent fistula. In such cases the treatment consists in devising an apparatus which will drain away the discharge and prevent it from soaking the clothes. A modification of Irving's suprapubic drainage apparatus is the best for this purpose (Fig. 32).

In purulent non-urinary fistulæ it will be sufficient to dissect out the fistulous track and expose the kidney by a free incision, opening up pockets and tracks and providing free drainage. Injection of a bismuth paste as in non-urinary perirenal fistulæ may be tried (p. 156).

Before undertaking radical treatment in urinary fistulæ it is necessary to know (1) if the ureter is patent, (2) the functional power of the fistulous kidney and of the second kidney. This information is obtained by catheterization of the ureter, by examination of the discharge from the fistula and that from the ureter of the fistulous kidney, and of the urine from the ureter of the second kidney, and by using the tests for the renal function.

If the ureter is found to be patent, Albarran recommends drainage by a catheter *en demeure* in the ureter. In order to get a large catheter into the ureter, he introduces, by means of the cystoscope, a long stilette (70 cm.) which is flexible for the first 6 cm. Over this stilette a catheter with a terminal eye is passed and ascends the ureter to the renal pelvis. The catheter is held in place and the stilette removed; the catheter is left in the ureter for four or five days and then changed after passing the stilette

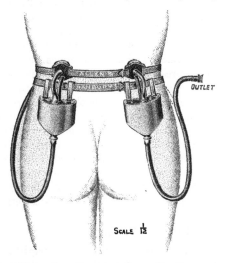

Fig. 32.—Watson's apparatus for collecting urine in permanent renal fistula.

as a guide. Eventually a No. 13 Fr. catheter may thus be passed. The renal pelvis is washed daily with silver nitrate solution (1 in 1,000). This continuous catheterization is maintained for three weeks (*see also* under Pyonephrosis, p. 151). Should it fail, a plastic operation should be performed upon the renal pelvis.

If the ureter is impassable and the kidney has been shown to retain a considerable part of its function, then also a plastic operation on the renal pelvis will be necessary. But should the functional value of the kidney be low, and that of the second kidney adequate, nephrectomy should be performed.

LITERATURE

Albarran, XII° Congrès franç. de Chir., Paris, 1898, p. 85.
Heitz-Boyer et **Moreno**, *Ann. d. Mal. d. Org. Gén. Urin.*, 1910, No. 11.
Pouquet, Thèse de Paris, 1901.

SURGICAL TREATMENT OF NON-SUPPURATIVE NEPHRITIS

ACUTE NEPHRITIS

In 1896, Reginald Harrison suggested operative interference in certain cases of acute nephritis. He operated on "cases of scarlatinal nephritis, nephritis complicating influenza, traumatic nephritis, and nephritis which had followed a chill." The operations were undertaken on account of one or more of the following symptoms, viz. diminished secretion of urine, pain, hæmaturia. He recommended operation in cases of acute nephritis where convalescence was delayed, and albumin and casts did not disappear from the urine; also in cases such as the malignant type of scarlatinal nephritis with suppression, and lastly where cardiac and circulatory complications were present. The operation was performed with the object of setting aside the dangerous symptoms and also of preventing the sequence of chronic nephritis. Harrison suggested incision of the renal capsule and puncture of the kidney to relieve the renal tension in these cases. Other observers (Pel and Rosenstein) recommended nephrotomy in acute nephritis when oliguria was present and medical treatment had failed. Confusion in regard to statistics has been caused by the publication of cases of suppurative nephritis in the same category as those referred to above.

All Harrison's cases recovered, but the after-history is unrecorded.

CHRONIC BRIGHT'S DISEASE

Acute exacerbations in chronic Bright's disease.— Edebohls, Pousson, Casper, and others have treated the acute exacerbations of chronic Bright's disease by operation. In these cases surgical interference is supplementary to medical treatment. Where there are symptoms of uræmia, diminished secretion of urine, and œdema, operation may be of service when medical treatment has failed. Cases with advanced cardio-vascular changes and pulmonary complications are unsuitable for operation.

Decapsulation and nephrotomy are the operations recommended. Except in the rare cases when the disease can be proved to be unilateral, decapsulation should be rapidly performed on both sides. Pousson recommends that nephrotomy be performed on one side, and only decapsulation on the other.

The immediate results give a mortality of 25 per cent. (Pousson), some part of which is due to the patient being moribund when the operation is performed. Of 92 patients who survived the operation, 8 were considered as cured. The others died after a temporary relief lasting from some months to one or two years in a few cases.

In my experience of decapsulation and nephrotomy in these cases and in large white kidney very striking improvement may be observed. Œdema and ascites disappear, and the patient, who has been rapidly losing ground under medicinal treatment, regains some measure of health and vigour. This improvement is, however, only temporary, and after some weeks or months relapse occurs and the disease pursues its course.

Chronic interstitial nephritis with hæmaturia. — These cases have already been discussed under the term Essential Hæmaturia (p. 59).

Chronic nephritis with pain.—Legueu described these cases as neuralgia of the kidney. In a few cases the renal condition is that of chronic Bright's disease, but in many cases there has been a renal calculus at some previous date, while in others there is a history of traumatism.

The kidney shows chronic nephritis, and there are thickening and adhesion of the fibrous capsule and fibrosis of the fatty envelope. The pain may be localized to the kidney, and be spontaneous, constant, and unaffected by movement, or there are attacks of renal colic. There may be a trace of albumin with hyaline and granular casts.

Nephrectomy, nephrotomy, capsulotomy, decapsulation, and simple freeing of the kidney from surrounding adhesions have been practised.

The operation, like that for hæmaturia in partial nephritis, usually takes the form of an exploratory nephrotomy, and to this decapsulation may be added.

The great majority of patients have been relieved by operation, and the relief is known to have lasted for some years. If there have been a diminution in the quantity of urine and albuminuria, these symptoms disappear.

Decapsulation in chronic Bright's disease. — In 1899 Edebohls suggested nephrotomy as a method of treatment of chronic nephritis in cases of chronic nephritis in movable kidney. Newman, of Glasgow, had previously treated two cases of this nature by nephropexy.

In 1901 Edebohls proposed decapsulation of the kidney with the object of curing chronic Bright's disease. He held that the thickened fibrous capsule prevented the establishment of a collateral circulation, and that if this barrier were removed a free flow of blood through the kidney, which the diseased vessels were unable to supply, was provided by anastomosis with the parietal vessels. By this means the increased interstitial tissue would be absorbed, pressure on the tubules removed, and a regeneration of renal epithelium take place.

Experimental inquiry into this hypothesis has shown that no damage is done to the kidney by decapsulation, and that although the fibrous capsule invariably re-forms in a few weeks the new capsule is composed of loose connective tissue which does not· compress the kidney. A parietal anastomosis has actually been observed, which was not strangled by contraction of the new capsule. On the other hand, Hall and Herxheimer have shown that a thick, strong connective tissue capsule is formed in from eight to fourteen days, and they did not find anastomotic vessels passing through the new capsule. Conflicting statements have been made in regard to the results found post mortem after decapsulation in human beings.

The kidney has also been transplanted into the peritoneal cavity and formed adhesions with the serous membrane or with the omentum.

Results.—Pousson gives a mortality of 5 per cent. Of 55 cases, 36 survived more than three months after the operation.

Of 10 cases of nephritis with nephroptosis, there were 9 greatly improved, 3 of which were said to be cured; while of 16 cases of nephritis without nephroptosis 3 were improved, 4 much improved, 4 greatly improved, and 5 cured. The 5 cases of cure were under observation for 11 years, $6\frac{1}{2}$ years, $5\frac{1}{3}$ years, 2 years, and 1 year.

It will be seen, therefore, that although the course of the disease is uninfluenced in a considerable proportion of cases, improvement is undoubted in some, and it is claimed that a cure has been brought about in a few cases.

The cases of movable kidney with albuminuria and tube casts should be carefully separated from the others, for the prognosis without operation is very different from that of chronic Bright's disease, and the effect of nephropexy alone is to cure most of these cases. In cases of chronic Bright's disease the results might be improved by operation performed at an earlier date than is usual.

LITERATURE

Edebohls, *Med. News*, April 22, 1899 ; *Med. Rec.*, May 4, 1901.
Hall and Herxheimer, *Brit. Med. Journ.*, 1904, i. 821.
Harrison, *Lancet*, 1896, p. 19.
Legueu, *Ann. d. Mal. d. Org. Gén.-Urin.*, 1891.
Lehmann, *Berl. klin. Woch.*, Jan., 1912, p. 158.
Newman, *Trans. Clin. Soc.*, 1897.
Pousson, *Chirurgie des Néphrites.* Paris, 1909.
Walker, Thomson, *Pract.*, June, 1903.

SURGICAL TREATMENT OF PUERPERAL ECLAMPSIA

Although the modern views on the pathology of puerperal eclampsia are not yet settled, it is undoubted that there are changes in the kidneys, amounting to great engorgement or even to acute nephritis, and symptoms are present which result from interference with the renal function.

On these grounds decapsulation of the kidneys and nephrotomy have been practised in this fatal malady, with the object of relieving the renal engorgement and allowing the escape of poisons.

In some cases the convulsions cease and the symptoms disappear, the secretion of urine becoming re-established. Kehrer collected 26 cases with a mortality of 36 per cent.

The general opinion is not, however, favourable to decapsulation. The state of the kidneys, de Bovis holds, plays but a secondary part in the disease, and even if the renal function is resumed it does not prevent the development of hepatic necrosis, or the petechial hæmorrhages of the encephalitis found in eclampsia. There may, however, he believes, be cases where the renal lesions exceed the other morbid changes in the body, and these cases explain certain striking successes which are too numerous to be mere coincidence.

LITERATURE

De Bovis, *Semaine Méd.*, Jan., 1912, p. 3.
Kehrer, *Zeits. f. Gyn. u. Urol.*, 1909, ii. 111.　　　　　[i. 561.
Pousson et Chambrelent, *Ann. d. Mal. d. Org. Gén.-Urin.*, 1906,

CHAPTER XII

HYDRONEPHROSIS

HYDRONEPHROSIS is chronic aseptic retention of urine in the kidney and renal pelvis due to obstruction.

Etiology.—Hydronephrosis is slightly more frequent on the right side and in the female sex. It is frequently bilateral when the obstruction is urethral, and occasionally when it is ureteral. Of 665 cases, 217 were unilateral and 448 bilateral (Newman). The obstruction may be ureteral or urethral.

1. **Ureteral obstruction** may be caused by—
   (a) Changes in the wall of the ureter, such as valves, folds, strictures.
   (b) Obstruction of the lumen by calculi, tumours, foreign bodies, clot.
   (c) Pressure from without by tumours, fibrous bands, purulent collections, an aberrant renal vessel.
   (d) Kinking of the ureter due to undue mobility of the kidney.
   (e) Torsion of the ureter.

2. **Urethral obstruction** may be caused by a congenital fold or diaphragm, or obliteration, or more frequently by stricture and enlarged prostate.

There are two principal categories into which the cases of hydronephrosis fall, namely :
   (1) Congenital.
   (2) Acquired.

1. By **congenital** hydronephrosis is understood cases of hydronephrosis occurring in the fœtus or new-born, or appearing soon after birth. Cases of hydronephrosis occurring in adults and ascribed to congenital malformation are not included in this category.

In congenital hydronephrosis one or both kidneys may be affected. When the condition is unilateral it is due to an abnormal renal artery, to valves or folds, or to stenosis of the orifice of the ureter, or bending or kinking of the duct, which is malplaced in the bladder, urethra, ejaculatory duct, seminal vesicle, vas deferens, vagina, or urethro-vaginal septum. More frequently congenital hydronephrosis is bilateral, and is due to obstruction in the urethra by a complete or an incomplete septum or imperforate portion, a cyst, torsion of the penis (Morris), or phimosis. In some cases no obstruction can be found, but the bladder, both ureters and kidneys are greatly dilated.

2. There are two classes of **acquired** hydronephrosis :

i. Hydronephrosis due to obstruction in the lower urinary organs or to disease in the pelvic organs. These cases are almost invariably bilateral. Those due to disease of the lower urinary organs occur most frequently in the male, and are due to urethral stricture and enlarged prostate, and less frequently to growths of the bladder.

Those due to disease of the pelvic organs occur more often in the female, and are caused by new growths of the uterus and ovaries less frequently by carcinoma of the rectum in either sex, or carcinoma of the prostate in the male.

In this group of cases the distension of the kidneys is seldom great, and may not be detected clinically. When the lower urinary organs are diseased, infection is frequently superadded and pyo-nephrosis may develop.

ii. Hydronephrosis due to obstruction of the ureter. In these cases the narrow point is usually situated at the upper end of the ureter, at the junction of the ureter and renal pelvis; less frequently the middle or lower end of the ureter is the seat of obstruction, and the ureter is dilated.

Pathology. 1. Hydronephrosis due to valves, folds, torsion, and stenosis.—The ureter and renal pelvis are developed as an outgrowth from the Wolffian duct. As development proceeds the new-formed tube rotates around the Wolffian duct, and, its lower end being fixed, becomes twisted upon its axis. This twisting is said to be the cause of torsion of the ureter, which has been described in rare cases. In the fœtus the ureter has a very irregular lumen, some parts being dilated and others contracted. The narrowing is due to folds formed either by the mucosa or by the mucosa and muscular layers; these are most common at the uretero-pelvic junction, at the vesical end of the ureter, and in the middle of its course. These folds are constant in the fœtus, and occur at the upper end of the ureter in 20 per cent. of new-born children (Wolfler). If anything interferes with the normal growth of the ureter, these valvules persist, and are the cause of hydronephrosis at a later date. (Fig. 33.) English found that of 65 ureteral strictures, 3 occurred in the middle, 34 at the upper, and 28 at the lower end—a distribution which corresponds very closely with that of the physiological valves in the fœtus.

Folds or valves of mucous membrane may be found at the uretero-pelvic junction in hydronephrosis developing in adult life, and may have a congenital origin or may result from other causes, such as stone or the drag of adhesions outside the pelvis and ureter.

Acquired stricture of the ureter may be caused by external injury, operations on the ureter or on the pelvic organs, lacera-

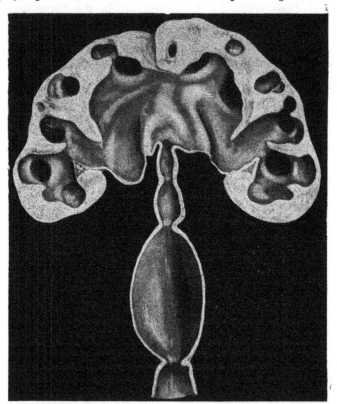

Fig. 33.—Hydronephrosis in boy of 7, due to multiple congenital strictures of the ureter. Nephro-ureterectomy specimen.

tion from the passage of calculi, or irritation from the presence of calculi or from chronic ureteritis.

2. **Hydronephrosis due to bands and adhesions outside the ureter.**—The most frequent site of obstruction is in the region of the uretero-pelvic junction. The bands may affect only the pelvis and ureter, or the ureter, or there may be adhesions between these structures and neighbouring organs.

In the most frequent form the ureter is bound down for the first inch or two of its course by fibrous adhesions to the surface of the distended pelvis (Fig. 34).   Occasionally there is narrowing of the lumen at the pelvo-ureteral junction (Fig. 35), and it is possible that the ureter may have become adherent to the already distended pelvis.   Usually, however, the lumen is found to be free

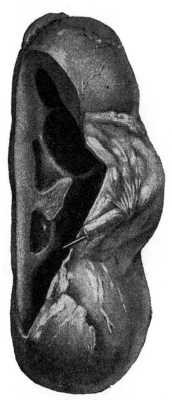

Fig. 34.—Hydronephrosis due to bands of adhesion between ureter and renal pelvis.

after dissecting away the bands which were evidently the cause of the obstruction.   The ureter is less often affected alone, but may sometimes show distortion from adhesions.

The cause of these adhesions may be obscure, as, except for the distension of the kidney and pelvis, there is no disease of that organ or of neighbouring structures.   In a few cases stone is present with extensive perinephritis and periureteritis.

Disease of neighbouring organs is sometimes present and is obviously the cause of the adhesions. In one case an early hydronephrosis was shown by pyelography (Plate 8, Fig. 2) to be due to adhesions around a spinal curvature. In another case the descending colon was adherent to the surface of a hydronephrosis binding the first 2 in. of the ureter down to the sac in a thick hard plaque the size of the palm of the hand. A fæcal fistula, lasting a week, followed dissection of this adhesion and nephrectomy.

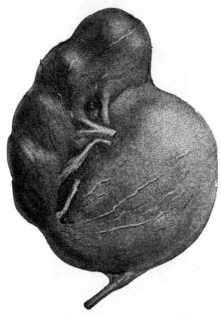

Fig. 35.—Hydronephrosis (pelvic type) due to stenosis of uretero-pelvic junction.

In other cases the bands apparently originated in appendicitis and perityphlitis or duodenal ulcer, or followed peritonitis.

3. Hydronephrosis due to abnormal blood-vessels.—The abnormal vessels which are important are those which pass to the lower pole of the kidney. Such an artery may be derived from the main renal artery or from the aorta, and it passes in front of or behind the ureter in the proportion of 3 to 1. The vessel may be as large as the radial artery. Mayo found that anomalous blood-vessels were present in 20 out of 27 cases of hydronephrosis, and the obstruction in each case was at the point at which the vessels crossed the ureter.

The importance of aberrant vessels as the cause of obstruction has been disputed, for in some specimens which have been described the dilatation commences above or below the aberrant vessel, and is evidently independent of it. The relation of the hydronephrosis to the vessels in these cases is said to be accidental. There are, however, cases in which no other cause for obstruction is present, and in which division of the vessels

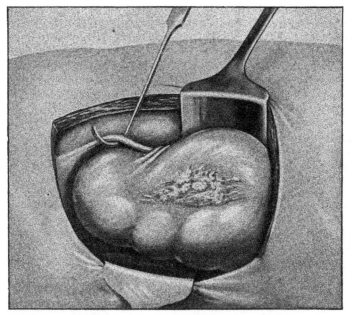

Fig. 36.—Hydronephrosis due to aberrant renal vessels.

Operation view : aneurysm needle under normal ureter.

suffices to relieve the obstruction. This was the case in a boy of 13, in whom I found an aberrant artery and vein the size of the ulnar vessels crossing in front of the uretero-pelvic junction to the anterior surface of the lower pole of the left kidney. The obstruction was caused not so much by the vessels as by the fibrous tissue around them, which formed a strong, flat band. (Fig. 36.) There was no stenosis or other cause of obstruction, and the condition was cured by section of the vessels and fibrous band.

4. **Hydronephrosis due to movable kidney.**—In a large number of cases of hydronephrosis the kidney is abnormally movable. In these cases the hydronephrosis is intermittent. The hydro-

nephrosis has been said to be caused by the undue mobility kinking a ureter which has become rigid from periureteral adhesions, but it is also held that the undue mobility is secondary to the increased size of the kidney, hydronephrotic from some other cause. The former hypothesis is probably the correct explanation of the origin of the dilatation.

4. Traumatic hydronephrosis. — Hydronephrosis may be found a few days after an injury to the loin, or it may develop several months or years after the injury. In the majority of the former the fluid collects around the kidney (pseudo-hydronephrosis) and not in the pelvis. Gardner points out that the severe pain caused by rapidly distending the renal pelvis is completely absent in these cases. In a few cases of tense hydronephrosis found soon after an injury the distension of the kidney has preceded the injury. Late traumatic hydronephrosis results from stricture caused by injury to the ureter.

5. Hydronephrosis due to calculus.—The degree of obstruction does not correspond to the size of the calculus. A very large calculus (7 in. by 1 in.), or numerous calculi (sixteen), may cause no dilatation, while a small solitary stone may cause a hydronephrosis.

The stone may be situated at the outlet of the pelvis, or it may lie at the vesical end of the ureter (Fig. 37). At the upper end of the ureter the calculus is often wedge-shaped, and usually fixed; at the lower end it is frequently round or oval, and freely movable upwards. Stenosis of the ureter on the vesical side of the stone usually becomes superadded if the case is of long standing.

6. Relation of diuresis to hydronephrosis.—Diuresis plays an important part in the production of hydronephrosis. There are many cases of congenital valves and narrowings of the ureter, of pressure of aberrant vessels, or of strictures following injury, in which the lumen is sufficient for the escape of the urine under ordinary conditions, but is too narrow to drain a sudden diuresis. From the comparative obstruction thus established hydronephrosis begins to develop, and the pressure it exerts upon the ureter increases the obstruction. It is only thus that I can explain the delay in the development of hydronephrosis until adult life, where the cause is evidently congenital. A young Canadian consulted me with regard to recurrent attacks of renal pain and enlargement due to the intermittent blocking of a congenitally narrowed pelvic outlet. Early in life he learnt that he could not take whisky or beer without inducing an attack.

A hydronephrosis is said to be "closed" when the obstruction is complete, and "open" when urine escapes.

Sudden complete obstruction such as is caused by ligaturing the ureter produces either shrinking and atrophy of the kidney or hydronephrosis in about an equal number of cases. According to Lindermann the accumulation of fluid depends upon the development of a compensatory anastomosis being established through capsular vessels as the intrapelvic pressure blocks the renal vessels.

The obstruction in hydronephrosis is only complete at inter-

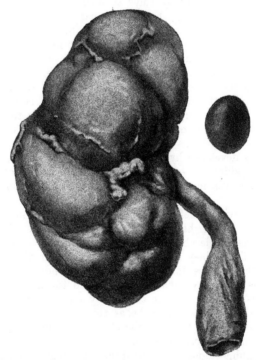

Fig. 37.—Hydronephrosis (renal type) with dilatation of ureter caused by smooth oval calculus. Nephro-ureterectomy specimen.

vals. Even in the largest hydronephrosis the obstruction is rarely complete. A small amount of fluid escapes, but a slightly larger quantity is secreted and the kidney is slowly distended. The tension never becomes sufficient to arrest the renal secretion. Where a very large hydronephrosis becomes completely closed atrophy does not take place, for the absorption from the sac is very slight.

In an open hydronephrosis there may be attacks of retention from kinking of the ureter, an excess of polyuria, or other causes, and the hydronephrosis is "intermittent." In the intervals the sac which disappears clinically is partly collapsed, and still contains a considerable quantity of fluid. When the attack of retention occurs the sac again becomes tensely filled with fluid. After a varying period the outflow is re-established.

Pathological anatomy.—In the early stage of hydronephrosis there is a slight increase in the capacity of the renal pelvis. The normal pelvis is said by Luys to hold from 2 to 3 grm. of fluid (about 30–50 minims); but Bazy regards a pelvis as normal that contains ten times this amount of fluid. According to Leguen a capacity of from 30–40 grm. (about 1–1½ oz.) indicates the first stage of hydronephrosis.

The kidney is not increased in size at this stage, but the pelvis is sac-like and the kidney hollowed. The apices of the pyramids are flattened and the calyces dilated. This stage is frequently met with at operations upon movable kidney, stone in the ureter, and in aseptic urethral obstruction. In the last the dilatation seldom passes beyond this stage.

In the fully developed hydronephrosis either the pelvis (" pelvic type ") or the kidney (" renal type ") may form the greater part of the sac, and even in advanced cases the pelvis and kidney are distinguishable.

When the pelvis is chiefly affected the subdivisions and branches of the normal pelvis have completely disappeared. (Fig. 35.) There is a large single chamber, one part of which is capped by the kidney. The kidney itself is hollowed, and, if viewed from the inside, the calyces form large round secondary chambers. The thickness of kidney substance is reduced to half an inch or less. There is a groove between the kidney and the dilated pelvis. The wall of the pelvic sac may be as thin as brown paper, and consists of fibrous tissue, the muscular elements having disappeared. The lining is smooth, opaque, white.

When the kidney alone is distended the pelvis is small and hidden by the cyst, and may contain a stone. (Fig. 37.) The surface shows rounded bosses corresponding to the sacs of the hydronephrosis. These are formed by the atrophy of the pyramids and destruction of the renal cortex. Between them are septa showing as depressions on the surface and formed by the sclerosed columns of Bertini. There is a small central cavity with numerous rounded chambers leading from it, often communicating laterally with each other. In the pelvis, or at the junction of the pelvis and ureter, will be found the narrowing, valve, kink, calculus, or other cause of the hydronephrosis ; occasionally no cause for obstruction can be discovered.

If the obstruction is situated at the lower end of the ureter this tube is dilated and tortuous, and its wall is thick and has lost its elasticity and contractile power.

There may be very little perirenal inflammation, but frequently there are tough adhesions between the hydronephrosis and its surroundings.

A partial hydronephrosis may be formed by the blocking of one segment of a double pelvis or the malformation of a calyx. Hydronephrosis has been observed in a horseshoe kidney; about a dozen cases are on record. Morley describes an interesting case operated on by Wright in which hydronephrosis was produced in one part of a horseshoe kidney by a papilloma at the uretero-pelvic junction.

In rare cases of extreme distension the kidney tissue has entirely disappeared from the wall, but there is usually a considerable layer of renal parenchyma, which shows an increase in the interstitial connective tissue, with scattered areas of round-cell infiltration. The tubules are distorted, and the lining cells partly or totally destroyed. The glomeruli are crowded together and sclerosed. The walls of the blood-vessels are considerably thickened.

The hydronephrosis may hold from 1 or 2 oz. to as much as 26 pints of urine of the specific gravity of 1005–1010, and containing traces of urea, phosphates, and chlorides. Occasionally as a result of injury, and sometimes spontaneously, the fluid becomes mixed with blood, and the cyst is transformed into a hæmatonephrosis.

The second kidney is usually normal and hypertrophied. Occasionally chronic inflammatory changes are observed in it. The secretion of this organ is often reflexly depressed, and complete anuria may supervene during a crisis of retention in the hydronephrotic sac.

Symptoms.—There are two clinical stages of hydronephrosis, (1) an early stage, before a tumour can be detected, and (2) a stage when an enlarged kidney is found. The first of these is the more important therapeutically.

1. **Early stage.**—When the enlargement of the kidney is not recognizable on palpation the hydronephrosis is latent. Thus, in a malignant growth of the prostate, bladder, or uterus, anuria may suddenly set in without any previous warning, and the kidneys are found dilated; or again, in urethral obstruction from enlarged prostate, or in a movable kidney, or in obstruction from valves, adhesions, aberrant vessels, etc., though there may be no symptoms directly pointing to dilatation of the kidney, yet dilatation is taking

place. In other cases symptoms are present at this early stage : they are pain and polyuria.

The pain is a constant dull aching, is situated at the costo-muscular angle over the lower pole of the kidney, and is bilateral or unilateral according to the cause. In movable kidney it is indistinguishable from the pain caused by constant dragging on the renal pedicle. In other cases there are recurrent attacks of renal colic.

Polyuria is an important sign. The specific gravity of the urine is diminished and the percentage of urea and salts reduced. In bilateral obstruction this may be very marked, but in unilateral hydronephrosis it is frequently obscured by the urine from the second kidney. The polyuria may, however, be remarkable in early unilateral hydronephrosis.

2. **Late stage.**—In the late stage the symptoms are tumour, pain, and changes in the urine.

The tumour is situated in the loin, or it may fill a large part of the abdomen. It is rounded and moves with respiration. If it is moderate in size the sensation of ballottement can be obtained, but if very large it will be in contact with the anterior abdominal wall and ballottement will be lost. Fluctuation cannot be obtained. The tumour is not tender. A partly tympanitic note can be elicited in front of the tumour, while the outer and lateral parts are dull on percussion. The collapsed colon can frequently be felt passing vertically over its anterior surface. Where the pelvis is greatly dilated a vertical groove may be felt, and even seen, between this and the enlarged kidney.

There are two clinical types of hydronephrosis :

1. Constant hydronephrosis.
2. Intermittent hydronephrosis.

1. In **constant hydronephrosis** the tumour varies little in size, the urine is normal in quantity or may be reduced, and, beyond some aching pain, there are no symptoms. The hydronephrosis in such cases is " closed."

2. In **intermittent hydronephrosis** there are periods during which the tumour completely or almost completely disappears. From time to time there are attacks of retention, during which the patient has severe pain in the kidney and sometimes renal colic, the urine diminishes in quantity and may become completely suppressed, the tumour can be felt and is large, tense, and sometimes tender. After some hours or some days the patient suddenly passes a large quantity of pale urine, the pain subsides, and the tumour rapidly vanishes. These attacks may follow some unusual exertion or the drinking of some diuretic such as tea, whisky, or beer.

Cystoscopy.—Where the obstruction is situated at some part of the ureter the ureteric orifice is unchanged. In the early stages of hydronephrosis when polyuria is present, contractions of the ureter are more frequent on the diseased side. In advanced cases when a small quantity of urine escapes there is a slower and less frequent contraction of the orifice on the diseased side. When the obstruction is complete, but some muscular power is retained by the renal pelvis and ureter, an occasional gaping movement of the orifice is seen at long intervals, although no efflux takes place. When the kidney and the muscular structure of the pelvis are completely destroyed the orifice is still, and there is no efflux. The injection of methylene blue or indigo carmine will assist in the observation of the efflux.

Catheterization of the ureters.—The catheter is arrested at some part of the ureter, but usually it will move on after gentle manipulation, and the urine passes in hurried drips, or it may spout from the catheter in a continuous stream. Pressure upon the hydronephrosis increases the stream. I have withdrawn 16 oz. from a tense hydronephrotic sac in this way. The quantity of urine which drains from the ureter of the diseased side is greater than that from the healthy side when polyuria is present. I have observed a secretion of 82·6 c.c. on the diseased side to 68·4 c.c. on the healthy side. In advanced cases a small quantity of urine is collected by the catheter from the diseased side. In one of my cases 45 c.c. passed from the dilated kidney and 213 c.c. from the healthy kidney. Finally, no urine at all may pass. In one case I observed 158·5 c.c. with 1·3 per cent. of urea, and in another 150 c.c. of urine with 2 per cent. of urea, from the healthy kidney, while no urine appeared on the diseased side. In an open hydronephrosis the elimination of methylene blue is delayed, diminished, and prolonged on the diseased side, and the glycosuria produced by phloridzin is reduced or suppressed.

After relief of the obstruction by operation the functional value of the kidney greatly increases, even when the outflow has been completely blocked.

Diagnosis.—Diagnosis in the early stage before the development of a tumour is important therapeutically. The symptoms may sometimes lead to a diagnosis. Occasionally, when a stone is situated at the lower end of the ureter, the X-rays will show the outline of a thickened dilated ureter and an enlarged kidney.

Recently other methods have been introduced for the early diagnosis of hydronephrosis :

1. **Estimation of the capacity of the renal pelvis.**—This is carried out by the passage of a ureteral catheter into the renal

pelvis. The urine is withdrawn and warm boric solution is slowly injected from a graduated syringe until pain is felt. The quantity of fluid injected shows the capacity of the pelvis. A capacity of 30 to 40 c.c. shows a slight degree of hydronephrosis. This method is open to some objections. It may be uncertain whether the fluid has reached the pelvis of the kidney, and some of it may flow back into the bladder alongside the catheter. If the fluid is coloured with methylene blue, the latter objection may be obviated. If more than 150 c.c. can be injected without pain, but little secreting substance remains (Braasch). There is frequently polyuria of the diseased kidney, so that the pelvis will be partly filled with urine, and the capacity is then under-estimated.

2. **Injection of metallic solutions and photography by the X-rays (pyelography).**—Völcker and Lichtenberg introduced this method. After passing a ureteral catheter to the pelvis of the kidney and allowing any accumulated fluid to run off, a warm solution of collargol (10 per cent.) is slowly injected with a syringe. A radiogram is now taken, and shows a shadow of the renal pelvis. If dilatation is present it is demonstrated by the shape and increased area of the shadow. (Plate 2, Fig. 3; Plate 3; Plate 4, Fig. 1.) There is usually pain in the renal pelvis, which may amount to renal colic. The fluid is aspirated off after examination, and the pelvis may be washed with warm boric solution. Völcker and Lichtenberg employed this method in 17 cases without harm resulting. They obtained 9 good shadows, 4 that were less defined, and 4 were failures. I have used this method in a large number of cases, and have found no difficulty in obtaining a clear outline of the pelvis and calyces. A catheter opaque to the X-rays, or one opaque in alternate half-inches, should be used. The fluid should not be injected, but is allowed to run in by hydrostatic pressure from a glass receptacle attached to the end of the ureteric catheter and held about 6 or 8 in. above the external meatus. The utmost gentleness should be used, and forced injection must be avoided. The injection is stopped whenever pelvic pain is felt. No morphia or other anæsthetic is used before or during the examination. The abnormalities that can be shown are kinking at the uretero-pelvic junction, dilatation of one or more calyces, hydronephrosis of pelvic or of renal type. Where an abdominal tumour is suspected to be a hydronephrosis, pyelography will demonstrate the position of the renal pelvis and its relation to the tumour.

3. I have recently introduced two methods of measurement of the X-ray shadow thrown by the kidney (Plate 9, Figs. 1 and 2), as follows :—

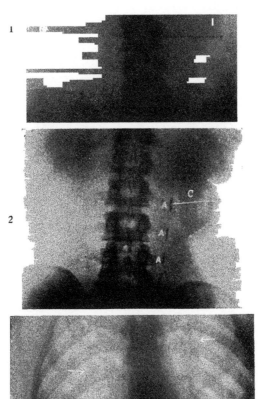

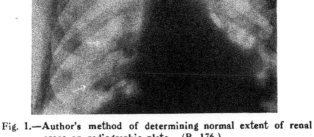

Fig. 1.—Author's method of determining normal extent of renal
areas on radiographic plate. (P. 176.)

Fig. 2.—Method of measuring shadow of kidney. A A A, opaque
½-in. segments of catheter; B, points in outline of kidney;
C, ½-in. shadow values placed across kidney shadow.
(P. 176.)

Fig. 3.—Shadows thrown by metastatic deposit in mediastinal
glands and in lungs in case of malignant growth of
kidney. (P. 199.)

PLATE 9.

(a) The narrowest transverse measurement of the body of the 1st lumbar vertebra is doubled and projected transversely from the middle of the outer edge of the vertebral body and a point is found. The same measurements are made in regard to the 2nd and 3rd lumbar vertebræ. By joining the three points the normal outer border of the kidney is roughly indicated.

(b) A ureteric catheter alternately opaque and translucent in segments of half an inch is passed up the ureter. On the plate the shadow value of half an inch is obtained, and by using this the shadow of the kidney can be measured.

Diseases that have been mistaken for hydronephrosis are appendicitis and gall-stones. The diagnosis depends upon the position of the pain and tenderness, the absence of fever and of jaundice, and the changes in the urine. If a tumour is present it has the characters of renal tumour. (See also p. 35.)

Course and prognosis.—These depend upon the cause. In urethral or vesical obstruction sepsis is frequently superadded, and the prognosis becomes very grave. In ureteric obstruction infection is less frequent and later. It may take place by the blood-stream, and a pyo-hydronephrosis is formed. Rupture of the sac spontaneously or from an injury is very rare. Carstair and Muir describe a fatal case of rupture of a hydronephrotic kidney followed by suppression. The second kidney was also hydronephrotic. Where the second kidney is hydronephrotic or otherwise diseased the ultimate prognosis is grave, suppression of urine eventually taking place.

Treatment. 1. Congenital hydronephrosis.—Congenital hydronephrosis is more frequently of interest to the obstetrician than to the surgeon, on account of the difficulty in parturition to which it may give rise.

The condition is frequently associated with other congenital malformations, such as hare-lip, imperforate anus, etc., and the child seldom survives birth for more than a few hours, but occasionally lives a few months and very rarely four or five years. Morris performed bilateral nephrostomy on a male child within twenty-four hours of its birth, and the child survived ninety-four days.

2. Hydronephrosis due to urethral, vesical, or pelvic obstruction.—In cases of urethral obstruction from stricture or enlarged prostate operations will be undertaken for the relief of the obstruction. The presence of dilatation of the kidneys in these cases and in cases of growths of the pelvic organs, such as uterine and ovarian tumours, increases the gravity of such operations. In growths of the bladder which involve one ureter

M

causing a moderate degree of hydronephrosis, but which are in other respects suitable for operation, removal of the growths with transplantation of the ureter to some part of the bladder should be undertaken. No direct operative treatment of the hydro-nephrosis will be necessary in these cases.

In nearly all these cases the formation of a hydronephrosis can be prevented by early operation, and this is especially true of cases of urethral obstruction and of bladder growth.

3. Movable kidney with hydronephrosis.—In cases where hydronephrosis is combined with undue mobility of the kidney the mobility is not always, at the time of the operation, the cause of the obstruction. Strictures, valves, and adhesions may be found, the removal of which is necessary for the relief of the obstruction. But in many instances the mobility is the direct cause of the ureteric obstruction. In cases of movable kidney hollowing of the organ with slight distension of the pelvis is fre-quently discovered. In these cases nephropexy will be sufficient to cure the hydronephrosis.

The early diagnosis of these cases is possible by the methods described, and early operation should be insisted upon in order to prevent destruction of the kidney tissue.

In more advanced cases, even when no sign of narrowing or adhesion or permanent kinking is found on exposure of the kidney, the renal pelvis must be opened and the patency of the outlet and the ureter examined. When a plastic operation has been found necessary in such cases, nephropexy must also be performed.

4. Hydronephrosis with calculus.—When calculus in the ureter or renal pelvis is combined with hydronephrosis the dis-tension of the kidney has frequently arisen from this cause, but n some cases strictures of the ureter are present, and have either preceded the formation of calculus or have developed secondarily. In addition to the removal of the calculus, the ureter must there-fore be examined for the presence of stricture.

5. Hydronephrosis with aberrant vessels.—In cases where an aberrant vessel is found, which bears no close relation to the point of obstruction, it need only be divided if it interferes with the plastic operation for the relief of the obstruction.

In other cases it lies in close relation to the point of obstruc-tion and is evidently the cause of the obstruction. If it is an unimportant vessel passing to the hilum or to the perirenal tissues, or an additional vessel arising from the aorta, it should be divided between two ligatures and the patency of the ureter then exam-ined, and if necessary a plastic operation performed. If, how-ever, the aberrant vessel is an important artery passing to the

lower pole of the kidney, and it is not proposed to perform nephrectomy, the vessel should be preserved and some form of plastic
operation carried out which will circumvent the obstruction caused
by it. Helferich divided such a vessel between ligatures, and
necrosis of a part of the kidney followed, necessitating nephrectomy.

In a case in which I divided an aberrant artery and vein of
considerable size the lower pole of the kidney at once became
blanched. Before the end of the operation, however, it had
become dark purple from the establishment of collateral blood
supply. No ill effects followed.

**Operations for congenital and acquired malformations
of the ureter and renal pelvis. 1. Operations which
modify the form of the
renal pelvis.** — i. *Nephropexy* in intermittent hydronephrosis. The kidney is not
only raised and fixed, but
the pelvis resumes its old
form, provided that the
distension has not been so
long established as to lead
to a weakening and sagging
of the sac wall.

ii. To remove the pouch-
ing Israel introduced an
operation, *pyeloplication,* by
which the redundant part
of the wall is folded inwards
after emptying the sac by
puncture. A row of Lem-
bert sutures fixes the fold.

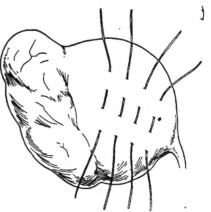

Fig. 38. — Pyeloplication (Israel's
operation) in pelvic type of hydronephrosis.

(Fig. 38.) In addition, an operation may be performed to correct
any malformations of the uretero-pelvic junction.

iii. My own plan is to resect a large triangular portion of the
posterior wall of the renal pelvis, the apex of the triangle being at
the uretero-pelvic junction and the base at the margin of the
kidney. A plastic operation for relief of any malformation of
the uretero-pelvic junction is then performed, and the wound
closed by Lembert's sutures. A flap of renal capsule is reflected
and stitched over the pelvic wound, the kidney drained through
a nephrotomy wound and fixed to the posterior abdominal wall.
(Fig. 39.)

iv. " *Orthopædic resection* " or " *capitonnage.*" — Albarran removes the pouch consisting of the portion of the pelvis and kidney which lies below the level of the outlet of the pelvis, and sutures the opening. (Fig. 40.)

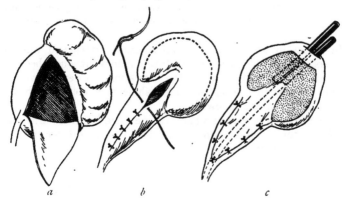

Fig. 39.—Resection of the renal pelvis (author's operation) in pelvic type of hydronephrosis.

a, Triangular flap of posterior wall of pelvis turned down. *b*, Triangular flap removed, closing wound in pelvis ; area of decapsulation marked with dotted line. *c*, Pelvic wound covered with flap of capsule and fatty tissue ; tubes draining kidney and in ureter through nephrotomy wound.

2. Anastomosis. i. *Uretero-ureteral anastomosis.*—This may be—

(*a*) End-to-end anastomosis with transverse or oblique section

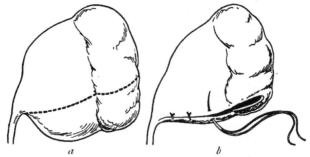

Fig. 40.—Orthopædic resection (Albarran's operation) in hydronephrosis.

a, Portion of pelvis and kidney below dotted line to be resected. *b*, Closing wound in pelvis and kidney.

of the ends, or by invagination of the upper into the lower end (Pozzi). (Fig. 41.)

(*b*) End-to-side anastomosis by ligaturing one cut end and

implanting the other end in a lateral slit below the ligature. (Fig. 41A.)

(c) Lateral anastomosis without section or after section of

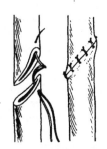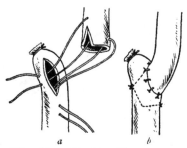

Fig. 41.—End-to-end anastomosis of ureter.

Ends cut obliquely.

Fig. 41A.—End-to-side anastomosis of ureter.

a, Two primary sutures in position; b, primary and secondary sutures tied.

the ureter. The edges of two lateral incisions are brought together by interrupted sutures. (Fig. 42.)

ii. *Pyelo-ureteral anastomosis.*—(a) Lateral anastomosis. This is the oldest plastic operation for hydronephrosis, and was performed by Trendelenburg in 1886. The ureter is split longitudinally on a level with the lowest part of the hydronephrotic sac, and a transverse incision is made in the sac wall. The edges of these wounds are sutured, and the kidney is then drained and fixed. (Fig. 43.)

(b) Transplantation of the ureter into the lowest part of the sac (uretero-pyelo-neostomy). The ureter is cut across transversely or obliquely, and in addition it may be split longitudinally to prevent stenosis. An incision

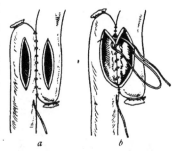

Fig. 42.—Lateral anastomosis of ureter.

a, One half of outer continuous suture in position; b, one half of inner continuous suture in position.

is made into the lowest part of the sac, a small triangular portion excised, and the ureteral mucous membrane is sutured to a pelvic mucous membrane. (Fig. 44.)

(c) Nephro-cysto-anastomosis. This is the direct anastomosis of a hydronephrotic sac with the bladder, and has been done in cases of displaced hydronephrotic solitary kidney. The operation is performed intraperitoneally. The sac is emptied by puncture, and the peritoneum over its lowest part incised and brought into contact with an incision in the upper posterior peritoneal surface of the bladder, and the edges sutured.

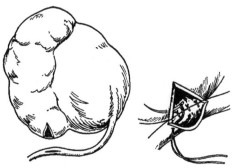

Fig. 43.—Lateral pyelo-ureteral anastomosis, showing incisions and details of stitching.

iii. *Plastic operations on strictures and valves.*—(a) Incision of a valve. This is performed through a nephrotomy wound or a large opening in the posterior wall of the dilated sac. The pyelo-ureteral opening is found, and one blade of a pair of scissors introduced into it. The valve is then cut downwards. If it is thin and formed only of mucous membrane, this will suffice; usually, however, the thickness of the pelvic and ureteral walls is cut through, and these are sutured to each other. (Fig. 45.)

(b) Uretero-pyeloplasty. This consists in making a longitudinal incision through a stricture at the ureteropelvic junction and uniting the edges of the wound transversely. It is similar to the operation of pyloroplasty for narrowing of the pylorus. The operation is frequently combined with one of the methods of reducing the sac of the hydronephrosis.

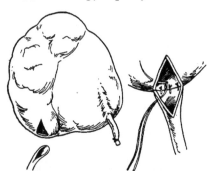

Fig. 44.—Uretero-pyelo-neostomy, showing details of stitching.

General observations. —1. These operations are performed on aseptic or on mildly infected hydronephrotic sacs.

2. When infection is present a preliminary nephrotomy with drainage for some weeks should be carried out.

3. The lumbar extraperitoneal route is used in all except nephrocystostomy.

4. Adhesions of the hydronephrotic sac and ureter should be removed before commencing the plastic operation.

5. Operations on the renal pelvis are performed on the posterior surface. The renal vessels are usually adherent to and stretched over the anterior surface.

6. Before commencing the operation a catheter should be passed up the ureter from the bladder to ascertain the position of the obstruction and assist in the operative measures.

7. The pelvic outlet may be examined through a nephrotomy or pyelotomy wound, and the examination is rendered simpler by everting this part of the sac through the wound.

8. The sac should be drained through a nephrotomy wound. Some surgeons leave a ureteric

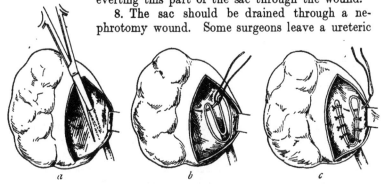

a   b   c

Fig. 45.—Plastic operation on a valve.

a, Section of spur consisting of pelvic and ureteral walls. *b*, Stitching cut edges of pelvis and ureter. *c*, Stitching completed.

catheter *in situ*, but this is not necessary, and may be a source of irritation.

9. Nephropexy is an important part of many of these operations.

10. Catgut should be used as suture material.

Functional value of a hydronephrotic kidney.—In the early stages of hydronephrosis the functional power of the kidney is impaired, but if the obstruction is relieved the organ will secrete urine almost as well as the normal kidney. The early diagnosis and operative treatment of hydronephrosis are therefore of extreme importance. In the fully developed hydronephrosis, where the layer of kidney tissue is reduced to half an inch, the organ still retains a considerable degree of functional power. I have operated on both kidneys for the relief of obstruction in bilateral advanced hydronephrosis, and the patient was well two and a half years later. There are cases of bilateral advanced hydronephrosis in which the patient has lived for many years, and there are other cases where a solitary kidney was converted into a hydronephrotic sac and yet carried on a function sufficient to maintain life. In the hydronephrotic sac the renal tissue, although greatly damaged, persists even when the wall is only a few milli-metres thick, and it very rarely completely disappears. After relief of the obstruction the kidney does not return to the normal state, and if regeneration takes place it is not the invariable rule.

Results of plastic operations.—Schloffer collected 86 opera-tions with the following results :—

	Operations		Deaths		Failures
Section of valves ..	.. 12	..	1	..	3
Uretero-pyeloplasty ..	.. 18	..	1	..	4
Uretero-pyeloneostomy	.. 19	..	2	..	6
Lateral anastomosis	.. 13	..	2	..	3
Plastic operations on renal pelvis	.. 1	..	—	..	1
Pyeloplication ..	.. 4	..	—	..	—
Orthopædic resection	.. 8	..	1	..	—
Combined operations	.. 11	..	—	..	—
Total	.. 86	..	7	..	17

To this I can add three personal cases treated by my method, with two successes, and one failure due to hæmorrhage into the resected pelvis. This patient was submitted to nephrectomy and recovered. I can also record a successful result in a case of pyelo-ureteral anastomosis. In a fourth case there was bilateral hydro-nephrosis, and the operation was performed on each pelvis with an interval of three weeks. The patient died two months later of renal failure, which had commenced some months previously and slowly progressed.

Nephrostomy.—Incision and drainage of the sac without any attempt to overcome the cause of the obstruction is some-times performed. This has been followed in between 30 to 45 per cent. of cases by re-establishment of the flow of the urine through the ureter and healing of the nephrotomy wound. In the remaining cases a fistula persists.

Nephrectomy.—Primary nephrectomy is only indicated when the sac is very large and its wall so thin and fibrous that no renal tissue is present, and only in cases when it can be proved that a second kidney is present and efficient.

Secondary nephrectomy is required when nephrotomy and plastic operations have failed.

LITERATURE

Albarran, *Bull. de l'Acad. de Méd.*, 1898, p. 59.
Albarran and Legueu, Congrès franç. de Chir., 1892, p. 561.
Braasch, *Journ. Amer. Med. Assoc.*, 1909, p. 1386.

LITERATURE—*continued*

Carstair and **Muir,** *Brit. Med. Journ.,* 1904, i. 136.
Gardner, *Ann. Surg.,* 1908, p. 575.
Helferich, *Deuts. Zeits. f. Chir.,* 1896, p. 323.
Israel, *Deuts. med. Woch.,* 1906, p. 22.
Krogius, *Centralbl. f. Chir.,* 1902, p. 686.
Küster, *Arch. f. klin. Chir.,* 1892, p. 850.
Lindermann, *Zeits. f. klin. Med.,* 1898, p. 299.
Luys, *Ann. d. Mal. d. Org. Gén.-Urin.,* 1906, i. 579.
Mayo, *Journ. Amer. Med. Assoc.,* 1909, p. 1383.
Morley, *Lancet,* June 11, 1910.
Schloffer, *Wien. klin. Woch.,* 1906, p. 50.
Trendelenburg, *Volkmanns Sammlung klin. Vortr.,* 1890, p. 355.,
Viertel, *Centralbl. f. Chir.,* 1896, p. 9.   .
Völcker und **Lichtenberg,** *Beitr. z. klin. Chir.,* 1907, p. 1.
Wagner, *Folia Urol.,* June, 1907.
Walker, Thomson, *Lancet,* Aug. 11, 1906, and June 17, 1911 ;
     Trans. Med. Soc. Lond., 1912.

CHAPTER XIII

TUMOURS OF THE KIDNEY AND URETER

TUMOURS OF THE KIDNEY

New growths are found in greater variety in the kidney than elsewhere in the body. Benign growths of the kidney are few and rare, but malignant growths are more common. Here as elsewhere, the border-line between innocence and malignancy is ill defined. Secondary growths in the kidney are infrequent. They occur as a part of a widespread metastatic deposit, and are of no surgical importance.

BENIGN GROWTHS

Benign growths form less than 7 per cent. of renal growths. They are more interesting from a pathological than from a surgical standpoint.

ADENOMA

Adenomas occur as small tumours, and may reach the size of a cherry. They are subcapsular, usually single, but may be multiple, round or nodular, greyish-white or pink in colour, and surrounded by a distinct capsule. They usually occur in kidneys which show chronic interstitial nephritis.

Two varieties are described—a papillary, which consists of acini lined with cylindrical epithelium and containing papillary formations; and an alveolar or tubular form, consisting of solid or hollow masses of cylindrical epithelium.

LIPOMA

Lipomas are usually small multiple tumours, situated underneath the capsule. (Fig. 46.) Very rarely a large lipoma has been observed.

FIBROMA

Pure fibromas are extremely rare. They have been found as small fibrous nodules in the cortex or medulla.

186

LEIO MYOMA

This is a very rare form of growth of the kidney, occurring as small nodules of smooth muscle fibres originating in the smooth muscle of the capsule of the kidney (*see* under Perirenal Tumours, p. 220).

Diagnosis of benign renal tumours.—The diagnosis of simple growths of the kidney is very difficult. Those of small size give rise to no symptoms and are found post mortem. Large

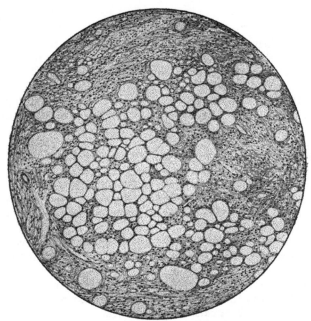

Fig. 46.—Microscopical section of lipoma of kidney.

growths are indistinguishable clinically from malignant growths, and, unless a positive diagnosis of simple growth can be made on exposing the kidney, nephrectomy should be performed.

MALIGNANT GROWTHS

The following varieties of malignant renal tumours are found :—

1. Carcinoma.
2. Sarcoma.
3. Hypernephroma.
4. Mixed tumours of embryonic type.

Of 434 cases recorded since 1903, 65 were carcinomas, 74 sarcomas, 45 mixed tumours, 218 hypernephromas, and 32 benign
or of unknown nature (Taddei).

A renal growth is most prone to develop at the two extremes
of life, the great majority of these tumours being found under
5 or over 40 years.

Küster found the following age-distribution :—

1- 5 years	128
6-10 ,,	41
40-50	125
51-60 ,,	128

The right kidney is more frequently affected than the left, and
bilateral renal growths are rare. Men are more frequently
affected than women in the proportion of 227 men to 73 women
(Albarran). Any part of the kidney substance may be the seat
of growth. Occasionally the tumour is situated immediately
beneath the fibrous capsule, or the growth may take origin
in the renal pelvis or in the tissues at the hilum or around the
kidney.

Etiology.—The large number of tumours found in childhood suggests that many renal growths are congenital, and the
structure of the mixed tumours found in infancy and childhood
supports this view. There is no direct evidence that injury is a
cause, but an injury to the kidney may draw attention to a new
growth which already exists.

Stone sometimes coexists with new growth of the kidney, but
such cases are too rare for this factor to play an important rôle in
the etiology.

In a few cases a new growth has been found in a movable
kidney. It is said that such kidneys are more exposed to trauma
and that this may be a cause of new growth.

Pathology and histology. 1. Carcinoma.—In recent years
it has been shown that carcinoma of the kidney is a rare form
of tumour, and that many of the growths formerly regarded as
carcinomas belong to the group known as hypernephromas.
Garceau states the frequency of carcinoma as 7 per cent. of
renal tumours. The new growth takes origin in the tubules of
the kidney. (Fig. 47.)

The following three varieties of histological structure are
found :—

    i. Diffuse infiltration of the interstitial tissue, tubules, and
        glomeruli by cancer cells. In parts the cells are
        arranged in masses or in alveoli.

XIII] RENAL CARCINOMA 189

   ii. Tubules lined with epithelium closely resembling the **structure of the normal kidney.**

   iii. Acini into which papillary growths project.

The first and second varieties are frequently found in the same tumour, and the name adeno-carcinoma is sometimes given to this type (Fig. 48). The third variety may form a characteristic tumour, and is then called papillary adeno-carcinoma.

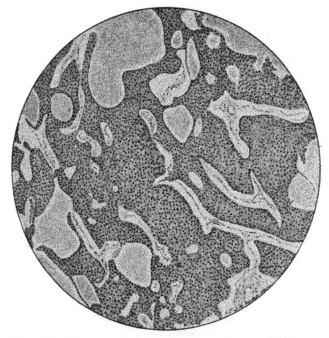

Fig. 47.—Microscopical section of carcinoma of kidney.

Garceau points out that the histological appearances may vary greatly in the same specimen, and that in some tumours which closely resemble renal carcinoma the metastases have the appearance of a hypernephroma.

The kidney may retain its natural outline in the infiltrating form of carcinoma. The growth is usually small, but occasionally reaches a large size. On section it is grey, yellow, or brown, and is broken up by tracts of connective tissue.

   2. **Sarcoma** (Fig. 49).—Sarcoma is more often bilateral than carcinoma, and is especially found in infants (82 adults, 80 infants —Albarran and Imbert). In adults the tumour is rarely larger

than an infant's head, but in children it may reach enormous proportions. A tumour of this nature weighing 33 lb. has been described by Van der Byl.

The growth increases rapidly in size, and quickly forms adhesions to the surrounding structures.

Some of these growths arise from the capsule of the kidney and others from the connective tissue surrounding the vessels at

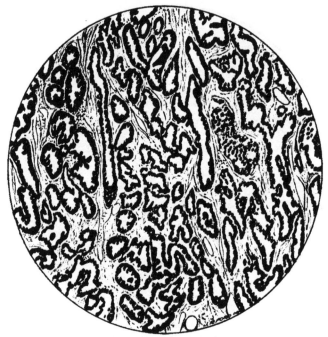

Fig. 48.—Microscopical section of adeno-carcinoma of kidney.

the hilum, but the great majority take origin in the substance of the kidney.

On .section the sarcoma has a greyish, brain-like appearance, and in parts an alveolar arrangement may be observed. It is limited on the surface by the fibrous renal capsule, and separated from the parenchyma by a fibrous capsule which may be ill . defined at parts. The histological varieties of sarcoma are the spindle-celled and small round-celled.

Angio-sarcoma of the kidney has been described, but these growths are now included in the group of hypernephromas, with which they are identical.

3. Hypernephroma.—Under this name are placed tumours of the kidney which resemble the suprarenal gland in their histological appearances. These tumours were described, in 1883, by Grawitz, who held that they took origin in small aberrant nodules of suprarenal tissue found in the cortex of the kidney, usually beneath the capsule. In the embryo the suprarenal gland surrounds the kidney, and portions of suprarenal tissue become included in the kidney in the process of development.

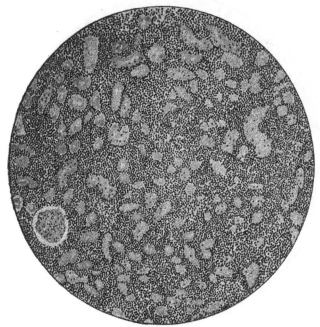

Fig. 49.—Microscopical section of kidney infiltrated by lympho-sarcoma.

Recent observations on the embryology of the suprarenal gland appear to show that it is formed from mesoblastic cells (Poll), and these new growths should therefore be looked upon as sarcomas. The point is not finally settled, and it is convenient to classify the growths separately under the name of hypernephroma.

Stoerk has recently disputed the suprarenal origin of these growths. He looks upon them as papillomatous in nature. According to this observer they are adenomas, or papilliferous cysts, or carcinoma, and take origin in the renal epithelium. Wilson and Willis hold that they arise in remains of the Wolffian body. The

tumours are most frequently found under the capsule, and have
no covering of renal tissue. · Küster found 80 situated in the
middle, 54 at the upper and 60 at the lower pole of the kidney.·
The medulla of the kidney may be the seat of a hypernephroma.·
The right kidney is more frequently affected than the left (82–77),
and male subjects more · often · than · female (102–71)—Garceau.
The tumour is very rarely bilateral. .

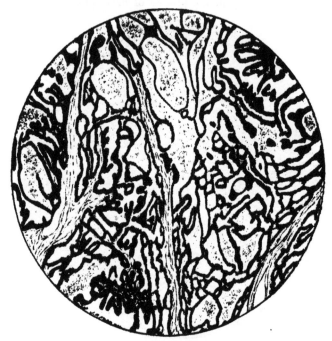

Fig. 50.—Microscopical section of hypernephroma of kidney,
papillary type.

This is the most frequent form of new growth in the kidney.
Of 102 tumours of the kidney 68 were of this nature (Israel).

The growth may become active and give rise to clinical symptoms at any age. Garceau's table of 176 cases shows 48 between
the ages of 40 and 50, 61 between those of 50 and 60, and 24
between those of 60 and 70.

·   The tumour consists of a rounded mass of varying size.· (Plate
10.)   On section it is surrounded by a capsule of firm fibrous tissue,
often of considerable thickness. The substance of the growth is
broken up by fibrous bands into nodules of different sizes. ·(Plate 11.)

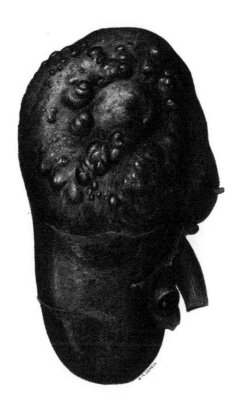

Hypernephroma of kidney; operation specimen;
surface view. Note renal vein distended with
growth, and aberrant renal artery passing to
upper pole. (P. 192.)

PLATE 10.

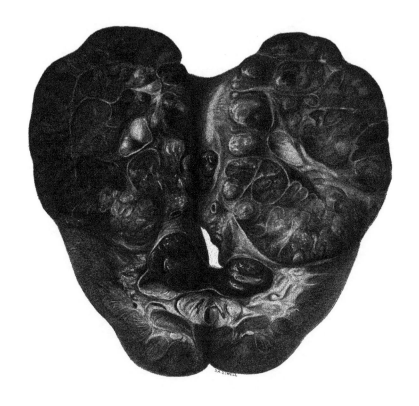

Section of hypernephroma of kidney. Note vein distended with growth. Same kidney as in Plate 10. (P. 192.)

PLATE 11.

These may, however, be absent, when the growth presents a more
uniform appearance. There is a characteristic yellow-red colour
which is found in most of these growths, and is due to the presence
of a large quantity of fat in the cells of a very vascular growth.
Patches of necrosis are not infrequently seen, and hæmorrhages
sometimes take place in the substance of the growth. The microscopical appearances resemble the cortex of the suprarenal gland.

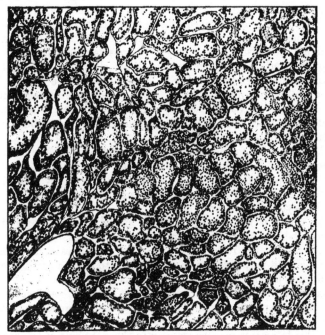

Fig. 51.—Microscopical section of hypernephroma of kidney,
alveolar type.

The growth consists of a network of capillary vessels, and set
directly upon these, without the intervention of connective-tissue
fibres, are the tumour cells. These are large polyhedral cells
with clear protoplasm containing a quantity of fat. There is a
large nucleus with a distinct nucleolus. The cells are arranged
around the capillary vessels in a single row or several rows.
Where a single row or relatively few rows of cells lie on the capillaries a papillary appearance is given (Fig. 50); when the spaces
between the capillaries are filled up with closely packed cells an
alveolar appearance is presented (Fig. 51). According to Garceau

N

the alveolar arrangement is more frequently seen in large growths than the papillary.

4. **Mixed tumours.**—These tumours are found during the first four years of life. They are formed of tissues arising from the three layers of the embryo. The basis of the tumour consists of connective tissue of a more or less embryonic type, the cells being round, oval, and spindle-shaped in varying proportions. In this are found striped muscle fibres in an embryonic stage of development, the fibres lacking sarcolemma and the nuclei lying at the side of the fibres. Non-striped muscle fibres, cartilaginous nodules, fatty tissue, elastic tissue, and epithelial elements in the form of tubules are also found. There is considerable variation in the proportions and arrangement of these elements. When the striped muscle fibres are present in large numbers the growth is termed a "rhabdo-myo-sarcoma." When the epithelial elements are numerous the name "embryonic adeno-sarcoma" is used. Bland-Sutton holds that when the striped cells are very abundant the tubules are, as a rule, absent.

These growths, as Bland-Sutton points out, arise in the tissues of the sinus of the kidney and distend the organ, so that a thin layer of expanded kidney tissue can be found covering the growth. Eventually the capsule is ruptured and the growth spreads beyond the organ.

The ureter is not usually invaded, and this accounts for the absence of hæmaturia which is noted in these cases.

Growth into the renal veins and inferior vena cava is almost invariable, and may give rise to embolism or to œdema and ascites. The disease is bilateral in about 50 per cent. of cases.

Extension and metastases.—Some forms of renal growth, especially hypernephroma and mixed growths, are prone to spread along the renal veins, and buds may extend into the vena cava. From this fragments may be swept into the right side of the heart and the pulmonary artery. This extension may give rise to difficulty in ligaturing the vessels, or to tearing of the renal vein at operation. Spread through the capsule of the kidney takes place in large growths. Examination of the perirenal adhesions and adipose tissue occasionally shows microscopic nodules of growth when nothing is seen with the naked eye. In the later stages neighbouring organs and nerves are invaded. Extension along the lymphatics to the lymph-glands lying alongside the aorta and vena cava usually occurs late. Lymphatic glands at the root of the neck and groin have been the seat of deposit in rare cases. The suprarenal capsule is very frequently invaded by tumours of the upper pole of the kidney. In the majority of adult cases the growth invades the pelvis, where rarely it forms a pedunculated tumour. In children the pelvis is usually free from growth. From the pelvis the growth may spread down the ureter and project into the bladder, or a portion may become detached and be held for a time at the ureteric orifice or engrafted on the ureter. Metastases may occur early in hypernephroma when the primary growth is still small, or the renal growth after a period of slow development may suddenly increase rapidly and form metastases. Hypernephromas are specially prone to form metastases in bones.

In children lymphatic glands may be affected late, but there is frequently no deposit apart from the kidneys.

The most common seats of metastatic deposit are the lungs, liver, lymph-glands, and bones, and more rarely the second kidney, pleura, omentum, suprarenal gland, and brain.

Concomitant diseases of the kidneys, such as stone, movable kidney, and tuberculosis, have been observed with new growth, but these conditions have no etiological value.

The kidney which is the seat of a new growth shows fibrous induration in the neighbourhood of the tumour, the result of compression. There is also epithelial and interstitial nephritis in this and in the second kidney, due to the absorption of toxins from the growth (Albarran). This diminishes the functional value of the second kidney, and may be the cause of death after nephrectomy.

Obliteration of the ureter by portions of growth or by compression may give rise to hydronephrosis, and accumulation of clots in the pelvis may produce a hæmatonephrosis. Chronic myocarditis from the circulation of toxins is frequently present, and is a cause of heart failure after nephrectomy (Israel).

Symptoms.—The cardinal symptoms of new growth of the kidney are hæmaturia and tumour.

Hæmaturia is the most constant symptom and usually the first to appear. In adults it is present in over 90 per cent. of cases, and is the first symptom in 70 per cent. In children it is much less frequent, occurring in only about 16 per cent. of cases, and it is rarely present until after an abdominal tumour is discovered. The first appearance of hæmaturia sometimes follows a strain or blow on the loin, but the initial attack and subsequent attacks are usually spontaneous. It is intermittent and capricious. Blood appears without cause, and lasts a day or a week or longer, and then disappears for an indefinite period, an interval of a week, a month, six months, or a year occurring before the next attack. Rest in bed may be followed by disappearance of the blood, but often it does not influence the attack.

The blood is well mixed with the urine, and may be dark purple, or bright red, or only a pink tinge. When the urine appears clear, blood cells may be found with the microscope.

Clots are frequently present, and slender worm-like clots 10 or 12 in. long are sometimes passed. (Fig. 52.) Israel describes a special form of clot found in new growth of the kidney. The clots are the size and shape of maggots, are red, pale yellow, or white, and are contracted at parts. They occur in a slightly bloody urine.

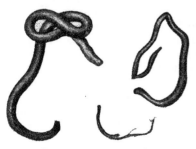

Fig. 52.—Ureteral clots in renal hæmaturia.

Clots may block the lumen of the ureter and give rise to attacks of ureteral colic, with sudden disappearance of the blood in the urine. Copious hæmorrhage may fill the bladder rapidly with clots and cause strangury.

The hæmaturia has no relation to the size of the growth. A small growth may cause copious and repeated hæmorrhages, while the hæmorrhage from a large growth may be scanty and occur at long intervals.

Hæmaturia occurs in all forms of renal growth. It is least frequent in the mixed sarcomas of children and infants.

Tumour is a very frequent symptom. It is present in the advanced stage of nearly all growths (84 per cent.—Albarran and Imbert). It is less often than hæmaturia the first symptom (23 per cent.—Heresco). In children, however, tumour is almost constant (140 in 142 cases—Walker), and is the initial symptom in about one-third of cases.

The kidney can usually be felt enlarged when hæmaturia first appears. When the new growth is situated at the upper pole it is not palpable until it has reached a large size. The kidney is, however, pushed down and can be felt lower than normal. Small tumours of the lower pole can be detected in favourable subjects. Israel felt a tumour the size of a nut in this position.

A large growth is easily felt, and has the characters of a renal tumour. (Fig. 53.) It forms a rounded mass occupying the loin. On percussion a dull note is given, and there is usually a resonant band formed by the colon on the surface of the tumour, or the flattened colon can be rolled under the finger. The colon may be distended with air to assist the examination. The tumour is rounded, and frequently smooth, and is firm and resistant. There may be nodular irregularities, and some parts of a large growth can occasionally be felt less resistant than others. The mass extends backwards into the loin, and can be felt here with the fingers below the 12th rib. When it is small the sensation of ballottement can be detected by projecting it forwards from the loin against the hand laid flat on the abdomen. In a large growth the mass is already in contact with the abdominal wall, and this sensation is lost. The tumour usually moves with respiration, and retains this character until it has reached a large size. If it is fixed, and

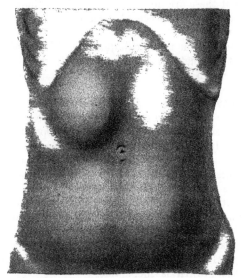

Fig. 53.—Visible tumour in case of large renal growth.

especially when the tumour is still small, adhesions have already formed.

When masses of enlarged glands lie along the aorta they may be continuous with the tumour on palpation, and a large irregular mass is felt.

Pain is a common symptom, and is due to a variety of causes. Attacks of ureteral colic are, as already mentioned, produced by the passage of clots along the ureter. Severe aching renal pain may be due to tension within the renal capsule, caused by engorgement of the kidney or hæmorrhage into the growth. Constant aching pain unaffected by movement, or by the variations in the hæmaturia, and only temporarily relieved by drugs, is the characteristic pain of renal cancer. It is caused by the spread of the growth beyond the kidney and the involvement of nerves. It may take the form of intercostal neuralgia, or may radiate to the genital organs or down the thigh. I have known constant sciatica-like pain precede by some months the onset of hæmaturia and the appearance of enlargement of the kidney.

Changes may be present in the urine apart from hæmaturia. Occasionally portions of growth are passed in the urine, the nature of which can be recognized by the microscope. Cancer cells are said to be present in the urine in some cases, but it is very doubtful if these are not cells derived from the epithelium of the renal pelvis. The absence of such formed elements has no diagnostic importance.

Albumin may be due to a small quantity of blood which cannot be detected with the naked eye, or it may be due to toxic nephritis. Pyuria is present in the rare cases where calculus coexists with growth.

The quantity of urine is frequently increased, the polyuria being due to the higher pressure in the renal vessels.

Varicocele is sometimes observed. It develops steadily, sometimes rapidly. It may be an early symptom, and may already be present when the first hæmaturia appears, but it usually develops late in the course of the disease. It is due to pressure either of enlarged glands or of the growth itself, or it may be produced by engorgement of the capsular veins which anastomose with the spermatic vein. It disappears after nephrectomy, and should not be considered a contra-indication of operation.

Hochenegg states that if the varicocele does not disappear in the genu-pectoral position, it is due to compression of enlarged glands and the growth is inoperable.

Cachexia occurs in the late stages. It is sometimes present, but is never a pronounced feature in the early stage of the growth.

Israel has described a *specific fever* in 8 per cent. of cases of new growths of the kidney which may occur early or late in the course of the disease, and may be remittent or recurrent, or there may be occasional attacks. It disappears after complete nephrectomy.

Hypertrophy of the left ventricle is frequently observed. Increased arterial tension has been observed by some authorities, and it is stated that these patients die of cerebral hæmorrhage. This has been attributed to the absorption of increased quantities of suprarenal secretion in cases of hypernephroma. An abnormally rapid pulse is not uncommon, and is said to be due to pressure on the lumbar sympathetic ganglia. This symptom is common to other large growths in the lower part of the body.

The X-rays give a dense shadow with indefinite outline in large growths of the kidney. Metastatic nodules in the lungs are clearly shown by the X-rays (Plate 9, Fig. 3), and this method of examination should be used before operation in every case. The symptoms of pulmonary metastases may be insignificant (Plate 9, Fig. 3).

Course and prognosis.—Symptoms are frequently present for a number of years before the patient is submitted to operation. Krönlein, Israel, and Loumeau operated on patients respectively eight, twelve, and fifteen years after the first symptom. The general health may remain unaffected for four, eight, or ten years.

Garceau found that the average duration of the disease from the appearance of the first symptom to the fatal issue in 32 cases was three and a half years. The course is rapid where metastases have appeared.

Diagnosis. 1. Cases where hæmaturia is the only symptom.—Here the character of the hæmaturia may assist, but cystoscopic examination during an attack of hæmorrhage is the only certain method of localizing the source of the bleeding. Beyond the localization of hæmaturia to one kidney it is seldom possible to go in these cases. The presence of cancer cells or of portions of growth in the urine is a rare and doubtful means of diagnosis. Exploration of the bleeding kidney is the only certain method, and this should be carried out in every case of unilateral renal hæmaturia in which the diagnosis cannot be clearly established.

2. Cases where tumour is the only symptom. — The characters of the renal tumour have been described. In moderate-sized tumours the diagnosis presents little, if any, difficulty, but in large growths there may be difficulty.

Tumours of the suprarenal gland, liver, gall-bladder, spleen, omentum, and colon are the cause of the most frequent mistakes. Sometimes an exploratory laparotomy may become necessary before the diagnosis is established.

3. Tumour with hæmaturia, without other symptoms. —No other disease of the kidney gives rise to this combination of symptoms. Stone has pain and pyuria in addition, and tuberculosis has pyuria and the tubercle bacillus is discovered. In congenital cystic degeneration of the kidney there is rarely hæmaturia. In this disease the bilateral tumour and the long and very slow development will suggest the true nature of the disease, which an exploratory operation will confirm.

It is rarely possible to make a diagnosis of the variety of growth before operation. In children the frequent growths are mixed sarcomas, but hypernephroma has been observed at the age of 1½ years (Cheeseman). The presence of metastatic deposits in bones is characteristic of hypernephroma.

Treatment.—Palliative treatment is adopted in cases which are unsuitable for nephrectomy. It consists in the administration of such drugs as ergot, adrenalin, opium, and calcium lactate to control hæmorrhage, and opium, morphia, bromides, aspirin, and phenacetin to soothe pain; and attention to the bowels, since the pressure and adhesions of the growth may cause obstinate constipation.

Calcium lactate should be administered with caution, as it encourages the formation of clots and may give rise to clot colic. Palliative operations, such as nephrectomy where there are secondary growths, or partial nephrectomy for pain, are seldom called for.

Radical treatment by total nephrectomy, performed as early as possible, is the only method which holds out a prospect of cure. Partial nephrectomy is unsuited to the treatment of malignant growth of the kidney.

Operation is contra-indicated where (1) the growth has spread beyond the kidney, (2) the second kidney is functionally inadequate, (3) the patient is weak and cachectic, (4) the heart is dilated and feeble.

It is therefore necessary to ascertain, before proceeding to nephrectomy, whether the growth has spread beyond the kidney. Where the kidney is still small the disappearance of movement on respiration is an important sign of spread beyond the kidney, but immobility in a large tumour has not the same significance. The extent of the growth can best be ascertained after exposure of the kidney.

In all large growths the peritoneum should be opened and the peritoneal aspect of the tumour examined. The upper pole of the kidney can at once be explored by this means, whereas it cannot be reached until a late stage of the operation if approached extraperitoneally. I have twice had to desist from nephrectomy on finding the peritoneum adherent and nodular over the highest part of the kidney in tumours which in other respects appeared to be suitable for removal.

The lymph-glands lying alongside the aorta or the vena cava should be examined by palpation, and if the peritoneum is opened a further examination should be made. The most frequent seat of secondary growths is the lungs, and a radiograph of the thorax should be obtained.   The liver should be examined by palpation and percussion.

The condition of the second kidney is ascertained by catheterization of the ureters and examination of the urine thus obtained, and the use of the tests for the renal function.   The presence of chronic nephritis does not contra-indicate operation if the renal function is adequately performed.

The ideal operation should remove the kidney and growth, the adipose capsule, the lymphatic vessels and glands and the fat in which they are embedded, and the suprarenal capsule. Nephrectomy may be performed by the abdominal (transperitoneal) or lumbar (retroperitoneal) route.

At the present day, in a considerable proportion of cases the operation commences as an exploration of the kidney for hæmaturia before any enlargement of the kidney can be detected, and the discovery of the growth leads to nephrectomy.   In such cases the operation commences as a retroperitoneal exploration of the kidney, and when the growth is discovered the adipose capsule has already been opened and the kidney incised.   The incision in the kidney should be closed with catgut sutures and nephrectomy performed.

The perirenal fat should then be dissected from the peritoneum and from the muscles of the posterior abdominal wall.   This should be carried inwards as far as the great vessels, preserving the spermatic vessels, and carefully removing the lymph-glands along the aorta or the vena cava.   The suprarenal glands should also be removed.

Where a diagnosis has been made before operation in larger growths abdominal nephrectomy will give a better approach, or the growth may be exposed by the lumbar retroperitoneal route and the peritoneum opened to the outer side of the colon.

Grégoire has described an operation which is to be recommended when a diagnosis of new growth has been made.

A firm pillow is placed under the diseased side as far as the vertebral column, and the body is curved backwards.

The incision runs in the anterior axillary line from the costal margin to the iliac crest, and each end of this is carried forwards for 4 or 5 cm. along the costal margin and iliac crest respectively. This is carried through the muscles, and the peritoneum, colon, and perirenal fascia are then displaced forwards from the muscles of the posterior abdominal wall as far as the vertebral column. The fascia of Zuckerkandl is incised 1 cm. behind the reflection of the peritoneum, and the peritoneum and colon are stripped forwards.   The upper pole of the kidney, with the suprarenal capsule, is separated, the renal vessels are ligatured, the ureter is tied, and the kidney removed. The adipose tissue; lymphatics, and glands are now dissected along the vena cava and aorta, preserving the spermatic vessels.

Dangers of nephrectomy for renal growth.—The immediate danger is hæmorrhage. The kidney is frequently surrounded by large, dilated, easily torn veins, and free venous hæmorrhage, difficult to control, may take place. Formidable veins are also met with at the upper pole, and are difficult to reach. They are controlled by a temporary packing during the operation. The renal vein is easily torn when it is filled with growth, and may give rise to severe hæmorrhage. The inferior vena cava has been torn, and lateral suture has been performed (*see* Nephrectomy, p. 297). Pulmonary embolism has been caused by the separation of a clot or portion of growth in the renal veins during operation.

The wound may be soiled with carcinomatous tissue, and as a result recurrence takes place in the scar.

Anuria may supervene from inadequate function of the second kidney. This danger should not arise in properly selected cases.

Cardiac failure may occur at the close of or soon after the operation, or it may be delayed. Chronic myocarditis predisposes to its occurrence.

Results.—The mortality of nephrectomy for renal growths has fallen during recent years from 76 per cent. (Minges, 1885) and 65·2 per cent. (Tuffier, 1888) to 22 per cent. (Albarran and Imbert, 1902). Schmieden's statistics of 329 cases show that the mortality during the first ten years of renal surgery was 64·3 per cent., in the second ten years 43·0 per cent., and in the third 22·0 per cent. in adults.

The high death-rate in the earlier operations was largely due to septic infection, and this also explained the higher mortality of transperitoneal nephrectomy as compared with the retroperitoneal operation.

In the transperitoneal operations previous to 1890 the mortality was 50 per cent., while the mortality of the retroperitoneal operation was 37 or 38 per cent. (Gross, Brodeur).

Operations performed after 1890 showed a mortality of 23 per cent. for lumbar and 21·1 per cent. for transperitoneal nephrectomy (Albarran and Imbert).

Death is due in these cases to septic infection, heart failure, shock, asthenia, and anuria.

Late results.—Recurrence takes place in 60 per cent. of cases, and in over 70 per cent. of these it appears within the first year. After the first year it is less common, and it is rare after the third or fourth year. Cases of late recurrence after three years have, however, been recorded by Bloch (three years), Helferich (three and a half years), Abbe (four and a half years), and Witzel (five years). The recurrent growth is most frequently found in the scar. It occurs also in the lymph-glands, lungs, and liver, and in these cases metastases have almost certainly taken place before the operation.

Forgue found that 28 cases (7 to 10 per cent.) had survived at the end of the fourth year without recurrence. Wagner found 21 cases remaining well after three years (16 adults, 5 children).

Results in children.—In children' the operative mortality is higher, and recurrence is more rapid and more frequent than in the adult. Walker states the general mortality from operation and recurrence at 93·22 per cent., while Albarran and Imbert give the mortality from operation as 25 to 30 per cent., and state that recurrence takes place in between 67 and 81 per cent. of survivals. Simon has collected 11 cases in good health a year after the operation, during which the longest were—Israel five years, Döderlein four years, Schmidt three years, and Shend and Rovsing each two years. The longest survival of which I have definite information is a case operated on by Mr. J. D. Malcolm, in November, 1892, which was well in February, 1911, eighteen years and three months after the operation. Abbe, of New York, recorded two cases of prolonged survival: in one the patient died of new growth in the remaining kidney four and a half years after operation; the other patient was alive and well over ten years after operation.

LITERATURE

Albarran et Imbert, *Les Tumeurs du Rein.* Paris, 1903.
Bland-Sutton, *Tumours, Innocent and Malignant.* 1911.
Forgue, VIᵉ Sess. de l'Assoc. franç. d'Urol., Paris, 1902.
Garceau, *Tumours of the Kidney.* 1909.
Grawitz, *Virchows Arch.,* 1883, p. 39.
Grégoire, Thèse de Paris, 1905; *Presse Méd.,* 1905, p. 49.
Heresco, Thèse de Paris, 1899.
Hochenegg, *Arch. f. klin. Med.,* 1907, p. 51.
Israel, *Nierenkrankheiten,* 1901; *Deuts. med. Woch.,* 1911, p. 57.
Poll, *Handbuch der vergl. und exper. Entwickelungslehre der Wirbeltiere,* p. 456. Jena.
Schmieden, *Deuts. Zeits. f. Chir.,* 1902.
Simon, Thèse de Paris, 1904.
Stoerk, *Zieglers Beitr.,* 1908, p. 393.
Taddei, *Folia Urol.,* 1908, pp. 303, 638.
Trotter, *Lancet,* 1909, p. 1581.
Wagner, *Handbuch der Urologie* (von Frisch und Zuckerkandl), 1905, ii. 273.
Walker, *Ann. Surg.,* 1897, p. 549.
Wilson and **Willis,** *Collected Papers of St. Mary's Hospital* (Mayo Clinic), 1911.

TUMOURS OF THE RENAL PELVIS AND URETER

The majority of growths of the kidney project into the pelvis. Primary growths of the pelvis arise apart from the kidney, and are very rare. Albarran collected 42 cases, and Israel found only 2 primary growths of the pelvis in 68 new growths of the kidney. Drew described a case of villous carcinoma of the renal pelvis and collected 8 others from the literature. I have performed nephrectomy on 2 such cases.

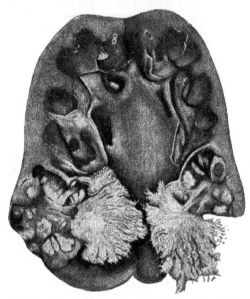

Fig. 54.—Papillomatous growth of renal pelvis, with malignant growth of kidney.

Etiology.—Calculi have been present in the pelvis in some cases, and the prolonged irritation caused by their presence may have been the cause of the growths. Drew found calculi in 4 out of 8 cases collected from the literature.

Pathology.—Epithelial tumours (papilloma and epithelioma) are most frequent, while mesoblastic tumours (sarcoma, myxoma, rhabdomyoma, lipoma) are rare.

Papilloma is the most frequent form of tumour (22 in 54—Albarran and Imbert). The tumour is situated at the junction of the pelvis and ureter, or in the ureter, usually at its lower end, or may extend along the ureter from the pelvis and may protrude into the bladder. The structure and appearance closely resemble papilloma of the bladder. These tumours are simple, but show a tendency to become malignant. The malignant form of papilloma is less frequent than the simple papilloma (16 in 54 cases—Albarran and Imbert), and has the same appearance; but on microscopical examination the tumour cells are found infiltrating the wall of the pelvis or ureter. The growth spreads to the kidney (Fig. 54) and along the ureter, and a graft may be implanted at the orifice of the ureter.

Columnar-celled carcinoma is less frequent and forms a nodular growth. Prolonged inflammation in the renal pelvis or ureter causes transformation of the epithelium into stratified squamous epithelium, and patches of leucoplakia are produced. In this squamous-celled epithelioma may arise. These tumours spread rapidly to neighbouring structures and the lymphatic glands, and form metastases.

When the growth is situated at the outlet of the pelvis or in the ureter the obstruction produces hydronephrosis, and if hæmorrhage occurs this becomes a hæmatonephrosis. Pyonephrosis results if this becomes infected. Wright and Morley record a case of hydronephrosis in a horseshoe kidney caused by a papilloma at the uretero-pelvic junction.

Symptoms.—The symptoms resemble those of growths of the kidney. There is hæmaturia of similar characters, together with pain and tumour. There are attacks of renal retention accompanied by intense renal and ureteral pain and rapid enlargement of the kidney. These variations in size are much greater than are observed in new growths of the kidney.

On cystoscopy a tumour may be seen projecting from the ureter or implanted on the lip of the orifice. When a detached portion is caught at the ureteric orifice it will be passed in the urine in a few days, and a later cystoscopy shows the orifice free from growth. Catheterization of the ureter shows an accumulation of blood and urine in the renal pelvis. Cells characteristic of the growth may be found in the fluid.

Portions of papillomatous growth may be passed in the urine after attacks of renal coho and temporary cessation of hæmorrhage. In a case under my care these fragments had been passed at frequent intervals for four years, and had been pronounced benign in character by an able pathologist. The kidney then began to increase rapidly in size, and I removed a large carcinomatous kidney with papillomatous growth in the pelvis.

Diagnosis.—Diagnosis may be difficult, and has very seldom been made before operation. The most important points are the recognition of an intermittent hæmatonephrosis without other renal symptoms, the demonstration of columnar or squamous epithelium in the fluid, and the discovery with the cystoscope of a tumour projecting from the ureteric orifice.

Where portions of papillomatous growth are passed in the urine after attacks of renal colic and the kidney is enlarged, the diagnosis is readily made.

Prognosis.—The prognosis is grave. Simple papillomas may become malignant, and the malignant growths very frequently recur after removal.

Treatment.—In tumours of the pelvis nephrectomy is indicated, whatever the nature of the growth, and, if the ureter appears to be affected also, nephrectomy should be combined with ureterectomy. When the growth is situated at the lower end of the ureter and the kidney is enlarged, nephrectomy followed by ureterectomy should be done. It may be necessary to remove the lower end of the ureter through the bladder after suprapubic cystotomy. A small growth at the ureteric orifice is removed in the same way as a vesical growth. When the growth in this position is extensive the portion of the bladder wall surrounding the ureterio orifice should be resected, and the ureter drawn into the bladder and cut across beyond the growth and implanted into the bladder wound. If the growth extends far up the ureter it may be necessary to approach it from the outside of the bladder and excise the diseased segment, and then implant the ureter high up in the bladder; and if the growth is still more extensive, nephrectomy should be performed.

Results.—Recurrence has taken place in nearly all the cases that have been followed after operation. Albarran and Giordano have each recorded cases well six years, and Fenwick a case five years, after operation in malignant growths.

LITERATURE

Drew, *Trans. Path. Soc.,* 1897, p. 130.
Heresco, *Ann. d. Mal. d. Org. Gén.- Urin.,* 1901, p. 655.
Legueu, *Traité Chirurgical d' Urologie.* 1910.
Morley, *Lancet,* June 11, 1910.

CHAPTER XIV

CYSTS OF THE KIDNEY

APART from retention cysts of the kidney due to obstruction in the renal pelvis (hydronephrosis, pyonephrosis), there are several varieties of renal cysts, some of which are of doubtful origin. These are as follows :—

Multiple cysts in chronic nephritis.
Dermoid cysts.
Polycystic kidney and congenital cystic kidney.
Solitary cysts or serous cysts.
Hydatid cysts.

Multiple cysts occurring in kidneys the seat of chronic nephritis possess no surgical interest.

DERMOID CYSTS

Dermoid cysts of the kidney are very rare, only 6 or 7 examples —those of Haeckel, Rider Thompson, Madelung, Walker, Biggs, Wyss, and Goldschmidt—being on record. The cases of Haeckel and Rider Thompson originated in the neighbourhood of the renal pelvis. Goldschmidt's case was subcapsular. In the cases of Madelung and Wyss the cysts were calcified and had replaced almost the whole kidney. In a case that came under my observation the patient had previously submitted to an incomplete operation of which I could obtain no details. There was extensive scarring, and a long sinus leading to the region of the left kidney. A large wisp of black hair and a quantity of pultaceous material were removed from a cavity in this region. Some fragments of squamous epithelium were identified in the scrapings from this cavity. The urine was normal, and the bladder and ureteric orifices healthy. The sinus closed.

LITERATURE

Biggs, *New York Path. Soc. Trans.,* vol. lxxxviii.
Goldschmidt, *Surg., Gyn., and Obst.,* 1909, p. 400.
Haeckel, *Berl. klin. Woch.,* 1902, p. 964.
Madelung, *Arch. f. klin. Chir.,* 1887.
Thompson, Rider, *Lancet,* 1906, ii. 1589.
Williams, *Lancet,* 1913, i. 561.

POLYCYSTIC KIDNEY AND CONGENITAL CYSTIC KIDNEY

In this condition the kidney is transformed into a collection of cysts, and has an appearance almost like a bunch of grapes.

Etiology.—Polycystic kidney is sometimes found in several members of a family, and there may be an ancestry of the same disease. In infants affected with polycystic kidney developmental errors have sometimes been noted, such as horseshoe kidney, hare-lip, etc. The disease may be present at birth, and occurs in infants and in adults. It is rarely found between infancy and the age of 21. In adult life it is most common between the ages of 40 and 50. Women are more frequently affected than men in the ratio of 7 to 5, and the left side is slightly more often affected than the right. The disease is bilateral in almost all cases, being more advanced in one kidney. Lejars found that only 2 out of 63 cases in adults were unilateral, and Richie only 2 out of 72 post-mortem examinations.

Pathology.—It is now almost universally held that the polycystic kidney of infants (congenital cystic kidney) and that of adults are identical.

The kidney reaches enormous proportions and may weigh as much as 16 lb. The characteristic outline of the kidney is preserved. The organ is converted into a mass of cysts of varying sizes, some being hardly visible to the naked eye, while others are the size of a cherry or a grape. On the surface the thin walls of the cyst are semi-transparent, and show the clear yellow or brown within. On section the cysts are spread throughout the substance of the kidney, being especially numerous in the cortex and at each pole. In some, fine septa are found, suggesting coalescence of smaller to form larger cysts. The kidney tissue lying between may be indistinguishable with the naked eye.

The cysts contain a clear yellow or sometimes brownish fluid which holds in suspension cortical and columnar epithelial cells, tube casts, red blood-corpuscles, leucocytes, and sometimes uric-acid and calcium oxalate crystals. Urea is present in small quantities, and albumin, phosphates, chlorides, and cholesterin are also constituents.

The kidney may be movable and is sometimes displaced. The renal pelvis is often deformed, and the pyramids are transformed into cysts. Calculi have been found in the pelvis. There may be double ureter, and sometimes small cysts are present on the mucous membrane ; these have also been found in the bladder. The wall of the kidney cysts is formed by connective tissue lined

with columnar cubical or flattened epithelium, which shows proliferation in parts, and the heaping up of epithelium gives the
appearance of papillary formations.

The tissue between the cysts is fibrous, and under the microscope shows tubules and glomeruli compressed and separated by
fibrous tissue. The larger cysts are surrounded by denser fibrous
tissue than that around the smaller.

Cystic changes in the liver are present in 18 per cent. of cases
of polycystic kidney. The liver cysts are due to dilatation of
biliary canals. They are not usually numerous, but occasionally the organ may be much enlarged.

Cystic changes have also been found in a few cases in the pancreas, spleen, thyroid gland, ovaries, uterus, and seminal vesicles.
Hypertrophy of the left ventricle of the heart and arterio-sclerotic
changes are frequently present.

Pathogenesis.—The following theories have been advanced
to explain the development of the cystic changes :—

1. Congenital theory.—The frequent occurrence of polycystic kidney in the new-born, and of concomitant malformations
such as hare-lip, etc., and the occasional appearance of the disease
in several members of one family, give support to this theory.
The congenital lesion has been held to be—

    (*a*) Degeneration of remnants of the Wolffian body.

    (*b*) Unusual feebleness of the tubules leading to dilatation
        by the normal intrarenal pressure.

    (*c*) Failure of union of the excretory canals with the con-
        voluted tubules.

Huber has shown that the excretory canals and convoluted
tubules are developed from separate structures. In the early
embryo there are a renal vesicle and a primary collecting tubule,
which are separate structures, and these become united to form
a single canal, which later becomes convoluted. Should this
union fail to take place, cysts will form from the renal vesicle.
It is significant that the early stage of polycystic disease is found
in the cortex of the kidney, where these developmental changes
take place. This is the most probable of the congenital theories.

2. Inflammation theory.—Virchow held that the cysts result from occlusion of the urinary tubules, caused by inflammation of the interstitial tissue in the papilla of the kidney.
Inflammation of the papilla is, however, seldom found, and experimental evidence shows that artificial papillitis is not followed by
the development of cystic kidney.

The presence of interstitial nephritis has been held to support this theory. It is generally believed, however, that this is

o

the result, and not the cause, of the cystic formation, a view which is supported by the greater density of the sclerosis round the larger than round the smaller cysts.

3. Neoplastic theory.—This theory is supported partly by analogy with cystic tumours elsewhere, and also by certain histological characters. There is excessive proliferation of the cells lining the cysts, and nuclear division is abundant. The tubules may be filled with young cells, and there are papillary ingrowths into the cysts. Transition stages between the solid masses of epithelial cells and the cysts are stated to exist.

At the present time the weight of opinion.appears to favour the congenital and neoplastic theories.

Symptoms.—The congenital form may give rise to difficult labour, on account of the size of the kidney or liver. The large size of the infant's abdomen attracts attention at birth and leads to discovery of the tumour. Death from uræmia takes place soon after birth.

The course of symptoms of polycystic kidney in the adult may be described in three periods :

1. Latent period.
2. Period of renal tumour with symptoms.
3. Period of renal failure.

1. The disease may remain latent or undiscovered until the kidney has attained a large size. The duration of this stage is difficult to estimate, but it may be several years.

2. This period commences with the discovery of the enlarged kidney and the development of symptoms.

Tumour.—Although the disease is almost always bilateral, it is more advanced in one kidney. In most cases, therefore (76 per cent.), the tumour is clinically unilateral.

The tumour may be of very large size. It has the position, contour, and percussion note of a renal tumour. In very thin subjects surface cysts may be recognized on palpation. The kidney is sometimes displaced or unduly movable. It is occasionally tender. Pain is present, but may be late in onset. It is a dull aching in the loin, and there may be attacks of ureteric colic due to the passage of clots.

Changes in the urine are constant. There may be polyuria, amounting to as much as 17½ pints in twenty-four hours. The polyuria may be interrupted by periods of oliguria, or even anuria. The specific gravity is low, and there is frequently, but not inevitably, a trace of albumin. Casts are rarely found. The quantities of urea and urinary salts are diminished. Hæmaturia occurs in 16 per cent. of cases (Luzzato), and is intermittent and slight.

The heart is hypertrophied and the arteries are sclerosed. Œdema of the feet, but not of the eyelids, occurs, and there is no ascites. Pressure upon the bowel produces constipation.

3. In the period of renal failure the urine becomes scanty, anuria supervenes, and symptoms of uræmia develop.

The patient is drowsy and suffers from severe headaches, dyspepsia, vomiting, and diarrhœa. The face is pale, sometimes bronzed, and the body emaciated. Convulsions occur, and the patient dies comatose.

Diagnosis.—When the tumour is bilateral and there are signs of chronic nephritis the diagnosis is easily made. When the tumour is unilateral the diagnosis is difficult. Hydronephrosis is excluded by the variation in size of the hydronephrotic tumour with catheterization of the ureter. A diagnosis of new growth of the kidney will probably be made, but it is impossible to differentiate between cancer, pararenal tumour, hydatid cyst, and polycystic kidney, unless a history of several years' duration, characteristic of polycystic kidney, can be obtained.

Prognosis.—The disease is invariably fatal, but the duration may extend over many years. Jossaud found that the age at death in 47 cases was between 50 and 60, in 17 cases between 60 and 70, in 11 between 70 and 80, and in 2 between 80 and 90.

Treatment.—The disease has been shown to be bilateral in all but the rarest cases, and nephrectomy is contra-indicated on this account. After nephrectomy the disease of the second kidney continues to develop, and the patient dies of renal failure. In polycystic kidney more than in any other disease of the kidney the period of existence of the patient is measured by the amount of active renal tissue, and the removal of a portion of this by nephrectomy can only be called for under the most exceptional conditions of severe pain or violent hæmaturia. The mortality of nephrectomy in 60 cases collected by Seiber was 32·7 per cent The longest survivals were 4 after three years, 1 after five years, 1 after six years, and 2 after seven years.

Nephrotomy with evacuation of the large cysts has been performed for pain, and may be tried in anuria.

LITERATURE

Huber, *Amer. Journ. of Anat., Supplement,* 1904–5, p. 17.
Lejars, Thèse de Paris, 1888.
Luzzato, *La Degenerazione cistica del Rein.* Venice, 1900.
Malassez, *Bull. Soc. Anat.,* 1877, p. 566.
Ritchie, *Lab. Repts. Roy. Coll. Phys. Edin.;* 1892, p. 213.
Seiber, *Deuts. Zeits. f. Chir.,* 1905, p. 495.
Stromberg, *Folia Urol.,* 1909, p. 541.

SOLITARY CYSTS

Large single cysts of the kidney are very rare. They have also been termed " serous " cysts—a misnomer, as in some cases urinary constituents have been found in the fluid contents.

Guinsberg in 1903 could only find 39 cases recorded in the literature. They are rarely (7 cases) bilateral, and each kidney is affected with equal frequency.

Pathology.—The cyst may be found at the upper or the lower pole, or in the body of the organ, and may arise in the cortex

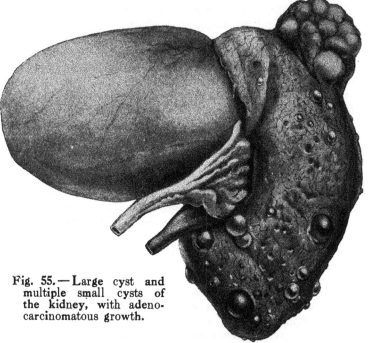

Fig. 55.—Large cyst and multiple small cysts of the kidney, with adeno-carcinomatous growth.

or the medulla. There is usually one cyst, but rarely two or three are present. It is usually the size of a fist or of an orange, but may be larger. A cyst observed by Morris weighed, with its contents, 16 lb., and measured 29 by 26 in. in diameter.

The cyst projects from the surface of the kidney, and its wall consists of a thin, transparent, fibrous membrane in which vessels course. The interior frequently shows the remains of septa indicating the fusion of smaller cysts to form a single large cyst. Occasionally the wall is thick and very hard. It has an incomplete lining of flattened or cubical epithelial cells. At the margin of attachment to the kidney a thin layer of kidney tissue passes for a short distance on to the cyst wall. Except in very rare cases, the cyst does not communicate with the pelvis or the calyces. The cavity contains clear fluid, amber or yellow, in which albumin, chlorides, phosphates, and traces of urea are found. Sometimes blood is mixed with the fluid.

The parenchyma of the kidney in the immediate vicinity of the cyst is compressed and fibrous, but the rest of the kidney is normal.

Cysts in all respects similar to these are found along with numerous small cysts in kidneys which are the seat of chronic interstitial nephritis. Fig. 55 is taken from a kidney removed post mortem from a man, aged 65, who had suffered from enlarged prostate. The kidney was moderately dilated and showed chronic interstitial nephritis with numerous small and one large cyst and an adeno-carcinomatous growth the size of a marble.

A calculus has been found in a solitary cyst (Roche).

Pathogenesis.—The cysts are generally held to be retention cysts, although the ultimate cause is not clear. The fact that large cysts indistinguishable from these solitary cysts are some times found in sclerosed kidneys, and the more frequent occurrence of small cysts in these kidneys, point to sclerosis as the initial lesion.

Brigidi and Severi hold that the cysts arise from the glomeruli or tubules and are due to obstruction caused by desquamated and degenerated cells, sometimes mixed with blood.

Symptoms and diagnosis.—Small cysts and even comparatively large cysts are unrecognized during life, and are found at autopsy.

Large cysts may give rise to pressure symptoms. There is frequently dull, aching, heavy pain in the loin. Récamier records a case in which there was sudden severe lumbar pain and vesical tenesmus caused by a large cyst at the upper pole of the kidney. Œdema of the lower extremities may be produced by pressure on veins, and the intestine may be compressed by a large cyst. The urine shows no change.

Large cysts are very difficult to recognize as originating in the kidney, and are frequently mistaken for ovarian cysts. Smaller cysts are more easily diagnosed as belonging to the kidney. They possess the characters of a renal tumour. Of renal tumours they are most likely to be mistaken for hydronephrosis or new growth, as they may form symptomless renal tumours. The fixed volume, the failure of catheterization of the ureter to empty the tumour, and the injection of collargol (pyelography) into the renal pelvis show that the kidney is not dilated.

Of 52 cases collected by Simon the correct diagnosis was only made in 4. The most frequent mistakes in diagnosis were ovarian cyst (9), movable kidney (5), renal growth (5), cyst of liver (4), and hydronephrosis (2).

Prognosis.—The cysts are benign and unilateral. By continned increase the kidney may be destroyed by compression. Suppuration may in rare instances occur.

Treatment.—After exposure of the kidney by the lumbar route the cyst may be incised and the wall brought up to the surface and stitched to the skin. A permanent fistula occurs in 50 per cent. of cases treated in this way.

Resection of the pouch should be carried out whenever possible. The part which projects beyond the kidney surface should be cut away, and the remaining portion of cyst wall in the substance of the kidney cauterized. This part cannot be dissected from the kidney without lacerating the kidney tissue and causing free hæmorrhage.

Partial nephrectomy consists in removing the part of the kidney containing the cyst. This can be performed when the cyst is situated at one pole, and if the renal pelvis is not opened the wound heals without a fistula. The results of this operation are good. Simon collected 10 cases of partial nephrectomy with 10 recoveries.

Nephrectomy is the usual treatment for large cysts. The results have recently much improved. In 1891 Tuffier found a mortality of 45 per cent. (11 in 24), while in 1903 Albarran found 7 cases of nephrectomy with 7 recoveries.

In large cysts the diagnosis will probably be doubtful and the transperitoneal route undertaken. In small cysts the kidney is approached by the lumbar route.

LITERATURE

Guinsberg, Thèse de Paris, 1903.
Morris, *Surgical Diseases of the Kidney and Ureter,* i. 634. 1901.
Roche, *Ann. d. Mal. d. Org. Gén.-Urin.,* 1895, p. 1139.

HYDATID CYSTS

Hydatid cysts represent the cysticercus stage of the tænia echinococcus, a cestode which inhabits the upper part of the intestinal tract of certain animals, notably the dog, sheep, ox, and pig.

The method of conveyance of the ova to the human being is as follows : The proglottis is shed and discharged with the fæces of the dog or other animal. The ova are then deposited on grass, vegetables, and in water, and may remain viable for a long time, even in the dry state. Uncooked vegetables, such as lettuce, parsley, or watercress, are most likely to convey the ova to the human intestinal tract, or dogs may convey the ova by licking the face or hands. The latter is not, however, a frequent form of contagion, for children are most likely to submit to this demonstration of affection, and they are very rarely affected with hydatid disease. On reaching the stomach the envelope which surrounds the egg is dissolved, and the embryo, by means of six small hooklets, becomes attached to and penetrates the mucous membrane, entering either the blood or the lymphatic stream. It is arrested in the capillaries of the liver in the majority of cases, but may be deposited in any part of the body. The kidney is affected in a very small proportion of cases. Thomas found only 2 renal cases in 307 cases of hydatid disease (0·065 per cent.) in Australia, and Cranwell and Vegas found 36 renal cases in 1,696 in Buenos Ayres (0·021 per cent.). When the embryo becomes arrested in a capillary vessel development of the hydatid cyst commences. The hooklets disappear, and a small cyst slowly forms, the wall of which consists of two layers, an outer fibrous and an inner germinal layer. Outside the cyst wall the reaction of the tissues forms a fibrous layer called the ectocyst. On the inside of the germinal layer groups of small vesicles called brood capsules are formed on narrow pedicles. Inside the brood capsules scolices are formed. The scolex is less than a pin-head in size, and is provided with hooklets and four sucking discs. These hooklets may become diffused in the fluid of the hydatid cyst. In addition to these scolices, daughter cysts resembling the parent cyst in every particular develop from the cyst wall, and may grow outwards or inwards into the cavity of the cyst. The daughter cysts become detached and may fill the parent cyst. They vary in size from a pea to a gooseberry.

The fluid contained in an hydatid cyst is opalescent, it has a specific gravity of 1005 to 1015, and contains albumin, sodium chloride, phosphates, sodium sulphate, succinic acid, and certain toxic bodies of unknown nature.

Etiology.—Hydatid disease is prevalent in some countries and rare in others. In Iceland, Australia, and the Argentine Republic it is common; in Germany, Russia, Austria, and France it is less common; in Great Britain and Ireland it is uncommon, and in the United States and Canada it is rare. In this geographical distribution it is noticeable that dogs are proportionally most numerous and live in most intimate relationship to human beings in Iceland. The disease occurs most frequently between the ages of 20 and 40; it is very rare under the age of 15. Men and women are affected in about equal numbers, and the right kidney as often as the left.

Trauma appears to have some influence in localizing the deposit of the hydatid embryo. Multiple hydatid cysts are very rare.

Pathology.—The embryo is arrested in the capillary plexus of the convoluted tubules, usually at one pole of the kidney. Rarely the cyst develops at the hilum. The growth is slow, but after reaching the size of the fist the cyst may increase rapidly to a large size.

In the neighbourhood of the cyst the kidney tissue is compressed and sclerosed; rarely a large part of the kidney tissue is destroyed by pressure. As the cyst develops it projects from the surface of the kidney and forms adhesions with the neighbouring structures and organs.

The cyst may continue to grow for twenty years or more, giving rise to pressure or other symptoms.

Active growth sometimes ceases and the cyst dies. When this occurs the cyst shrinks, its walls become calcified, the fluid is gradually absorbed, and the contents of the cyst are converted into a putty-like mass. A large cyst may rupture. This most frequently takes place into the pelvis of the kidney, and the contents are discharged down the ureter, the daughter cysts being passed in the urine. The cyst may now collapse and give no further trouble; more commonly, however, it fills up again, and the rupture is repeated after an interval of some years.

Rupture of the cyst into the stomach, the bowel, or the lung may take place. Rarely the contents are discharged into the peritoneal cavity.

Suppuration of the cyst without rupture is very exceptional; it frequently follows rupture, and is a grave complication.

Symptoms.—The first intimation is the discovery of a painless tumour in the lumbar region. The tumour is globular and occupies the position of the kidney. In a favourable subject the kidney may be detected attached to the tumour. There is no movement with respiration. Percussion shows a resonant band on the anterior surface of the tumour if the cyst is of moderate size, but in large cysts the colon is pushed aside and the note is dull. Fluctuation can seldom be detected. A tensely filled cyst is hard like a solid tumour. A hydatid thrill can be elicited in a small number of cases (2 in 30—Houzel). It is obtained by placing one hand flat on the tumour and tapping it sharply with the other.

A sensation of weight and discomfort in the lumbar region is common. In large tumours there may be pain caused by dragging on adhesions or by pressure upon nerves.

Severe colic along the line of the ureter occurs when the cyst ruptures into the renal pelvis and the daughter cysts are discharged into the bladder. The urine is normal except where rupture into the renal pelvis has occurred.

Rupture into the renal pelvis occurs very frequently (104 out of 161 cases—Nicaise). It is accompanied by severe pain in the region of the kidney, and coho along the line of the ureter. There are vomiting and collapse. The urine becomes turbid and alkaline and contains small hydatid cysts, complete or ruptured, scolices, hooklets, fat droplets, and sometimes blood. There may be difficulty in passing the cysts through the urethra, causing frequent micturition, straining, and sometimes retention of urine. These symptoms may continue intermittently for several days, and then cease. Sometimes the cyst is completely emptied and spontaneous cure is established; usually, however, the cyst refills, and recurrence of the rupture and its attendant symptoms takes place after a year or more. Boeckel found that 6 cases out of 29 recovered after rupture into the renal pelvis. More frequently inflammation with suppuration follows the rupture. Rupture may also take place into the stomach or intestine, with subsequent suppuration of the sac.

Rupture into the peritoneal cavity is usually the result of external violence. Acute peritonitis may immediately result and prove fatal, or a more chronic form of peritonitis may supervene. Multiple secondary cysts are sometimes formed in the peritoneum, arising directly from scolices which have been disseminated. Rupture of a hydatid may be followed by symptoms of toxæmia which are believed to result from the absorption of toxins contained in the hydatid fluid. The temperature is high, and there is general urticaria. In severe cases there are convulsions.

Suppuration in the hydatid cyst occurs after rupture into the pelvis or elsewhere.

Diagnosis.—The diagnosis is that of other renal tumours. When the tumour is small the diagnosis is easily made, but with large tumours it may be extremely difficult.

When the tumour has been localized to the kidney, the differential diagnosis from a solid growth or from other cystic conditions of the kidney is also attended with great difficulty. The hydatid tumour is of very slow growth, and is unaccompanied by attacks of pain, nor does it show variations in size or changes in the urine, which would point to hydronephrosis. Catheterization of the ureters and pyelography further exclude dilatation of the kidney.

From polycystic kidney or a large solitary cyst the diagnosis is more difficult. Polycystic kidney may be bilateral clinically, while hydatid and solitary cysts are unilateral. The patient may have been exposed to contagion, a hydatid thrill may be detected, and, if the cyst has ruptured into the renal pelvis, cysts and hooklets are found in the urine.

The blood in cases of hydatid cyst may show an eosinophilia amounting to 40 per cent.

Recently the reaction known as "fixation of the complement" has been employed for the diagnosis of hydatid cysts, and has given important results.

Course and prognosis.—The disease may last for twenty years or more, giving rise only to symptoms of pressure on neighbouring organs. Spontaneous cure occurs rarely. The slow destruction of renal tissue is compensated by hypertrophy of the second kidney, and does not affect the prognosis unless, as has exceptionally occurred, the hydatid cyst develops in a solitary kidney.

Suppuration of the cyst and rupture are serious and often fatal complications.

Treatment.—Only operative measures need be considered.

Nephrectomy.—This should only be performed when it is impossible to adopt more conservative measures. The cases suitable for nephrectomy are those in which the kidney is totally or almost totally destroyed by a large cyst, and those in which the cyst develops in the hilum of the kidney, involving the renal vessels and making the removal of the cyst alone a more dangerous proceeding than nephrectomy. Where suppuration of the cyst has extended to the kidney, nephrectomy may be advisable; and where the cyst has ruptured into the intestine, peritoneum, or lung, the kidney should be removed.

The operation may be rendered extremely difficult by widespread adhesions, and it is sometimes wiser, on account of the danger of hæmorrhage, to be content with less radical measures.

In 42 nephrectomies Nicaise found a mortality of 19 per cent. due to the operation. Lumbar nephrectomy was less fatal than transperitoneal.

Resection, or partial nephrectomy.—This operation is applicable only in small cysts situate at the poles or on the convex border. The kidney is exposed by a lumbar incision, the renal vessels are controlled by pressure, and the kidney is incised immediately outside the ectocyst, cutting through kidney tissue.

When the cyst has been removed the raw surfaces are stitched together with catgut. Nicaise collected 14 cases with 3 deaths.

Nephrostomy, or marsupialization.—The cyst is exposed by a lumbar incision, and part of the fluid is aspirated so that the flaccid wall of the cyst can be drawn through the wound. The cyst is opened and washed out, and as much as possible of the wall clipped away. The edges are then sutured to the skin and a drain introduced. The pouch is washed out daily with iodine or other antiseptic solution. The drain should be removed about the fourth day, and the wound allowed to heal. The mortality of this operation, according to Nicaise, is 6·12 per cent.

In order to minimize the risk of suppuration after an operation such as nephrostomy, Delbet suggests that as much as possible of the cyst wall should be removed and the opposing surfaces stitched together with catgut. The edges of the ectocyst are then brought together and sutured.

LITERATURE

Boeckel, *Étude sur les Kystes Hydatiques du Rein.* Paris, 1887.
Cranwell and Vegas, *Revista de la Sociedad Medica Argentina,* 1904,
Finsen, *Arch. Gén. de Méd.,* 1869, i. 29. [xii. 215.
Gardner, *Intercolon. Quart. Journ. Med. and Surg.,* 1894-5, i. 147.
Houzel, *Rev. de Chir.,* 1898, xviii. 703.
Kermisse, *Arch. Gén. de Méd.,* 1883, ii. 516.
Marchat, Thèse de Paris, 1901.
Nicaise, Thèse de Paris, 1905.
Thomas, *Lancet,* 1879, i. 297.

CHAPTER XV

PERIRENAL AND SUPRARENAL TUMOURS

PERIRENAL TUMOURS

THESE tumours are of rare occurrence, but they present a very large variety of structure. Many of them are tumours developing in the retroperitoneal tissue, and their relation to the kidney is accidental. Others develop from vestigial remains around the kidney, and some arise in the kidney capsule.

Pathology.—The tumours are solid or cystic. Of the solid tumours, the varieties of lipoma are most frequently observed. These are pure lipoma, fibro-lipoma, myxo-lipoma, fibro-myxo-lipoma. There are also fibroma and fibro-myoma developing in relation to the fibrous capsule of the kidney, which contains non-striped muscle fibres. These tumours are usually small, but in rare cases attain a large size.

Fig. 56 is drawn from a large fibro-myoma or leio-myoma which I removed together with the kidney from a woman aged 56. The tumour springs from the tissues in the hilum of the left kidney. The patient was alive and well three years after the operation.

Sarcoma occurs as pure sarcoma or fibro-sarcoma, angio-sarcoma, and some other varieties. The sarcomas early form adhesions with neighbouring structures.

Mixed tumours are rare, only a few cases being on record. The structure resembles that of mixed tumours of the kidney. They arise in remains of the Wolffian body.

Cysts may be unilocular or multilocular. Unilocular cysts contain clear yellow fluid, in which urea and uric acid are some-times found. A cyst communicating with the renal pelvis has been observed. Polycystic tumours have been described. The cystic tumours are believed to arise in the remains of the Wolffian body, or, according to Rambaud, in detached portions of the embryonic peritoneum which have become included in the peri-renal tissues.

Perirenal tumours may acquire a large volume. When they arise from the fibrous capsule of the kidney they are firmly adherent to the kidney. Those originating in the fatty capsule are not adherent to the kidney, but the organ is buried in the growth. Atrophy of the kidney from pressure and obstruction of the ureter may occur. Cysts rarely form adhesions to surrounding struetures, but sarcomas and fibromas become early and densely adherent to the peritoneum and intestine. Necrosis with false cyst formation, fatty degeneration, and calcification may take place in the solid tumours. The colon is pushed forwards by the

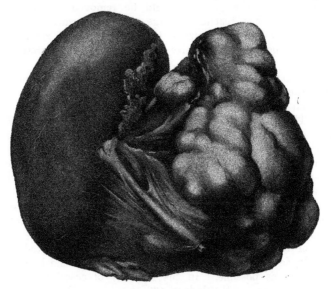

Fig. 56.—Fibro-myoma arising from hilum of kidney.
Operation specimen.

growth, the bulk of which may be either internal or external to the large bowel.

Symptoms.—Tumour is the only constant symptom. It is of very slow growth in all except the sarcomas. Situated in the loin, the tumour has the colon in front of it. The contour is irregular. The consistence depends upon the nature of the growth. Fibromas are hard, while lipomas are soft and frequently give a sensation of fluctuation.

Pain may be present, but is inconstant. Constipation results from pressure on the colon, and œdema, ascites, and varicocele from pressure on veins.

The urine is normal unless nephritis be present as a complication.

Diagnosis.—The slow, painless growth and the position in the loin and relation to the colon, together with the absence of urinary symptoms, are the points on which the diagnosis rests.

The nature of the growth cannot be diagnosed, with the exception of sarcoma, which is of extremely rapid growth.

The growths are most likely to be mistaken for malignant tumours of the kidney or suprarenal gland, hydronephrosis, ovarian tumours, or tumours of the liver, mesentery, or pancreas.

Treatment.—The growth should be removed in the early stage before it has reached a large size and formed extensive adhesions. In smaller growths the lumbar route should be chosen ; in those of larger size a transperitoneal operation is necessary.

In the latter operation the surgeon exposes the tumour by incising the peritoneum on the outer side of the colon, so that there is no interference with the blood supply of this part of the bowel. The colon is then dissected inwards off the growth. The tumour is usually limited by the perirenal fascia, and the dissection is more easily carried on within this. The chief danger is hæmorrhage, which may result from injury to the renal vessels, the spermatic vessels, or the superior or inferior mesenteric vessels, all of which, at some part of their course, lie within the perirenal fascia. The growth is most readily attacked from the lower end, which is less vascular, while its relations are less complicated. Portions of the growth may be removed to allow of easier dissection of the remainder. The kidney should be isolated and, if possible, saved. In any case the renal vessels should be identified as soon as possible. In the majority of cases it is found necessary to remove the kidney (66 per cent.—Hartmann and Lecène).

Sarcoma and fibroma form dense adhesions ; on this account they are more difficult to remove than cysts, which shell out with greater facility.

The mortality of the operation has been reduced in operations performed since 1890 to 6 per cent. The after-results depend upon the nature of the growth. Pure lipomas, fibromas, and cysts do not recur, but mixed tumours and sarcomas recur within a short time.

LITERATURE

Adler, *Berl. klin. Woch.*, March 20, 1893.
Albarran et **Imbert,** *Les Tumeurs du Rein.* Paris, 1902.
Bork, *Arch. f. klin. Chir.*, 1901, p. 928.
Hartmann et Lecène, *Travaux de Chir. Anat. Clin.*, Paris, 1903.
Rambaud, Thèse de Toulouse, 1903.

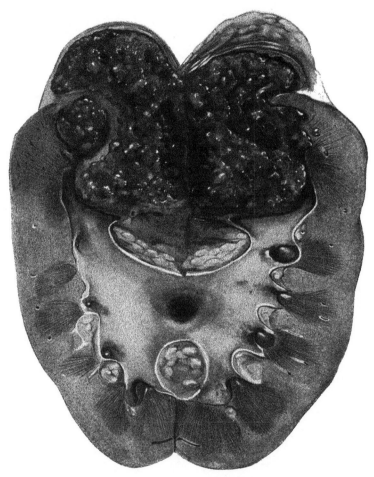

W. THORNTON SHIELLS.

Hypernephroma of suprarenal capsule invading kidney; operation
specimen. (P. 223.)

PLATE 12.

TUMOURS OF THE SUPRARENAL GLAND

Growths arising in the suprarenal gland are rare, and are slightly more frequent in the adult male than in the female.

The nomenclature of these tumours is in a state of confusion. For the purpose of clearness, and in order to avoid nomenclature which implies an origin of the growths in one or other of the embryonic layers, the term hypernephroma will be used for those growths which resemble the suprarenal gland in structure, and terms such as adenoma, carcinoma, sarcoma, will be eschewed. Isolated examples of the following tumours have been described, viz. glioma, neuroma, glio-fibro-myoma, angioma, lymphangioma, lipoma, and cysts.

The most common form of new growth in the suprarenal gland has the histological characters of the gland. (Plate 12.) Both benign and malignant hypernephroma are described, the latter showing a great preponderance.

These hypernephromas have the histological character of the cortex of the gland. There is a framework of capillary blood-vessels upon which polygonal cells are directly set. The cells adjacent to the capillary wall are regularly arranged, those more distant are irregularly packed together. In the meshes of the vascular network the cells become arranged in alveolar form or in long columns. The cells are large and polygonal in shape, and have a large nucleus, and the protoplasm is frequently vacuolated, the vacuoles having originally contained fat. Rarely, melanotic granules are found in the protoplasm. The tumours are single or multiple. They are rounded, and possess a fibrous capsule which sends supporting septa into the interior of the growth. They have the characteristic yellow colour of suprarenal tissue, and frequently show hæmorrhages in the tumour substance.

The benign tumours are small in size, and may be single or multiple. The cells are smaller, more uniform in size, and more regularly arranged in long, narrow columns.

The cells of the malignant hypernephroma are less uniform and may show great irregularity in size, shape, and arrangement. They may attain the size of a small melon. Metastases take place by the blood stream, and deposits are found in the lungs, bones, and liver.

In the malignant growths portions may be observed which have the appearance described as characteristic of the benign growths, and transition forms are found.

Etiology.—New growths of the adrenals are found both in

adults and in children. About one-third occur in infancy and childhood. Garceau gives a list of 25 cases in children, 19 of which occurred in infants and children of 4 years and under. Females are more frequently affected at this age, and the left side more often than the right. .

Symptoms.—The symptomatology consists in certain general symptoms and the appearance of an abdominal tumour. Hæmaturia is very rare (2·9 per cent.—Ramsay), and when it occurs is due to passive congestion of the kidney from involvement of the renal vein.

Progressive emaciation is the most characteristic feature of the disease. There are loss of strength and weight, and profound anæmia. Anorexia, vomiting, constipation, and sometimes œdema are observed.

The pigmentary changes characteristic of complete destruction of the adrenal tissue as seen in tuberculous disease are very rarely observed. Ramsay found bronzing of the skin in 3 out of 37 cases, but in 9 others there was brownish discoloration of the skin.

In children there is the same emaciation, and there may also be an arrest of mental development, the child being dull and stupid.

Certain changes in regard to growth and development are of extreme interest. There may be unilateral hypertrophy. Hutchinson has recorded the case of a male child of 4 years in which there was hypertrophy of the left thigh, leg, and arm, and of the paired organs on the same side. Precocious puberty is a frequent characteristic of hypernephroma in children. In Garceau's list it occurred in 10 out of 25 cases. There is excessive growth of hair on the face, pubes, and elsewhere. Early and excessive development of the genital organs occurs in either sex, and abnormal development of the clitoris may lead to an erroneous diagnosis of hermaphroditism.

In the earlier stages a tumour is not detected, as it lies high up under the ribs. Later a tumour can be detected in the hypochondriac region. The bowel lies in front of it, and gives a tympanitic note. The kidney may sometimes be recognized pushed down by the growth, and occasionally a distinct groove between the kidney and growth may be detected. The tumour appears at the level of the 8th and sometimes the 7th costal cartilage, and extends towards the middle line.

Extreme mobility of the tumour is, according to Morris, a diagnostic point of some importance.

Pain is usually present, and is referred along nerves, and sometimes to distant parts of the body.

In a considerable proportion of cases there are no symptoms directly pointing to the seat of growth, which may remain unsuspected, and only be revealed by post-mortem examination.

In children the first sign may be a secondary growth in the bones, the orbit being frequently affected.

Diagnosis.—The majority of cases, when a tumour appears, have been diagnosed as renal growths.

The most characteristic features of suprarenal growths are the absence of changes in the urine, the early and extreme emaciation, pigmentary and developmental changes, and the appearance of the tumour at the level of the 7th or 8th costal cartilage and its growth towards the middle line, whereas growths of the kidney appear at the costal margin between the 9th and 11th costal cartilages. The lower border of the suprarenal growth, fused with the kidney, is broad and almost horizontal; suprarenal tumours are very mobile. The injection of collargol into the renal pelvis and subsequent radiographic examination (pyelography) is a very important means of distinguishing between suprarenal and renal growths. Rarely suprarenal growths have been mistaken for tumours of the liver or gall-bladder.

Prognosis.—The growth of hypernephroma is rapid, and metastases take place early. The average duration of life after the first onset of symptoms is from six to ten months (Ramsay).

Treatment.—Early removal of the tumour, together with the kidney, is the only radical method of treatment. There is danger of severe hæmorrhage and of opening the pleural cavity during the separation of adhesions.

Morris collected 11 cases of removal of suprarenal tumours with 5 deaths and 6 recoveries. Of the latter only one patient was known to be alive eighteen months after the operation, and most of them died in a few months from recurrence. In children the operation is peculiarly fatal.

LITERATURE

Bulloch and Sequeira, *Trans. Path. Soc. Lond.*, 1905, lvi. 157.
Ferrier et Lecène, *Rev. de Chir.*, 1906, xxvi. 325.
Garceau, *Tumours of the Kidney.* 1909.
Hutchinson, *Quart. Journ. of Med.*, 1907, i. 33.
Israel, *Deuts. med. Woch.*, 1905, xxxi. 746.
Linser, *Beitr. z. klin. Chir.*, 1903, xxxvii. 296.
Morris, *Surgical Diseases of the Kidney and Ureter*, ii. 14. 1901.
Ramsay, *Johns Hopkins Hosp. Bull.*, 1899, p. 25.

CHAPTER XVI

INFECTIVE DISEASES

TUBERCULOSIS OF THE KIDNEY AND URETER

TUBERCULOSIS of the urinary organs may occur without other active foci of tubercle being present in the body, or it may be secondary to active tuberculosis of the genital system, or to tuberculosis of some other organ such as the lung.

The combination of genital and urinary tuberculosis is very frequently met with in the male, rarely in the female.

Tuberculosis of the kidney is said to be primary or secondary. In the strict sense primary tuberculosis of the kidney does not occur as it does in the lung. There is always a focus in some other part of the body. The term is used in the narrower sense that the kidney is the primary focus in the urinary system.

Renal tuberculosis occurs (1) as a part of an acute miliary tuberculosis, both kidneys being strewn with miliary tubercles; (2) as a tuberculous infiltration of the kidney

Miliary tuberculosis occurs in early childhood and as an insignificant part of a general tuberculous infection. It has no surgical interest.

Tuberculous infiltration of the kidney forms about 10 per cent. of tuberculous infections.

Method of infection.—The tubercle bacilli reach the kidney by one of three paths :

    1. Ascending.

    2. Hæmatogenous.

    3. Lymphatic.

1. Ascending infection (*secondary renal tuberculosis*). — Ascending infection was long regarded as the usual method of infection of the kidney. This view was based upon the occurrence of early symptoms of cystitis and supported by some postmortem examinations and the results of experiments.

Albarran produced tuberculosis of the kidney by injecting tubercle bacilli into the ureter after ligature of the duct, and Wildbolz more recently obtained similar results without ligature. On the other hand, Giani could not produce ascending tuberculosis by introducing tubercle bacilli into the bladder, and Brongersma has shown clinically that vesical tuberculosis may remain limited to the bladder, without ascending to the kidney, during a period of twelve years. Hallé and Motz have been unable to find a single clinical or pathological example which proved that ascending infection had taken place. It is, therefore, doubtful if ascending infection takes place at all. Within the kidney itself, according to Ekehorn, ascending may be found along with descending lesions. From a single focus of hæmatogenous origin in the renal tissue the bacteria enter the canaliculi, cause ulceration of the papillæ, and spread upwards towards the base of the pyramid along the lymphatics.

2. **Hæmatogenous infection** (*descending infection, primary infection*).—Experiments by Albarran show that if tubercle bacilli are injected hypodermically and the ureter of one kidney is ligatured, tuberculosis develops in this kidney; and this has been confirmed by other observers.

Clinically, tuberculosis of the kidney is very frequently found without vesical tuberculosis, and the after-history of cases of nephrectomy shows that the original focus was in the kidney. Pathological specimens also show primary tuberculosis of the kidney without any other lesion of the urinary organs.

3. **Lymphatic infection.**—Brongersma holds that lymphatic is more probable than hæmatogenous or ascending infection. He believes that the primary tuberculous focus is situated in the thorax. In 62 out of 71 cases of renal tuberculosis there were symptoms of tuberculosis of the lung or pleura on the same side as the affected kidney. Infection of the kidney takes place through the mediastinal lymphatic glands, and by a retrograde lymph current produced by pleural adhesions the bacilli pass to the renal lymphatics. This, he believes, explains the unilateral distribution of renal tuberculosis.

The more frequent occurrence of bilateral caseous tuberculosis in children is explained by the occurrence of bilateral tuberculous thoracic glands in children and the comparatively large size of the lymphatic vessels.

A history of bygone pleurisy is certainly frequently obtained in cases of renal tuberculosis, but I have not seldom found that the pleurisy was on the side opposite to the renal tuberculosis.

Of the three paths of infection there is more evidence in favour of the hæmatogenous than of the others. The ascending form, although it has been proved experimentally to be possible, is very rare clinically, if indeed it occurs at all.

Etiology.—Renal tuberculosis is most frequent between the ages of 20 and 40. It is uncommon in childhood and rare in old age. Women are more frequently affected than men in the proportion of 33 to 15 (Kümmel).

Renal tuberculosis is unilateral in the earlier and very frequently bilateral in the late stages. This accounts for some discrepancy between the statistics of different observers. Krönlein states that 92 per cent. and Leguen 85 per cent. of cases are unilateral, and clinical evidence obtained by catheterization of the ureters and the results of nephrectomy certainly supports this view. Such statements must always be subject to the qualification that they apply to the early stage of the disease. In the late stage the disease in a large proportion of the cases is bilateral, although Hallé and Motz found 89 unilateral out of 131 postmortem examinations, which may be taken to represent the late stage of the disease.

Experimental evidence goes to show that injury to a kidney will determine the development of tuberculosis in that organ. This is not borne out by clinical experience. Although a few patients may give a history of a blow on the loin, it is not certain that the disease was not already present; and, further, the development of tuberculosis in a kidney which is known to have been ruptured is very rare, nor do I know of any instance in which a kidney that has been explored by nephrotomy and found healthy has afterwards developed tuberculosis.

The right kidney is rather more often affected than the left, and this, together with the fact that women are more liable to the disease, and that the right kidney in the female is more frequently movable, has led to the supposition that undue mobility may have damaged the kidney and led to the deposit of tubercle. The proportion of movable tuberculous kidneys is, however, very small (5 per cent.—Küster).

The tubercle bacillus is present alone in the majority of cases, but there may be secondary infections with the bacillus coli, the streptococcus, or the staphylococcus albus.

Pathological anatomy.—A large number of types of tuberculous kidney have been described, most of which are merely stages of development of the same process without any fundamental difference. The following have outstanding features which permit of their being described as varieties of tuberculous kidney:

1. **Miliary tuberculosis.**—Apart from the acute bilateral miliary tuberculosis which is of no surgical interest, some authors have described a chronic unilateral miliary tuberculosis in which the kidney is strewn with small greyish-yellow tubercles. In a

W. THORNTON SHIELLS.

Tuberculosis of kidney, ulcero-cavernous type; operation specimen. Disease confined to upper branch of pelvis; ulceration of apices of pyramids, with secondary miliary tubercles in cortex. Note great fibrous thickening and contraction at neck of branch of pelvis, an attempt to shut off this segment. (P. 229.)

PLATE 13.

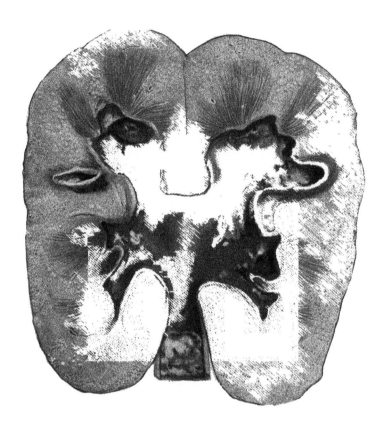

Acute tuberculosis of kidney with mixed infection; operation
specimen. Ulcero-cavernous form affecting whole of pyramids,
also pelvis and ureter; extensive secondary miliary tuberculosis.
(P. 229.)

PLATE 14.

large proportion of the ulcero-cavernous form there are miliary tubercles in varying numbers in the cortex or the medulla, and this is the only form of miliary tuberculosis of the kidney which is seen surgically.

2. **Ulcero-cavernous form.**—This is the most common form of surgical tuberculosis of the kidney. It consists essentially in progressive destruction by ulceration from the pelvis outwards towards the surface of the kidney substance, and the organ is not enlarged.

In the earliest form there is intense congestion and commencing ulceration at the apex of a pyramid (Plate 13) at the upper or lower pole. The ulceration progresses from apex to base of pyramid until the pyramid is entirely scooped out. Several pyramids may be attacked, and the tissues between either become thickened so as to produce separate pockets, or are broken down to form a larger cavity. (Plate 14.) The cavity is lined with an irregular caseous layer, outside of which is a narrow greyish layer, and beyond this a zone of intense congestion. In the cortex corresponding to these pyramids, and sometimes also in the columns of Bertini between them, solitary grey tubercles or groups of tubercles are dotted: There may be a single group, or the whole cortex may be strewn with them. The area of ulceration usually corresponds to the area over which the tubercles are distributed. In some examples of this form of kidney these tubercles are absent.

In almost all kidneys thus attacked examination will show an attempt to shut off the tuberculous area from the rest of the pelvis by fibrous thickening and contraction of the mouth of a calyx or of a large branch of the pelvis into which several ulcerated calyces open (Plate 13), or of the pelvo-ureteral junction. The communication between the diseased part of the pelvis and the remaining part may be very narrow. It may be completely obliterated, and a partial or total hydronephrosis results.

Commencing ulceration may be found at the apex of a pyramid at the lower pole, with advanced ulceration at the upper pole. Microscopically the wall of the cavity shows an inner layer of caseous material, a middle layer of tubercles with giant cells, and an outer layer of renal tissue infiltrated with round cells. The whole kidney, or one pole only, may be much enlarged. On the surface the diseased part is seen as rounded bosses, which are soft to the touch. In the early stage the kidney may appear normal on the surface, or there may be a group of small yellow tubercles immediately under the fibrous capsule.   •

· 3. **Caseous or massive tuberculosis of the kidney.**—This is a much less common form. The kidney substance is replaced by large irregular or rounded masses of yellowish-white caseous material of putty-like consistence. The tissue separating these is fibrous, and bacilli are rarely found. This is an obsolete, very advanced form of the ulcero-cavernous type, and is a variety of tuberculous hydronephrosis. -(Plate 17.)

4. Tuberculous hydronephrosis.—Where the thickening and contraction of the wall of one segment of the pelvis or of a single calyx continues to the point of obliteration, or where the same process develops at the outlet of the ureter, a partial or total tuberculous hydronephrosis results. (Plate 15.) The fluid contained in the pockets is pale, and turbid with flakes of tuberculous débris. The lining of the cavities is irregular and of greyish-white colour, and beyond this, separating the pockets and enclosing the whole, is a dull greyish-brown fibrous wall. (Plate 15.) When a partial hydronephrosis develops, the rest of the kidney may be the seat of the ulcero-cavernous type of disease.

Both this and the preceding form (3) are " closed," i.e. shut off from the rest of the urinary tract, so that there may be no clinical evidence of renal tuberculosis.

Infection of the tuberculous hydronephrosis will produce a pyonephrosis.

A polycystic renal tuberculosis in which the renal substance is transformed into very numerous small cysts separated by sclerosed renal tissue has been described, but is very rare.

5. Toxic lesions of the kidney.—Acute nephritis, parenchymatous nephritis, interstitial nephritis, and waxy disease of the kidney are observed in the kidneys of tuberculous patients. These lesions are due to the action of the toxin of the tubercle bacillus on the kidney. They may be found in the kidneys when the tuberculous focus is elsewhere in the body, or may be present in the non-ulcerated and non-caseous part of the tuberculous kidney, or in the second kidney.

It has recently been shown by Lecène that a fibrous form of nephritis may be directly caused by the tubercle bacillus, with the production of giant cells, but without any trace of caseation.

6. Lesions of the renal pelvis and ureter.—The pelvis of the kidney becomes involved in all cases. Inflammation of varying severity, with ulceration, extends from the part of the pelvis draining the diseased segment of the kidney to the general cavity. One or more calyces 'of the pelvis may be affected and the rest be apparently normal, the disease reappearing at the upper end of the ureter and extending down that duct. Again, there may be a small portion of the upper part of the pelvis affected and the rest healthy, except a single calyx at the lower pole.

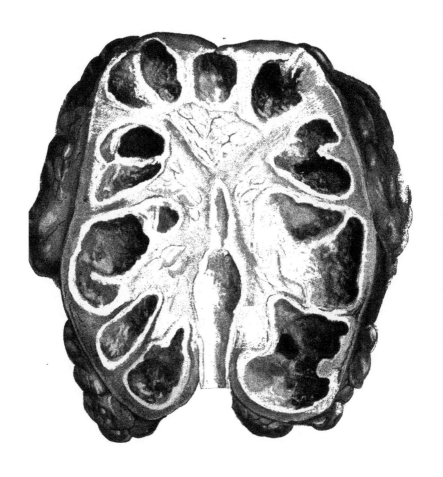

Tuberculosis of kidney, final stage : tuberculous hydronephrosis.
(P. 230.)

PLATE 15.

The whole pelvis may be ulcerated and inflamed.

When one branch of the pelvis is affected, the wall may become greatly thickened and cartilaginous at the outlet of the diseased into the healthy portion, and the communication between these may be very narrow. Further narrowing will cause a partial hydronephrosis. Stenosis of the upper end of the ureter causes distension of the pelvis and kidney, and complete tuberculous hydronephrosis, which is completely shut off from the bladder. The fatty tissue around the pelvis becomes greatly increased, sclerosed, and adherent.

7. **Lesions of the ureter.**—The ureter is infected with tubercle bacilli conveyed by the urine. Superficial ulcers of the mucous membrane may be found scattered along the lumen of the tube. More frequently, however, there are extensive changes in the wall of the duct. It is thickened to the size of the little finger, hard and rigid. On section there is a thick, hard, fibrous ring, and inside this the diseased mucous membrane, which shows extensive ulceration. The lumen is small and filled with tuberculous débris. Sometimes the lumen is completely blocked with masses of caseous material. The ureter is adherent to the peritoneum. There may be one or more patches of tuberculous ulceration in the course of the ureter, and the rest of the tube normal.

8. **Lesions of the perirenal tissues.**—The fatty capsule is greatly thickened, coarse, fibrous, and densely adherent to the surrounding structures. The fat at the hilum and along the renal vessels, and along the aorta and inferior vena cava, is also fibrous and adherent, and occasionally enlarged glands, discrete or in masses, are found adherent to these vessels.

On microscopical section giant-cell systems are found in the perirenal fat (Leguen).

9. **Condition of the second kidney.**—Bilateral tuberculosis is found in a certain proportion of cases (see p. 228). The infection may very rarely reach the second kidney by ascending from the bladder which has become tuberculous. The usual method is by the blood stream.

Where the second kidney has not become infected by the tubercle bacillus, toxic lesions may be present (see p. 230).

Symptoms. 1. Vesical symptoms. — The symptoms of tuberculosis of the kidney, through nearly the whole course of the disease, may be entirely confined to the bladder.

It is a frequent experience, when examining patients whose only trouble has been cystitis of a mild grade, to find one kidney, and occasionally both, the seat of advanced tuberculosis.

The symptoms of cystitis commence insidiously with gradually increasing frequency of micturition. At first there is increased frequency and urgency of micturition during the day only, but later there is nocturnal frequency, and this increases until the patient passes water during the night as often as, or more frequently than, during the day. Finally, there may be nocturnal incontinence. Bazy regards this nocturnal frequency as a very important sign of inflammation of the kidney. There is some scalding on micturition, and often pain towards the end of the act. Occasionally there is a slight terminal hæmaturia.

2. **Changes in the urine.**—*Polyuria* is an early symptom of tuberculosis, and it may be proved, by ureteral catheterization, to exist only on the diseased side. It is said to be more marked at night. The urine is very pale and opalescent, faintly acid or neutral, and hazy with a small amount of well-mixed pus. It is lacking in pigment to a greater degree than one would expect from the amount of the polyuria. *Hæmaturia* is a variable symptom. It may be entirely absent or only present in microscopic quantities. There may be slight persistent terminal hæmaturia with vesical symptoms, and here the blood emanates from the bladder. In some cases there is an outburst of hæmorrhage at the beginning of the illness, occasionally before other symptoms have appeared. I have observed an attack of hæmaturia as long as two years before the onset of other symptoms. This initial hæmaturia was probably due to congestion of the organ; occasionally it is due to a focus of tubercle which becomes temporarily shut off from the pelvis. Severe hæmaturia may also occur during the course of the disease, and usually follows some strain or injury. It may be the dominant symptom and necessitate operation. *Albuminuria* may be present before the appearance of pyuria, when the urine is still clear (Bazy). This premonitory albuminuria may come from the sound kidney as well as from the diseased organ (Leguen). The urine contains pus and sometimes blood corpuscles, and tube casts may also be present. The percentage of urea and chlorides is reduced.

3. **Pain.**—There may be no history of pain in a kidney which is completely destroyed by tuberculosis. Aching pain is sometimes complained of, and the patient may not be able to lie on the affected side.

Reno-ureteral coho is sometimes present from the passage of clots or débris, or from the blockage of a ureter by further swelling of a thick mucous membrane. Pain at the neck of the bladder and at the tip of the penis at the end of micturition, and scalding along the urethra, are due to cystitis.

Examination of · kidney and ureter.—On examination of the abdomen the kidney is not usually enlarged. If it can be felt it is sometimes hard and somewhat irregular. The kidney is frequently tender. In the late stages the kidney may be small and shrunken so that it cannot be detected. The organ is occasionally felt to be enlarged. In this case ·there is usually hypertrophy from destruction of the second kidney, or partial or complete hydronephrosis.

There is frequently tenderness along the line of the ureter, and the duct can be felt as a thick cord on deep palpation of the abdomen.· Per rectum in the male a thick tender cord can be felt above the prostate, and passing outwards and upwards to the side of the pelvis. In the vagina the thick tuberculous ureter can readily be detected passing outwards from near the middle .of the anterior vaginal wall, and it can be rolled beneath the finger on the lateral wall of the vagina.

·The second kidney in unilateral tuberculosis may be enlarged, painful and tender from hypertrophy, with or without commencing tuberculosis.

· There is usually progressive loss of weight and lassitude, which are partly explained by the disturbed sleep consequent upon the frequent micturition.

Course and prognosis.—The onset of symptoms of uncomplicated tuberculosis of the kidney is insidious and the course slow. When the symptoms have become fully established, fluctuations are frequently observed. For months the symptoms abate, and the patient may apparently improve, only to relapse later. These fluctuations are due to external influences such as climate, surroundings, and diet, and in a measure also to the tendency to which I have pointed for the disease to become partly shut off by fibrous contraction from the rest of the renal pelvis. In some cases the symptoms cease and the pus and tubercle bacilli disappear from the urine. Recurrence of symptoms takes place after some months or even several years (in one case after eleven years), and may follow a blow or some exciting cause. On the whole, however, there is gradual advance of the disease until death takes place several years (four to seven or even ten) after the first symptoms. It is generally accepted that spontaneous cure of tuberculosis of the kidney can only occur in the most exceptional cases, and that the disease progresses until the organ is completely destroyed.

· Where septic infection is superadded the progress is much more rapid. Infection may be hæmatogenous, but most frequently follows infection of the bladder, the result of sounding or of irrigation. Fever appears, and the ureter may become blocked and pyonephrosis develop.

The dangers of renal tuberculosis are that it may spread to the bladder, that the second kidney may become affected with tuberculosis or nephritis, that the tuberculous infection may involve other organs, or that septic infection may follow.

Death takes place from anuria when both kidneys are invaded, or from exhaustion when septic infection is superadded.

Diagnosis.—It is necessary first to make a diagnosis of tuberculosis of the kidney and then to examine the extent of the disease.

Type I : symptoms of cystitis with pyuria and detection of the tubercle bacillus in the urine.—This is the most frequent clinical type. The symptoms of cystitis appear insidiously in a young patient, are persistent and increasing. A bacteriologist accustomed to the examination of urine for the tubercle bacillus seldom fails to discover the bacillus, which may be present in very small numbers or may be abundant and sometimes in chain-like form.

The bacillus may be found in the urine of tuberculous patients without urinary tuberculosis being present. The existence of pyuria and hæmaturia and of other signs is sufficient to differentiate these cases from those of tuberculous bacilluria. The tuberculin reaction obtained by subcutaneous injection or by rubbing tuberculin into an excoriation, or the ophthalmic reaction of Calmette, may be useful, but I have seldom obtained any help from these methods where any real doubt existed.

One kidney may be enlarged or tender, and the ureter is thick and tender.

Cystoscopy may show that the bladder is healthy and that the vesical symptoms are reflex. On the other hand, there may be cystitis, and the examination is then more difficult. A general cystitis may be found without typical appearances of tuberculosis, or there may be tubercles or tuberculous ulceration. The changes at the ureteric orifice are important. There may be cystitis and thickening of the lips of the ureter with inflammation around it, and sometimes greyish tubercles on the lips or in the immediate neighbourhood, or tuberculous ulceration (Plate 16, Fig. 2). The lips of the ureter may be ulcerated and eaten away, and surrounded by grey tubercles. There may be one or two or a collection of tiny cysts around the orifice. In an advanced stage the ureter is open and trumpet-shaped, with extensive ulceration around. In old-standing tuberculosis of the kidney with thickening and shrinkage of the ureter the ureteric orifice is dragged upwards and outwards (Plate 16, Fig. 3) and appears like a tunnel (Fenwick).

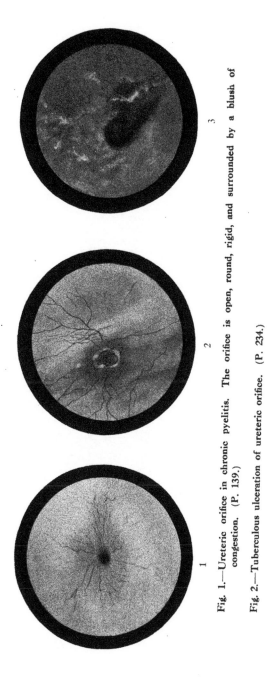

Fig. 1.—Ureteric orifice in chronic pyelitis. The orifice is open, round, rigid, and surrounded by a blush of congestion. (P. 139.)

Fig. 2.—Tuberculous ulceration of ureteric orifice. (P. 234.)

Fig. 3.—Dragged-out ureter in chronic tuberculous ureteritis. (P. 234.)

PLATE 16.

The urine of each kidney should be obtained and examined separately. Separators are difficult to use, and give fallacious results when the bladder is affected. Catheterization of the ureters is the only reliable method. When cystitis is present in a moderate degree no great difficulty is experienced, but when there is extreme sensitiveness of the bladder the operation may be difficult. It may be necessary to make more than one attempt, and sometimes to wait for some weeks until an acute cystitis has subsided under treatment before the catheterization can be done successfully. Where catheterization of the ureter has failed it has been suggested that the ureter be catheterized after opening the bladder suprapubically, or even that a temporary ligature be placed upon the ureter in order to obtain the urine from the other. It is better to wait until the acute symptoms have subsided, and to give a course of tuberculin (T.R.) before again attempting the catheterization; and these measures failing, the supposed healthy kidney should be explored by lumbar nephrotomy and carefully examined.

Where one ureter is obviously diseased, only that of the supposed healthy kidney need be catheterized, since that is the organ concerning which information is desired. If both ureters appear healthy, catheterization of both is necessary. The following is the report of the urines drawn by catheter from both kidneys in a case of tuberculosis of one organ :

Right Kidney (Tuberculous)	*Left Kidney (Healthy)*
95 c.c.	180 c.c.
Neutral.	Sharply acid.
Sp. gr. 1007.	Sp. gr. 1024.
Albumin—moderate amount.	Albumin absent.
Blood present.	Blood absent.
Sugar absent.	Sugar, 0·729 grm. (phloridzin glycosuria).
Urea, 0·55 per cent.	Urea, 2·4 per cent.
A fair amount of pus.	No pus.
Tubercle bacilli fairly numerous.	No tubercle bacilli.

Without examination of the unblended urines of the two kidneys it is impossible to form a reliable judgment as to the state and functional power of the second kidney.

Type 2 : enlargement of the kidney.—Enlargement of the kidney usually occurs in the late stage when other signs of tuberculosis are present.

Rarely a tuberculous hydronephrosis may be completely shut off from the bladder. I have observed such a case when a hydronephrotic movable tuberculous kidney was present. There was no change in the urine, but the ureter on the diseased side was dragged out of place and very thick. In other cases there is no change at the ureteric orifice.

There is a danger of mistaking a large hypertrophied and recently infected kidney for the only diseased kidney when the other kidney has been quietly destroyed. Only catheterization of the ureters and examination of the separated urines will demonstrate the true state of the kidneys.

The X-rays usually show enlargement of the renal shadow and an increase in the opacity of the organ. Occasionally caseous masses throw a dense defined shadow (Plate 17), and this may be so sharp in outline as to resemble a calculus or a collection of calculi.

Type 3 : hæmaturia.—This may occur in the form of initial hæmaturia above described. Where the tuberculous foci are buried in the substance of the kidney it may be impossible to obtain the bacillus in the urine or to find any change apart from the hæmaturia.

In such a case there is nothing to distinguish the condition from a small new growth or from hæmorrhagic nephritis, before exploration of the kidney which is bleeding.

TREATMENT

The treatment of renal tuberculosis is dependent upon the exact diagnosis of the extent of the disease. Before considering the question of operation it is necessary to have information on the following points :—

Is there tuberculous cystitis ?

Is there a second kidney, and, if so, is it healthy or diseased ?

Are there tuberculous foci elsewhere in the body ?

This is obtained by the methods already described.

The following methods of treatment will be discussed :—

Tuberculin treatment.

Medicinal and climatic treatment.

Operative treatment.

Tuberculin treatment. 1. Tuberculosis of one kidney alone.—It is impossible to speak with certainty in regard to the effect of tuberculin upon the early stage of renal tuberculosis when one organ only is affected, for extensive observations on the subject are wanting. I have used it in a number of cases where operation has for some reason been impracticable. In some of these cases, after treatment for one or two years, tubercle bacilli and all signs of inflammation have disappeared from the urine

Shadow thrown by caseous tubercle of left kidney.
Each segment represents a calyx filled with putty-
like material. The upper arrow points to a fibrous
septum, the lower to a caseous mass. (Pp. 230,
236.)

PLATE 17.

and there have been no further symptoms. The tuberculous focus in these cases has been shut off and is apparently quiescent. It is not certain, however, that this is permanent, as sufficient time has not yet elapsed since the symptoms disappeared. In other cases the symptoms continued and the tuberculosis progressed. The results of early nephrectomy in unilateral renal tuberculosis are so good that, in order to justify the adoption of tuberculin as a routine treatment, a series of cases known to be cured by tuberculin must be shown. This has not up to the present time been done.

The cases of unilateral renal tuberculosis that may be selected for tuberculin are those where operation has been refused. An exception may perhaps be made in renal tuberculosis in children. The frequency with which the disease is bilateral in the early stage in young children is much greater, and the difficulties in accurate diagnosis by modern methods are more formidable. In such cases tuberculin may be used in place of operation.

2. **Tuberculosis of both kidneys.**—In such cases operative interference is contra-indicated, and tuberculin should be tried.

I have not met with a cure, or any case approaching a cure, in cases of this class. There has, however, been undoubted improvement after the institution of the tuberculin treatment. When the disease is so extensive a considerable period of time might be expected to elapse before the full effect of the tuberculin is obtained. Such a period, unfortunately, is seldom afforded in these cases before death takes place from intercurrent infection or renal failure.

The treatment should be commenced with very small doses and carried on with great caution, for there is some danger of blocking of the already obstructed ureters if a reaction and swelling of the mucous membrane take place.

If the injections are followed by renal pain or by a rise of temperature, or an increase of fever already present, they should be stopped, or the dose much reduced.

3. **Tuberculosis of one kidney with tuberculous foci in other parts.**—A frequent combination is renal and genital tuberculosis. Tuberculin treatment is often of service in these cases, either in combination with nephrectomy or apart from operation.

After nephrectomy tuberculin treatment of the genital tuberculosis is likely to be successful. Tuberculosis of the kidney may occur with active tuberculosis of the lungs, bones, or joints. My experience of tuberculin in these cases has not been encouraging. There was improvement in the renal disease in some of the cases, but the extrarenal foci were unaffected or even appeared to increase under the treatment. When the extrarenal disease was quiescent it could be ignored in the treatment of the renal tuberculosis.

Tuberculin treatment should be commenced with a dose of $\frac{1}{10000}$ mg. to $\frac{1}{5000}$ mg. (T.R.), and the injection given once a week or once a fortnight, and cautiously increased. If a reaction occurs a longer interval and a smaller dose should be used. The treatment extends over one or several years, and the tuberculin may be given continuously, or in courses of two or three months with an interval of one or two months.

Progress is measured by the increase or decrease of body weight, the general feeling of vigour, the effect on pain, frequency of micturition, tenderness, enlargement of the kidney, and hæmaturia. Where vesical symptoms are present the amelioration of these frequently provides a most striking demonstration of improvement. The specific gravity and pigmentation of the urine increase as the renal condition improves. The quantity of pus and the presence and numbers of tubercle bacilli are critical tests of progress.

Climatic and medicinal treatment.—A warm climate without great variations in temperature is most suitable (Egypt, Morocco, South Africa). Nourishing diet with plenty of milk and fats should be recommended. Urotropine is unnecessary unless septic infection is present, and it may irritate the hypersensitive bladder. Sandal-wood oil soothes the vesical irritation.

Washing the bladder should be interdicted. It is useless therapeutically, and there is very great danger of introducing sepsis.

Operative treatment.—The operations which may be performed for tuberculosis of the kidney are partial nephrectomy, total nephrectomy, and nephrotomy.

Partial nephrectomy.—This operation consists in removal of the diseased part of the kidney. It has been practised in isolated cases by Israel, Watson, Morris, Godlee, and others, and has been recommended in the early stage of renal tuberculosis. In practice, however, it is found that at this early stage it is impossible to make certain how much of the kidney is affected. On surface inspection the organ may appear normal, or one pole may appear tuberculous and the rest of the kidney healthy when the disease has already affected both poles. For this reason partial nephrectomy has not been widely adopted, and the opinion is practically universal at the present time that total nephrectomy is the only radical operation that should be practised for tuberculosis of the kidney.

Nephrectomy.—Nephrectomy in the early stage of renal tuberculosis is the only method by which a cure can be assured, and the operation is indicated whenever the diagnosis of unilateral renal tuberculosis is made.

Nephrotomy is reserved for certain cases that are unsuitable for nephrectomy, and is a purely palliative operation.

The indications for and against nephrectomy are as follows :—

1. *Bilateral tuberculosis.*—When both kidneys are proved to be tuberculous nephrectomy cannot be recommended.

The disease is always more advanced in one kidney than in the other, and it may be open to discussion whether the removal of the organ in which the disease is more advanced will not prolong life. If we set aside general tuberculosis, which is a rare accident in tuberculous disease of the kidney, and is not likely to be affected by the removal of one of two tuberculous organs, the dangers to which a patient with bilateral renal tuberculosis is exposed are two: (i) toxæmia due to absorption from the tuberculous foci ; (ii) anuria from destruction of the renal tissue.

In so far as the general health is suffering from the absorption of toxins from the diseased area, considerable benefit will accrue from removal of one focus of disease, and it is also certain that the second and functionally the more active kidney will be relieved of the irritation caused by the excretion of toxins from the blood. But, on the other hand, the period of life remaining to the patient is also measured by the quantity of active renal tissue which he possesses. By nephrectomy of the more diseased organ some functional renal tissue is removed, even when the tuberculous inflammation is far advanced. The whole work of secretion is thus thrown upon the remaining kidney. In some cases the removal of even this small amount of renal tissue leaves the patient with too little active secreting tissue, and anuria follows the operation. In other cases the patient survives the operation, but after a short period death from anuria takes place.

Unless it is proved by the examination of the urine obtained by the ureteric catheter and by the various tests of the renal function that the disease of the second kidney is in a very early stage, and unless it is obvious that the health of the patient is suffering to a marked degree from the absorption of toxins from the first kidney, nephrectomy of the more diseased kidney in bilateral tuberculosis is contra-indicated.

2. *Non-tuberculous nephritis of the second kidney.*—A slight degree of chronic nephritis is very frequently present in the second kidney. This is shown by the presence of albumin and granular and hyaline tube casts in the urine, and is due to the excretion of toxins. It does not, however, contra-indicate nephrectomy of

the tuberculous kidney unless the nephritis is advanced. The urine from this kidney must be examined, and the tests for the renal function carried out, in order to ascertain the extent of the renal disease. Should these prove satisfactory, nephrectomy should be performed.

3. *Tuberculous lesions of the bladder.*—Tuberculous cystitis does not contra-indicate nephrectomy if it is proved that the second kidney is healthy. The removal of the tuberculous kidney has usually a most beneficial effect upon the disease of the bladder. The cystitis may subside without further local treatment.

The use of tuberculin after nephrectomy in these cases has given most satisfactory results in my hands. Where the tuberculous infection has become mixed with colon-bacillus or other infections the prognosis is not, however, so good.

4. *Tuberculous lesions of other organs.*—Obsolete tuberculous foci, such as spinal curvature, ankylosed joints, healed tuberculous disease of bones or glands, do not contra-indicate nephrectomy, although for anatomical reasons the operation may be rendered more difficult.

In active tuberculous disease of the genital system nephrectomy may be performed if the genital disease is not widespread. In a case where both epididymes, both seminal vesicles, and the prostate are affected, nephrectomy would be contra-indicated, but in less extensive lesions, such as unilateral tuberculous epididymitis, nephrectomy and epididymectomy may be performed. When renal tuberculosis is complicated by active spinal caries, psoas abscess, tuberculous arthritis, pulmonary phthisis, and other such serious lesions, nephrectomy is contra-indicated.

5. *The general state of the patient.*—It is occasionally necessary to refuse primary nephrectomy on account of an enfeebled general state, apart from any of the complications above described. Secondary nephrectomy may sometimes be possible in these cases after nephrotomy.

Technique.—The retroperitoneal route is invariably chosen for the removal of a tuberculous kidney. An oblique lumbar incision gives the most satisfactory access.

The operation is simple or complicated, according to the absence or presence of perinephritic inflammation.

Nephrectomy in an early stage of renal tuberculosis, before the perinephritic fat has become dense and sclerosed, presents no difficulties or unusual features. On exposing the organ the outward appearance may not suggest that it contains any disease, and palpation does not detect any change in consistence. In such a case the value of the previous examination of the urine from each kidney becomes evident. The kidney is removed without being incised, and the danger of infecting the wound with tubercle is avoided. The ureter is first isolated and carefully examined. Whether thickened or not, it should be cut across between two ligatures, and each end seared with the cautery or touched with pure carbolic acid. The pedicle is ligatured, and the kidney removed. Leguen recommends that the perirenal fat be dissected away, as there are frequently tuberculous deposits in it.

When there has been perinephritis the fatty capsule is transformed into a thick, firm, adherent fibro-fatty mass, and a subcapsular nephrectomy becomes necessary. The kidney is exposed and stripped from its capsule with the forefinger, great care being taken not to rupture the tuberculous cysts, the walls of which are thin and easily torn. If the kidney is converted into a large pyonephrosis it may be advisable to tap it, and so reduce the size and diminish the possibility of rupturing the wall of the sac during the enucleation. This is seldom necessary, however, and if it is done the most stringent precautions must be observed to prevent soiling of the wound with the escaping tuberculous material. The puncture is made with a trocar and cannula after protecting the wound with large gauze swabs, and the puncture wound is closed by pressure forceps over gauze during the remaining stages of the operation. After removal of the kidney the cavity must be drained.

Treatment of the ureter.—When the ureter is normal in appearance it is ligatured and dropped into the wound. When it is thickened and tuberculous, one of three courses may be pursued :

    1. The upper end may be fixed in the lumbar wound.

    2. The upper end may be ligatured, cauterized, and dropped into the retroperitoneal space after removing the kidney.

    3. The ureter may be excised.

    1. The fixation of the upper end of the tuberculous ureter in the lumbar wound has been done with a view to ureterectomy at a later date. A tuberculous sinus results; and in one case in which I did this the lumbar wound became extensively infected with tubercle and only healed after some months.

    2. When the upper end is dropped into the retroperitoneal space after being ligatured and cauterized, the tuberculous process in the majority of cases becomes quiescent and the tube is gradually transformed into a fibrous cord.

Zuckerkandl found that a sinus followed nephrectomy more frequently where the ureter had been left intact.

Occasionally tuberculous cystitis appears to be kept up by the persistence of tuberculosis in such a ureter.

    3. In order to excise the ureter the oblique lumbar incision is

Q

prolonged forwards beyond the anterior superior iliac spine and runs parallel to Poupart's ligament and about 1½ in. above it to about the middle of its extent. The patient should be placed in the Trendelenburg position in order to reach the pelvic portion of the ureter. The thick rigid tube is easily traced down into the pelvis. The adhesions may give rise to some difficulty in isolating it. In the male subject the ureter can be traced to the bladder and there ligatured and cut across. In the female, the pelvic portion of the ureter is concealed in the broad ligament and the tube must be cut across behind this. Kelly has removed the lower portion of the tuberculous ureter and a portion of the bladder wall through the vagina.

The advisability of performing an extensive operation for the removal of the ureter at the end of nephrectomy will depend upon the state of the patient and the duration of the nephrectomy. The ureterectomy should only be performed if the nephrectomy has passed off smoothly and the patient's strength is well maintained. Most authorities are content to remove " as much as possible " of the ureter, which means that the ureter is traced over the brim of the pelvis and cut across in the descending part of its pelvic course, leaving the remaining portion of the pelvic ureter. This operation occupies less time and necessitates less extensive dissection than the more complete removal of the ureter; it protects the lumbar wound against the possibility of infection from the ureter, and the small stump does not give rise to any further trouble. On these grounds it is to be recommended.

Instead of carrying the lumbar incision forwards, a second small vertical or transverse incision may be made above Poupart's ligament, the peritoneum pushed aside, and the thickened ureter seized, drawn out, and ligatured as low as possible.

Immediate mortality of nephrectomy for primary tuberculosis.— The following figures are given by Brongersma :—

Surgeon	Nephrectomies	Deaths from operation	Per cent.
Albarran	108	3	2·77
Brongersma	58	3	5·17
Casper	19	2	10·52
Israel	97	11	11·34
Krönlein	34	2	5·88
Kümmel	69	3	4·35
Pousson	20	2	10·00
Rafin	40	5	12·50
Rovsing	47	3	6·38
Zuckerkandl	23	3	13·04
	515	37	

This gives an operative mortality of 7·18 per cent. in 515 cases. There has been a steady and rapid decrease in the mortality of nephrectomy for tuberculous disease of the kidney, as the following figures show :—

1885 (Gross)	..	..	.. 90·00	per cent.
1893 (Vigneron)		..	.. 38·40	,,
1896 (Israel)	..	..	.. 18·00	,,
1908 (Brongersma)	..	..	7·18	,,

The improvement in the statistics was due in the earlier years to more complete asepsis and to improved methods of treating surgical shock and more perfect technique, as well as to experience in the selection of cases suitable for operation. Recently the great advance in the methods of early diagnosis and examination of the renal function afforded by catheterization of the ureters and the use of the phloridzin and other tests has led to further reduction of the mortality.

As Brongersma points out, when from the list of operations only the statistics of surgeons who use modern methods of diagnosis as a routine measure are taken (the operations performed previous to the introduction of these methods being excluded), the mortality falls to 2·85 per cent.

A more recent series of statistics was published in 1911,[1] from which the following are selected :—

Surgeon	Cases	Immediate mortality	Remote mortality
		Within six months :	Up to two years :
Israel ..	{1,023 collected 170 personal}	12·9 per cent.	10–15·0 per cent.
Wildbolz ..	139	2·8 ,,	15·0 per cent.
			Up to four years :
Asakura ..	70	5·7 ,, .	7·1 per cent.
André ..	57	3·5 ,,	15·0 ,,
von Frisch..	100	10·0 ,,	9·0 ,,

After-results.—The after-history of 369 patients on whom nephrectomy was performed for primary tuberculosis shows that death occurred after a considerable interval in 56 cases (15·2 per cent.). In these cases the interval varied from one or two to fourteen or sixteen years. In the great majority of the fatal cases the patients died within the first two years. Thus, in 329 cases of nephrectomy, 35 (10·6 per cent.) of the patients died

III. Kongress der deutschen Gesellschaft für Urologie, Sept., 1911.

during the first two years. In these cases the fatal result would be due to a spread of the tuberculous process.

Of 184 patients surviving two years after nephrectomy for tuberculosis, only 6 (3·2 per cent.) died of tuberculosis later.

It may be stated, therefore, that there is a risk amounting to 10·6 per cent. of the patient dying of tuberculosis during the first two years, and a risk of 3·2 per cent. of a fatal result from tuberculosis after this.

Nephrotomy.—Nephrotomy is a preliminary or a palliative operation in tuberculosis of the kidney, and is indicated under the following conditions :—

1. Where it is impossible, from the state of the bladder, to catheterize the ureter and obtain information in regard to the state of the second kidney, the obviously tuberculous organ is drained. After an interval the cystitis subsides and the examination can be carried out.

Casper has recommended that in these very rare circumstances the diseased kidney should be exposed, its ureter compressed, an injection of indigo carmine given, and the urine collected from the bladder by a catheter. By this method the functional power of the second kidney is tested.

2. Nephrotomy of the supposed healthy kidney is performed when other methods of examination have failed to give satisfactory evidence of the presence or absence of disease.

3. As a preliminary operation to nephrectomy where the general condition of the patient is much enfeebled. Secondary nephrectomy is performed some weeks later when the patient has regained strength.

In late stages, when the frequent and painful micturition are very distressing, it has been suggested that one kidney should be removed and the ureter of the other brought to the surface of the loin.

4. Where both kidneys are tuberculous, to relieve (a) a collection of tuberculous material, (b) excessive hæmorrhage or severe pain, (c) profound toxæmia.

The mortality of nephrotomy is high. Pousson, in his personal statistics, found an operative mortality of 27·5 per cent. for nephrotomy and 6·54 per cent. for primary nephrectomy. A fistula persists during the lifetime of the patient. In a few cases the fistula has closed after the kidney has been entirely destroyed.

LITERATURE

Albarran, *Ann. d. Mal. d. Org. Gén.-Urin.*, 1908, p. 81.
Brongersma, Ier Congrès de l'Assoc. Internat. d'Urol., Paris, 1908, p. 533.
Casper, *Deuts. med. Woch.*, 1905, p. 98 ; *Semaine Méd.*, 1908, p. 288.

LITERATURE—*continued*

Garceau, *Boston Med. and Surg. Journ.,* 1902, ii. 13.
Hallé et Motz, *Ann. d. Mal. d. Org. Gén.- Urin.,* 1906, i. 162.
Krönlein, *Folia Urol.,* 1908, p. 245.
Kümmel, *Arch. f. klin. Chir.,* 1906, p. 270.
Legueu, *Rev. de Chir.,* 1909, p. 86.
Lichtenstein, *Zeits. f. Urol.,* 1908, p. 219.
Pousson, *Ann. d. Mal. d. Org. Gén.- Urin.,* 1905, i. 801.
Rochet, *Ann. d. Mal. d. Org. Gén.-Urin.,* 1909, p. 1226.
Tendeloo, *Münch. med. Woch.,* 1905.
Walker, Thomson, *Pract.,* May, 1908.
Zuckerkandl, *Zeits. f. Urol.,* 1908, p. 97.

ACTINOMYCOSIS OF THE KIDNEY

Actinomycosis affects the kidney either as a metastatic deposit or by direct continuity. The number of cases on record is comparatively small. In an excellent chapter Garceau collects the known facts regarding the disease in the kidney.

In the early condition there are miliary pale-yellow tubercles in the cortex of the kidney. These have a radiating structure at the edge, due to the characteristic clubbed bodies closely set together. Around these bodies there is inflammation and softening, and small abscesses form containing the actinomycotic masses as yellow granules. The abscesses are numerous, and the intervening kidney tissue shows chronic interstitial inflammation. The abscesses may discharge into the pelvis, and the urine contains pus and yellow granules.

The metastatic form is derived from a focus in some internal organ such as the intestine or appendix.

A perinephritic abscess may form, and there may be rupture on the surface of the body. Amyloid degeneration is frequently present in the kidneys when actinomycosis affects some other organ, and it may also be observed when the kidney itself is the seat of actinomycosis.

Where the disease is confined to the kidney the symptoms are those of suppurative pyelonephritis of a mild type.

In a young man of 35 operated upon by Israel an exploratory nephrotomy had previously been performed for hæmaturia. A year later there was pyuria with pain, and the hæmaturia reappeared. High fever and rigors followed. Improvement took place, but three years later the scar broke down and pus with yellow granules was discharged. Israel removed the kidney, the upper two-thirds of which was the seat of actinomycosis, while the pelvis contained a stone.

When other organs are seriously involved the metastatic deposit in the kidney forms an insignificant part of the disease. Nephrectomy is justifiable only when the disease of the kidney is the sole or the most important focus of disease. Iodide of potassium should be given in as large doses as the patient will tolerate, and arsenic may also be administered. Iodides have not been so successful in the treatment of actinomycosis as was at one time anticipated.

LITERATURE

Ammentorp, *Centralbl. f. Chir.*, 1894, xxi. 1074.
Garceau, *Tumours of the Kidney.* 1909.
Israel, *Berl. klin. Woch.*, 1889, Nos. 7, 8 ; *Münch. med. Woch.*, 1899, xlvi. 49.
Ruhrah, *Ann. Surg.*, 1899, p. 417.

BILHARZIOSIS OF THE KIDNEY AND URETER

Bilharzial lesions of the kidney are very rare. In a few cases the ova have been found in the renal pelvis and in the substance of the organ. Grebel found them in the kidneys in advanced pyelonephritis, and other lesions such as interstitial nephritis, subcapsular cysts, etc., have been observed. Ruffer discovered calcified ova of bilharzia in the straight tubules of the kidneys in two Egyptian mummies of the Twentieth Dynasty (1250–1000 B.C.).

In the pelvis there are hæmorrhages and ulcerations ; a calculus may form with the bilharzial ova as a nucleus. The mucous membrane may be covered with grey-yellow plaques formed by blood pigment, urie-acid crystals, and ova.

The bilharzial lesions most frequently affect the lower part of the ureter, but the whole length of the duct may be involved. Lesions similar to those observed in the bladder are found. According to Kartulis, annular striæ of the mucosa are characteristic of bilharzia of the ureter. The lumen may be contracted and obliterated, and dilatation of the ureter and hydronephrosis result.

LITERATURE

Debove, Achard, et Castaigne, *Maladies des Reins.* 1906.
Madden, *Bilharziosis.* 1907.
Ruffer, *Brit. Med. Journ.*, Jan. 1, 1910.

SYPHILIS OF THE KIDNEY

1. Nephritis due to *secondary* syphilis is very rare. The lesions are bilateral, and take the form of the large white kidney. The microscopical lesions are principally epithelial. In old-standing lesions interstitial nephritis with changes in the glomeruli and blood-vessels are found.

In slight cases there is a trace of albumin in the urine and

slightly marked œdema. In severe cases there are oliguria, pronounced albuminuria, with red cells, epithelial casts, and a few
leucocytes in the urine; nausea, vomiting, anasarca are observed;
uræmia may supervene, and the patient dies in spite of treatment.
In those who recover, chronic nephritis frequently persists.

2. *Tertiary* syphilis may affect the kidney in the form of nephritis
or gummata.

Syphilitic nephritis in the tertiary stage takes the form of
subacute or chronic interstitial nephritis, or, less frequently, of
parenchymatous nephritis. The disease is frequently unilateral,
and may affect one part of the kidney. Scarring of the kidney
is sometimes found. In a man aged 50, who had contracted
syphilis fifteen years previously, and had suffered from severe
hæmaturia with ureteral clots for ten months, the left kidney was
non-adherent, and on the convex border near the lower pole there
was a depressed scar with a thickened adherent fibrous capsule
over it. On microscopical section of a wedge of kidney tissue at
this part there was fibrosis of the capsule, and areas of fibrosis
were scattered through the cortex. The hæmaturia ceased after
the operation.

Gummata are single or multiple, and may be associated with
tertiary lesions of other organs. There may be as many as twenty
or more small pea-sized gummata, or a single large mass. The
gummata commence in the interstitial tissue, and have a yellowish
colour. Their characters are those of gummata found elsewhere.
The rest of the kidney substance may be the seat of nephritis.
A large gumma replaces the renal tissue, so that the kidney is
enlarged, hard, and irregular. Such kidneys have been mistaken
for malignant growth or tuberculous disease and operated upon.
Bowlby and Israel have performed nephrectomy under these
conditions.

Amyloid degeneration occurs in tertiary syphilis, and may
coexist with gummata of the kidneys or other organs.

3. *Congenital* syphilis may affect the kidney during fœtal life
and, as Stoerk has shown, cause arrest or delay of development,
so that at birth the outer layer of the cortex contains imperfectly
formed tubules and glomeruli.

During infancy and childhood acute or chronic interstitial
nephritis is the usual form of the disease. The condition is most
frequently bilateral, but one kidney or a part of one kidney may
be affected.

Treatment.—The diet and general management of these cases
differ in no way from those of other forms of nephritis. Salvarsan
should be avoided; mercury should be given in small doses and

with caution. 'Some authorities believe that mercury is harmful. In tertiary lesions it should be combined with iodides.

Nephrectomy has been performed under a mistaken diagnosis, but has proved successful in large gummata.

LITERATURE

Bowlby, *Trans. Path. Soc.*, 1897, p. 128.
Carpenter, *Brit. Journ. Child. Dis.*, 1908, p. 93.
Delamore, *Gaz. des Hôp.*, 1900, p. 553.
Guthrie, *Lancet*, Feb. 27 and March 13, 1897;
    Brit. Journ. Child. Dis., 1908, p. 90.
Israel, *Deuts. med. Woch.*, 1892, No. 1.
Nádor, *Deuts. med. Woch.*, 1911, p. 838.
Stoerk, *Wien. med. Woch.*, 1901.
Sutherland and Thomson Walker, *Brit. Med. Journ.*,
    April 25, 1903.

CHAPTER XVII

RENAL CALCULUS

STONES formed in the kidney may remain lodged in a calyx or in the pelvis, or they may enter the ureter and either become arrested in the duct or pass into the bladder.

Etiology.—A urinary calculus is an agglomeration of crystals held together by a cement substance. In discussing the origin of calculi it is therefore necessary to consider (1) the presence of crystals in the urine, and (2) the nature and origin of the cement substance.

1. **Presence of crystals in the urine.**—The crystals which form calculi are the crystalline form of substances normally found in solution in the urine. The urine is something more than a watery solution of certain salts, for it has the power of holding a greater proportion of some salts in solution than has distilled water. Thus, uric acid is soluble to a greater extent in urine than in distilled water. This property is due to the presence of certain colloid bodies such as mucin and urochrome.

Precipitation in crystalline form of certain salts occurs as a result of their presence in excessive quantities, or of changes in reaction, or of bacterial action. In this way crystals of phosphates, of oxalate of lime, and of uric acid are deposited in the urine.

Phosphaturia may be due to general or to local causes which are described elsewhere. The form of phosphatic deposit in the urine which is important in the formation of stone is that caused by bacterial decomposition of the urine. This occurs in chronic septic pyelonephritis, and " secondary calculi " are formed.

In *oxaluria* (p. 47) there is a deposit of crystals of calcium oxalate, and this condition is frequently associated with the deposit of uric acid. The oxalates in the urine are derived partly from the food and partly from the tissues, and are kept in solution in the urine by acid phosphates of sodium and magnesian salts. Oxaluria is due less to the ingestion of excessive quantities of oxalates in the food than to derangements of digestion and assimilation.

The *uric acid* in the urine is derived from the nucleins of the food and as a product of metabolism in the body. The conditions which produce an increase and deposit of uric acid are excess of nitrogenous foods and alcohol, want of oxidation from leading a sedentary life, hepatic congestion, gout, and the gouty form of diabetes mellitus. Uric acid is held in solution by the salts of the urine as urates and by the pigmentary colloids. Deposit of uric acid may be due to an increase in the total quantity, or to a reduction of the salts or pigment, or to an increase in the acidity of the urine. Uric acid is excreted in the form of urates of sodium, potassium, calcium, and magnesium, which are soluble in the urine. If the urine is highly concentrated the urates are deposited when the fluid cools. This is frequently observed after excessive exercise, in tropical heat, in fevers, and in derangements of the liver and stomach.

In infants " renal infarcts " composed of urates and uric acid are frequently found in the convoluted tubules soon after birth. These disappear when the flow of urine is fully established. They may remain to form the nucleus of a true calculus.

Cystinuria is an hereditary and family disease, due to an abnormality in metabolism. The tissues are unable to complete the oxidation of the cystin normally formed in the breaking down of protein. Cystin contains 25·5 per cent. of sulphur, and in cystinuria about 0·5 grm. is excreted in twenty-four hours. The health is not impaired.

The precipitation of these bodies in crystalline form is not alone sufficient to form a calculus, but it is one factor in the production of a calculus.

2. Colloid substances.—The second essential factor in the formation of a stone is the presence of a colloid cement substance. Colloid bodies are present in the normal urine in the form of mucin and urochrome. But these colloid bodies are not sufficient to produce a stone. Phosphaturia, oxaluria, etc., may be present for years without a calculus being formed. In cystitis mucin is in excess, and large quantities of triple phosphates are thrown down and are entangled in the masses of mucin. Plugs of this material are formed and are passed in the urine. They are of slimy consistence, rarely approaching the firmness of putty, and are readily broken up between the fingers. These masses do not, even after the lapse of months, form calculi.

Schade has pointed out that the colloids found in the urine vary in nature. They may be " reversible," for, after once having passed out of solution, they may under changed conditions of reaction, etc., be again taken into solution. Or they may be

" irreversible," i.e. when once precipitated they are insoluble. For the formation of a calculus an irreversible colloid is necessary.

Irreversible colloids do not occur in normal urine, but are present in pathological conditions. Fibrin, formed from fibrinogen, is the characteristic representative of the group of irreversible colloids. It appears in the urine as a result of hæmorrhage or of inflammation; it occurs also in a very rare state of the urine known as fibrinuria. Schade suggests that fibrinuria in a very slight form may occur more frequently than is supposed. It is of extreme interest to note that bodies having the shape and appearance of calculi, but composed almost wholly of fibrin, are sometimes found in the renal pelvis or in the bladder. The ultimate cause which leads to the presence of fibrin or other irreversible colloids in the urine where there has been no injury is at present doubtful. The passage of quantities of crystals in the urine may itself excite mild inflammation in the urinary tract. It is known that bacteria and toxins are constantly being absorbed into the circulation from the throat and bowel (especially in constipation), and excreted by the kidneys, without causing gross inflammatory changes, but it is not unlikely that lesser degrees of reaction may be induced.

General factors in etiology.—Heredity plays an undoubted although ill-defined rôle in the production of renal calculus. A history of calculous disease in one or several members of the patient's family in different generations can frequently be obtained. I have twice had under my care a father and son afflicted with renal calculus. That this is not due to external influences is shown by the record given by Leroy d'Étiolles of eight brothers suffering from stone, who lived in different parts of Europe under varying conditions of hygiene and climate. Heredity is most marked in uric-acid calculus.

Renal calculi occur most frequently in mid-adult life. Watson found the average age in fifty-four cases was 38 years. Operations for renal calculus is rarely necessary in children under 10, or in adults over 60. It is not unusual, however, in young adults to obtain a history of symptoms dating back to infancy or childhood. Men are slightly more liable than women. Each kidney is affected with equal frequency. In the later stages renal calculi are usually bilateral, but at an early period they are unilateral. Küster found bilateral renal calculi in 11·78 per cent., and Israel in 27 per cent. of operated cases. With earlier diagnosis by the X-rays these figures may now be further reduced. Post-mortem evidence, representing the final stage of the disease, shows that calculi are bilateral in over 50 per cent. of cases.

Food and drinking-water play an important part in the production of calculi. The effect of foods on the increase in uric acid and oxalates in the urine has already been mentioned. Hard water influences the production of calculus by supplying an excessive quantity of calcium salts. Deposits of calcium oxalate or calcium phosphate in the urine are thus encouraged. Sedentary habits causing deficient oxidation of nitrogenous bodies and inaction of the liver increase the uric-acid output in the urine and predispose to calculus.

Calculous disease is very irregularly distributed. It is common in India, and occurs both in Europeans and in natives—in the latter more frequently than in the former. Here the effect of tropical climate is held to influence the production of stone. The concentrated urine is believed to cause such irritation as will produce the colloid necessary for the formation of a calculus.

In Europe, Central Russia, Hungary, Holland, Italy, Northern Germany, Western France, and the Eastern Counties of England calculus is especially prevalent. According to Preindlsberger, stone cases in Bosnia and Herzegovina are confined to a strip of land which for the most part consists of limestone of the Dinaric Alps, and in this area Christians are much more frequently affected than Mohammedans. On the authority of Küster, Jews are stated to be more frequently affected than other races in North Germany. The reason for this geographical distribution is unknown. Neither climate, geological formation such as chalky soil and drinking-water, nor race is a common factor. In secondary phosphatic calculi, stasis of urine from obstruction is frequently present and is an important predisposing cause.

Structure and chemical composition.—In the centre of the calculus is a nucleus, and disposed around this are concentric laminæ of varying composition. In infants the nucleus usually consists of urate of ammonia, in adults of uric acid, and after the age of 40 of oxalate of lime. Rarely a fragment of blood clot forms the nucleus; and the ova of bilharzia have been found. The laminæ are formed of crystals or amorphous material bound together by cement substance. Alternate layers of uric acid and oxalate of lime, or, if the urine is alkaline, a covering of triple phosphates and calcium carbonate, are deposited.

The substances that enter into the composition of renal calculi are—

> Uric acid.
> Ammonium and sodium urate.
> Calcium oxalate.
> Calcium phosphate.

Calcium carbonate.
Ammonium and magnesium phosphate.
Cystin.
Xanthin.
Indigo.
Blood.

The phosphates and carbonates are found in alkaline urines, all the others in acid urines.

Calculi are said to be primary when they arise in a previously healthy urinary tract, and secondary when they result from changes in the urine due to infective processes.

They are rarely composed of one salt. In the great majority of stones several substances are present. Thus, uric acid and calcium oxalate frequently occur in alternating layers in the same calculus. If the urine becomes alkaline a deposit of phosphates takes place on the surface of the stone.

Hitherto it has been customary to name calculi uric-acid or uratic when these bodies were present, without reference to the possibility that they might form only a small fraction of the total calculus. In this way uric-acid calculi have been looked upon as being much more common than any other form of calculus. Beneki found that 479 out of 649 urinary calculi in the Hunterian Museum, or about 74 per cent., contained uric acid or urates, and Dickinson found about the same proportion (70 per cent.) in renal calculi. In calculi removed by operation, however, where minute. fractions of salts are not taken into account, oxalate of lime is much the most frequent component. Of 77 calculi collected by Morris the composition was as follows :—

Oxalate of lime	..	...	34	..	..	44·15 per cent.
Uric acid ..	..	..	17	..	..	22·07 ,,
Phosphates..	..	..	13	..	..	16·88 ,,
Cystin	..	..	2	..	..	2·6 ,,
Calcium carbonate	..		1	..	..	1·3 ,,
Mixed calculi	..	..	10	..	..	13·0 .,
			77·			

Oxalate calculi are therefore much more common than was at one time believed. Moore has corroborated this view from an analysis of 21 renal and ureteral calculi removed by operation, all of which contained calcium oxalate in large amount, in more than two-thirds of them over 70 per cent.

Renal calculi vary in appearance and consistence according to their chemical composition.

Oxalate-of-lime calculi are usually single. They are very hard, dark-brown or black, with a nodulated surface or covered with fine crystals or coarse, clear, crystalline spicules. Oxalate-of-lime calculi sometimes take the form of multiple small polished brown or black seed-like bodies. They are laminated on section, and are found in acid urine. *Uric-acid* calculi are single or multiple, hard, smooth, sometimes highly polished, and yellow or red-brown in colour. They occur in acid urine, and show a laminated cut surface. Calculi composed of *ammonium* and *sodium urate* occur in children. They are small, soft, and friable, and of a pale fawn colour. *Calcium-phosphate* calculi are greyish-white, hard, with an irregular and sometimes crystalline surface. They may become coated with triple phosphate. On section they are laminated. They are found in a neutral or slightly alkaline urine. Calculi of *mixed phosphates* (fusible calculus) are whitish-grey, mortar-like, friable masses, which increase in size with great rapidity. There is no lamination. They may be covered with crystals of triple phosphate. They occur in ammoniacal urine. *Cystin* calculi are yellow, smooth, and soft. After removal they assume a greenish, waxy appearance. On section they have a radiating structure. They are very rare. *Xanthin* calculi, too, are very rare. They form smooth, hard, reddish, cinnamon-coloured stones. *Indigo* calculi are also very rare, only two examples being known. The calculus is blue-black with a grey polished surface on section, and it leaves a blue mark on white paper. *Blood* calculi or *fibrin* calculi are of extreme rarity. In 1907 I explored the left kidney of a woman aged 58 for two attacks of hæmaturia, pain, and undue mobility of the organ. In the renal pelvis were packed six greyish-brown masses, the size of a small marble, shaped like gall-stones with facets. They had a putty-like consistence, and became darker brown on exposure to air. On section the masses were laminated and composed of fibrin coated on the surface with blood and some crystals of uric acid. Gage and Beal have collected a few similar cases from the literature.

Size, shape, and number.—Most calculi removed by operation are single, but it is not unusual to find multiple calculi. (Plate 18 and Fig. 57.) As many as 200 have been removed from a kidney. Two or three small round calculi may be formed in a small pouch of the pelvis or calyx, and passed down the ureter at intervals, and this process may be repeated at intervals during many years. Slightly larger solitary calculi in the pelvis are rounded or oval and are freely movable, or they may be wedge-shaped and fixed. Larger calculi are moulded into an exaggerated form of the renal pelvis and have sometimes fixed branches which fill the calyces, or there may be facets with which smaller calculi that lie in the calyces articulate.

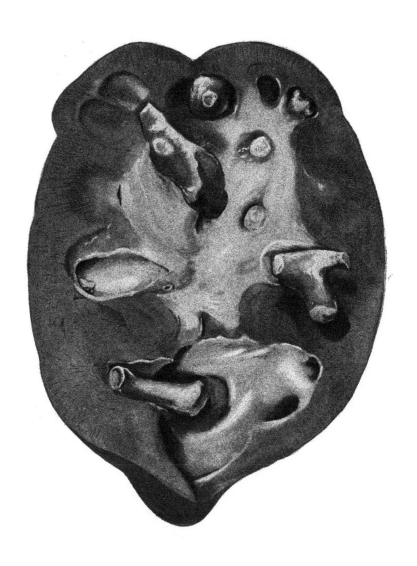

Multiple calculi of kidney. (P. 254.)

PLATE 18.

Very large calculi are sometimes found.   Shield records one of
1½ lb. having a circumference of 10 in., and Le Dentu one weighing
over 3 lb.

Small calculi usually lie in the renal pelvis, or they may be
wedged into a calyx.   The communication with the pelvis of a
calyx containing a calculus may be very narrow.   A large calculus
is lodged in the pelvis, and the branches in the calyces.   A branch

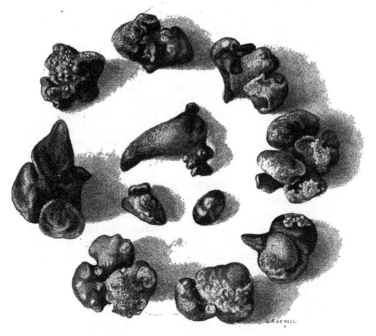

Fig. 57.—Calculi removed from one kidney.

may have a neck which is firmly gripped in the narrow communication between pelvis and calyx.

It is said that a calculus has rarely been found embedded in
the substance of the kidney and unconnected with the calyces
I have not met with such a case.

Changes in the kidney.   1. Aseptic lesions.   i. *Diathetic
nephritis.*—Albarran has shown that all calculous kidneys are
found, on microscopical examination, to bear the lesions of
nephritis.   Even when the organ appears normal to the naked eye,
microscopical examination shows that chronic nephritis is present.

These lesions depend upon the original cause of the lithiasis, and when once the calculus is formed they are aggravated by its presence.

Diathetic nephritis consists of a diffuse nephritis probably commencing in epithelial lesions and accompanied by interstitial nephritis. At first the kidney may appear normal or increased in size. Later it contracts and becomes granular. The capsule becomes adherent, and small cysts form. The condition is that of granular contracted kidney.

ii. *Lesions consecutive to the presence of a calculus in the kidney or renal pelvis.*—When the calculus reaches a certain size or lies in a position to cause obstruction, changes in the kidney are added to those already existing. The following conditions may be found :—

(*a*) The kidney appears almost normal. There is a slight condensation of the fatty capsule, the fibrous capsule is slightly more adherent, and the organ appears a little large. The pelvis contains one or several stones. There is a little thickening of the pelvic wall, and slight distension of the calyces and pelvis. The microscope shows the lesions described by Albarran as *néphrite diathésique.*

(*b*) There is advanced interstitial nephritis with atrophy, or occasionally the kidney may have previously been enlarged as a hydronephrosis and then have shrunk till it is small and atrophied.

(*c*) Perinephritis leading to a great increase in the perirenal fat has already been described. In the majority of cases it results from calculus of the kidney, and may be found either in aseptic or in septic calculus. The kidney may be surrounded by a large mass of adherent fibro-fatty tissue. The circumrenal fatty tissue invades the hilum and spreads along the blood-vessels into the substance of the kidney, compressing and eventually completely destroying it. (Plate 19.) The kidney retains its normal contour.

(*d*) Hydronephrosis is a comparatively common complication of renal calculus, and results from the impaction of a small calculus at the outlet of the renal pelvis. Rarely a calculus may plug the outlet of a single calyx or of one branch of a dichotomous pelvis, and a partial hydronephrosis results.

Hydronephrosis due to calculous impaction differs from other forms in the presence of ureter o-pyelitis caused by the irritation of the calculus. This leads to thickening and narrowing of the duct at a later time. In calculous hydronephrosis also the aseptic nephritis above described is already present when dilatation commenees, and changes in the kidney substance are much more advanced in the earlier stages of distension than in other forms of hydronephrosis.

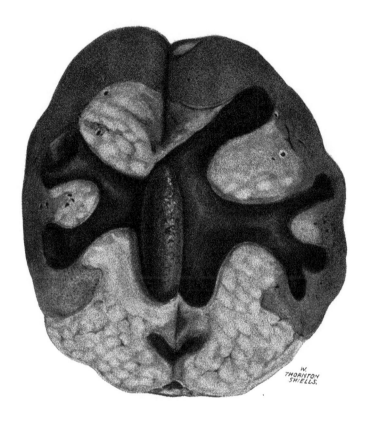

Renal calculus; dilatation of renal pelvis and pyelitis; invasion and destruction of kidney by hypertrophy of fat in renal sinus. (P. 256.)

PLATE 19.

2. **Infective lesions.**—Infection of the calculous kidney may take place by the blood stream (*hæmatogenous infection*), or the infection may ascend the urinary tract after the passage of instruments (*ascending infection*).

In the great majority of cases the infection is hæmatogenous, and has taken place before any instrument has been passed. Hæmatogenous infection may, however, be supplemented by an ascending infection after the passage of an infected instrument. The infection may, in quiescent calculus, obscure the presence of the stone. On the other hand, secondary calculi may develop in an infected kidney.

i. *Pyelonephritis.*—Acute pyelonephritis without obstruction does not occur frequently when calculi are present. Subacute and chronic septic pyelonephritis are much more common. Pyelitis is very seldom found without nephritis being superadded.

ii. *Pyonephrosis and uro-pyonephrosis.*—Calculous pyonephrosis is much more common, and may reach a large size. In the dilated calyces calculi of varying sizes lie, and may be tightly grasped by the narrow neck of the calyx. (Fig. 58.) At the outlet of the pelvis lies the plugging calculus, which may be of moderate size, and is often roughly conical in shape. Many calculi may be present, and there is sometimes a quantity of mortar-like secondary phosphatic deposit.

In uro-pyonephrosis the content is either cloudy or purulent urine.

iii. *Perinephritis and perinephritic abscess.*—Fatty and fibro-fatty perinephritis are more frequent and extensive in septic calculi than in aseptic. Large masses may thus be produced, and dense adhesions with the peritoneum, bowel, vena cava, and other neighbouring structures are formed, which render removal of the whole mass dangerous. The kidney may be easily stripped from its fibrous capsule inside the fatty mass. Suppurative perinephritis sometimes develops, and a calculus may be found in the abscess, having escaped from the kidney.

Rupture of the abscess has led to the discharge of a calculus on the surface of the buttock or in Scarpa's triangle.

iv. *Malignant growth of the renal pelvis.*—In a small number of cases a calculus has been found coexisting with a malignant growth of the renal pelvis, and in these cases the new growth is believed to have resulted from the prolonged irritation of the calculus. Drew found calculi in 4 out of 8 cases of villous growth of the renal pelvis collected from the literature. Others have been recorded by Israel, Hartmann, Kundrat, Ransohoff, and Porter.

R

3. Lesions of the second kidney.—Of 78 cases collected by Leguen, there were lesions of the second kidney in half the number. In 21 cases there was sclerosis or atrophy.

Of 22 cases of death from anuria after operation for renal calculus, I found that the second kidney contained calculi in 12, and that hydronephrosis had resulted in 2 of these, pyonephrosis in 3,

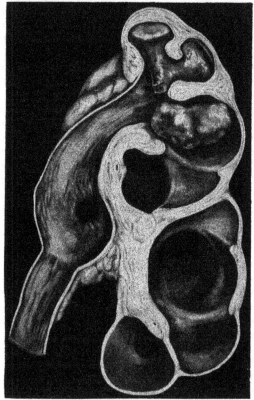

Fig. 58.—Calculous pyonephrosis with dilatation of ureter.

and atrophy in 2. There was atrophy without calculus of the second kidney in 4, hydronephrosis in 2, amyloid degeneration in 1, interstitial nephritis in 1, and fatty degeneration in 2 cases.

i. Compensatory hypertrophy of the second kidney occurs if the parenchyma of the calculous kidney is widely destroyed.

ii. Stone is present in the second kidney in over 50 per cent. of cases in late stages, but in only about 11 per cent. in the early stage.

iii. Interstitial nephritis is present in many cases even where the kidney appears healthy to the naked eye.

iv. Ascending pyelonephritis occurs as a fatal complication in some cases where cystitis is present. It may follow an operation for calculus of the bladder.

Symptoms.—In the majority of cases renal calculus gives rise to a distressing train of symptoms from which the patient demands relief.

Quiescent calculus.—Occasionally a calculus lies quiescent for many years, and the patient is unaware of its existence. Two varieties of quiescent calculus have come under my observation. In one variety there are no symptoms to attract the attention of the patient ; there may have been symptoms during childhood, or no symptoms at any time. In the second variety there are persistent symptoms of cystitis, but none of renal disease. In a man aged 45, from whom I removed the stones shown in Fig. 57, there had been cystitis for twenty-seven years, with attacks of hæmaturia on exertion, but no pain or other symptom pointing to the kidney until a few weeks before I saw him.

There are cases of unsuspected calculi with high temperature and great mental prostration, which present the features of severe acute pyelonephritis due to the bacillus coli. When the acute symptoms have subsided, calculi are discovered in the kidney.

The cardinal symptoms of renal calculus are pain and hæmaturia.

Pain.—Pain is present in over 70 per cent. of cases, and is felt in the posterior renal area at the costo-muscular angle. If the pain is severe it can also be felt at a spot on the front of the abdomen about 1½ in. below and internal to the tip of the 9th rib.

There are three varieties of pain in renal calculus—(1) fixed renal pain, (2) renal colic, and (3) referred pain.

1. *Fixed pain.*—The pain is felt in the positions described above. It is a constant dull ache, of varying intensity. It is increased by movement or jarring. Walking, especially over rough ground, jumping, driving, or motoring, and especially horse-riding and bicycling, aggravate the pain and may be the cause of intense suffering. The patient is most comfortable in bed, but even in the recumbent position must turn carefully, and may be unable to sleep on the diseased side when the pelvis is inflamed (Fenwick). In walking the patient may bend the body towards the diseased side ; in lying, the thigh may be flexed to relax the psoas muscle. Extreme flexion of the body may produce great

pain. I saw an actor who, with a stone in his right kidney, had to give up playing the part of a hunchback on account of the intolerable pain he suffered on bending the body.

Where the renal pelvis is inflamed the pain becomes intense and is provoked by slight movements.. The pain corresponds in some degree to the size and character of the · stone. A large stone gives little or no severe pain, but may cause dull aching. A small stone fixed in a calyx is unlikely to give much pain. A small round or oval stone with rough crystalline surface free in the renal pelvis is accompanied by the most severe pain.

2. *Renal colic.*—Renal colic commences in the anterior or posterior renal-pain area (Fig. 59) and shoots downwards, following the line of the ureter on the surface of the body, or a line lower

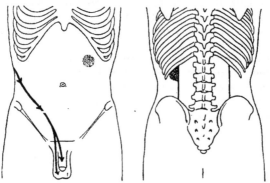

Fig. 59.—Line of right renal colic : anterior and posterior renal-pain areas in renal calculus.

down almost at the level of Poupart's ligament. The pain passes to the external abdominal ring; it may end there, or may be continned along the cord into the testicle of the corresponding side, or may shoot along the urethra to the tip of the penis. It may radiate down the front of the thigh, or along the sciatic nerve, or across the abdomen. Renal colic never shoots directly across or upwards.

An attack of renal colic is usually initiated by some exertion or jar, such as a stumble, or by a sudden twist or turn in bed;. or it may commence during sleep. The patient sits writhing or rolls in agony, the face is pale, the skin clammy and sweating, and vomiting frequently occurs. The testicle on the painful side is retracted and intensely tender. The abdominal muscles are rigid, the thigh is flexed.

There may be an intense and urgent desire to micturate, and.

repeated attempts are made at short intervals. The quantity of
urine secreted during an attack of renal coho is small, and no
urine may be passed for several hours.

If unrelieved by treatment the attack may last for one or for
several hours. It frequently ceases quite suddenly, but may
subside more gradually. After an interval a quantity of blood-
stained urine is passed. Some hours, or several days, afterwards
a stone may be passed from the urethra with the urine.

3. *Referred pain.*—With the slighter constant pain of renal cal-
culns there may also be pain referred to a distant part. (Fig. 60.)

Persistent pain is occasionally felt in the sole of the foot or

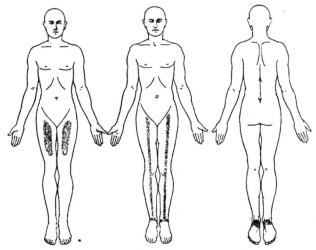

Fig. 60.—Areas of referred pain in renal calculus.

heel. It is felt also in the thigh or leg, and sometimes in the
testicle or labium. Rarely the testicular pain is more prominent
than the renal pain, and may even exist apart from it. Bladder
pain with frequent and urgent micturition is sometimes present
in renal calculus when the bladder is quite healthy. The most
important reflex pain is that in which pain is referred to the second
kidney (reno-renal reflex). Thornton stated that pain in one
organ might be caused by a calculus in the other, the calculous
kidney being painless. This has frequently been disputed, and
it has been held that aching pain may be felt in the second
kidney, but that the referred pain does not occur in a healthy
kidney without severe pain being present at the same time in
the diseased organ. I have, however, seen two cases where the

referred pain was present without pain in the calculous kidney, and there are a few similar cases on record.

Since the introduction of the X-rays in the diagnosis of renal calculus and the use of methods for the examination of the urine of each kidney, this question of referred pain has lost much of its importance.

Hæmaturia.—Less than half the cases of renal calculus suffer from hæmaturia. The hæmaturia is not usually severe. Blood corpuscles are often found with the microscope· in cases in which the blood cannot be detected with the naked eye. Hæmaturia frequently occurs with renal còlic, and may continue after the coho has ceased. It is intimately connected with movement and exertion. Occasionally it is the only symptom. There may be persistent hæmaturia lasting many months, and unaffected by rest or movement. Like pain, it is more apt to be present, and is more severe, if the surface of the stone is rough and irregular.

Pyuria.—Pus may be found in the urine in · small amount from slight pyelitis caused by the irritation of the calculus. When the kidney becomes infected the urine is cloudy and purulent to the naked eye. It remains acid, and the pus settles in a solid layer at the bottom of the vessel. Occasionally, when decomposition of the urine has taken place in the kidney, the urine passed is alkaline and decomposing.

Other changes in the urine.—Hyaline casts and an excessive quantity of urine may be present and indicate changes in the kidney substance. Crystals of calcium oxalate or uric acid may be present. Phosphaturia sometimes occurs with renal colic, without other changes in the urine.

In the later stages of renal calculus, and especially where both kidneys are the seat of calculus and are extensively destroyed, the urine is pale, very abundant, and of low specific gravity, and the total amount of urea excreted is reduced. Calculous anuria will be discussed later (p. 278).

Examination of the kidney and ureter.—On **palpation** of the abdomen the tips of the fingers may detect rigidity of the muscles on the side of the calculus.

If the kidney is large and contains many stones, it forms an abdominal tumour. If the patient is thin, this may be seen in the recumbent position as a prominence in the lumbar region about the level of the umbilicus or a little below. In the erect posture the prominence disappears. Palpation shows the kidney greatly enlarged and tender. In cases in which the patient is thin and the stones are large and covered with a thin layer of renal tissue they can be felt on palpation as irregular, very hard, craggy masses,

and grating may be detected. With smaller calculi no enlargement of the kidney is felt in uncomplicated cases. The kidney
is, however, frequently tender on palpation. Jordan Lloyd has
pointed out that in renal calculus a stabbing pain may be elicited
by prodding deeply with the finger-tips over the kidney.

Cystoscopic examination.—In cases in which hæmaturia is
the only symptom the bleeding is seen to come from one ureteric
orifice, and the observation will lead to the further examination
and eventual exploration of that kidney. When the urine is
purulent it can be seen as a cloudy efflux, with flakes, coming from
one ureteric orifice. The efflux is ejected vigorously, and is rapidly
repeated in pyelitis. In old-standing pyelitis due to calculus or
to other cause, a solid pipe of pus may be seen to be slowly expelled
from the ureteric orifice and glide down the slope of the ureteric
ridge like a worm, or break up into short segments. The appearance of the ureteric orifice gives little information in the early stage
of renal calculus. There may be a blush of congestion and inflammation round the ureteric orifice and basal cystitis if infection of
the renal pelvis is present. In long-standing pyelitis and ureteritis
from calculus or other cause the ureteric orifice is round, open,
and rigid.

Should nephrectomy be required, the ureter of the second
kidney should be catheterized and the urine examined, and the
function of the kidney tested.

Radiography.—The examination of the kidneys by the
X-rays is discussed at p. 38. (Plate 20.)

Course and complications.—Renal calculus may exist for
many years and give rise to very slight inconvenience. The
symptoms may only be excited by movement, and the patient
gradually curtails his exercise until he lives in comparative com-
fort. Often, as the stone increases in size, the pain and attacks
of colic diminish and occur less frequently. The general health
is unaffected.

Certain complications may supervene:

1. **Migration of the calculus.**—The passage of the calculus
along the ureter is accompanied by renal colic, and has already
been described (p. 260).

2. **Obstruction.**—Obstruction gives rise to suppression of
urine (calculous anuria) or to hydronephrosis.

3. **Infection.**—Infection of the kidney and renal pelvis may
precede the formation of a calculus, or it may be superimposed on
a renal calculus. The symptoms due to the infection may completely obscure those caused by the calculus, which may remain
unsuspected.

The infection of a primary calculus is almost invariably hæma-togenous. It may take the form (a) of pyelitis, (b) of pyonephrosis, or (c) of perinephritis.

(a) *Calculous pyelitis.*—The pain of the calculus becomes greatly intensified, and the kidney is very tender on palpation, without being enlarged. There is acid pyuria with polyuria, most marked at night.

(b) *Pyonephrosis.*—General symptoms become evident. There are fever and emaciation. The kidney is enlarged and may vary in size, the variations coinciding with an increase or decrease of pus in the urine.

(c) *Perinephritis and perinephritic abscess.* (*See* pp. 111, 112.)

Prognosis.—An untreated renal calculus destroys the kidney in which it is lodged, by causing sclerosis and atrophy if it is aseptic, and by suppuration when it is infected. The second kidney becomes affected with calculus in over 50 per cent. of cases, and is eventually the seat of other disease in a still larger proportion. The prognosis of renal calculus is therefore grave unless early operation is performed.

Diagnosis.—Radiography has revolutionized the diagnosis of renal calculus, and has replaced exploratory operations upon the kidney in cases of suspected calculus. So certain and precise has this means of diagnosis become in the hands of one practised in the radiography of urinary disease that there is a tendency to use the method as a short cut to diagnosis without duly weighing the symptoms. Disappointment and a tendency to cavil at the limitations of radiography are thus engendered. In any case the proper reading of a radiographic plate of good quality may over-ride an opinion based upon symptoms ; but there are few, if any, cases in which the work of the radiographer is not rendered easier and more valuable by a knowledge of the clinical symptoms.

Diagnosis in renal calculus presents itself as a number of different problems:

1. Cases with pain and hæmaturia.—These cases are some-times attended with difficulty in diagnosis.

In typical cases the pain predominates and the hæmaturia occurs with the pain. Both symptoms are initiated or increased by movement or jarring. The passage of a calculus at a previous date and the discovery of numerous crystals in the urine are of great importance in the diagnosis.

In movable kidney the pain is also closely associated with movement, and hæmaturia, although it is rare, may occur. The discovery of a movable kidney should not be accepted as exclud-ing calculus. Radiography should be used, and when nephror-

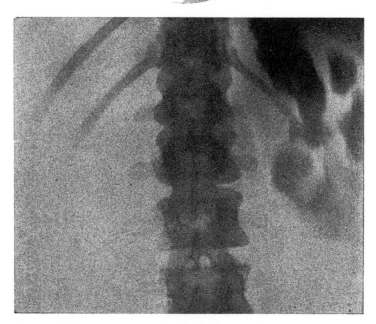

Fig. 1.—Shadows of large branching calculus and of two smaller calculi
(arrows) in kidney. (Pp. 39, 263.)

Fig. 2.—Shadow of calculi in right kidney, with clear field in left kidney
area. (Pp. 39, 263.)

PLATE 20.

rhaphy is performed the kidney should be thoroughly examined for stone.

New growths of the kidney with hæmaturia and clot colic may resemble renal calculus. In such cases the hæmaturia is profuse, and occurs for the most part without any pain; it is capricious in its onset and duration, and is little affected by rest or exercise. Colic does not occur apart from an attack of hæmaturia. It co-incides with the sudden disappearance of blood from the urine, and as it subsides the hæmorrhage reappears and ureteral clots are found in the urine. When a tumour is palpable there is little difficulty, for its characters do not resemble those of a pyo- or hydronephrosis, and the condition of the urine is different.

In cases of hæmorrhagic nephritis with pain there may be difficulty, and the X-rays, and eventually exploration of the kidney, may be necessary before a diagnosis is made.

Patients passing a highly acid concentrated urine with uric-acid or calcium-oxalate crystals may suffer from renal colic, fre-quent micturition, and hæmaturia, and there may be a small quantity of mucus or even a trace of pus in the urine. In such cases the symptoms quickly disappear on alkaline diuretic treatment.

2. **Cases with hæmaturia as the only symptom.**—These are rare, and if a radiogram is not obtained the presence of a stone will certainly be overlooked. The hæmaturia is initiated and increased by exertion. New growths of the kidney or ureter and hæmorrhagic nephritis are the conditions most likely to be con-fused with these cases. Very rarely portions of growth are found in the urine, and occasionally numerous tube casts and albumin may be met with in the intervals between attacks of hæmaturia in nephritis. In rare instances cystoscopy shows a portion of growth projecting from the ureter.

3. **Cases with pyuria alone.**—Tuberculous disease should be excluded by examination of the urine for the tubercle bacillus, and by cystoscopy. Non-calculous pyonephrosis may be dis-tinguished by the history of an initial attack of acute pyelo-nephritis or other cause.

4. **Cases with renal pain as the principal symptom.**— The most frequent cause of renal coho is calculus in the kidney or ureter, but it may also be due to the passage of clots, of pus and débris, or to acute ureteritis without a calculus. Hepatic colic without jaundice is said to resemble renal colic. The dis-tribution of the pain is, however, different. Hepatic colic com-menees over the gall-bladder and radiates inwards towards the umbilicus or transversely, while renal eolie frequently commences

in the posterior renal area, and always shoots downwards either along the line of the ureter or lower down in the groin. It passes to the testicle or penis, and is accompanied by retraction of the testicle.

In nephritis dolorosa there is renal pain which may be severe. These cases were at one time described as renal neuralgia. It has been shown, however, by Israel, Albarran, and others that microscopical evidence of interstitial nephritis can always be obtained. The pain is seldom so severe as renal colic, and does not radiate along the ureter. It is unaffected by movement. Where hæmaturia is present also, diagnosis without the X-rays is impossible.

Raynaud has shown that the crises of locomotor ataxy may be indistinguishable from renal colic. When the possibility of such a cause of confusion is remembered, the only difficulty that can arise is in the irregular cases of tabes (*formes frustes*) where the classical symptoms may be wanting.

Morris has recorded cases of hysteria in which difficulty in diagnosis from renal calculus was experienced. Persistent and sometimes severe pain in the posterior renal area is sometimes caused by osteo-arthritis of the lumbar vertebræ. Rigidity of the vertebral column and the appearance of lipping of the vertebral bodies in a radiogram suffice for the diagnosis.

Calculus in the ureter causes the same symptoms as renal calculus. There may, however, be fixed pain at some spot in the line of the ureter, the calculus may be felt per rectum or per vaginam, symptoms of vesical irritation may be very marked, and cystoscopy may show changes at the ureteric orifice, or the stone itself may be seen projecting into the bladder.

5. **Cases with symptoms of cystitis.**—Persistent cystitis may be present with latent renal calculus and lead to an erroneous diagnosis. I have already referred to a case of this nature.

The diagnosis is made by the examination of the ureteric orifices and the efflux with the cystoscope, and, if necessary, by examination of the urine drawn from each kidney by catheter. The X-rays may show a large stone shadow.

Even where a stone is found in the bladder it must not be concluded that no stone is present in the kidney, and radiography should be employed to exclude renal and ureteric calculi in these cases.

Diagnosis of the presence and health of a second kidney. —The most frequent disease of the second kidney is calculus, and a clear renal area in a radiographie plate will exclude this. In addition to radiography the only reliable methods of diagnosis are cystoscopy, chromocystoscopy, and examination of the urine drawn from the second kidney by means of the ureteral catheter.

Treatment. Prophylaxis.—This consists in the treatment of oxaluria, phosphaturia, and lithiasis, and the removal of local conditions which may assist the formation of stone. The treatment of oxaluria and phosphaturia has been discussed elsewhere (pp. 48, 51). The local conditions which assist in the formation of stone are urinary infection and obstruction, of which the treatment is considered at pp. 134 and 119. When a patient passes highly acid concentrated urine containing uric-acid crystals the treatment should be directed to reducing any excess of uric acid which may be derived from the food, assisting the complete metabolism of nitrogenous bodies, and preventing the crystallization of uric acid in the urine.

Diet.—In prescribing diet it should be remembered that there is a daily excretion of nitrogenous bodies, uninfluenced by the diet, which is sufficient to form calculi should other conditions be favourable. The patient's strength should therefore not be reduced by too rigid a regimen. It is advisable to limit the quantities of nitrogenous foods, but it is unnecessary to prohibit meat altogether. Beef and mutton should be taken sparingly. Cellular organs, such as brain, sweetbreads, kidney, and liver, contain excessive quantities of nuclein, from which uric acid is derived, and they should be avoided. White meat is less harmful than red, but veal and pork are unsuitable articles of diet. Duck and goose, among poultry, and high game should be avoided. Fish may be taken, except salmon, mackerel, lobster, and crab. Bread and all the cereals, all the roots and fruits and green vegetables in abundance, and salads, should form part of the diet. Butter and milk and eggs may be taken.

Tea and coffee should be avoided, or drunk very weak. Sugar and fats are harmful and should only be taken sparingly. It is better to avoid wine altogether, but should it appear necessary to permit some wine, the lighter Moselle and white French wines, or a light claret, should be selected. Heavy wines such as Burgundy, Australian and Californian wines are especially harmful. Port and champagne should be interdicted. New port is slightly less pernicious than old. Whisky may be allowed in very small amount.

Careful attention should be paid to regular action of the bowels, and a course of waters containing sulphates of soda and magnesia, such as Hunyadi or Friedrichshall, is beneficial. Half a tumblerful or more should be taken on waking, followed by a tumblerful of hot water. Courses of three or four weeks, with intervals of several weeks, may be prescribed. Watson speaks highly of calomel given in doses of $\frac{1}{6}$–$\frac{1}{4}$ gr. at night for a week at a time.

The urine should be diluted and its acidity reduced. A large . glass of hot water should be taken in the early morning and at night. Aerated distilled waters, such as Salutaris, are beneficial. Alkalis, and especially those with a diuretic action, are useful. The citrate and acetate of potash should be given in doses of 30–60 gr. four times daily, or the carbonate or citrate of magnesium or lithium. The boro-citrate of magnesia in doses of 15 gr. thrice daily is well borne.

Alkaline mineral waters, such as Contrexéville (Pavillon), Vittel (Grande Source), and Evian (Cachet), should be given, and a visit to one of these spas is often beneficial. The most powerful effect is obtained by drinking the water after fasting. For this reason a large draught should be taken in the early morning, and another in the late afternoon.

Uric-acid "solvents" should be administered by the mouth. Of these the following is a selection, viz.: piperazine, 4–15 gr.; sidonal, 7$\frac{1}{2}$ gr.; hexamethylenetetramine (synonyms urotropine, formin, cystamine, cystogen, metramine, uritone), 5–15 gr.; helmitol, 15 gr.; hetralin, 7$\frac{1}{2}$–30 gr.; cystopurin, 30 gr.; chinotropine, up to 90 gr.; uricedin, 15 gr.; uraseptin, 4 drachms. Turpentine may sometimes be administered with benefit in doses of 10 minims in capsule thrice daily for a week or ten days.

Regular graduated exercise in the open air, bathing and Turkish baths, massage, and radiant heat baths are important adjuncts to treatment.

Treatment of certain symptoms. (a) *Renal colic.*—The pain in renal coho varies greatly in severity. In severe attacks the patient is placed in a hot bath and a hypodermic injection of morphine sulphate ($\frac{1}{4}$–$\frac{1}{2}$ gr.) with atropine sulphate ($\frac{1}{100}$ gr.) given. On his return to bed hot fomentations or poultices are applied over the loin and abdomen. . The pain usually subsides half an hour after the injection. Occasionally it is necessary to repeat the injection after some hours. Very rarely chloroform has to be administered and the patient kept lightly under its influence for an hour or more. If this becomes necessary and the stone is known to be lying at the upper end of the ureter, a ureteric catheter may be passed and the stone pushed back into the renal pelvis. The injection of a small quantity of sterilized oil into the ureter has facilitated the passage of a descending calculus (Schmidt).

(b) *Renal hæmaturia.*—Hæmaturia is seldom severe in renal calculus, but there may be profuse hæmorrhage after exertion or a fall or blow. The patient should rest in bed with an ice-bag over the kidney. A hypodermic injection of morphia should be given and 10 or 15 gr. of calcium lactate administered by mouth every four hours. Ergotin may be given hypodermically, but is of doubtful value. For persistent and severe hæmaturia operation is necessary.

(c) The treatment of *calculous anuria* is discussed later (p. 282).

Operative treatment.—When a diagnosis of renal calculus is made the stone should, unless in some exceptional cases, be removed without delay. It is unwise to wait in expectation of a small stone passing down the ureter, for it is impossible to judge from the size and shape of the stone whether its position in the pelvis or calyx will permit of its descent. Moreover, there are the dangers of dilatation of the kidney and hæmatogenous infection while it remains in the kidney, and the same dangers and that of calculous anuria during its descent along the ureter. The danger of nephrolithotomy in experienced hands is very small.

Cases that are *unsuitable for operation* are (a) those of extensive bilateral calculous disease, either aseptic with signs of progressive failure of the renal function, or when there is widespread sepsis and uræmic symptoms are present or are easily induced by exposure or other causes ; (b) those in which small calculi are frequently passed and the X-rays do not show a large single shadow or a collection of small shadows in the kidney. Operation in cases of this kind is followed by a recurrence of the stone formation without any prolongation of the interval. They are suitable for diuretic and spa treatment.

Before commencing the operation for removal of a stone the following information should be in possession of the surgeon :—

1. *The position and number of calculi.*—The whole urinary tract must be examined by the X-rays. The assistance of an opaque bougie in the ureter is sometimes necessary to distinguish doubtful shadows. The bladder must be examined with the cystoscope.

2. *The presence of a second kidney and its functional state.*— This is ascertained by examination of the ureteric orifice and the observation of an efflux, by chromocystoscopy, and by the examination of the urine drawn from each kidney by the ureteral catheter and the use of tests for the renal function. This information is absolutely necessary where there is a possibility of nephrectomy being done.

The operations which may be performed are—

1. Nephrolithotomy.
2. Pyelolithotomy.
3. Nephrectomy.

1. **Nephrolithotomy.**—In nephrolithotomy the kidney is exposed by a lumbar incision and separated from its fatty capsule as far as the hilum. It is then carefully palpated for a hard nodule which would indicate the presence of a stone. The pelvis is also examined and the finger pressed into the sinus of the kidney. The further procedure will depend upon whether a hard nodule is discovered or not. If a nodule is felt in the substance of the kidney, it should either be exposed by an incision on the convex border of the organ, or, if it is near the anterior or posterior surface, it may be cut upon directly.

Needling the kidney for a nodule felt in its substance is an unnecessary procedure, for the reason that if the nodule is a stone it must be cut upon; and if it is not a stone, and also if no nodule can be felt, the surgeon cannot rest content with the meagre information afforded by passing a needle into the kidney substance, but will proceed to explore the organ by a free incision.

If nothing is felt, the kidney should be explored. The ureter

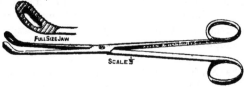

Fig. 61.—Author's stone forceps.

is first separated from the vessels at the hilum, which are compressed with the finger and thumb. An incision is made in the convex border of the kidney, 4 mm. behind the most prominent line. The incision is placed in the middle of the organ and extends for 2 in. or more. The cut surfaces are separated, and the finger introduced into the renal pelvis, and with this and a metal sound a careful search is made for the calculus. Instead of making a single large incision a slightly smaller incision may be made into each pole of the kidney, and by this means the extremities of the organ are searched and the portion intervening between the incisions is easily examined. If a stone is felt in the pelvis or one of the calyces the incision should be extended so that it is exposed. By means of forceps or a fine scoop and the forefinger the calculus is removed.

In some cases in which there is a short pedicle, or in a stout or muscular patient with a narrow loin, the kidney can only be partly brought into the wound. In such cases I use long fine forceps with an angled grasping extremity which can be passed along the forefinger and seize the calculus just beyond its tip. (Fig. 61.) Occasionally the end of a calculus can be felt, the remaining portion being connected with it by a narrow neck tightly grasped by the opening from the calyx into the pelvis; and in larger stones the branches of the calculous mass are tightly grasped in the calyces. The kidney must be freely incised and the calculus gradually freed by working with the finger-tip, with forceps, and with elevators, and by incising the constrictions and bands which bind it down. The search for multiple calculi should be carefully pursued. The large calculus should be examined for facets, for each of which a calculus must be found. A good radiogram is of great assistance, and should be before the surgeon at the operation. In isolated scattered calculi it is of especial value.

A number of small stones lying close together frequently appear as a single shadow. Small seed-like calculi or soft phosphatic material are removed by a copious stream of warm lotion from an irrigator after packing the perirenal space with gauze.

The stones having been removed from the kidney, the ureter should be carefully examined. The upper portion is easily palpated with the finger as far as the brim of the pelvis. A long fine gum-elastic bougie of even calibre is now passed down the ureter into the bladder. Should this be arrested at any part of the ureter the finger is passed along the outside of the ureter, and at the end of the bougie a calculus may be discovered. A complete radiographic examination of the urinary tract, together with sounding the ureter before the operation is decided upon, will shorten this part of the operation.

After removal of the calculi the kidney wound should be closed with sutures. Soft catgut sutures are most suitable. Catgut preserved in iodine and chromic catgut are too hard, and cut out. The sutures are introduced with round-bodied straight needles, and are passed about an inch from the edge of the wound. They are placed about half an inch apart, and five or six interrupted sutures usually suffice. They are tied slowly, and not too tightly, lest they cut out through the friable kidney substance. When the kidney substance has not been destroyed these sutures will suffice, but occasionally it is necessary to introduce a mattress suture to control bleeding from a large vessel. If mattress sutures are used a second row of interrupted sutures should be introduced near the edge of the wound, as otherwise the lips become everted.

When the kidney substance has been much reduced there is more difficulty in closing the wound satisfactorily. The thin lips become everted or inverted, and there is some danger of the sutures tearing out. In the cases in which severe hæmorrhage persists after nephrolithotomy the bleeding usually arises from a suture having penetrated into a dilated calyx, and either cut out and allowed a vessel to bleed, or torn through a vessel from being tied too tight.

When there is sepsis with dilatation of the kidney, drainage of the intrarenal cavity is necessary, and this is provided by a rubber tube of moderate size, which is retained in the kidney cavity by a catgut stitch passed through the edges of the kidney incision. The perirenal space should also be drained.

Dangers of nephrolithotomy.—The dangers of nephrolithotomy are hæmorrhage and septic infection.

Cases have been recorded in which, at the end of the operation of nephrolithotomy, very severe hæmorrhage occurred from a large vessel and necessitated nephrectomy. These cases are, however, very rare, and there is usually no difficulty in controlling the hæmorrhage by sutures so long as the fibrous capsule is intact. If the capsule has been stripped from the kidney the sutures cut out very readily.

Bleeding may, however, commence after the operation, the blood escaping into the pelvis and causing hæmaturia. This postoperative hæmaturia may assume serious proportions, and clotting may occur in the bladder, or it may persist and cause profound anæmia and even death.

When postoperative hæmaturia is moderate, treatment by absolute rest and the application of an ice-bag, together with small doses of morphia and the administration of calcium lactate, 10–15 gr. every four hours for two days, may be tried. Should this fail to arrest the bleeding, operation should not be too long delayed; and further, if the hæmorrhage is alarming from the first, operation should be performed at once.

The kidney should be rapidly exposed and the previous incision opened. Usually a quantity of blood escapes under tension. A stream of hot lotion should be directed into the cavity, and then a medium-sized rubber tube introduced into the renal pelvis. Round the tube long strips of aseptic gauze are packed. The patient may be infused on the table, and continuous rectal infusion commenced on returning to bed. This treatment usually suffices to control the hæmorrhage, and after three days the packing is removed, or, if necessary, renewed.

Sepsis may arise from a kidney already infected, or may be introduced at the operation. Septic pyelonephritis sometimes follows nephrolithotomy, and frequently causes severe hæmaturia. Postoperative hæmaturia when combined with elevation of the temperature is usually due to this cause. Perirenal suppuration may occur. The infection usually subsides, and only very rarely is there an infection of the lumbar wound necessitating opening it up.

Results.—The results are influenced by the presence or absence of sepsis previous to the operation. Some authorities, notably Morris, regard as cases of nephrolithotomy only those in which the kidney is healthy and there is no infection. Most surgeons look upon all cases of removal of calculi from the kidney as cases of nephrolithotomy.

The results of nephrolithotomy in cases uncomplicated by sepsis or dilatation show a very low death-rate. Watson collected 135 such cases with 3 deaths (2·2 per cent.); Rovsing, 115 cases of nephrolithotomy in non-infected cases with 7 deaths (6·08 per cent.).

In infected cases the mortality is high. Schmieden collected 211 cases with 43 deaths (20·3 per cent.), and the statistics of Küster show 251 cases with 50 deaths (19·9 per cent.).

The causes of death are septicæmia or toxæmia, anuria and uræmia, and hæmorrhage.

A patient under my care died of gangrene of both lower extremities after the removal of several large stones from the left kidney. At the operation a large, hard, inflammatory mass was found around the aorta, and thrombosis had probably spread from this.

After nephrolithotomy the wound usually heals rapidly, even where mild infection has been present. In infected cases a fistula may persist, and this is occasionally due to calculi having been left in the kidney, or to ureteral or pelvic obstruction. In Schmieden's cases (infected) a fistula followed the operation in 22·2 per cent. In Watson's collection (infected and non-infected) there were fistulæ in 8·0 per cent.

2. **Pyelolithotomy.**—By this term is understood the removal of a calculus through an incision in the pelvis of the kidney.

The kidney is drawn out of the lumbar wound. The organ is grasped in the left hand of the operator and turned forwards and upwards so that the posterior aspect of the pelvis is exposed. The fat covering the pelvis is removed with dissecting forceps. A posterior branch of the renal artery lying immediately within the renal sinus and irregular vessels must be avoided. If a stone is felt in the pelvis it is made prominent by pressure of the fingers on the front of the pelvis, and a longitudinal incision is made upon it through the posterior wall. The stone is then removed with forceps.

If a stone is not felt, the kidney is given to an assistant to hold, and a longitudinal incision is made in the pelvis about ¾ in. in length, a fine catgut suture passed through each lip, and the wound held open by these sutures. A probe is now introduced, and the

s

pelvis and calyces are explored. (Fig. 62.) If a calculus is now felt, the probe is held in position and a pair of forceps slipped along it, the stone grasped and removed.

After removal of the stone the edges of the wound in the pelvis are brought together by interrupted stitches of fine catgut. Over this a row of Lembert's sutures may be inserted.

Since 1905 I have covered all wounds in the renal pelvis with a flap of the fibrous capsule turned down from the kidney and stitched in place. This has proved very successful in preventing the escape of urine and promoting primary healing. Mayo recommends a flap of fatty tissue for the same purpose.

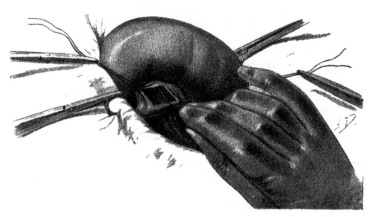

Fig. 62.—Pyelolithotomy.

The left kidney is delivered from the lumbar wound and turned forwards. The pelvis has been opened, and the edges of the wound are held apart by catgut sutures. The calyces are being sounded with a fine probe.

A drainage tube is placed behind the kidney and the lumbar wound closed. Usually there is no escape of urine, but occasionally some urine leaks for a few days. Rarely this continues for a fortnight or longer, and a urinary fistula may become established.

The cases which are suitable for pyelolithotomy are those of small unbranched stones lying in the pelvis.

As a method of exploration of the kidney for stone, pyelotomy is usually considered inferior to nephrotomy. The relative merits of these operations will be discussed later.

Results.—In Schmieden's statistics there are 54 cases of pyelolithotomy, of which 36 (66·7 per cent.) were completely healed. There were 12 (22·2 per cent.) recoveries with fistula, and 6 (11·1 ·

per cent.) died. These operations were performed on uncomplicated cases only.

In my experience the percentage of fistula following nephrolithotomy and pyelolithotomy given in the statistics quoted is much too high.

Nephrolithotomy and pyelolithotomy compared.—By nephrolithotomy all calculi which are not so extensive or so fixed as to require nephrectomy can be removed. Pyelolithotomy can only be performed for small or moderate-sized calculi occupying the renal pelvis or calyces, and it is only in regard to these cases that the relative merits of the two operations can be discussed. In cases where there is a short pedicle and a deep loin, pyelolithotomy may be impossible, while nephrolithotomy presents no insuperable difficulty. In nephrolithotomy the incision through the renal tissue produces some destruction of the tissue, and the sutures introduced to control hæmorrhage cause further damage. Each suture is a sclerotic centre, and fibrosis may extend for some distance around it. In pyelolithotomy there is no destruction of renal tissue by incision, tearing, or suture.

In nephrolithotomy there is some immediate and remote danger of hæmorrhage. In pyelolithotomy a retropelvic vessel may be wounded, but there is little probability of severe hæmorrhage. In an exploration of the kidney for stone which cannot be felt in the pelvis, pyelotomy, as already mentioned, is looked upon as inferior to nephrotomy. In a single large pelvis (ampullary pelvis) Leguen looks upon the two operations as being equally efficient.

When there is a branched pelvis, nephrolithotomy is the better operation, as it is difficult to explore all the calyces satisfactorily with an instrument, and the small calibre makes the introduction of the finger impossible. The exploration in nephrolithotomy is also difficult in many cases. After incising the kidney the finger may pass through the wound into the sinus of the kidney without entering the pelvis at all, and a probe appears at the hilum alongside the pelvis. The sounding of each calyx by an instrument, when the pelvis is much branched, is less likely to be successful through a nephrotomy than through a pyelotomy wound. In cases where a small radiographic shadow is present and the stone is not felt in the renal pelvis, and the kidney can be brought out of the wound, I usually explore the kidney first by pyelotomy and sounding with a probe, and, if this fails, open the kidney and explore the calyces through both incisions simultaneously.

Urinary fistula is stated to occur more frequently after pyelolithotomy than after nephrolithotomy, and the statistics of a number of cases support this view.

The danger of a fistula following pyelolithotomy has been over-stated. The probability of postoperative fistula is slight if care be taken to remove any obstruction to the flow of urine along the ureter and there be accurate suturing of the pyelotomy wound. In cases of moderate-sized unbranched calculi in the renal pelvis, and for many small concealed stones in the calyces, pyelolithotomy is preferable to nephrolithotomy, for it is more easily performed, there is no danger of hæmorrhage, and the kidney is not damaged.

3. Nephrectomy.—Primary nephrectomy is rarely practised for calculus. Under the following conditions it may become necessary :—

1. Severe uncontrollable hæmorrhage during nephrolithotomy.
2. Where the kidney is atrophied or destroyed by suppuration or dilatation.
3. Where calculi are so numerous and large that they cannot be removed without destroying the kidney.
4. A malignant growth has been found with renal calculi and necessitated nephrectomy.

Secondary nephrectomy may be called for in—

1. Urinary fistula causing great discomfort irremediable by other means.
2. Recurrence of stone with an atrophied kidney.
3. Prolonged renal suppuration.

The operation may be very difficult on account of extensive adhesions to the peritoneum, colon, liver, aorta, and vena cava. An intracapsular operation is often impossible from the adhesion of the kidney to the capsule, or a portion of the kidney may be shelled out while the rest of the organ is firmly adherent.

Watson collected the following statistics :—

Primary nephrectomy, 136 cases, 41 deaths (30·1 per cent.).
Secondary „ 33 „ 6 „ (18·1 „).

Bilateral calculi.—It is unwise to remove the stones from both kidneys at the same operation. The better kidney should first be operated on, in case it may become necessary to perform nephrectomy on the second kidney later. Pyelolithotomy should be performed on both sides whenever possible. Where a small stone is present in one kidney and a large stone in the other, the small stone should be removed without delay, as the conditions favourable for calculous anuria are present.

Küster collected 20 double operations and found 10 successful cases, 3 recoveries with fistulæ, and 7 deaths, due in most cases to uræmia.

Calculus in a solitary kidney.—A conservative operation

is here a necessity. Pyelolithotomy is preferable to nephro-lithotomy whenever possible. Both operations have been successfully practised.

The same limitation applies to calculus in a horseshoe kidney.

LITERATURE

Albarran, *Traité de Chirurgie* (Le Dentu et Delbet).

Badin, Thèse de Lyon, 1908.

Bevan and **Smith,** *Surg., Gyn., and Obst.,* 1908, p. 675.

Brödel, *Johns Hopkins Hosp. Bull.,* 1901, p. 10.

Drew, *Trans. Path. Soc.,* 1897, p. 130.

Faltin, *Folia Urol.,* 1908, H. 3, 4.

Fenwick, *Ureteric Meatoscopy in Obscure Diseases of the Kidney.* 1903.

Freplin, *Arch. f..klin. Chir.,* 1904, p. 868.

Gage and **Beal,** *Ann. Surg.,* 1908, p. 378.

Israel, *Arch. f. klin. Chir.,* 1900.

Kümmel, *Zeits. f. Urol.,* 1908, p. 193.

Küster, *Berl. klin. Woch.,* 1894, p. 35.

Legueu, *Traité Chirurgical d'Urologie,* 1910 ; XIᵉ Sess. de l'Assoc. Franç. d'Urol., 1908, p. 561.

Mayo, *Surg., Gyn., and Obst.,* April, 1910.

Moore, *Brit. Med. Journ.,* 1911, p. 737.

Morris, *Surgical Diseases of the Kidney and Ureter.* 1901.

Newman, *Lancet,* 1909, p. 8.

Robinson, *New York Med. Journ.,* 1904, p. 1113.

Schade, *Münch. med. Woch.,* 1909, No: 1.

Shield, *Lancet,* 1904, p. 1074.

Stewart, *Amer. Journ. Med. Sci.,* Aug., 1905.

Preindlsberger, *Wien. klin. Rundschau,* 1900, No. 46.

Watson, *Diseases and Surgery of the Genito-Urinary System,* vol. ii. 1909.

CHAPTER XVIII

CALCULOUS ANURIA

Etiology.—Calculous anuria may occur at any age. It is rare in children, although cases have been described. It is most frequent between the ages of 40 and 60. Men are more often affected than women.

The calculus which causes the anuria is usually small and single. The immediate cause is not infrequently violent exercise, shaking or jarring such as is produced by riding in an omnibus or jumping; but anuria may supervene without any apparent exciting cause.

Pathology.—Suppression of urine may be caused not only by impaction of a calculus, but also by the gradual destruction of the renal tissue from the action of calculi until it is insufficient to carry on the renal function. This is the last phase of long-standing bilateral renal calculi.

By calculous anuria is understood sudden suppression of urine from obstruction caused by the impaction of a calculus at the outlet of the renal pelvis, in the ureter, or very rarely in the bladder.

On the obstructed side there is the arrest in the pelvis or ureter of a calculus, usually of small size, with complete obliteration of the lumen of the duct. There is usually only one calculus, which is most frequently arrested at the upper part of the ureter. Rarely, several calculi are present. Donnadieu gives the situation of the calculus in 61 cases as follows: in the upper part in 34 cases, in the lower part in 16 cases, and in the middle in 6 cases.

The obstructed kidney is large and deeply congested, with ecchymoses on the surface and in the substance, and the pelvis contains 2 or 3 drachms of blood-stained urine under considerable tension.

The condition of the second kidney varies. It is generally agreed that the second kidney is always the seat of some organic change. A few cases have been recorded in which the second kidney was apparently healthy, but Leguen, and most authorities with him, holds that some lesion of the second kidney is invari-

able, and that if the kidneys which were supposed to be intact
had been examined histologically some lesion such as nephritis
would have been found. In most cases atrophy or sclerosis is
present.

In a few cases (12 in 43 cases—Donnadieu) this ureter is also
blocked by a calculus, and more rarely the second kidney is wanting (6 in 43 cases—Donnadieu).

The effect of the impaction of the calculus on the kidney of
the same side is sudden and complete obstruction and suppression
of its function, and the effect on the opposite kidney is reflex
suppression. Reflex anuria may be observed when the second
kidney is normal, but it is of temporary duration, and the secretion
is re-established when the first effect of the impaction has passed
off. When, however, the second kidney is diseased the secretion
remains suppressed and anuria results.

The pathological conditions under which calculous anuria supervenes may be summed up as follows :—

1. The ureter of a single functional kidney is blocked by stone.
The second kidney is absent, atrophied, or completely destroyed
by disease.

2. The ureters of two functional kidneys are simultaneously
blocked by calculi.

3. The ureter of one functional kidney is blocked by stone,
and the function of the second kidney is suppressed by reflex
influences (uretero-renal reflex). The second kidney is always
diseased, and this renders it more susceptible to reflex influences
and less able to re-establish the secretion when this has once been
suppressed.

Symptoms.—The kidney on the recently affected side is
frequently enlarged and tender, and there is rigidity of the abdominal muscles, especially marked on this side. There may be
tenderness along the line of the ureter and of the lower end of
the ureter per rectum. The calculus is occasionally detected
by the finger in the rectum or vagina. On cystoscopic examination the ureteric orifice on the recently diseased side may be congested or even ecchymosed. Rarely, a calculus has been found
projecting from the orifice.

Morris describes two clinical types of calculous anuria, namely,
the gouty, fat, and apparently robust adult past middle age ; and
the thin, nervous, dyspeptic individual.

Anuria may commence without pain or other symptoms, or
there may be indefinite aching, so slight as to be forgotten by the
patient, who is unable to indicate one side as having been recently
affected. More often there is a definite and sometimes severe

attack of renal coho accompanied by strangury,· and the urine is diminished in quantity or at once suppressed. As the attack passes off, the secretion, which may have continued in small quantity, ceases altogether and anuria becomes established. There is a period of tolerance during which no symptoms are present, and a period of intoxication.

1. **Period of tolerance.**—This period lasts a varying time, the average duration being five or six days. It may be as short as twenty-four hours or may be prolonged to ten or even to sixteen days. During this time the urine may be absolutely suppressed, not a drop being passed. Frequently, however, some urine is secreted. There may be a few drachms or ounces of urine containing blood, or the anuria may be interrupted by one or more intervals of copious polyuria. Many pints of pale, limpid urine, of 1006 or 1008 specific gravity, and with very small quantities of urea and urinary salts and colouring matter, are secreted. The polyuria ceases as suddenly as it commenced, and anuria is again complete. Several intermissions of polyuria may be observed,. and life may be prolonged in these cases ; in a case recorded by Weber the patient lived for thirty days.

During the tolerant stage the patient may feel in his usual health, and is able to conduct his business and get about in apparently good health. After some days digestive disturbances usually appear. The appetite fails, and there are nausea, constipation, and flatulence. The patient becomes sleepless and irritable, and suffers from headache and lassitude.

2· **Period of intoxication.**—The signs of intoxication set in usually about the fifth to the seventh day. The patient becomes heavy and drowsy, at first at intervals, and later continuously. He can be roused, but quickly relapses again. There is often restlessness, and later there are hallucinations and muttering delirium. The pupils are contracted, and there is usually twitching of muscles. Convulsions do not occur. The patient may complain of inability to move one or both legs, and the knee-jerks are slow or abolished. The pulse is slow (40 or 50 per minute); the respiration is slow and increasingly irregular, and may assume the Cheyne-Stokes type. The temperature is subnormal (97°–98° F.). Œdema of the feet and ankles may be observed, but is frequently absent. Hiccough is an occasional symptom, but is more likely to occur in cases where pyelonephritis is the cause of anuria than in calculous anuria. Vomiting appears at first after food, and later becomes frequent and exhausting. The bowels are constipated. Attacks of dyspnœa occur, and the patient usually dies suddenly in one of these; or there may be increasing coma and gradual heart failure. Uræmic symptoms may set in at any time. Death sometimes takes place suddenly without any symptoms of uræmia having appeared.

Diagnosis.—There are two important points in diagnosis : (1) What is the cause of the anuria ? (2) Which side is affected ?

1. The cause of the anuria.—In calculous anuria there may have been previous attacks of renal colic, or the passage of calculi or gravel, or calculi may have been removed from the kidney or bladder by operation. One kidney may be enlarged and tender, and a calculus may be detected by the finger at the lower end of the ureter. Cystoscopie examination may assist in the diagnosis.

The absence of fever excludes such forms of anuria as that caused by acute pyelonephritis. From other forms of obstructive anuria calculous anuria is diagnosed by exclusion. The bladder is examined for evidence of new growth, and for this diagnosis the cystoscope may be necessary. I have seen a case of obstructive anuria due to malignant growth of the bladder where the patient had suffered from slight symptoms of cystitis for five months and suddenly developed anuria. There was no enlargement of the kidneys. Other forms of obstruction, such as cancer of the uterus or prostate, and other pelvic tumours, must be excluded. Hydronephrosis may develop in these forms of obstruction, but may be absent.

Postoperative and traumatic anuria are excluded by the history. Toxic anuria due to such drugs as cantharides, mercury, lead, etc., is gradual in its onset, and is accompanied by other characteristic symptoms.

Anuria occurring in the course of acute or chronic nephritis is preceded by symptoms which leave little doubt as to the cause of the suppression of urine. The œdema and cardio-vascular symptoms, and the prominent place which headache, convulsions, and coma take in the symptomatology, usually suffice for a diagnosis. Anuria is the last phase of such conditions as tuberculosis and polycystic disease, but the previous history provides sufficient evidence on which to base a diagnosis.

2. The side affected.—The patient sometimes gives a history covering many years of pain and attacks of renal colic on one side, with a recent attack of colic on the other side. The side of the recent pain is that of the active kidney and recently blocked ureter. The abdominal muscles are rigid on the affected side. The kidney is tender and may be enlarged, and there is tenderness along the line of the ureter and at the lower end of the ureter, felt from the rectum or the vagina. Radiography, if it is available, may give important information. Extensive shadows in one kidney will point to the organ having been inactive or feebly functional, and a shadow in the line of the opposite ureter will indicate and localize the cause of the anuria.

Cystoscopy may show an open congested or œdematous or ecchymosed ureter on the diseased side, and an efflux of bloody urine may be observed if some urine is still being secreted.

Catheterization of the ureter has demonstrated the affected side and the position of the stone, and Krebs has by this means displaced a calculus and obtained relief from the anuria. The position of the calculus will frequently be discovered in making the diagnosis; should it not be found at the operation, time should not be spent in looking for it.

Prognosis.—If the anuria is untreated by operation, death occurs in 71 per cent. of cases according to Leguen, and in 67 per cent. according to Donnadieu. It takes place usually about the tenth or twelfth day, after two or three days of the intoxication stage. In cases which recovered, the date of the spontaneous relief was the third day in 1, the fifth to the tenth in 10, the thirteenth in 1, the fourteenth in 1, the fifteenth in 1, and later than the fifteenth in 2.

Treatment.—Operation should be performed at the earliest possible moment in all cases of calculous anuria. It has been held that operation may be delayed until the fifth or sixth day, as uræmic symptoms rarely supervene before that time. This delay could only be justified by a large proportion of spontaneous recoveries, and such does not exist. Death, if it takes place, is a result not of the operation but of the condition for which the operation is performed.

Huck's statistics show that the mortality rises each day that operation is delayed. Before the fourth day there is a mortality of 25 per cent., before the fifth day of 30·7 per cent., and before the sixth day of 42·1 per cent. Operations should therefore be performed as soon as anuria is established and the diagnosis clearly made. The presence of uræmic symptoms does not contra-indicate operation. Successful cases of operation under these conditions have been recorded.

In addition to operation, other measures should be employed to re-establish the secretion of urine. Diuretics such as Contrexéville or Evian water, tea, theocin sodium acetate in doses of 4 gr. combined with digitalis, every four hours, should be administered. Infusion of normal saline solution into a vein acts as a powerful diuretic; two pints should be given during or after the operation, or a solution of 2¼ or 5 per cent. of glucose may be used (*see* under Anuria, p. 19). A purge should be administered, and every means taken by hot packs and vapour baths to obtain a free action of the skin.

Nature of the operation.—This will to some extent depend upon the position of the obstructing stone, the possibility of accurately localizing it, and the ease or difficulty with which it can be removed. The operation for calculous anuria is one of emergency performed under the worst possible conditions, and it should be realized that it is more important to relieve the obstruction and do it quickly than to carry out an operation for the removal of calculus of the ureter. Nephrotomy should be performed where the stone is localized to the pelvis, where no accurate localization of the stone has been possible, or where the stone has been localized to the ureter but its position is such as to necessitate a prolonged operation which the patient is considered unfit to undergo.

If the stone is found it should be removed; if it is not found a large drainage tube should be placed in the pelvis and the wound in the kidney lightly packed with gauze. After the anuria has been relieved an operation for the removal of the obstructing calculus will be undertaken.

Pyelotomy may be substituted for nephrotomy where the stone is easily reached and removed through a pelvic wound.

Ureterotomy should be performed where the obstructing calculus has been accurately localized and is easily accessible, as in the lateral vaginal fornix or in the middle or upper segments of the ureter.

The nature of the operation in 46 cases collected by Morris was—nephrotomy 34, pyelotomy 5, ureterotomy 7.

Watson suggests that where a diagnosis of the side affected has not been made previously to operation, and the kidney on exposure does not appear to be adequate to carry on the renal function, the second kidney should at once be exposed and incised.

Results.—Watson collected 205 cases of calculous anuria, and found the following results of treatment :—

Treated without operation, 110; deaths, 80; mortality, 72·7 per cent.
Treated by operation, 95 ; ,, 44; ,, 46·3 ,,

Huck has shown that the mortality of cases operated upon before the fourth day is 25 per cent.

The results are capable of great improvement if the necessity for early and rapid operation is fully realized.

LITERATURE

Donnadieu, Thèse de Bordeaux, 1895.
Huck, Thèse de Nancy, 1904.
Krebs, *Petersb. med. Woch.,* 1903, No. 52.
Legueu, *Ann. d. Mal. d. Org. Gén.-Urin.,* 1895, p. 865.
Morris, *Surgical Diseases of the Kidney and Ureter,* ii. 145. 1901.
Watson and **Cunningham,** *Diseases and Surgery of the Genito-Urinary System,* ii. 193. 1909.

CHAPTER XIX

OPERATIONS ON THE KIDNEY

THE indications for operation upon the kidney are discussed under each disease for which it may be required. Only the technique need be considered here.

Preparation.—Careful preparation of the bowel is important, for a distended colon interferes greatly with the ease with which a kidney operation is performed, and there is a tendency to distension of the colon following the operation, which is increased when the bowel is already filled with flatus. A mild aperient should be given on two successive nights, and then the patient allowed to sleep without further purgation on the night previous to the operation, but an enema is given three hours before the patient enters the theatre. Violent purgation should be avoided. The diet should be light for two days before operation, and the patient should have an abundant supply of fluids up to two hours before it is done. The latter direction is especially important where there is a possibility of suppression of urine taking place from advanced renal disease. I prefer chloroform, given by an experienced anæsthetist, to other forms of anæsthesia.

The preparation of the skin will vary with the individual surgeon. An efficient method is to wash the skin of the field of operation, the evening before operation, with soap-and-water and ether soap, and, after drying it thoroughly, to paint it with a solution of iodine in rectified spirit (2 per cent.), and apply a dry aseptic dressing. At the time of the operation the field is again painted with the iodine solution. The field should extend to the middle line anteriorly and beyond the spines of the vertebræ posteriorly, as high as the level of the nipple and as low as the pubes.

The methods of approach are lumbar or extraperitoneal, and abdominal or transperitoneal. The lumbar route is that commonly used, transperitoneal operations being reserved for large growths or cases where it is important first to explore the abdominal cavity.

Lumbar operations.—In addition to the instruments required:

284

for any major operation, bone forceps, necrosis' forceps, and a periosteum elevator should be provided in case resection of a rib may be required. Two pairs of pedicle clamps and a pedicle needle are necessary where nephrectomy is proposed, and round-bodied needles, straight and curved, are used for stitching the kidney in nephrotomy or nephropexy. The patient is placed on the sound side (Fig. 63) with a firm pillow under the loin—a round sausage-like air cushion of large size is most convenient for this purpose—or there may be a special elevating apparatus attached to the table. The lower knee is drawn well up and the upper one fully extended, and the legs are steadied by a sand pillow. The

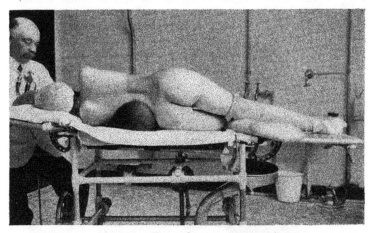

Fig. 63.—The "kidney position."

Note the air-cushion under the loin, the lower leg flexed and the upper leg extended.

lower shoulder and the pelvis should rest on the table. Too great elevation of the loin by the pillow permits the patient to roll back-wards or forwards. In this position the distance between the iliac crest and the costal margin is increased to its utmost. There is a tendency for the uppermost arm to fall across the chest and impede the breathing, and in order to obviate this Carter Braine's arm-rest is used, and the arm placed horizontally upon it. (Figs. 64, 65.) In stout, heavy subjects the upper shoulder tends to roll upwards and interfere with the breathing, and it may be necessary to have the shoulder controlled by a nurse.

The prone position is sometimes used, the patient being placed upon his face with a pillow beneath the upper part of the abdomen, but the lateral decubitus is that almost universally adopted.

The incision is oblique, extending from the angle between the 12th rib and the erector spinæ mass of muscle downwards and forwards towards the anterior superior iliac spine for a distance varying according to the build of the patient and the magnitude of the operation upon the kidney. (Fig. 66, A A'.) The upper end of the incision may be with advantage made to curve vertically upwards so as to cross the 12th rib, and a somewhat curved incision passing almost vertically from the 12th rib along the outer border of the erector spinæ muscle and curving forwards an inch above the crest of the ilium is sometimes preferable to the strictly oblique incision. (Fig. 66, B B'.) When the ilio-costal space is narrow the incision will be more transverse, as little is to be gained by obliquity in such a case.

A vertical incision along the outer

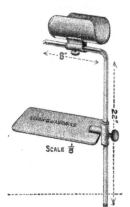

Fig. 64.—Carter Braine's arm-rest for kidney operations.

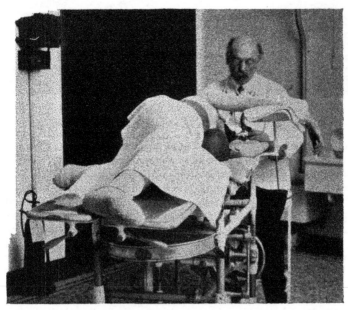

Fig. 65.—Showing arm-rest in use, to allow expansion of thorax.

border of the erector spinæ muscle from the 12th rib to the iliac
crest is sometimes used for simple procedures such as nephropexy.
(Fig. 66, D D'.)   For this incision the patient lies prone with a
pillow beneath the abdomen.   The modern incisions are the out-
come of the following incisions, which possess an historical interest,

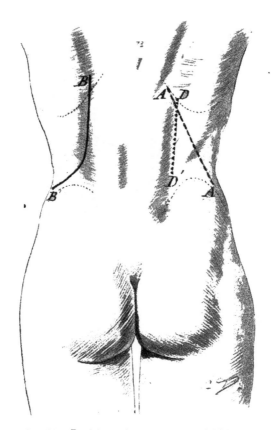

Fig. 66.—Incisions for exposure of kidney.

A A', Usual oblique incision.   B B', Curved incision with long vertical limb carried
over 12th rib.   D D', Vertical incision.

viz.: vertical incision along the outer edge of the erector spinæ
mass of muscles, used by Simon and Czerny; horizontal incisions,
used by Péan and Küster; and oblique incisions, used by von
Bergmann and Guyon.

Before the incision is commenced the skin should be scratched

with a needle so that there is a series of scratches crossing the
line of the proposed incision transversely and about an inch apart.
These serve to show the proper relation of the upper and lower
lips when the wound comes to be closed.

The skin, subcutaneous fascia and fat are incised, and the

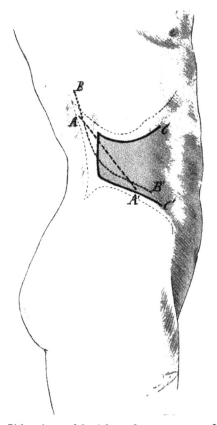

Fig. 67.—Side view of incisions for exposure of kidney.

A A', Oblique incision. B B', Curved incision. C C', Grégoire's incision.

latissimus dorsi and posterior part of the external oblique exposed.
The latissimus dorsi is cut through, and some fibres of the serratus
posticus superior, the 12th rib, the edge of the erector spinæ muscle,
the transversalis or lumbar fascia, the external oblique, and below
this the internal oblique, are exposed. The incision is carried

through the external oblique muscles and some fibres of the internal
oblique, and then the lumbar fascia is incised in the line of the
skin wound, and the fascia of Zuckerkandl comes into view. In
making this incision the 12th dorsal vessels and nerve are encountered. If possible, they should be turned aside, but they usually
intersect the line of the incision and must be cut across. The first
and second fingers of the left hand are inserted beneath the muscles
of the abdominal wall and the peritoneum pushed backwards.
With scissors the remaining muscles (internal oblique and transversalis) are severed, cutting between the fore and middle finger

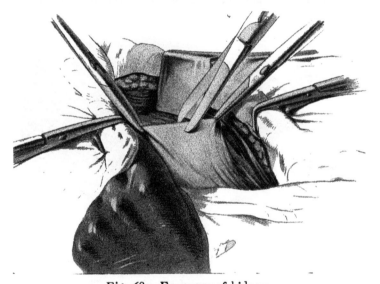

Fig. 68.—Exposure of kidney.

Cutting through the posterior layer of perirenal fascia (Zuckerkandl's fascia).

of the left hand to the full extent of the wound. At the upper
angle of the wound the lower border of the 12th rib is freely exposed by cutting some fibres of the serratus posticus inferior and
the external arcuate ligament. Before cutting the latter the
finger should be slipped up internally to it, so as to protect the
pleura, which sometimes descends to this level. Bleeding may
follow from cutting the last intercostal vessels, which should be
tied. The fascia of Zuckerkandl is picked up in forceps and incised (Fig. 68), and the lemon-yellow fat of the fatty renal capsule
exposed. The edges of the fascia are seized and the kidney exposed by stripping with the forefinger. A stronger band of fibres

containing the perirenal fat is frequently found at the lower pole of the kidney, and by traction on this the organ is brought into view and may be raised into the wound. Where there are adhesions and increase in the fat around the kidney there may be considerable difficulty in freeing the kidney. This is done partly by blunt dissection with the fingers and partly by cutting with scissors. Where a strong band of adhesions is met with, this is clamped and cut, and a ligature placed upon it. The hand is inserted beneath the ribs, and the upper pole of the kidney isolated and finally brought down into the wound. (Fig. 69.)

The peritoneum may be wounded when the perineal fascia

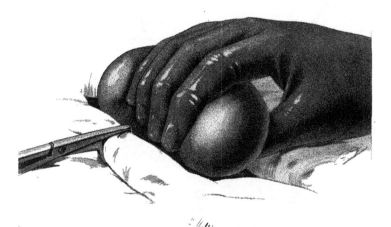

Fig. 69.—Delivery of the kidney from the lumbar wound.

is opened, or during the isolation of the kidney. The extremities of the peritoneal wound are immediately picked up in forceps and the rent closed by means of a continuous catgut suture. Occasionally a rent very high up under the liver in a prolonged and difficult nephrectomy must be left unsutured. I have never had aftertrouble from wounds of the peritoneum even in septic diseases of the kidney.

Nephrotomy and nephrostomy.—When *exploration of the kidney* is the object of the operation the kidney is incised along its convex border. The surgeon grasps the vascular pedicle of the kidney between the thumb and forefinger of the left hand, and incises the kidney in the exsanguine line of Hyrtl, parallel to and a little behind the curved border. (Fig. 70.) The knife is entered vertically to the surface, and the size of the incision varies.

The object of the nephrotomy is to examine the kidney substance and also to explore the calyces. It is necessary, therefore, to open the calyces, and for this purpose I prefer two incisions, one at the lower pole and the other at the upper pole, to a single larger incision in the middle of the kidney. This double incision is suited for the exploration of the bifid form of renal pelvis. Keeping up pressure on the renal pedicle, the lips of the wound are parted and the kidney tissue is examined. The forefinger is inserted and

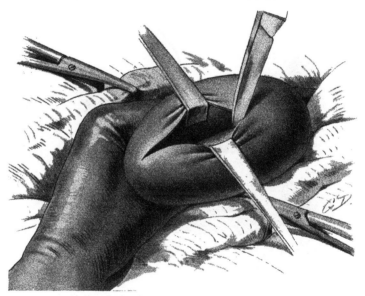

Fig. 70.—Nephrotomy.

The left hand is grasping the pedicle.

carefully explores the calyces, care being taken not to rupture the attachment of the pelvis to the kidney by rough manipulation.

In short, thick-set individuals, in whom the renal pedicle is short and inelastic, it may be difficult or impossible to bring the kidney into the wound or to deliver it on the loin. In such cases full use must be made of the additional space given by detaching the muscles and arcuate ligament from the lower border of the 12th rib. It may further be necessary to excise a portion of this rib, or to cut it with bone forceps and mobilize it. The kidney must be incised *in situ*, and the operation becomes much more difficult.

The nephrotomy wound is closed by means of thick catgut

sutures (No. 3 or 4) on round-bodied needles. One or even two mattress sutures may be required where the bleeding is profuse; they are placed 1 or 1½ in. from the edge of the incision, and tied carefully so as not to cut the kidney capsule and tissue. The wound is closed with interrupted catgut sutures, three or four in number. (Fig. 71.)

The kidney is returned to its fatty bed and a drainage tube placed in the upper extremity of the lumbar wound. Before commencing to suture the muscles, the skin and subcutaneous

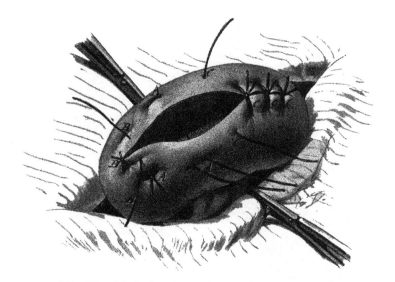

Fig. 71.—Methods of suturing nephrotomy wound.

A, Mattress sutures. B, Superficial sutures to bring edges of wound together over mattress suture. C, Interrupted sutures deeply placed.

fat should be freed for an inch or so from the cut edge of the muscles. The muscular wound is closed by means of a single or a double row of interrupted sutures of thick catgut. The sutures are all introduced, and clipped with artery forceps. The air is now allowed to escape from the cushion under the loin, and the edges of the wound fall together. The sutures are then tied. The skin wound is closed with interrupted silkworm-gut sutures, care being taken that the upper lip, which slides forwards as much as an inch or more on the lower one, is brought into its proper position. The scratches made before commencing the incision indicate the proper relations of the two lips.

In *nephrostomy* the kidney is drained temporarily or permanently. This is performed usually for hydronephrosis or pyonephrosis. The kidney is exposed, but is not raised from its bed. The most prominent part is incised with a · knife, and a large drainage tube inserted, a stitch being introduced through the kidney tissue and the tube. A second tube may be placed alongside this to drain the perinephritic tissue.

When permanent drainage is desired, an apparatus for collecting the urine is applied (*see* p. 159).

Lumbar nephrectomy.—When nephrectomy is proposed

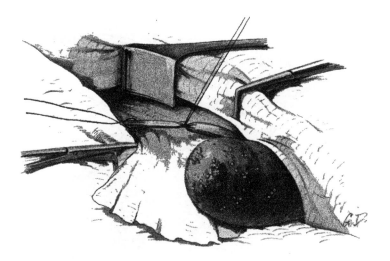

Fig. 72.—Lumbar nephrectomy.

Ligature of ureter previous to section.

the preliminary steps are the same as those already described. The incision may be prolonged as far as the anterior iliac spine, and it may occasionally be necessary to excise the 12th rib in order to gain access to the upper part of the kidney and to the renal pedicle. In doing so care must be taken to avoid damaging the pleura. Wounds of the pleura have frequently been recorded, but they do not appear to have been followed by collapse of the lung or other untoward results.

In operating for malignant growths of the kidney which are adherent at the upper pole it is wise to open the peritoneum outside the colon, and introduce the hand in order to palpate the upper pole of the kidney and ascertain whether the growth has spread to the peritoneum and surrounding structures, and is therefore inoperable.

Modifications of the operation in malignant growths are described elsewhere (pp. 200-2).

In lumbar nephrectomy for stone, tubercle, growth, or other disease, the separation of adhesions may be a long and tedious process. The adhesions are clamped and tied as the operation proceeds. The ureter is cut across between two ligatures (Fig. 72), and the lower pole of the kidney moves more freely. The kidney is freed on its posterior and convex surfaces and the upper pole

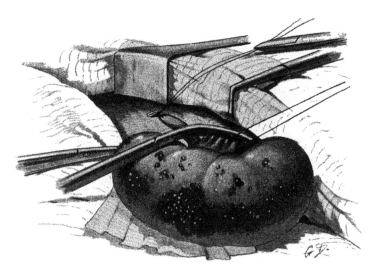

Fig. 73.—Lumbar nephrectomy.

The ureter has been ligatured and cut, the vascular pedicle clamped, and ligatures are being placed on each vessel separately.

reached. The pedicle is now reduced by dissection to its vascular elements, the pelvis being freed from its posterior surface. A clamp is placed on the pedicle close to the kidney but avoiding the pelvis. The kidney is cut away, leaving the pedicle in the grasp of the clamp.

Attention is now turned to the ligature of the pedicle (Fig. 73). If the vessels are readily separated by dissection a strong catgut suture is placed upon each and the clamp carefully removed. In some cases it is impossible, from the short, thick, rigid condition of the pedicle resulting from chronic inflammation, to do this, and the pedicle must be transfixed with a double silk thread

(No. 4 or 5) and tied in two portions, care being taken to draw the knots tight and to place the ligatures as far behind the clamp as possible. The clamp is now cautiously removed, the stump being held with a pair of Kocher's forceps until it is evident that all is secure. Difficulty in dealing with the pedicle may arise from the unexpected discovery of tuberculous or malignant glands adherent to it and to the aorta or vena cava. Careful dissection is required in such cases.

The treatment of the perirenal fat and lymphatic area and of the ureter is described under the different diseases for which nephrectomy is required.

A large rubber tube is placed in the upper angle of the wound and leads to the neighbourhood of the stump of the pedicle, and another leads downwards into the iliac fossa. These tubes are removed on the fourth day.

The wound is closed in the same manner as in nephrotomy.

Subcapsular nephrectomy.—Where there is excessive perinephritis with the formation of dense adhesions and a large mass of fibro-fatty tissue the kidney may be removed by subcapsular nephrectomy.

The incision is carried down to the perirenal fat, which is freely incised in a vertical direction, grasped with sponge forceps and held aside. The forefinger is now introduced between the kidney and the capsule, and swept first round the lower pole and then round the upper. A broad pedicle is isolated, consisting of the renal pelvis, vessels and a mass of fibro-fatty tissue. This is clamped and the kidney removed.

The broad pedicle may now be tied in sections with stout silk and the clamp cautiously removed. Great care is taken to get a good grasp with the ligatures. If the pedicle is not too broad it should be transfixed and tied in two portions. Another method which may be successful is to make an incision in the capsule round the pedicle and isolate it beyond the fibro-fatty mass.

Nephrectomy by morcellement.—This is seldom required, but it may be necessary in removing a kidney the seat of long-standing suppurative pyelonephritis. The organ is removed in portions, large clamps being used to control the bleeding. These should be placed as near the pedicle as possible, and will usually have to be left *in situ*. They are removed in forty-eight hours, the wound being rapidly and firmly packed if bleeding should follow their removal.

Partial nephrectomy has been advocated in the treatment of tuberculosis and new growths of the kidney, but has now been abandoned as it is impossible to define the limits of these diseases and remove the whole disease by this method.

Ligature of the renal vessels.—In a few cases, where nephrectomy has been judged too formidable an undertaking owing to previous unsuccessful operations and to extensive adhesions, transperitoneal ligature of the renal artery and vein has been practised as a substitute for nephrectomy. According to Kellock, who has recorded a case and has made observations on the cadaver, the operation on the right side is more difficult than that on the left, owing to the position of the duodenum and pancreas. Aberrant arteries may give rise to difficulties.

Difficulties in lumbar operations.—The chief difficulties encountered in lumbar operations on the kidney are—(1) great adipose development; (2) narrow ilio-costal space, which is found in short, thick-set individuals; (3) high position of the kidney and short vascular pedicle; (4) adhesions and excessive development of the perinephritic fat; (5) distension of the colon due to over-purgation or to want of preparation; (6) deformities of the spine or hip-joint.

Abdominal nephrectomy.—The patient lies on his back. A vertical incision is made either in the semilunar line on the affected side or through the rectus sheath parallel to the median line. In the latter case the rectus muscle is displaced towards the median line, and the posterior layer of the sheath and the peritoneum are incised. The colon is exposed and the small intestine packed off. An incision is made through the outer layer of the mesocolon, and the bowel displaced inwards. The kidney is exposed by incising the anterior layer of perinephritic fascia.

The procedure is now similar to that adopted in the lumbar operation. After removal of the kidney a stab wound is made in the loin and a large rubber drain passed through it. The wound in the mesocolon and the abdominal wound are then closed.

Dangers of nephrectomy.—Wounds of the pleura and peritoneum have been referred to. They are treated by immediate suture, and do not give rise to further trouble.

Shock.—Shock is the most frequently fatal complication. It occurs in a pronounced degree in kidney operations compared with operations on other organs. Traction on the renal pedicle during removal of the kidney has an immediate and powerful effect on the pulse and respiration. In prolonged operations the shock may be profound. It may commence towards the end of the operation or after the patient is returned to bed, and it·is frequently observed three or four hours after nephrectomy. Saline subcutaneous infusion may be administered during the operation if the pulse begins to fail. Rectal saline infusion (enteroclysis) should be commenced when the patient is returned to bed, and continued for several hours, and repeated if necessary. Brandy or strong coffee may be added to the rectal infusion. Hypodermic injections of strychnine ($\frac{1}{60}$–$\frac{1}{30}$ gr.) and intramuscular injection of camphor ($\frac{1}{2}$–3 gr.), or of camphor ($\frac{1}{2}$ gr.) with ether (17 min.), may be required.

Hæmorrhage.—During the operation hæmorrhage may be due to a number of causes. An aberrant artery may be torn during separation of perirenal adhesions. These arteries enter the upper or lower pole of the kidney, and may give rise to severe hæmorrhage. Care should be taken to clamp all suspicious bands before cutting them across. Long artery forceps are useful for seizing the artery when it has been inadvertently torn. The inferior vena cava has been torn during the removal of a malignant growth. The tear is usually lateral, and is followed by very serious venous bleeding. When the wound is small and can be picked up with a pair of forceps a lateral ligature should be placed on it, and this has resulted in recovery in several cases. When the wound is more extensive lateral suture has been practised, and where a severe transverse tear has been produced double circular ligature of the vena cava below the renal veins is recommended.

Hæmorrhage from the pedicle during the operation is frequently due to carelessness or flurry in tying the ligature, resulting in the ligature, from being too loosely applied, slipping after removal of the clamp. A renal vein may be injured in passing the ligature through the pedicle. Good exposure, careful dissection, and care in tying the ligature prevent such accidents.

Should bleeding occur, the pedicle is at once seized with pressure forceps and the individual bleeding-point, if possible, secured, or a new ligature placed more firmly around the whole pedicle. Finally, in a difficult case where the condition of the patient does not permit of much time being spent in again securing the pedicle, a clamp should be applied, and left in position for three days, when it is cautiously removed.

Hæmorrhage after the operation may be due to oozing from unligatured vessels or to slipping of the pedicle ligature. If it is severe the wound must be opened up, the clots removed, and the bleeding-point secured, or, this failing, the cavity is firmly packed with strips of gauze, which are removed in two days.

Anuria.—Anuria may occur immediately after nephrectomy, or there may be gradual failure of the renal function. This is due to inadequacy of the second kidney. Before nephrectomy the state of the second kidney should be examined by catheterization of the ureters and the use of the tests for the renal function. The value of these methods in discriminating cases which are inoperable is strikingly demonstrated by the statistics of nephrectomy for tuberculosis of the kidney previous to their use, and recent statistics since these methods have been employed.

Anuria and oliguria are treated according to the directions given at p. 19.

Remote dangers are **sepsis** and **pulmonary embolism.** Sepsis is avoided by care in preventing the soiling of the wound with pus or tuberculous material when cutting the ureter and removing the kidney, and in general aseptic technique. Should the muscular layers of the wound be infected, this may necessitate the opening up of the wound and entail a prolonged and tedious convalescence. Peritonitis is a danger in transperitoneal operations for septic diseases of the kidney.

The operations of nephrolithotomy, pyelotomy, pyelolithotomy, nephropexy, and decapsulation are described in other chapters.

PART II.—THE URETER

CHAPTER XX

SURGICAL ANATOMY—PHYSIOLOGY EXAMINATION

Surgical anatomy.—The ureter extends from the pelvis of the kidney to the bladder. The upper end commences at the lower pole of the kidney at the level of the 2nd lumbar vertebra, and there is a slight narrowing as it joins the renal pelvis. From this point the ureter passes vertically downwards to cross the iliac vessels at the brim of the bony pelvis, descends into the pelvis, and turns forwards and then inwards to pierce the wall of the bladder. (Fig. 74.)

The ureter has several curves (Fig. 75). The first or lumbar part is vertical, inclining slightly inwards at the upper part. It forms a slight, very long curve with a postero-external concavity. There is a second, more pronounced curve, with the concavity postero-external, as the ureter crosses the iliac vessels and drops into the pelvis; a third, wider but well-marked curve, with the concavity forwards; and finally the duct curves inwards towards the middle line to pierce the wall of the bladder. At the upper end the ureters are about 10 cm. apart, at the level of the iliac crests 7 cm., at the level of the brim of the pelvis 5 cm., at the widest part of the pelvic curve they lie 10 cm. apart, and at the point of entry into the bladder wall 4 cm.

The ureter is 30 cm. (12 in.) long, and has a varying calibre. Gelatin casts show that there are certain narrow points in the normal ureter. According to Poirier there are two types. In the first there are two contractions—the first at the junction of the ureter and pelvis, the second at the point of entrance into the bladder. In the second type there is, in addition to these narrow points, a third contraction at the brim of the pelvis. Between these points there are two " dilatations "—the lumbar dilatation, which is the larger, and the pelvic dilatation.

299

The relations to the skeleton as seen in radiography are very important, and are fully described in the section dealing with examination of the ureter.

Relations of the ureter.—The lumbar portion of the ureter lies upon the sheath of the psoas muscle and crosses the genito-crural nerve. Anteriorly it lies in close relation with the peritoneum, and is crossed by the spermatic or ovarian vessels at the level of the 3rd lumbar vertebra. On the left it is crossed by the

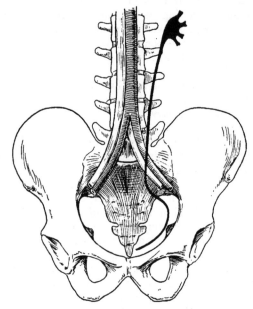

Fig. 74.—Diagram of renal pelvis and ureter, showing relation to spine, pelvic girdle, and great vessels. Drawn from radiograms.

left colic and sigmoid branches of the inferior mesenteric artery, and on the right by the right colic and ilio-colic branches of the superior mesenteric artery. If the vermiform appendix passes upwards and inwards it crosses in front of the lower part of this segment of the ureter.

At the brim of the pelvis the duct crosses the common iliac vessels near their bifurcation, or the external iliac vessels, and is covered by peritoneum. The ureters are intimately related to the peritoneum, and when this membrane is raised the duct remains attached to it.

Internally the right ureter is in contact with the inferior vena cava; the left ureter is in relation to, but not in contact with, the aorta.

The relations of the pelvic portion vary in male and female.

In the male the ureter crosses the brim of the pelvis and passes downwards, backwards, and a little outwards, lying in front of the spine of the ischium and crossing in front of the internal iliac vessels. External to it is the parietal layer of the pelvic fascia covering the obturator internus, and it crosses internally to the obliterated hypogastric artery and the obturator vessels and nerve. Internally it lies in relation to the peritoneum. The duct now turns forwards and inwards on the upper surface of the levator ani and beneath the peritoneum, and is crossed by the vas deferens before it enters the muscular wall of the bladder.

In the female the relations of the first part of the pelvic portion are the same as in the male, except that the ovarian vessels and the ovary lie in relation to it. The second part turns inwards on the upper surface of the levator ani and crosses beneath the broad ligament and alongside, and then in front of, the lateral fornix of the vagina and the cervix uteri, and enters the wall of the bladder. In this part of its course it is surrounded by a dense plexus of veins belonging to the uterine and vaginal plexuses, and it crosses below and behind the uterine artery. The ureter opens into the bladder at the level of the upper one-third with the lower two-thirds of the vagina, and it is adherent to the vaginal wall at the lateral fornix.

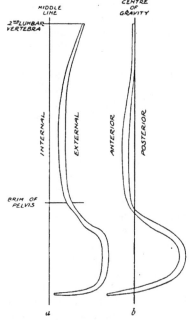

Fig. 75.—Diagrams showing curves and dilatations of ureter.

a, Lateral curves ; *b*, antero-posterior curves.

The ureters pass very obliquely through the muscular wall of the bladder, lying beneath the mucous membrane for some part of this intramural, course, which extends altogether for ¾ in. The ureteric orifices open from ¾ to 1 in. apart as fine slit-like orifices on a low muscular ridge.

Blood-vessels.—The sources of the arterial supply are numerous. From above downwards the ureter receives branches from the renal artery, the spermatic or ovarian, the aorta, the common iliac, the hypogastric, the uterine in the female and the vesical in the male. The arterioles anastomose along the whole length of the duct. The veins empty into the renal, spermatic or ovarian, and hypogastric veins.

The blood supply of a small area of vesical mucous membrane surrounding the orifice of the ureter is intimately connected with the ureteric vessels. The area is inflamed in ureteral inflammations, and congested when obstruction to the ureteric vascular drain is present.

The nerves are derived from the renal, spermatic or ovarian, and hypogastric and vesical plexuses.

Physiology.—The urine descends from the renal pelvis to the bladder, propelled by waves of vermicular contraction which pass down the ureter. The exposed ureter can be stimulated to contract by touching it with a pair of forceps or other instrument. Two forms of contraction are observed—a contraction of the circular muscle fibres, and a writhing movement due to contraction of the longitudinal muscle. The natural waves of contraction are initiated by contractions which commence in the renal pelvis and sweep the whole length of the duct, and are further stimulated by the passage of the urine along the duct. If the ureter is blocked or fistulous at its upper end, so that no urine travels along it, only a feeble contraction reaches the bladder. If the fistula is low down near the bladder the contraction at the vesical orifice is as powerful as if urine were discharged. These facts show that the passage of the urine along the tube is not necessary for the contraction, but that the stimulus of the passing urine greatly increases its vigour.

Continuity of the duct is necessary for the passage of the wave of contraction. If the tube is partly severed and fistulous the contraction passes on to the vesical end ; but if it is completely severed the lower segment no longer contracts.

The oblique insertion of the vesical end in the bladder wall gives it a valve action and prevents the regurgitation of fluid from the bladder. When the bladder becomes distended the trigone is pushed downwards and the rest of the bladder wall is stretched. As the lower end of the ureter is inserted into the trigone the ureter becomes stretched and more oblique. As a result the anterior and posterior walls are approximated, and the intravesical tension presses the anterior against the posterior wall, further occluding the lumen.

Examination. 1. **Inspection.**—I have once seen a greatly distended ureter form a swelling on the abdominal surface (Fig. 76). The patient was a girl of 9, admitted to my ward as a case of intussusception. The abdomen was not distended or rigid, and on the left side, extending from the left lumbar into the iliac region and disappearing in the hypogastric region, was a large sausage-like swelling, very evident on inspection and easily traced on

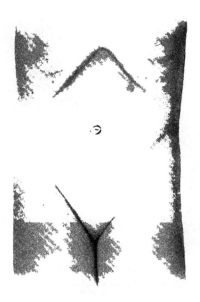

Fig. 76.—Prominence on surface of abdomen in a child caused by greatly distended left ureter.

palpation upwards into the left hypochondrium and downwards into the pelvis. On rectal examination a large tense mass bulged into the rectum. On opening the abdomen a swelling was found to the outer side of the descending colon, and proved to be the greatly distended and thickened left ureter, leading to a small hydronephrosis. The ureter was drained, and a nephro-ureterectomy performed later.

2. **Palpation.**—(a) On *deep palpation of the abdomen* in a favourable subject a thickened ureter can be felt lying alongside the spinal column. It is most readily detected as it crosses the

brim of the pelvis.   In order to palpate the abdominal portion of
the ureter (Fig. 77) the surgeon stands on the same side of the
patient and places the hands flat on the abdomen, the lower hand
reaching as low as the line between the umbilicus and the middle of
Poupart's ligament, the upper one above this hand.   The patient
may lie flat, or with the knees flexed, and respires slowly and
deeply.   With each expiration the fingers sink into the abdomen
in the line of the ureter, and at inspiration they hold the ground
already gained.   After two or three expirations the fingers have
sunk to the back of the abdomen and are slowly drawn outwards,

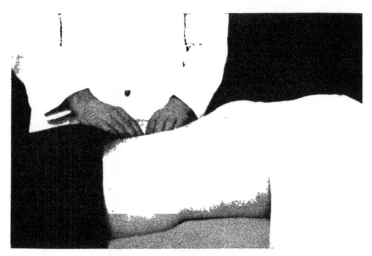

Fig. 77.—Palpation of right ureter.

The fingers are sunk deeply into the right side of the abdomen and are palpating the
ureter at the brim of the pelvis.

palpating the structures which roll under them.   No attempt
should be made to plunge or poke the fingers into the abdomen
against the inspiration of the patient.

The ureter is most readily felt in tuberculosis of the duct, when
it may resemble a leaden gas-pipe, and can be felt alongside the
vertebral bodies and traced over the brim of the pelvis.   Occasionally, after an attack of renal colic, it can be felt thick and very
tender, and when it is dilated and thickened in urethral obstruction it may be felt on careful palpation.

(b) On *rectal palpation in the male* the ureter is felt above and ·
outside the base of the prostate, and can sometimes be hooked
down with the tip of the. finger.   The finger is pushed far up

beyond the base of the prostate and then passed outwards towards the lateral wall of the pelvis.

(c) In the *female* the ureter may be felt in the *vagina* in the normal state, but frequently it cannot be detected. It commences near the middle line on the anterior vaginal wall and passes along the lateral wall at the junction of the middle and upper thirds of the vagina. About 3 in. of a thickened ureter may thus be palpated. The tuberculous ureter is readily felt as a thick, hard, and tender cord which can be rolled beneath the fingers, and it may also be felt in other conditions of chronic ureteritis.

3. Cystoscopy.—On cystoscopy the vesical end of the ureter can be examined and important information obtained.

The vesical mucous membrane surrounding the orifice, the shape and appearance of the orifice itself, the condition of the lips, the absence or presence of ureteric contractions and their frequency and character, the presence of an efflux and its characters, should all be noted. An account of these will be found in the sections dealing with Cystoscopy (pp. 58, 364).

4. Catheterization and sounding of the ureters. — By passing a catheter up each ureter into the renal pelvis, the urine derived from the corresponding kidney is obtained without blending with that of the other kidney and without passing over the surface of a diseased ureter or bladder. The tests for the function of each kidney can be carried out, and the urines examined for changes due to disease or loss of functional power.

The ureter may be sounded by passing a ureteric catheter or a wax-tipped bougie. Information in regard to the presence or absence of stricture or calculus is thus obtained. When a stone is present the catheter may be arrested, or it may hesitate and then pass on. The size of the calculus is not important in regard to the passage of the instrument; a very large calculus may permit the catheter to slip past, while a small calculus may arrest it. Wax-tipped bougies are only useful in the female subject, in whom Kelly's open cystoscopic tubes can be used. These methods are referred to in the chapter on Stone in the Ureter (p. 328).

5. Radiography.—The X-rays may in rare cases show the shadow of a greatly distended and thickened ureter.

Calculi in the ureter throw a shadow in the line of the duct. It is very important to define the course of the ureter in cases of suspected calculus, and this is done by passing up the ureter a bougie opaque to the X-rays, and obtaining a radiogram.

The line of the ureter shown by radiography.—In examining the ureter by the X-rays it is of the utmost importance, as Ironside Bruce has shown, to use a fixed position of the relations of the

U

patient to the source of light. For this there are two reasons:
(1) The line of the ureter is shown in its relation to the bony
skeleton, and variation in the position of the source of light causes
changes in the relations of the shadow of the ureter with those
of the bones. (2) When a stone is descending the ureter slight
changes in the position can only be detected by reproducing with
mathematical exactness at subsequent visits the previous positions of the patient and of the source of light.

The fixed positions suggested by Ironside Bruce are—(1) In
the abdominal and sacral segments "the anode of the X-ray
tube is placed immediately below the spine of the 2nd lumbar
vertebra." (2) In the pelvic and sacral segments the source of
light is opposite the upper border of the pubic symphysis.

There are three segments of the ureter which are important
in reading a radiographic plate :—

1. The abdominal segment, which extends from the renal pelvis
to the upper border of the shadow cast by the bones of the pelvis,
here the lateral mass of the sacrum.

2. The segment in the broad band of shadow thrown by the
lateral mass of the sacrum.

3. The pelvic segment of the ureter.

1. *Abdominal segment.*—The ureter commences in the renal
pelvis at the tip of the transverse process of the 2nd lumbar vertebra. From this point the duct passes inwards and downwards
upon the psoas muscle, crossing the tip of the transverse process
of the 3rd lumbar vertebra and inclining inwards to cross the
transverse process of the 4th lumbar vertebra near its base and
the transverse process of the 5th lumbar vertebra close to the
body. (Plate 21, Fig. 1.)

2. *Sacral segment.*—The ureter then passes vertically along the
lateral mass of the sacrum as it crosses the brim of the pelvis,
well internally to the sacro-iliac synchondrosis.

3. *Pelvic segment.*—After crossing the brim the ureter curves
outwards across the outer border of the sacrum, and now lies
within the ring of the shadow thrown by the brim of the pelvis.
It crosses the tip of the spine of the ischium and, keeping just
internally to the shadow of the pelvic ring, swings inwards. It
may then become hidden behind the horizontal ramus of the
pubic bone, but more frequently it passes above the upper border
of this bone, and reaches almost to the middle line. (Plate 21,
Fig. 2.)

This is the appearance most commonly found, but there are
cases where the course is different. This variation in the course
of the ureter as shown in a radiogram does not depend upon

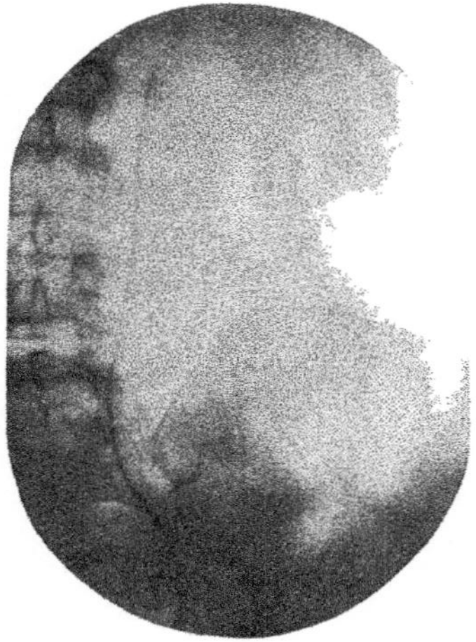

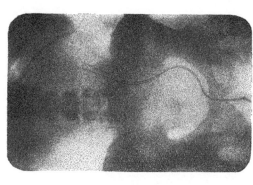

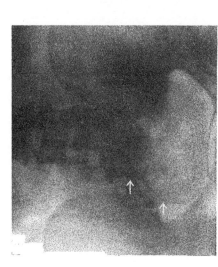

Fig. 1.—Opaque bougie in ureter, crossing sacrum and transverse processes of 5th, 4th, 3rd, and 2nd lumbar vertebræ. (P. 306.)

Fig. 2.—Shadow of calculus in ureter at brim of pelvis. The upper arrow points to long shadow of stone lying in shadow of sacrum, the lower arrow to opaque bougie in ureter. (P. 306.)

Fig. 3.—Shadows of opaque bougies lying in double ureter. (P. 312.)

PLATE 21.

changes in the position of the source of the rays or the patient, as these radiograms were taken in the "fixed position."

(i.) The ureter may lie nearer the middle line, and is partly obscured by the shadow of the vertebral bodies. (ii.) It may lie farther out beyond the tips of the transverse processes and pass outwards from the shadow of the psoas muscle at the level of the 3rd lumbar vertebra. (iii.) It passes upwards and outwards away from the vertebral column at the level of the 4th lumbar vertebra.

These variations may be partly accounted for by an abnormally placed or movable kidney, and it is likely that the less pronounced changes in the line of the ureter result from temporary outward displacement of the kidney by the compressor used during the radiography. The varying tilt of the pelvis also slightly affects the radiographic position of the pelvic ureter.

CHAPTER XXI

INJURIES OF THE URETER

FROM its protected position and the comparative thickness and elasticity of its wall the ureter is less liable to injury by violence than the kidney or other abdominal organs. In 1901, Morris could find only 12 probable cases in the literature, and but 3 of these were actually proved to be ruptures of the ureter.

With the progress of modern surgery a new and more numerous class of cases has appeared, namely, injury to the ureter during surgical operations upon the ureter or on neighbouring structures.

1. SUBCUTANEOUS INJURIES AND PENETRATING WOUNDS

Etiology.—Compression between hard bodies, kicks, falls on the loin, and being run over by a wheel are the forms of violence which have caused rupture of the ureter. Rowlands records the case of a young man who, walking with his left hand in his pocket, fell upon the left elbow and ruptured the left ureter at its upper end. Impaction against the transverse processes of the lumbar vertebræ and overstretching of the ureter are the mechanisms which are believed to produce the rupture. Only a few cases of bullet wounds and punctured wounds by a rapier are on record.

Pathology.—In 1 out of 12 cases the peritoneum over the ureter was ruptured (Morris).

The ureter may be bruised and cicatricial contraction follow; or it may be torn longitudinally, or be torn across.

If the ureter be partly or completely torn an accumulation of urine forms in the retroperitoneal space, which may later rupture into the colon. If the peritoneum be torn, urine leaks into the peritoneal cavity.

Symptoms.—If the ureter alone be injured there is slight hæmorrhage, or this may be completely absent. There are pain and tenderness, which, however, are difficult to distinguish from those which may follow a blow without rupture of the ureter, and which usually pass off in a few days. If the patient survive the injury a swelling forms in the loin. This may appear a few days after the injury, or it may be delayed for several weeks. It is rounded or elongated and well defined, and may assume a large size. This is due to accumulation of urine and blood in the retro-peritoneal tissues. Suppuration takes place, and the symptoms of extensive suppuration develop.

It is impossible to diagnose between rupture of the ureter and rupture of the renal pelvis. If the patient recovers after receiving a penetrating wound of the ureter a urinary fistula forms.

Prognosis.—When early operation is performed the prognosis is good. When the peritoneum is ruptured it is more serious.

Treatment.—In most of the cases recorded, puncture of the swelling and incision and drainage were the methods of treatment adopted. The real difficulties are met with in making an early diagnosis and in finding the ruptured ureter in a large mass of inflammatory tissue. A swelling of the loin following an injury in this region should be freely exposed by a lumbar or a lumbo-abdominal incision, when the presence of urine in the fluid will lead to a careful examination of the renal pelvis and ureter. Should the history of hæmaturia, however slight, or the position of the swelling have led to a suspicion of the nature of the injury, a catheter should be passed up the ureter before the operation, and will help in the identification of the tube. When the ruptured ends are found, one of the methods of ureteral anastomosis should be practised.

In a case recorded by Vaughan of a gunshot wound of the ureter, an implantation of the end of the ruptured ureter into the bladder was successful.

Nephrectomy may be required in rare cases for septic com-plications or for the cure of an intractable fistula.

LITERATURE

Allingham, *Brit. Med. Journ.*, 1891, i. 699.
Barker, *Lancet*, Jan. 17, 1885.
Morris, Hunterian Lectures, 1908.
Page, *Ann. Surg.*, 1894.
Rowlands, *Med. Press Circ.*, April 21, 1909.
Vaughan, *Amer. Journ. Med. Sci.*, 1905, p. 499.

2. Surgical Wounds

Injury to the ureter is occasionally caused by forceps during delivery, but the most frequent form of surgical wound of the duct is made during pelvic operations, and above all in gynæ-cological operations. The removal of malignant growths of the uterus by the extensive operations now in vogue is a prolific source of accidental wounds of the ureter.

The ureter may be partly or completely cut, or its wall or blood supply may be damaged by extensive stripping or by pressure or by rough handling, so that it sloughs and a fistula forms after some days. The fistula may open in the vagina, or, if a subtotal excision of the uterus has been performed, in the cervix or on the skin surface at the abdominal wound.

Spontaneous closure of such a fistula has taken place, but it is so rare as not to be looked for.

Treatment.—The treatment of such accidents is either immediate at the time of the operation, or remote when a fistula has formed. The treatment of fistula will be described later.

1. *Partial laceration or incision of the ureter.*—The ureter heals well if the blood supply has not been damaged by extensive stripping and rough handling. The edges of the wound should be carefully sutured with fine catgut. A ureteral catheter may be passed up the ureter to the renal pelvis from the bladder, and retained for a week. A covering of fatty or areolar tissue or even of peritoneum should be applied over the ureter wound to assist healing. Provision should be made for drainage of the urine should leakage occur. If there be an irregular tear of the ureter it is better to resect a portion of the tube and perform one of the operations for anastomosis.

2. *Complete laceration or section of the ureter.*—Ureteral anastomosis should be carried out.

The varieties of anastomosis are as follows :—

(1) End-to-end anastomosis. (a) The ends are cut transversely (Schopf) ; (b) the ends are cut obliquely (Bovée). The objection to this is that it leaves a ridge in the lumen which promotes stricture formation.

(2) End-to-end anastomosis with invagination (Poggi). This is facilitated by splitting one end and invaginating the other (D'Antona).

(3) The employment of a button (Boari) or a tube of magnesium over which the ends are drawn and invaginated. The tube is dissolved by the urine in twenty days (Taddéi).

(4) End-to-side anastomosis, in which one end is ligatured and the edges of the other end sutured to the edges of a longitudinal wound in the lateral wall of the first, or cut obliquely and invaginated into it (Van Hook).

(5) Lateral anastomosis, in which both ends are ligatured and the edges of a longitudinal lateral wound in each ureter are united in a manner similar to that used in intestinal anastomosis (Monari).

The peritoneum should be closed outside the junction to prevent extraperitoneal extravasation. The junction may be covered with a flap of peritoneum or a graft of omentum. A ureteral catheter may be passed from the bladder up the ureter, but this is likely to cause irritation and is better omitted.

When a portion of the ureter has been torn away, one of the following procedures may be carried out :—

(1) Uretero-cysto-neostomy, the upper end of the ureter being implanted into some part of the bladder. Here the rupture must be low down and the upper segment sufficiently long to reach the bladder (Novaro).

(2) Uretero-ureteral anastomosis, the two ureters being exposed by reflecting the peritoneum on the front of the promontory, and the end of the damaged ureter ligatured and brought across the middle line and united to the uninjured ureter by lateral anastomosis (Bernasconi and Colombino).

(3) The formation of a cutaneous fistula by suture of the severed end to the skin.

(4) Implantation into the intestine.

(5) Immediate nephrectomy.

(6) Ligature of the upper end of the ureter has been suggested, with the object of causing atrophy of the kidney.

Results.—Alksne collected all the published records of ureteral anastomosis since 1886, and found 43 complete recoveries in 60 cases, 9 recoveries after temporary fistula, and 8 deaths (11·6 per cent.).

Poggi's invagination method gave the best results, yielding 12 per cent. of fistulæ in 28 cases, while the circular method gave 24 per cent. of fistulæ.

LITERATURE

Alksne, *Folia Urol.*, 1908, p. 280.
Baja, Thèse de Paris, 1908.
Bernasconi et **Colombino,** *Ann. d. Mal. d. Org. Gén.- Urin.*, 1905, ii. 1361.
Boari, *Il Policlinico,* July 15, 1899 ; *Ann. d. Mal. d. Org. Gén.- Urin.*, 1908, ii. 1761.
Bovée, *Ann. Surg.*, 1900, p. 165.
Hein, *Jahresb. d. Urogen. Apparates*, 1906, ii. 126.
Markoe and **Wood,** *Ann. Surg.*, 1899.
Poggi, XIXᵉ Congrès de Chir., Paris, 1906, p. 188.
Scharpe, *Ann. Surg.*, 1906, p. 687.

CHAPTER XXII

CONGENITAL ABNORMALITIES OF THE URETER
PROLAPSE—FISTULA

CONGENITAL ABNORMALITIES

Anomalies of number.—The ureter is sometimes divided so that there are two ducts, and this may extend from the pelvis to the bladder (Fig. 78). The two tubes may unite to form a single lumen just before entering the bladder, or two distinct ureters may pierce the bladder wall and open separately. The ureter which drains the upper part of the kidney usually crosses that from the lower part and opens lower on the trigone. In such a case there are two physiologically separate kidneys on one side, although no anatomical division may be apparent. Sometimes a deep groove on the surface of the organ indicates the division. One portion of the kidney may be diseased and the other remain normal.

In routine cystoscopy the discovery of two ureteric orifices lying side by side on the horn of the trigone is comparatively frequent (Fig. 79), and an efflux may be seen from each opening. An opaque bougie can be passed up one, or sometimes both, and the double ureter demonstrated by means of the X-rays. The illustration of a double ureter (Plate 21, Fig. 3) was derived from a patient who had been treated for a urethral stricture, and subsequent cystoscopy revealed the double ureter. The frequency of double ureter is about 4 per cent. of cases (Lessig). Calculus is often found in kidneys which have a double pelvis and ureter. Bilateral double ureters are less frequent than unilateral.

Five or even six ureters have been observed in one individual. Absence of a ureter is combined with absence of the kidney. In a case of fused kidney with two ureters one duct may cross the middle line and open on the opposite side of the trigone.

Abnormalities of position.—When a single ureter is present and opens into the bladder the orifice is frequently misplaced, usually towards the middle line. I have seen a single ureter, in the lower end of which a stone was impacted, open in the middle line of the trigone. The ureter may open into the prostatic urethra

312

in the male or the urethra in the female. It has been found to
open into the seminal vesicles, the vagina, or the rectum. The
displaced opening is frequently that of a supernumerary ureter.

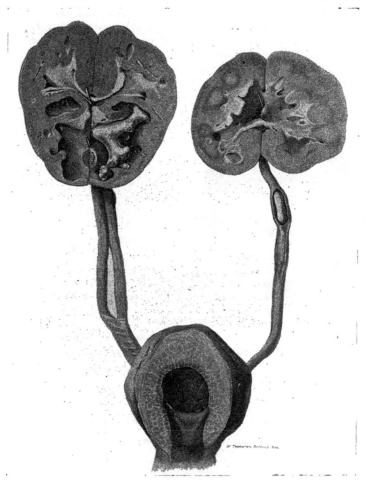

Fig. 78.—Double right ureter draining upper and lower halves
of kidney.

Case of septic pyelonephritis complicating vesical, ureteral, and renal calculi ; chronic cystitis and
hypertrophy of bladder. Lower half of right kidney destroyed by calculus, upper half shows recent
pyelonephritis ; calculus in left ureter ; commencing distension of left kidney.

Out of 9 cases recorded by Schwarz where the ureter opened
into the prostatic urethra, there were double ureters in 7. The

abnormally placed orifice is frequently narrowed so as to cause dilatation of the ureter and corresponding kidney. Sometimes a misplaced ureter ends blindly in the bladder wall and forms a cyst. Nebel has recorded the termination of the ureters on the surface of the abdomen between the umbilicus and the pubes. According to Schwarz the diagnostic sign of a ureter opening into the female urethra is incontinence of urine—the urine dribbling away from the urethra, while the patient can pass a quantity of urine voluntarily. The ureter has been transplanted into the bladder in such cases.

Congenital narrowing of the ureter.—I have observed congenital narrowing of the ureteric orifices in a man whose urinary system was otherwise normal. The finest ureteric catheter or bougie would not pass through the orifices. The lumen of the ureter may be narrowed or completely blocked by a valve or congenital stricture. As a result, either hydronephrosis develops or atrophy of the kidney ensues. Rarely the ureter immediately above the stricture dilates without distension of the renal pelvis and kidney. The ureter may be compressed by an artery or vein which takes an abnormal course (*see* under Hydronephrosis, p. 168).

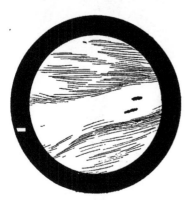

Fig. 79.—Double ureteric orifice on left side.

LITERATURE

Blumer, *Johns Hopkins Hosp. Bull.*, 1896, p. 175.
Israel, *Berl. klin. Woch.*, Feb. 27, 1900.
Lessig, *Charité Ann.*, xxx. 452.
Lewis, Brandsford, *Med. Rec.*, 1906, p. 521.
Meyer, *Virchows Arch.*, 1907, p. 408.
Schwarz, *Beitr. z. klin. Chir.*, 1895, Bd. xv.
Walker, Thomson, *Renal Function in Urinary Surgery.* 1908.
Zondek, *Zur Chirurgie der Ureteren.* Berlin, 1905.

PROLAPSE OF THE URETER

Under the term prolapse of the ureter two conditions are included which it is impossible to distinguish clinically. In one there is prolapse of the whole thickness of the ureteral wall, analogous to prolapse of the rectum ; in the other there is prolapse of the mucous membrane alone.

Pathology.—The tumour is a globular or sausage-shaped cyst attached by a narrower base in the position of the ureteric orifice. It varies in size from a pea to a walnut, or even larger. The cyst consists of a double layer of mucous membrane, the bladder mucosa externally and the ureteral mucosa internally. At some part of the surface, usually the summit of the swelling, the ureteric orifice can be found. It is small, and may be stenosed or completely obliterated. In some cases one or several small calculi have been found in the cavity. The cyst is usually single, but Portner found that of 40 cases 5 were bilateral. I have examined two cases with the cystoscope; in one both ureteric orifices were affected, one to a greater degree than the other, and in the second case the condition affected both orifices equally. (Plate 22, Fig. 1.) In some cases the cyst has prolapsed into the urethra and appeared at the external meatus in the female. Neelsen described a case in which the cyst was strangulated by the vesical sphincter and became necrotic. The condition may result from a congenital narrowing of the ureteric orifice or an acquired stenosis from ureteritis. Calculi may be present in the cystic ureter. In a number of cases there has been a double ureter on the diseased side.

Symptoms.—The symptoms are irregular. In some cases renal symptoms have been present, such as lumbar pain and pain in one or both ureters. More frequently there are symptoms of vesical irritation or obstruction, such as frequent micturition, scalding pain along the urethra, terminal hæmaturia, difficult micturition, and occasional intermittent passage of urine or attacks of complete retention. Attacks of hæmaturia may be the only symptom. The ureter and kidney are frequently dilated on the affected side. Infection of the kidney may supervene. The condition may be latent for a considerable period. The cyst may appear at the external meatus in the female, and can be distinguished from prolapse of the bladder by passing a catheter into the bladder and drawing off the urine.

The **diagnosis** is made with the cystoscope. In the position of the ureteric orifice a rounded, globular, or sausage-shaped swelling is seen, pink and semi-translucent in appearance. In a prolapse of the mucosa alone delicate blood-vessels can be seen coursing over the cyst, while in a prolapse of the whole thickness of the wall the vessels are abruptly arrested at the base (Kapsammer). In two cases that I have seen, the cysts gradually filled up under observation, becoming pale and more transparent until they reached a large size, and then slowly subsiding like an air balloon; and this was repeated in slow, regular rhythm.

In one of these cases the condition was equally developed on both sides, the left cyst being covered with small translucent cysts. On removal of the cysts I found both ureters dilated.

Treatment.—Before operation the kidneys and ureters should be searched with the X-rays for stone.

The pouch is cut off at the base with scissors and removed, with any calculi it may contain.

Operation by the urethra with cutting forceps or the cautery in the female has been successful. Removal by suprapubic cystotomy is preferable.

LITERATURE

Englisch, *Centralbl. f. Krankh. d. Harn- u. Sex.-Org.,* 1898, ix. 7.
Fenwick, *Obscure Diseases of the Kidney.* 1903.
Freyer, *Trans. Roy. Med. and Chir. Soc.,* 1897.
Grosglik, *Zeits. f. Urol.,* 1901, p. 577.
Kapsammer, *Zeits. f. Urol.,* 1908, p. 800.
Kolisko, *Wien. klin. Woch.,* 1889, No. 48.
Portner, *Monats. f. Urol.,* 1904, ix. 5.

FISTULA OF THE URETER

Fistula may follow an operation for stone in the ureter, the external opening being in the scar of the operation. Uretero-vaginal fistula is more common. Rarely it is congenital; frequently it is acquired and follows parturition, in which case it involves the bladder, ureter, and vagina (uretero-vesico-vaginal fistula); or it may result from a surgical operation on the uterus and involve the ureter and vagina only, the opening in the ureter being at some distance (5 cm.—Bazy) from the bladder. The ureter may be partly or completely severed. On the vesical side of the fistula there is almost invariably stenosis of the ureter. Above the fistula the ureter may be dilated, and the kidney is also dilated. The fistula very rarely closes spontaneously.

Infection of the fistula, ureter, and kidney is the rule.

Before operating upon a ureteral fistula it is necessary to ascertain—

(1) *Is the duct partly or completely severed ?* On examination of the bladder with the cystoscope the ureteric orifice shows no movement where the ureter is completely severed, but there is rhythmic contraction of the ureteric orifice if the ureter is only partly severed.

(2) *Is the fistula vesical or ureteral ?* By injecting methylene-blue solution into the bladder the blue fluid escapes by the fistula if the fistula communicates with the bladder, but not if the fistula is purely ureteral.

Examination with the cystoscope will show a healthy bladder when the ureter is fistulous.

(3) *Which ureter is fistulous?* Where the ureter has been completely severed, cystoscopic examination will show one ureter motionless and without efflux, and the subcutaneous injection of 4 c.c. of a 4 per cent. solution of indigo-carmine is followed by the appearance of a coloured efflux at the healthy ureter and no efflux at the other. Regular powerful contractions of the ureteric orifice are observed when the fistula is low down and the duct is not completely severed. There is, however, no efflux from the orifice.

(4) *What is the position of the fistula?* This is ascertained by sounding the ureter with a bougie opaque to the X-rays. The bougie is arrested at the stricture below the fistula, and the distance from the bladder ascertained by observing the markings on the bougie and by obtaining a radiogram.

Treatment. 1. Introduction of a catheter *en demeure.*— This is impossible in a large proportion of cases on account of the stricture of the ureter. It has been practised in a few cases, but the ultimate result has not been successful. The stricture recontracts and the fistula opens after the catheter has been removed, or the fistula may heal permanently and the recontraction of the stricture brings about atrophy of the kidney.

2. Suture of the ureter.—This is not feasible. The patent segments of the ureter are widely separated by a mass of fibrous tissue, and it is impossible to approximate them.

3. Transplantation of the ureter. i. *Implantation into the bladder (uretero-cysto-neostomy).*—This may be done by a transperitoneal operation or by the extraperitoneal route. Leguen recommends that the abdomen be opened and the position of the ureter ascertained. The peritoneum is then closed and the operation performed extraperitoneally. The urine is invariably infected in these cases, so that the extraperitoneal route is to be preferred.

The ureter is followed downwards as low as possible and cut across above the fistula. An opening is made in the most accessible part of the bladder, and the union of the ureter and bladder made at this point. It is essential that no traction be exerted on the newly formed union, and the ureter and bladder should be freed. Ricard sutures the wall of the bladder to the pelvic peritoneum to prevent traction. Many varieties of implantation have been used (p. 339).

Results of uretero-cysto-neostomy.—Primary union is occasionally obtained, but frequently there is leakage of urine. A few cases have been recorded in which by catheterization of the implanted ureter a successful result has been confirmed after considerable periods, but in other cases the kidney has been found atrophied post mortem.

ii. *Implantation into the bowel.*—On the right side the cæcum or ascending colon is selected, on the left the pelvic portion of the colon. (For a description of the operation, *see* p. 342.)

Results of implantation into the bowel.—Successful results have been published. The mucous membrane of the colon does not resent the action of the urine, and the fluid is passed with the fæces.

The dangers of the operation are shock, peritonitis, and ascending pyelonephritis from infection.

Papin found a mortality from the operation of 58 per cent. where bilateral implantation was performed, and 29 per cent. where one ureter only was implanted. A few cases have been recorded in which the patient continued in good health, but many patients die within a comparatively limited period of ascending pyelonephritis.

iii. *Lateral anastomosis of the upper segment of the injured ureter with the opposite ureter* has been performed experimentally by Bernasconi and Colombino for injuries of the ureter. The ureters are exposed by reflecting the peritoneum over the promontory, and lateral anastomosis carried out. The method has not yet emerged from the experimental stage.

4. Where the fistula opens high up in the vagina an operation may be performed which **turns a small portion of the vagina into the bladder.** The fistula is enlarged, and an opening made into the bladder close to it. This part of the vagina is then closed off so that the fistula and bladder become continuous.

5. **The vagina may be obliterated** after first establishing a large vesico-vaginal fistula.

6. **Ligature of the ureter** with the object of producing atrophy of the kidney was suggested by Guyon.

7. **Nephrectomy** has until recently been resorted to by a large number of surgeons. It should not be performed until a plastic operation has been tried, or unless septic pyelonephritis is present.

LITERATURE

Bernasconi et **Colombino,** *Ann. d. Mal. d. Org. Gén.-Urin.* 1905, ii. 1361.
Boari, *Ann. d. Mal. d. Org. Gén.-Urin.,* 1909, ii. 1232.
Budinger, *Arch. f. klin. Chir.,* 1894, p. 639.
Legueu, *Traité Chir. d' Urol.,* 1910, p. 1172.
Payne, *Journ. Amer. Med. Assoc.,* 1908, p. 1321.
Scharpe, *Ann. Surg.,* 1906, p. 687.
Tuffier et **Lévi,** *Ann. de Gyn. et d'Obst.,* 1895, p. 382.

CHAPTER XXIII

STONE IN THE URETER

THE great majority of calculi in the ureter are formed in the renal pelvis and passed into the ureter. Very rarely a calculus is formed in the ureter itself. In a man from whose right ureter I had removed a calculus impacted at the brim of the pelvis, I closed the ureteric wound with fine silk. Six months later he passed a smooth oval calculus with one silk suture and a facet, and after another six months he passed a second calculus articulating with the first and containing the remaining three silk sutures I had placed in the ureter. (Fig. 80.) Primary calculi have also been found on other forms of foreign body, such as a catheter or a pin (Boyer), or on an ulcerated surface.

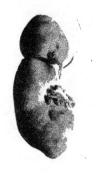

The etiology of secondary ureteric calculus is that of renal calculi (p. 249).

Fig. 80.—Two articulating ureteral calculi formed on fine silk sutures introduced after ureterolithotomy.

Pathology.—Ureteral calculi are either impacted or migrating. A stone migrating from the renal pelvis may pass without halting, and sometimes with little pain, into the bladder. It may pass after repeated attacks of renal colic, having remained in the ureter for a considerable time. It may be arrested in the ureter, and, in spite of repeated attacks of colic, remain impacted. (Plate 23, Figs. 1, 2.)

The calculus becomes arrested in the ureter on account of its large size, irregular shape, or rough surface, or from a part of

319

the ureter being too narrow, or from the presence of a fold or valve, or of a stricture caused by injury from the previous passage of a calculus, or from laceration or rupture of the ureter, or from the pressure of a tumour from without.

Position of impaction.—The calculus is usually arrested at one of the three narrow parts of the ureter, namely, at the outlet of the renal pelvis, at the brim of the bony pelvis (Figs. 81, 82, 83, 84), or at the entrance of the ureter into the bladder (Fig. 86).

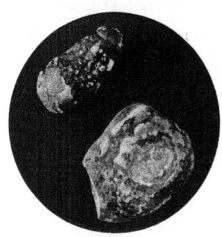

Fig. 81.—Faceted ureteral calculi removed from ureter at brim of pelvis (upper stone) and at vesical end (lower stone). Actual size. (*See* Plate 23, Fig. 1.)

Out of 204 collected cases, Jeanbrau found the calculus in the lumbar portion of the ureter in 46 (22·8 per cent.), in the iliac portion (just above the iliac vessels) in 15 (7·4 per cent.), in the pelvic portion in 105 (52 per cent.), and in the intramural portion in 36 (17·8 per cent.).

In rare cases the position of the calculus changes with the position of the patient. In a patient on whom I operated, a round calculus the size of a marble travelled from the lower part of the pelvic ureter, in which position it was radiographed, into the lumbar segment of the

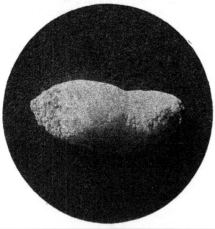

Fig. 82.—Calculus removed from pelvic portion of ureter. Actual size. (*See* Plate 25, Fig. 2.)

ureter at the level of the iliac crest, on the patient being placed in the

Trendelenburg position. (Fig. 87.) In another patient two stones threw shadows, one at the pelvic brim and the other at the bladder, and were found in this position at operation; they were faceted and articulated with each other. (Fig. 81.)

Number, shape, and size of calculi.—There is usually only one calculus (90 per cent.), but there may be two, three, or as many as twenty-seven. The calculi are bilateral in a small number of cases (3·6 per cent.).

In shape they resemble a date or olive-seed, or a coffee-bean, or they may be round, or, when large, oval or sausage-shaped.

The surface may be smooth and polished, or granular, or covered with small bosses, or very frequently they show a spiculated surface of sharp, glistening crystals.

Large calculi have been removed from the ureter. Bloch removed one weighing 816 gr., Carless one weighing 803 gr., and Federoff one of 780 gr. In composition they resemble renal calculi. A small calculus impacted in the ureter increases in size by deposits which are greatest at its upper end—that nearest

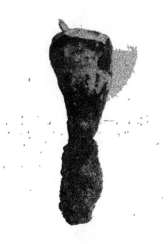

Fig. 83.—Calculus removed from ureter at brim of pelvis.

Note original calculus at lower end.

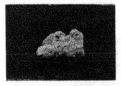

Fig. 84.—Calculus removed from ureter at brim of pelvis (actual size) previous to formation of calculi shown in Fig. 80.

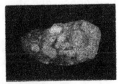

Fig. 85.—Ureteral calculus removed by operation.

the kidney—and the nucleus will be found at the lower or vesical end of a large stone. (Fig. 83.)

The wall of the ureter may be unchanged, or there may be a

v

stricture below the stone, or a diverticulum in which the stone
lies. In old-standing cases the ureter above the calculus is dilated

Fig. 86.—Ureteral calculus.
The small cone-like end projected into the
bladder, and the narrow neck was grasped
by the ureteric orifice.

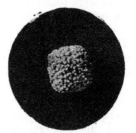

Fig. 87.—Calculus which
travelled up a dilated
ureter.

(Fig. 87) and the walls are greatly thickened, so that the duct
is the size of the small intestine.

When the stone occupies the intramural portion of the ureter

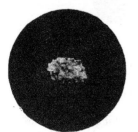

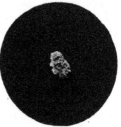

Fig. 88.—Types of ureteral calculi.

it forms a rounded swelling in the bladder to the outer side of
the ureteric orifice, and it may project into the bladder. (Fig. 86,
and Plate 22, Fig. 5.) The stone may ulcerate through this part of

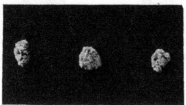

Fig. 89.—Oxalate-of-lime calculi passed from kidney.

the ureter into the bladder, leaving a ragged opening to the outer
side of the normal orifice. The edges of this eventually become

smooth and rounded, and act as the functional ureteric orifice. (Plate 22, Fig. 7.) Rarely a prolapse of the ureter is caused

In the corresponding kidney there are calculi in 13 per cent.

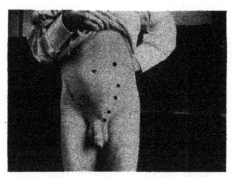

Fig. 90.—Areas of fixed pain in slowly descending ureteral calculus.

The uppermost spot represents anterior renal pain; the lowest spot, pain when the calculus had reached the lower end of the ureter. The intervening spots were pain areas at intervals of from six months to one year.

of cases, and there are bilateral renal calculi in 3 per cent. (Jean-brau). Hydronephrosis occurs in 11 per cent., pyelonephritis and pyonephrosis in 12 per cent. In rare cases the kidney becomes sclerosed and atrophied.

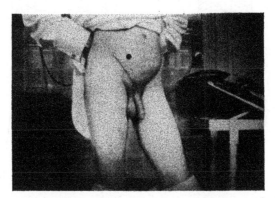

Fig. 91.—Position of pain in ureteral calculus at brim of pelvis, marked by black spot.

The scar of operation for extraperitoneal removal of the calculus is visible.

Symptoms.—In some cases of ureteric calculus there is a history of the passage of a calculus at some previous time. When a stone descends into the ureter there is an attack of renal colic, and this is repeated either at frequent or at long intervals. The colic has the same character and distribution as that caused by

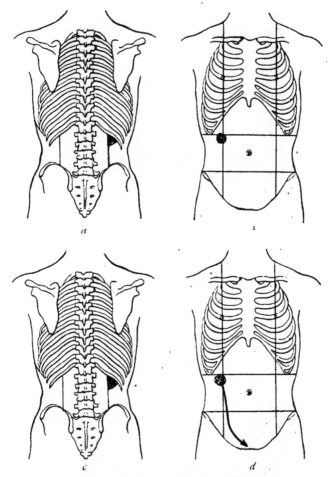

Fig. 92.—Pain-history in case of ureteral calculus which became impacted at brim of pelvis.

a, b, Severe fixed anterior and posterior renal pain, August, 1901.
c, d, Attacks of renal colic, October, 1901.

a stone in the renal pelvis, and there may be nothing to distinguish the two conditions. Frequently the colic commences at some spot lower than the kidney, and shoots downwards. There may be attacks of pain which does not radiate, at some spot in the line of the ureter. (Figs. 90, 91, 92, 93.)

Apart from the attacks of colic, there may be fixed pain of a

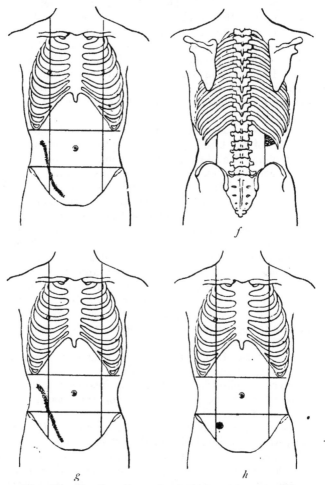

Fig. 93.—Continuation of pain-history (*see* Fig. 92).

e, Discomfort, 1901 to 1903. *f, g,* Attacks of pain, June, 1904. *h*, Fixed pain, July, 1904.

dull aching character over some part of the line of the ureter on the anterior surface of the abdomen. Occasionally there is fixed pain in the back just above the crest of the ilium and outside the erector spinæ mass of muscles. The fixed pain is worse on movement or straining, and is increased by taking diuretics.

The attacks of colic may be frequent and severe until the calculus is expelled into the bladder. The patient frequently feels something drop into the bladder, and the pain ceases. After an interval of one or several hours or of a few days the calculus is expelled, either easily or with pain and strangury. In other cases, after a period of frequent attacks of renal colic the attacks become less frequent and less severe, and may entirely cease. During the attacks of colic there may be frequent attempts at micturition and very little urine passed, or the bladder may remain undisturbed.

When the stone has descended to a point just outside or within the wall of the bladder, certain symptoms are often superadded. Symptoms of bladder irritation become prominent. There is frequent micturition day and night with strangury and pain referred to the end of the penis. Genital symptoms also appear. There are painful nocturnal emissions, pain at the moment of ejaculation, hæmospermia, and intermittent pain in the corresponding testicle. Genital symptoms are explained by the relations of the lower end of the ureter to the seminal vesicles (Young). There is also constant pain in the rectum, aggravated during defæcation. These symptoms, however, are often entirely absent.

Changes in the urine are very common. Hæmaturia may be pronounced, and in rare instances is the only symptom. It usually follows an attack of renal colic, and lasts a few hours or one or two days, and is aggravated by movement. It may, however, be absent or microscopic.

During an attack of colic there may be temporary diminution or complete suppression of urine. Under certain circumstances anuria becomes established. Sometimes an increased quantity of urine is passed after the crisis is over, or the quantity may gradually return to normal.

In rare cases there may be continuous polyuria. In a man of 38 years, with a small calculus in the pelvic portion of the left ureter, the quantity of urine varied from 120 to 165 oz. in twenty-four hours, with a specific gravity of 1006. After ureterolithotomy the quantity of urine fell to from 40 to 50 oz. in twenty-four hours, with a specific gravity of 1010 to 1024. (Chart 16.)

The urine may contain pus and bacteria, crystals, and tube casts. Phosphaturia may occasionally be present without other changes in the urine.

Course and prognosis.—In addition to calculous anuria, which is a rare accident, two complications occur, both of which

are almost inevitable in an impacted calculus; they are infection
and chronic urinary obstruction. Infection is usually hæmatogenous in origin, but may be introduced by a sound or catheter.
Pyelonephritis or pyonephrosis results. Obstruction takes place
insidiously, and may not cause pronounced symptoms until a
large hydronephrosis is found.

Examination of the patient. 1. Palpation. — There may
be tenderness on palpation at some part of the abdomen along

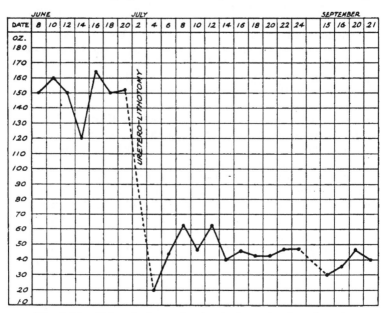

Chart 16.—Polyuria in ureteral calculus, showing drop to
normal quantity after uretero-lithotomy.

the line of the ureter. If this is due to a stone in the right
ureter at the level of the brim of the pelvis the tender spot is
close to the appendix, and may lead to confusion.

A stone is seldom of sufficient size to be palpable in the abdominal part of the ureter.

On rectal examination in the male a stone at the lower end
of the ureter may be felt above and outside the base of the
prostate as a small, buried, tender nodule.

A large stone is distinctly felt alongside the rectum. In a
favourable subject I have felt a stone as high as the brim of the
pelvis on rectal examination. In the female subject a small stone

:can usually be felt in the lower end of the ureter by the finger in the vagina.

2. **Cystoscopy.**—The symptoms may be similar to those of vesical calculus, and the X-rays throw a shadow in the bladder area when the stone is still in the lower end of the ureter.

By cystoscopy the presence of a calculus in the bladder is excluded.

In descending calculi the ureteric orifice may show no change even where the stone is large and low down. More frequently, however, changes are observed: the ureteric area is congested, the lips are thick and the orifice is gaping (Plate 22, Fig. 2). There may be fine ecchymoses around the orifice, or a flame-like hæmorrhage outside the opening (Plate 22, Fig. 3). In some cases one or both lips are bright-red and partly everted. When the stone has reached the lower end of the ureter, but has not entered the intramural part of the duct, the orifice may be open and puckered and surrounded by heaped-up, dark, velvety mucous membrane (Plate 22, Fig. 6), or the mucous membrane at the mouth of the ureter may be converted into a rosette of beautifully transparent œdematous bullæ or into delicate transparent clubs.

Sometimes the œdema spreads to the base of the bladder, and large œdematous fingers and bosses hide the trigone from view. In other cases the stone has reached the intramural portion of the ureter, and appears as a rounded swelling to the outer side of the ureteric orifice, which is red and gaping.

The brown or white tip of the stone may project from the ureteric orifice (Plate 22, Fig. 5). Sometimes it is crystalline and sparkles in the cystoscopic light.

When the stone has passed into the bladder a mushroom-shaped projection of mucous membrane may prolapse into the viscus (Plate 22, Fig. 4) like a prolapse of the rectum, or the orifice is open and lacerated.

The efflux when a calculus is descending may be rapid and forcible, and may be tinged or stained with blood or cloudy with pus. With an impacted stone low down in the ureter the movements at the orifice are frequently slow and lazy, and the efflux feebly wells out.

3. **Sounding the ureter.**—The ureter may be sounded by a ureteral catheter or solid ureteral bougie passed by means of a catheter cystoscope. The bougie may be arrested by the calculus, or it may hitch and then pass on. Stenosis of the ureter, or sometimes a fold of mucous membrane, or angling of the ureter from a loaded rectum or a poorly filled bladder, may block the passage of the catheter, and the value of this method, if used alone, is

Fig. 1.—Prolapse of ureters. The partly distended prolapse of right ureter and a small part of prolapse of left ureter are seen. (P. 315.)

Fig. 2.—Right ureteral orifice in descending ureteral calculus (infected). The orifice is open and the lips are rigid, thickened, and warped. (P. 328.)

Fig. 3.—Descending ureteral calculus (non-infected). Round open left ureteral orifice with ecchymosis near edge. (P. 328.)

Fig. 4.—Eversion of ureteral orifice twenty minutes after expulsion of calculus into bladder. (P. 328.)

Fig. 5.—Uric-acid calculus partly extruded from ureteral orifice (P. 328.)

Fig. 6.—Acute ureteritis in descending calculus. Note œdema of ureteral orifice and patch of ecchymosis. (P. 328.)

Fig. 7.—False ureteral orifice produced by ulceration of calculus from ureter into bladder. True ureteral orifice seen on right. (P. 323.)

PLATE 22.

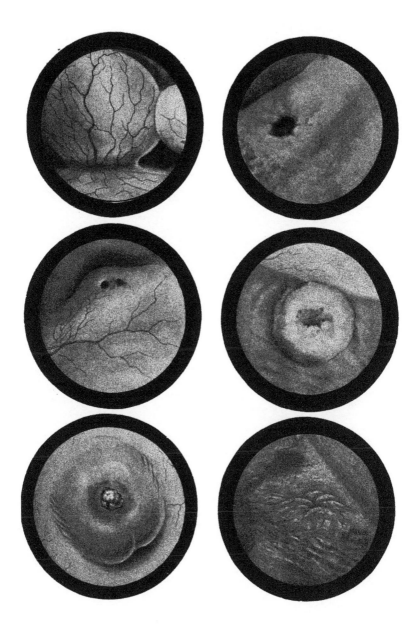

limited. Kelly has used wax-tipped ureteric bougies, which are passed up the ureter and may show scratches on the surface of the wax if a calculus is present. The method can only be used in the female and with a Kelly's tube, as the bougies do not pass freely along the tunnel of the catheter cystoscope, and are scratched by the rigid orifice of-the instrument. Newman has introduced a fine metal sound, which is attached to a small air balloon, and this to an ear-piece. The contact of the point of the sound with a calculus is heard by the operator. The application of this method is limited to female patients, and only a calculus in the lower end of the ureter could be safely reached with the metal sound.

Separation of the urines of the two kidneys by the separators or by the ureteral catheter will show changes such as blood, pus, casts, etc., on the diseased side, but does not give information in regard to the diagnosis of stone.

4. **Radiography.**—Radiography is the most accurate and reliable method by which ureteric calculus is diagnosed. The radiographer may be unable to show very small calculi or those formed entirely of uric acid, but stones the size of a split pea or even less can be demonstrated. Pure uric-acid calculi without the admixture of oxalates or phosphates are very rare. It is necessary that the whole urinary tract should be examined in every case, irrespectively of symptoms localized to a point in one ureter. A negative should always be obtained and examined: the screen is not sufficient.

A ureteric calculus throws a shadow in the line of the ureter (Plate 23, Figs. 1, 2, and Plate 25, Figs. 2, 3). This line crosses several bone shadows—the transverse processes of the 3rd, 4th, and 5th lumbar vertebræ, the sacrum internally to the sacro-iliac synchondrosis, the spine of the ischium, and frequently the horizontal ramus of the pubes—and in a doubtful case these parts should be carefully searched, and, if necessary, several plates taken at slightly different angles, as well as stereoscopic photographs. In small stones the shadow is usually oval, with the long axis in the line of the ureter, and they are generally single. Large calculi form round, or elongated rod-like, or sausage-shaped shadows.

Shadows thrown by other conditions may lead to difficulty in diagnosis of the shadow. Of these the most important are calci- fied lymph-glands (Plate 24, and Plate 25, Fig. 1), appendices epiploicæ, atheromatous patches in arteries, phleboliths, calcareous deposits in old scars or chronic inflammatory tissue or on ligatures from a previous operation, or calcareous deposits in the seminal vesicles, intestinal contents such as scybala, foreign bodies in the bowel (Blaud's pills, etc.), fæcal matter coated with bismuth, calculi in the appendix, and enteroliths. A differential diagnosis is made by the position of the shadow, the shape, the numbers, by stereoscopic photographs, and by the clinical history (*see also* p. 305).

Radiography with an opaque bougie as a guide.—Although a shadow, from its size, shape, and density, falls within the supposed path of the ureter, some further method of diagnosis will be necessary should the clinical symptoms not clearly point to the presence of a calculus. This is provided by the passage up the ureter of a bougie opaque to the X-rays. These instruments may be obtained in the form of a solid bougie or a catheter. Lead and antimony are metals frequently used in their manufacture. The method of introducing an opaque bougie into the ureter and obtaining a radiogram in order to define the position and trace the course of the duct was first used in the living subject by Tuffier (1897). Tilden Brown published observations on the method in 1898, but it was first placed on a certain and practical basis by an important article by Kolischer and Schmidt in 1901. In 1905, Fenwick drew attention to the value of the method in ureteric calculus. The bougie may be arrested by the stone, and the radiogram shows the stone shadow at the tip of the bougie shadow ; or the bougie may hitch and pass on, and the close relation of the two shadows is then evident. The combination of this method with stereoscopic radiograms gives very accurate information. (Plate 25, Figs. 2, 3, and Plate 26.)

Radiography and the injection of collargol.—In the life-history of a ureteral calculus there comes a time when dilatation of the kidney commences, and from this time onwards the renal tissue is steadily destroyed by expansion. The clinical symptoms give no indication as to when expansion is commencing, and when the kidney is found large and hydronephrotic the renal tissue is already destroyed. By the passage of a ureteric catheter and the injection of collargol (10 per cent.) a shadow of the contour of the renal pelvis is obtained and early dilatation is diagnosed (*see* p. 176).

Treatment. 1. Diuretic treatment.—The cases suitable for diuretic treatment are those of small stones recently engaged in the ureter with recurring attacks of renal colic, and especially where a calculus has previously been passed. Potassium citrate and acetate (15 or 20 gr. thrice daily), theocin sodium acetate (3–8 gr. twice daily), Contrexéville (Pavillon), Evian, and Vittel water, are some of the diuretics which may be given. Antispasmodies may be administered at the same time, such as atropine and belladonna. A visit to one of the spas, such as Contrexéville or Vittel, may prove successful when diuretic treatment at home

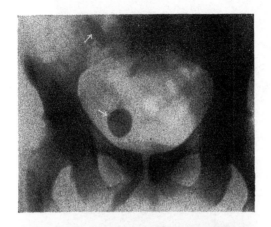

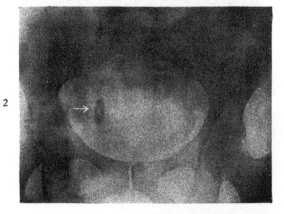

Fig. 1.—Two calculi in right ureter. The lower round calculus lies just outside the bladder, the upper long oval calculus lies obliquely in the shadow thrown by the sacrum and ilium, and was impacted at the brim of the pelvis, lying upon the iliac vessels. (Pp. 319 and 320, Fig. 81.)

Fig. 2.—Oval calculus in pelvic segment of right ureter. (P. 329.)

PLATE 23.

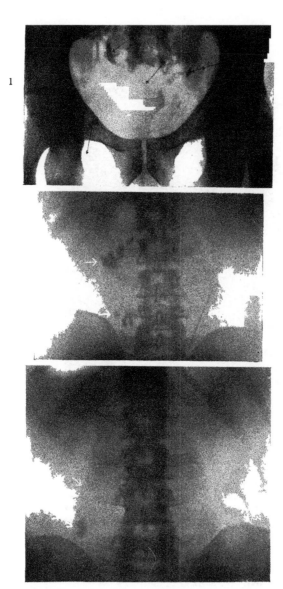

Fig. 1.—Shadows in pelvis due to calcareous glands. There is also a calculus in left ureter (double arrow). (P. 329.)

Fig. 2.—Shadows thrown by calcareous glands in region of pelvis and ureter on right side (arrows). Opaque catheter in left ureter (arrow). (P. 329.)

Fig. 3.—Shadow thrown by calcareous gland (lower arrow) outside line of right ureter. Edge of psoas muscle shown by upper shadow. (P. 329.)

has failed. The treatment should be limited to four or six months, at the end of which time an operation should be recommended if there is no sign of the stone passing. If collargol examination of the renal pelvis and calyces shows commencing dilatation, or bacteriological examination of the urine shows infection to have occurred, immediate operation should be undertaken.

2. **Instrumental treatment.**—The passage of a bougie up the ureter is sometimes followed by the expulsion of the stone. Oil has been injected and eucaine introduced along a ureteric catheter to assist expulsion and relieve spasm.

Nitze and Jahr have passed a ureteric catheter with a membranous balloon which, when distended, dilated the ureter below the calculus.

These methods are only successful in a small number of cases, and safe only in the most expert hands.

3. **Operative treatment.**—Operation is indicated—

i. In calculous anuria (*see* p. 278).

ii. When medicinal treatment has failed.

iii. When infection has occurred.

iv. When dilatation of the kidney is commencing.

When the calculus is situated in the lumbar segment of the ureter it is exposed by an oblique lumbar incision similar to that used for exposing the kidney, and the ureter found at the lower end of the kidney and traced down to the stone.

When the stone is impacted at the brim of the pelvis the ureter is exposed by a curved incision commencing at the level of the anterior superior iliac spine and passing downwards and inwards parallel to Poupart's ligament and about 2 in. above it. The incision passes through the abdominal muscles, care being taken at the inner end not to wound the veins of the spermatic cord. The deep epigastric artery is ligatured. The transversalis fascia is carefully divided to the full length of the wound, and the patient is then placed in the Trendelenburg position. The peritoneum is now reflected along the external iliac vessels. The ureter adheres to the peritoneum, and should be searched for at the level of the bifurcation of the iliac artery. An opaque line or a leash of vessels on the peritoneum will show its position if the stone cannot at first be felt. The ureter is separated by blunt dissection (Fig. 94), but should not be extensively isolated or roughly handled. A fine catgut suture is introduced before removing the stone, and the incision in the ureter should be accurately longitudinal. The ureteral wound is closed with fine catgut on fine rounded needles. The abdominal wound is very carefully closed with stout catgut and a rubber drainage tube introduced, care being taken to keep the tube high up to avoid contact with the iliac vessels.

Calculus of the pelvic portion of the ureter may be removed by several methods.

By an extraperitoneal route, using the Trendelenburg position and the same curved incision, and tracing the ureter over the brim into the pelvis. In a small movable calculus the ureter

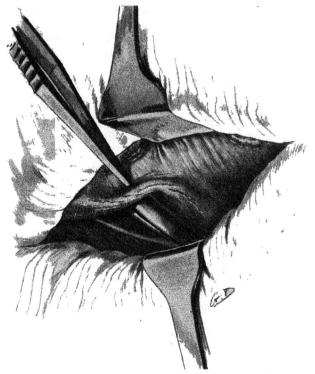

Fig. 94.—Operation view of exposure of ureter at brim of pelvis.

The ureter is being detached from the peritoneum by blunt dissection.

should be opened above the iliac vessels, and a fine scoop (Fig. 95) or long ureteral forceps passed down and the calculus removed. A large fixed stone must be removed by an incision through the ureter directly over it, the abdominal muscles being strongly retracted inwards, and a good light being directed into the wound from a head-lamp.

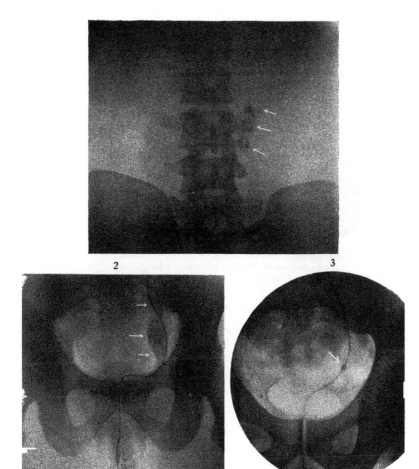

2

3

Fig. 1.—Shadows thrown by calcareous glands below and internally
to left kidney. (P. 329.)

Fig. 2.—Shadow of large oval calculus in pelvic segment of left
ureter, and opaque bougie lying beside it. At lower end
of calculus is seen denser shadow of nucleus. This calculus produced the hydronephrosis seen in Plate 4,
Fig. 1. (Pp. 329, 330.)

Fig. 3.—Calculus in pelvic segment] of ureter (arrow), and opaque
bougie lying in ureter. (Pp. 329, 330.)

PLATE 25.

2

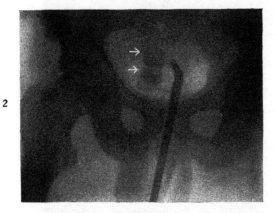

Fig. 1.—Ureteral calculus lying in pelvic segment, cystoscope in bladder, and opaque bougie in ureter.' (P. 330.)

Fig. 2.—Two calculi lying at lower end of right ureter (arrows). Cystoscope is seen in position, and opaque bougie passed into ureter and arrested by calculi. (P. 330.)

PLATE 26.

Other methods of exposing the ureter are described in the Chapter on Operations on the Ureter (Chap. xxiv.). For stone in the pelvic portion of the ureter the sacral, the transperitoneal, the vaginal, or the transvesical route may be used.

Calculus in the intramural portion of the ureter is removed from within the bladder after suprapubic cystotomy. The bladder must be drained by a tube in the suprapubic wound.

After all operations on the ureter for stone the duct should be examined by passing a bougie downwards into the bladder to search for other stones or for stricture. If a stricture be present it should be incised in the long axis of the duct, and if the lumen be much contracted it may be necessary to perform a plastic operation. Dr. R. Dos Santos has introduced a ureterotome which consists of a concealed knife in a flexible ureteric catheter. This is of use in cases of stricture of the ureter.

Apart from cases of calculous anuria, extraperitoneal ureterolithotomy has an operative mortality of under 2 per cent. (1·66

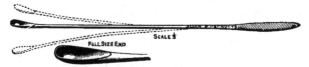

Fig. 95.—Author's pliable scoop for ureteral calculus.

per cent.—Jeanbrau). When other operations are combined with uretero-lithotomy the mortality rises to 13·11 per cent. Transperitoneal uretero-lithotomy has a mortality of 5·5 per cent.

Late results.—Urinary fistula results from stenosis of the duct, and is rare (3 per cent.). Recurrence is, I believe, also rare (*see* p. 319). Patients on whom I have operated have remained well seven years, five years, three years after the operation.

In the early stage of dilatation of the kidney the organ may completely recover, but in the later stage recovery of the renal tissue is only partial.

LITERATURE

Bloch, *Folia Urol.*, April, 1909.
Carless, *Proc. Roy. Soc. Med.*, Jan., 1910.
Dos Santos, *Med. Contemp.*, Dec. 31, 1911.
Fenwick, *Obscure Diseases of the Kidney.* 1903.
Jeanbrau, *Des Calculs de l'Uretère.* 1909.
Kelly, *Operative Gynæcology*, vol. i. 1898.
Kolischer and **Schmidt,** *Journ. Amer. Med. Assoc.*, Nov. 9, 1901.
Morris, *Surgical Diseases of the Kidney and Ureter.* 1901.
Rigby, *Ann. Surg.*, Nov., 1907.
Tuffier, *Traité de Chirurgie* (Duplay et Reclus), 1899, vii. 418.
Young, *Trans. Amer. Assoc. Gen.-Urin. Surg.*, 1907, vol. ii.

CHAPTER XXIV

OPERATIONS ON THE URETER

AN operation upon the ureter may be required to complete some operation upon the kidney or upon the bladder, or it may be called for to remedy some injury or disease of the duct itself. In operating upon the ureter the greatest delicacy and gentleness in manipulation is necessary. The muscular wall of the tube is easily torn, the blood supply readily damaged. The penalty of rough handling is the formation of stricture and fistula of the ureter, and the ultimate fate of the kidney is often nephrectomy.

If present, sepsis of the bladder and urethral obstruction should be effectually treated before the operation is embarked upon. In some cases cystotomy may be necessary for the purpose of drainage, apart from any question of intravesical operation upon the ureter.

Renal sepsis usually takes the form of pyonephrosis, which should be treated by temporary nephrostomy before the plastic ureteral operation. When the infection is mild this may not be required, but in such cases, and even when no infection is present, the question of draining the kidney as a temporary measure to spare the line of union in plastic operations on the ureter should be considered. Extensive stripping of the ureter is to be avoided. The adhesion to the peritoneum should be preserved as far as is compatible with the freedom required for a plastic or other operation. This is especially important when the duct is to be or has been cut across, and the continuity of the anastomosis of blood-vessels severed. The ureter can be cut across, or it may be stripped for a considerable distance, without any untoward result; but if it is both cut across and stripped, sloughing is likely to follow. In manipulating the ureter delicate-toothed forceps should be used, and care taken not to include in the grip the blood-vessels, which are usually quite evident.

Incisions into the tube should be made longitudinally. If the tube is to be cut across it is usually best to cut it obliquely, so as to obtain a larger.lumen, although this is not necessary in a dilated ureter.

The finest round-bodied needles should be used if the ureter is of normal size. A cutting needle causes a considerable amount of damage to the wall.

Fine soft catgut which is not impregnated with strong antiseptics such as iodine, or stiffened with chromic acid, should be used for suturing. Silk, even of the finest size, should be avoided, as a stone will form on the suture (*see* p. 319). It is seldom possible to suture the wall without including mucous membrane, nor do I consider that this matters in the least if proper catgut be used. Stitches should not be placed too near together, and should not be tied too tightly, lest the line of suture slough. Wherever it is possible some covering for the line of suture should be provided. A fold of peritoneum or a tag of fatty tissue is invaluable as soldering material for the wound. A drain should be placed as near the line of suture as possible, with the view of avoiding accumulation of urine should leakage take place.

A leak during the first two or three days does not mean failure of the suture line, and perfect union may follow if no accumulation of urine be permitted.

Exposure of the Ureter

The ureter may be exposed by a transperitoneal or an extra-peritoneal operation.

The four regions in which the ureter is exposed are the lumbar or abdominal, at the brim of the bony pelvis, in the pelvis, and in the wall of the bladder.

1. **Extraperitoneal exposure of the lumbar segment of the ureter.**—This operation is generally part of an operation upon the kidney. The usual oblique kidney incision is made and the lower pole of the kidney exposed. This is pushed up under the ribs, making the ureter tense, and the retroperitoneal surface of the colon is displaced forwards. In the areolar tissue behind or to the inner side of the colon the ureter is found and is isolated by blunt dissection.

By carrying the lumbar incision forwards just above the anterior superior iliac spine the ureter can be traced as far as the brim of the pelvis where it crosses the iliac vessels.

2. **Extraperitoneal exposure of the whole length of the ureter.**—Extraperitoneal exposure of the ureter commences as an oblique lumbar incision at the angle between the erector spinæ muscles and the last rib, and sweeps round the anterior superior iliac spine about 1 in. above and internally to it. The incision then runs parallel and about 2 in. above Poupart's ligament to

the outer border of the rectus muscle near its insertion. In this incision the epigastric vessels are ligatured and cut.

The incision has been used for ureterectomy, especially in tuberculous disease of the ureter. It is not, however, necessary to make so extensive an incision. If the upper wound be carried almost to the anterior superior iliac spine, a second small incision may be made above and parallel to Poupart's ligament and the pelvic portion of the ureter treated through this.

The mutilation of the abdominal wall is much less by this method, and a more satisfactory scar is obtained.

3. Extraperitoneal exposure of the ureter at the brim of the pelvis and in its pelvic portion.—An incision about 4 in. in length is made 1½ in. above and parallel to Poupart's ligament, commencing a little internally to the middle of that ligament, and curving upwards at its outer extremity to pass 1 in. internally to the anterior superior iliac spine.

The muscles are partly cut through and partly split, and the transversalis fascia exposed. This is incised for the whole length of the wound, and the extraperitoneal fat and peritoneum are exposed. In the male, care should be taken at the inner end of the incision to avoid the veins of the spermatic cord. The deep epigastric vessels usually require ligature. After exposure of the peritoneum the patient is placed in the Trendelenburg position and the peritoneum raised. The external iliac vessels are followed and the ureter searched for at the level of the bifurcation of the common iliac vessels, about 4 in. from the surface in an average body.

The ureter lies on the peritoneum and is raised up with it. If it be normal it may be difficult to find. A faint whitish track on the peritoneum or a fair-sized blood-vessel pursuing a long straight course may be the only guide. (Fig. 94.) The spermatic or ovarian vessels should not be mistaken for those around the ureter. The normal ureter cannot be detected on palpating the peritoneum. Good retraction and a powerful head-light are important aids to the search. When the ureter is dilated it is found as a large greyish tube, sometimes the size of the small intestine, with a tough wall ; but even when it is of considerable size it may not present more than a greyish band on the peritoneum until a few strokes of the dissecting forceps make it stand out. I have had great difficulty in exposing a ureter in this position in a case where there had been chronic appendicitis with retroperitoneal adhesions. A hard tuberculous ureter or a ureter containing a stone can be readily detected by the touch.

Having been exposed by blunt dissection, the ureter may be

followed over the brim of the pelvis, and the pelvic portion explored. The portion of the duct below the pelvic brim alongside the rectum may be difficult to reach. Beyond this the ureter passes forwards and is more easily accessible until it approaches the bladder, when it is surrounded by numerous vessels and in the female runs below the uterine artery.

After the operation a rubber drain is placed in the iliac fossa, and great care should be taken to keep it from touching the iliac vessels. It must not be allowed to lie over the brim into the pelvis, for it will certainly press upon the iliac artery and cause sloughing and hæmorrhage from that vessel. Several fatal cases of this accident are on record.

If the ureter has been opened in the pelvic segment the lower end of the bed should be raised, so that any leakage of urine may pass into the iliac fossa and be drained by the tube. I have not had any trouble with pelvic cellulitis even in septic cases. Should a doubt exist in the case of a female patient, a small incision should be made through the vaginal wall and a tube placed in it for a few days.

The route indicated in this section is the safest and most satisfactory for operation upon this part of the ureter.

4. Transperitoneal exposure of the ureter at the brim of the pelvis and in its pelvic segment.—A median incision is made, commencing just above the symphysis pubis; the peritoneum is opened, the patient is placed in the Trendelenburg position, and the intestines are packed off.

The ureter is seen appearing just internally to the cæcum, and passes over the brim of the pelvis, crossing the bifurcation of the iliac vessels. It can be traced in the pelvis until it disappears beneath the broad ligament in the female and the seminal vesicles in the male. By incising the peritoneum over it the duct is exposed in any part of the pelvic course.

The intraperitoneal route has the disadvantage that in septic cases there is a grave danger of infecting the peritoneum.

5. Parasacral extraperitoneal route for exposure of the pelvic segment of the ureter.—A number of operations have been described by Delbet, Cabot, and others for the exposure of the portion of the ureter by a sacral route. That used by Morris will be described.

A straight incision 5 in. in length is made 1 in. from and parallel with the median line, commencing 2 in. above the border of the gluteus maximus muscle, and extending nearly to the level of the anus. The edges of the gluteus maximus and great sciatic ligament are divided, the rectum and vagina are pushed aside,

w

and the ureter is found as it crosses the tip of the spine of the ischium.

The advantages claimed for this incision are the absence of bleeding, the avoidance of the peritoneum, and the dependent drainage. Morris advocates it especially in women. The disadvantage is the narrow, cramped field of operation.

6. **Vaginal route.**—An incision is made transversely through the upper part of the lateral vaginal wall. The ureter is exposed by blunt dissection and isolated, care being taken to avoid the uterine artery, which crosses above and close to it. The ureter is incised, the stone removed, and the wound closed with catgut sutures.

The vaginal route is used when a stone can be felt in the ureter and the exposure of the duct is made without difficulty. When the duct is not thickened or contains a stone, it may be very difficult to find. An unduly large percentage of urinary fistulæ have followed this operation, due probably to mistakes in technique.

7. **Vesical route for calculi in the intramural portion of the ureter.**—Suprapubic cystotomy is performed and the patient placed in the Trendelenburg position. The edge of the ureter is seized with long forceps, the mucous membrane slit up with long curved scissors, and the stone removed. The bladder should be drained suprapubically, and not closed, as there is a danger of ascending pyelonephritis even in a mildly infected bladder.

8. **Transvesical route for calculi lying in the lower two inches of the ureter outside the bladder wall.**—I have performed the following operation where great difficulty was experienced in exposing the lower part of the ureter by the iliac extraperitoneal route.

After suprapubic cystotomy the patient is placed in the Trendelenburg position and the wound well retracted. A curved incision with the concavity towards the trigone is made 1½ in. outside the ureteric orifice on the affected side. A flap of bladder wall is turned down, and by pulling on this the ureter is made tense and exposed. It is surrounded by a number of blood-vessels which may require ligature. After removal of the stone the duct is stitched, and the curved wound in the bladder closed with catgut stitches on a rubber tube which drains the extravesical space and is brought out of the cystotomy and suprapubic wounds. The bladder is also drained.

A perineal route has been used, but this and the rectal route have both been abandoned.

Choice of route.—For the lumbar segment of the ureter the lumbar extraperitoneal route is the only one available. To expose the ureter at the brim of the pelvis the iliac extraperitoneal route is the best, and this route is also the most satisfactory for the great majority of cases in which the pelvic portion of the ureter is to be exposed. The transperitoneal route may be useful in some cases for the pelvic segment of the duct, and the transvesical for difficult cases of impacted stone lying just outside the bladder. The vaginal route is also a useful method of approach, but rough handling should be avoided and the ureter carefully stitched.

URETERECTOMY

Partial ureterectomy.—This may be performed as part of the operation of nephro-ureterectomy. The kidney with a part of the ureter is removed for tuberculous or other disease (*see* p. 293).

The operation may in rare instances be required for the treatment of stricture or other disease of the ureter. Here a portion of the ureter is resected, and the ends of the tube are united by one of the methods of anastomosis.

Total ureterectomy.—This is part of the operation of nephro-ureterectomy which is described elsewhere. It is performed for tuberculosis of the kidney and ureter, suppuration and dilatation of the ureter, and new growths.

The ureterectomy may be carried out at the time of the nephrectomy (primary ureterectomy), or it may be deferred to a later date (secondary ureterectomy). In the latter case the upper end may have been fixed in the lumbar wound, or it may have been returned to the retroperitoneal space.

In primary ureterectomy, after the renal pedicle has been tied, the patient is turned on his back and the lumbar wound continued forwards so as to form the ilio-lumbo-iliac incision already described. The ureter, with the kidney attached, is stripped from the peritoneum and traced into the pelvis. It may be difficult to remove the last two inches of the duct, and this is usually ligatured and left, no harm resulting. The surgeon may, however, persist if the condition of the patient warrants it. The patient is placed in the Trendelenburg position, and the ureter traced up to the wall of the bladder and ligatured there. In the female subject Kelly has employed an incision in the vaginal wall to expose and remove the lower end of the ureter. Separate lumbar and iliac incisions may be made (*see* p. 336).

PLASTIC OPERATIONS ON THE URETER

1. **Anastomosis of ureter and kidney.**—These operations are used in hydronephrosis, where the seat of the obstruction at the renal pelvic outlet is inaccessible owing to adhesions or

perinephritic fat, or where the obstruction is irremediable. The operations consist in lateral anastomosis, transplantation of the ureter into the lowest part of the sac.

Incision of valves and uretero-pyeloplasty are methods of dealing with obstruction at the outlet of the renal pelvis. These operations are described under Hydronephrosis (p. 182).

2. **Uretero-ureteral anastomosis.**—This operation is used when the ureter has been torn or cut across, or when a portion of the tube has sloughed as a result of blows, stabs, injuries during childbirth, or when it has been injured during pelvic operations. Immediate suture should be performed. If a portion of the tube be damaged it should be excised before commencing the anastomosis.

The methods of performing uretero-ureteral anastomosis are described at p. 180.

3. **Anastomosis between ureter and bladder.**—This operation is performed for fistula of the ureter near its lower end, usually caused by injury during a pelvic operation such as hysterectomy or ovarian operations in the female, and removal of the rectum by the abdomino-perineal method in the male. It is also necessary in resections of portions of the bladder wall for malignant growth when the operation involves the lower end of the ureter. In cases of fistula following extensive pelvic operations the relations of the pelvic organs are usually completely changed, and there may be very extensive development of scar tissue. On this account the transperitoneal method of approach is preferred to the extraperitoneal route.

The operation is facilitated by passing a catheter up the vesical end of the ureter by means of the catheter cystoscope. The abdomen is opened, the patient is placed in the Trendelenburg position, and the intestines are packed off. The ureter is defined at the brim of the pelvis and traced downwards to the seat of the fistula if possible. Should there appear to be a prospect of obtaining union of the two ends of the severed tube, a ureteral anastomosis should be carried out. If this be not feasible, the upper end of the ureter should be dissected free for as far as is necessary and implanted in the bladder.

An incision is made in the bladder, and the tube pushed through and stitched from the inside of the bladder to the mucous membrane. A second set of sutures is introduced between the outer surface of the bladder and the ureter, and the first inch of the ureter buried by folding the bladder wall over it by means of a row of Lembert's sutures.

All traction on the sutures must be avoided, and Ricard stitches the bladder to the parietal peritoneum on the side of the anastomosis, to prevent tension. The bladder should be drained suprapubically by a large rubber drain.

There are many variations in the implantation of the ureter. Ricard turns back a cuff of ureter after splitting the tube, and stitches it. A portion of the ureter is made to project into the bladder, and the bladder and ureteral wall are sutured above this. Payne splits the ureter to form two flaps. A U-suture is introduced through each flap and carried through the vesical wall from the inside.

Transvesical operations are sometimes used, but are rarely successful. In a case in which the abdomino-perineal operation for rectal carcinoma had been performed by another surgeon a urinary fistula followed, arising from the right ureter about 2 in. from the bladder. After opening the bladder I made a free incision in the bladder wall near the right ureteric orifice, and stitched a large drainage tube through this at the lower end of the upper segment of the severed ureter, in the hope that a permanent fibrous track would result and form a new communication between the ureter and the bladder. For a few weeks this worked admirably, but contraction took place, and eventually nephrectomy became necessary.

The operations for implantation of the ureter in the bladder in resection of the bladder wall will be described in connection with malignant growths of the bladder (p. 481).

4. Implantation of the ureter on the skin (dermato-ureterotresis.—This operation is chiefly employed where the urine must be diverted in cystectomy. It may also be used when a ureter is injured and ureteral anastomosis is impracticable in a case where the second kidney is absent or inadequate.

The ureter is exposed in the loin and isolated. It is cut across, and the lower end tied and dropped into the retroperitoneal tissue. The upper end is brought up to the surface of the skin, care being taken not to kink or twist it. The cut end is split, and the flaps are stitched to the skin at the edge of the wound, supporting stitches being placed at the level of the subcutaneous fascia. A rubber tube is placed alongside the ureter and pierces the abdominal wall. This forms a weak spot in the wall and obviates the strangulation of the ureter which sometimes takes place. The results of this operation are rather better than those of implantation of the ureter into the intestine, but stenosis of the orifice and ascending pyelonephritis cause a very high late mortality. An apparatus similar to that worn in nephrostomy is used.

5. Implantation of the ureter in the intestine. — The operations performed for extroversion of the bladder are described elsewhere (p. 398). The following operations are suitable for cases of ureteral fistula, as a preliminary to total cystectomy, or for wounds of the ureter: The ureter may be implanted into the cæcum, the pelvic colon, or the ascending or descending colon. In the majority of cases the transperitoneal method is used, but in a .few cases the operation may be performed extraperitoneally. The abdomen is opened either in the middle line or over the portion of bowel in which it is proposed to implant the ureter. The ureter is exposed by cutting through the peritoneum over it, and, the peritoneum being protected from the septic urine, is cut across and the lower end ligatured and cauterized. The upper end is cut obliquely if it be of normal calibre. The extraperitoneal aspect of the bowel is exposed and the obliquely-cut ureter implanted into it.

This may be done by a double layer of continuous catgut sutures, the first layer uniting one half of the outer layer of the ureter to that of the intestine, and the next the whole circumference of the mucous lining, and then the second half of the outer layer in a manner similar to that used in intestinal anastomosis. A third row of sutures may be inserted for additional security.

In order to prevent the actual contact of fæcal matter with the ureteric orifice, Fowler has introduced the following method : The peritoneum is split and the ureter dissected up and divided. The upper end is displaced towards the bowel beneath the peritoneum and fixed to the surface of its wall by a few stitches. A rectangular flap of the bowel wall is now raised, and the mucous membrane dissected from the muscular coat. The flap of mucous membrane is doubled on itself and stitched so that a fold with a mucous covering on both sides is formed. Between this and the rectangular flap of the muscular wall the end of the ureter is placed and secured in position. The muscular flap is now replaced and stitched.

Uretero-appendicostomy. — In a case of very extensive papilloma of the bladder which recurred after four operations I made an anastomosis between the right ureter and the appendix. An incision similar to that for appendicectomy was made, and extended for 4 in. The patient was placed in the Trendelenburg position, and the appendix found lying close to the dilated ureter at the point at which it crossed the iliac vessels. The peritoneum over the ureter was incised and the duct freed for 2 in. and then cut across between two ligatures. A longitudinal incision was made in the upper segment. The appendix was cut across obliquely and two catgut stitches were passed through its wall and up inside the ureter, drawing about an inch of appendix into its lumen through the longitudinal opening. The sutures were passed through the wall of the ureter from within outwards, and tied. The longitudinal incision was carefully closed around the appendix, and sutures united the serous surface to the surface of the ureter. A flap of fat from the meso-appendix was stitched over the line of suture, and the wound in the peritoneum closed.

For three days the urine passed by the colon, but sloughing occurred, and the patient died of ascending pyelonephritis.

PART III.—THE BLADDER

CHAPTER XXV

SURGICAL ANATOMY AND PHYSIOLOGY

Surgical anatomy.—The adult bladder is a pelvic organ when it is empty or moderately full; when distended, it is partly abdominal.

The physiological capacity of the bladder is from 8 to 10 oz., but it may be so distended as to contain several pints, or even quarts.

There are an anterior, a posterior or postero-superior, and two lateral walls, a base, and an apex.

The apex is the highest, conical portion of the bladder, and to this is attached the urachus.

The extent of the base is indefinite. It is frequently looked upon as the portion of the lower segment of the bladder which is uncovered by peritoneum. In cystoscopy the term is used to indicate the trigone and an undefined area of bladder wall around this. The lateral walls are concave, and a recessus lateralis on each side is sometimes described.

The internal meatus of the urethra is on a level with and about 2 cm. behind the middle of the symphysis pubis. This is the most fixed part of the bladder.

The peritoneum covers the postero-superior wall, and descends to cover half the seminal vesicles within 1 cm. of the prostate. On each side it covers the greater part of the lateral wall. When the bladder is empty the peritoneum passes directly from the abdominal wall on to the bladder; when the viscus is full the postero-superior wall is pushed up to form the apex, and the peritoneum dips down on the front of the bladder for a short distance.

The area of bladder wall uncovered by peritoneum above the level of the symphysis pubis is about 1 or 1½ in. with moderate distension of the bladder (10 to 12 oz.); frequently it is less, and with the bladder fully distended the peritoneal fold may be found as low as the upper border of the symphysis pubis. The peritoneum is loosely attached to the bladder by areolar tissue, and is readily stripped from its anterior surface. At the apex around the attachment of the urachus and at the upper part of the posterior wall it sometimes adheres firmly; but below this and on the lateral walls it is readily detached. In front of the bladder, behind the symphysis pubis, is a space filled with areolar tissue, the space of Retzius.

Relations of the bladder.—The moderately distended bladder lies behind the symphysis pubis and pubic bones, and above these it comes in contact for a very short space with the posterior surface of the anterior abdominal wall.

The posterior wall in the male is covered with peritoneum, and in relation to this are coils of small intestine. The lateral wall is in relation to peritoneum as low as the obliterated hypogastric arteries, ahd below this it comes into relation with the obturator internus muscle covered by the parietal layer of pelvic fascia, and then with the levator ani muscle covered by the visceral layer of pelvic fascia.

The base in the male is in relation to the prostate, which extends rather more than half-way from the urethra to the base of the trigone, and passes out laterally beyond the ureteric orifices.

Behind this the ampulla of the vas deferens is in relation to the bladder wall on each side, and then to the peritoneum of the pouch of Douglas.

The base of the female bladder is in relation to the anterior vaginal wall, which extends backwards for more than an inch behind the base of the trigone. The trigone is firmly adherent to the vaginal wall, but above this the vagina and bladder are loosely attached. The bladder wall then comes into relation to the anterior surface of the uterus almost to the apex. At the apex the peritoneum covers it for a short distance before being reflected on to the uterus.

" In the new-born child the orifice of the urethra is about the level of the upper border of the pubic symphysis. In front of this orifice the bladder extends forwards and slightly upwards in close contact with the pubis until it reaches the anterior abdominal wall, against which it lies until within about 1 cm. of the umbilicus " (Symington). The anterior surface is entirely uncovered by peritoneum, which posteriorly reaches as low as the level of the orifice of the urethra. At birth the organ is described as being essentially an abdominal organ. According to Symington, however, if a line be drawn from the promontory of the sacrum to the upper edge of the symphysis, fully one-half of the bladder will be found below this line, or, strictly speaking, within the cavity of the true pelvis. The organ is pear-shaped; it has no base and no lateral recesses. As the child grows older the bladder dilates and sinks into the pelvis, so that at the age of 10 it is a pelvic organ with the same relations as in the adult.

The **bladder wall** consists of three coats—mucous, muscular, and serous.

In the contracted male bladder the posterior wall is thicker than the anterior. There are an outer and an inner longitudinal muscular layer and a middle interlacing layer. In the lateral walls the longitudinal muscle is less developed or absent.

The trigone is a separate structure from the rest of the muscular wall of the bladder. From the internal longitudinal layer of one ureter muscular bundles pass to join those from the other ureter, and these form a muscular ridge called the interureteric ridge or bar of Mercier. Other strands of longitudinal muscle pass from the ureters towards the urethra, and flow over the posterior edge of this orifice to join the internal longitudinal muscular layer of the urethra. These form the sides of the trigone. In the centre of the triangular space the muscle bundles interlace irregularly.

The **sphincter** of the bladder is formed as follows : Beneath the surface layer of the trigone is a thick layer of non-striped muscle lying on the upper surface of the prostate. This is continuous with the circular layer of bladder muscle, but distinguished from it by being thicker and the bundles being more closely set. As this layer approaches the urethra it becomes thicker and forms a thick wedge behind the opening of the internal meatus. Thence it is continued as a thin layer of circular muscle surrounding the urethra. Along the front wall of the prostatic urethra is a thick band of circular muscle similar in its compact arrangement to that lying upon the base of the gland, and extending as a gradually thinning layer to the apex of the prostate. The sphincter of the bladder is a fan-shaped muscle the posterior part of which is formed by the deep circular layer of the trigone muscle, while the anterior part is spread out along the anterior surface of the prostatic urethra. The mucous membrane consists of transitional epithelium, the superficial cells of which are characteristic, having several nuclei, and protoplasm which stains less deeply on the surface than on the deeper layer. The surface is smooth and rounded ; the deep aspect shows prickles. There are no papillæ.

In the normal submucous tissue there are round cells either diffusely distributed or grouped in nodules, and it is unsettled whether or not these represent lymphoid tissue.

Lendorf describes glandular structures around the urethral orifice and at the base. These are solid or hollow epithelial downgrowths and glands consisting of from one to five lacunæ which open into a single excretory duct. In the body of the bladder only the epithelial ingrowths are found, and the apex is free from glandular structures. The mucous membrane is smooth and delicate, and freely movable upon the underlying muscular layer over the whole bladder surface. Over the trigone it is coarser and firmer, and is adherent to the underlying structures.

At each angle of the trigone, set on the ureteric ridge, is the opening of a ureter, which appears as a fine pink slit.

In the mucous membrane at the apex there is frequently a trace of the urachus in the form of a dimple.

The urethral orifice is a half-moon-shaped slit, concave backwards. The shape is due to the prominence of the uvula vesicæ on the posterior lip, which passes down into the postmontanal ridge and to the verumontanum.

Arteries.—The arterial supply is derived from branches of the internal iliac arteries. The superior vesical and middle vesical are derived from the unobliterated portion of the hypogastric artery; the inferior arises from the anterior division of the internal iliac, frequently in common with the middle hæmorrhoidal. The superior supplies the apex and upper part of the body of the bladder, the middle supplies the rest of the body and base of the bladder, and the inferior supplies the trigone.

The branches perforate the muscular wall and form a submucous plexus from which proceed fine branches that penetrate the mucosa.

On the surface of the mucous membrane fine twigs can be seen with the cystoscope. They penetrate the mucosa at irregular intervals and break up into fine branches. There is no regular arrangement of these vessels, and they vary very considerably in numbers in healthy individuals. When the vessels are engorged from some pathological cause the fine branches can be seen to anastomose with each other and with branches of neighbouring vessels. In many bladders deep-blue branching vessels, three or four times the breadth of the surface vessels, are seen coursing deeply in the mucous membrane. The fine surface vessels cross these. One of these large vessels may be seen rising to the surface and splitting into two or more fine surface vessels. One or two vessels emerge from the ureteric orifice and pass outwards and backwards, breaking up into fine branches. In an area the size of a threepenny-piece around the ureteric orifice the circulation is intimately connected with that of the ureter. In health there is no indication of this, but in many diseases of the ureter this area shows a halo of congestion. The vascular supply of the trigone, as seen with the cystoscope, is distinct from that of the rest of the bladder. The vessels, which are much larger, run for the most part in a fan shape from the urethra backwards over the trigone area, overlapping it a little at each side and at the base. The fine twigs on the surface anastomose, and at the angles of branching there are frequently small dilatations.

Veins.—The vesical veins do not correspond to the arteries. Numerous veins pass downwards on the surface of the front of the bladder (anterior vesical veins) and join the large veins which pass backwards on each side at the base of the prostate. The posterior vesical veins collect the blood from the apex and peritoneal surface of the bladder by a vertical trunk, and by a horizontal trunk which collects the blood from the lateral wall and communicates with the anterior plexus. These veins form several large trunks which communicate with the hæmorrhoidal plexus and open by a single trunk into the internal iliac vein. The veins of the trigone pass into those of the prostatic urethra.

Lymphatics (Fig. 96).—No lymphatics have been described in the mucous membrane. In the submucous tissue there is a network of lymphatic vessels from which numerous branches pass into the muscular coat vertically to the surface, with free lateral anastomoses. From this network spring large trunks. On the posterior surface two parallel trunks course from the apex to the base and drain the lateral walls. The basal lymphatics communicate with those of the prostate and seminal vesicles in the male, and the anterior vaginal wall in the female. On the anterior face of the bladder there are one or two collecting trunks situated on each side of the middle line. A few small lymphatic glands are found on the outer surface of the bladder.

The lymphatics from the anterior surface pass to glands along the external iliac, those of the upper part of the bladder pass to the external iliac and to the hypogastric glands, while those of the lower part of the posterior wall pass alongside the rectum to the sacral ganglia lying at the bifurcation of the aorta.

Nerves.—From the 3rd, 4th, and 5th lumbar nerve roots nervi communicantes pass to the sympathetic chain and run without interruption by the three mesenteric branches to the inferior mesenteric ganglion. From this ganglion the two hypogastric nerves emerge, forming the hypogastric plexus, and pass to the wall of the bladder. A second set of nerves originate in the 2nd and 3rd sacral nerves (nervi erigentes or sacral nerves), and pass to the hypogastric plexus, where they are interrupted by ganglia, from which they pass to the fundus, anterior part, and neck of the bladder.

Physiology.—In the healthy individual the urine collects in the bladder and is passed four or five times during the day, and not at all at night. About 8 or 10 oz. are passed at each act of micturition.

Zuckerkandl and Frankl-Hochwart have shown that in normal individuals there is slight desire to micturate when 100–500 grm. of fluid are introduced into the bladder and the pressure varies

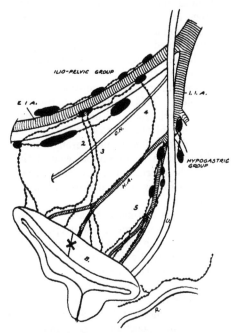

Fig. 96.—Lymphatics of bladder.

E.I.A., External iliac artery; I.I.A., internal iliac artery; O.N., obturator nerve; H.A., hypogastric artery; U, ureter; B, bladder; R, rectum; X, apex of bladder when distended; 1 to 6, lymphatic trunks.

from 10 to 30 cm. of water. When 400–700 grm. are introduced there is a powerful impulse and the pressure rises to from 13 to 53 cm. of water.

When the bladder is slowly filled the intravesical pressure very gradually rises, apart from any contraction of the bladder, giving a pressure of from 3 to 4 cm. In the living subject the gradual rise is followed by a rapid increase synchronous with a contraction of the bladder. The urine is retained in the bladder partly by mechanical conditions and partly by the tonic contraction of the vesical sphincter. In the cadaver fluid does not escape from the bladder when in the recumbent or the erect posture, and a considerable quantity can be injected into the bladder through the ureter without any escape from the urethra. Some amount of force is required to separate the elastic walls of the urethra at the vesical orifice.

. The compressor urethræ forms a second sphincter, partly voluntary and partly involuntary. After suprapubic prostatectomy the vesical sphincter does not resume its function in 50 per cent. of cases, and the compressor acts as the sphincter.

Micturition is performed by relaxation of the sphincter and contraction of the detrusor muscle. Two theories are advanced to explain the initiation of the act :

1. It is said to arise in gradually increasing waves of contraction caused by distension. This can be demonstrated by artificially distending the bladder with fluid. When the distension reaches a certain point contraction of the detrusor takes place.

If during the expulsion of the fluid through the urethra fluid is run in as rapidly through a suprapubic wound the contraction is not prolonged, but the detrusor relaxes after a regular period of contraction, and this is followed by an interval of relaxation and then another contraction.

2. When the bladder is distended to a certain degree, contractions of the wall occur which force a few drops into the sensitive prostatic urethra, from which the reflex is initiated. The reflex can be produced artificially by injecting a few drops of silver nitrate solution into the prostatic urethra, which produces intense desire to micturate. The injection of cocaine into the prostatic urethra may cause retention of urine when the bladder is fully distended. On the other hand, I have shown that the prostatic urethra is removed in the operation of suprapubic prostatectomy and the act of micturition is unimpaired.

The act of micturition consists in the accumulation of urine, with slow rise of intravesical pressure to 15 cm. of water (Starling), followed by rhythmical contractions of the bladder increasing in force. Afferent impulses pass to the spinal centre, and efferent impulses cause contraction of the bladder with rise of intravesical pressure to 20 or 30 cm. of water, when the sphincter resistance and adhesion of the urethral walls are overcome and the urine is discharged. The act of micturition can be voluntarily initiated by relaxing the perineal muscles, and perhaps also the sphincter of the bladder, and contracting the abdominal muscles.

The passage of the urine can be voluntarily interrupted by contraction of the voluntary perineal muscles, and perhaps also of the sphincter vesicæ.

There is a centre for micturition in the lumbar spinal cord which in the adult is subject to control from the cerebrum.

Reflex micturition can be carried on when the cord is cut across above this centre.

Complete destruction of the lumbar centre is followed at first by retention of urine and overflow, and later the bladder acts reflexly and is continent. The reflex centres here are apparently the inferior mesenteric and hypogastric plexuses of the sympathetic.

Finally, some power of causing contraction is possessed by the scattered nerve ganglia in the bladder wall itself. When the organ is completely isolated from the nervous system, stimulation will produce contraction of its wall.

LITERATURE

Frankl-Hochwart und **Zuckerkandl,** *Die Nervösen Erkrankungen der Blase.* 1898.
Goltz und **Treusberg,** *Pflügers Arch.,* vols. viii., ix.
Goltz und **Ewald,** *Pflügers Arch.,* vol. lxiii.
Jarjavay, *Recherches Anatomique sur l' Uretère de l' Homme.* Paris, 1856.
Kalischer, *Die Urogenitalmuskulatur des Dammes.* Berlin, 1910.
Lendorf, *Anatomie.* 1901.
Müller, *Deuts. Zeits. f. Nervenheilkunde,* 1901, S. 886.
Rehfisch, *Virchows Arch.,* Bd. cl.
Symington, *The Anatomy of the Child.* 1887.
Walker, Thomson, *Journ. Anat. and Phys.,* April, 1906, vol. xl.
von Zeissl, *Wien. med. Blätt.,* 1902, Nr. 10.
Zuckerkandl, E., *Handbuch der Urologie* (von Frisch und O. Zuckerkandl), Bd. i., 1904.

CHAPTER XXVI

EXAMINATION OF THE BLADDER

1. **Inspection.**—When the bladder becomes greatly distended it forms a prominent rounded swelling between the pubes and the umbilicus. When the patient is standing there is only a general prominence; when he is lying on his back the rounded swelling appears. (Fig. 97.)

2. **Palpation.**—With the patient lying on his back, the shoulders raised and the knees drawn up, the surgeon places his hand flat upon the suprapubic region. The distended bladder is felt as a firm rounded swelling rising out of the pelvis. The apex can be distinctly felt. Sometimes a large diverticulum can be recognized on palpation, especially when it is surrounded by inflammatory thickening. The distended bladder is dull on percussion; pressure upon it usually gives a heavy aching sensation in the perineum or at the end of the penis.

3. **Rectal examination.**—Examination of the rectal surface of the bladder is made with the patient in the knee-elbow position on a couch, or in the lithotomy position. The portion of the male bladder which can thus be examined is about $1\frac{1}{2}$ in., commencing just behind the interureteric bar. In front of this the seminal vesicles and prostate intervene between the finger and the bladder base. With the fingers of the other hand above the pubes a bimanual examination is made.

The distended bladder fills up the space above the prostate and bulges downwards so as almost to bury the gland. This may be simulated by a collection of pus in the peritoneal pouch of Douglas. Thickened ridges of hypertrophied bladder muscle can sometimes be felt. The thickening of an advanced infiltrating growth at the base of the bladder can be felt in this situation. Calculi are very seldom detected by this method of examination, but a very large calculus may be felt on bimanual examination.

The lymphatics of the bladder base pass out along with those of the prostate at the upper and outer angle of the prostate. A sling containing blood-vessels and lymphatics can be felt on each side in this position. In this lie the first lymph-glands of the

chain which passes to the internal iliac vessels. Enlargement of
these glands can be detected on rectal palpation.

4. **Vaginal examination.**—The short urethra can be felt in
the anterior vaginal wall, extending backwards from the outlet of
the vagina for 1½ in., when it expands into the trigone.

The trigone can sometimes be detected on palpation of the
anterior vaginal wall, and the ureters may be felt passing outwards from each lateral horn. Behind the trigone the bladder
base can be palpated in the anterior fornix.

5. **Examination by catheters and sounds.**—The passage of
a catheter is required to withdraw the urine in atony of the bladder
or obstruction of the urethra. It may be necessary in order to

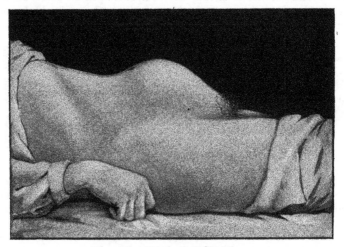

Fig. 97.—Distended bladder.

ascertain the presence and quantity of residual urine after the
patient has passed all he can voluntarily, or it may be used to
obtain a specimen of urine from the bladder for examination so
as to avoid contamination by the urethra or the external genital
organs. Occasionally it may be necessary to drain the bladder
continuously by tying the catheter in position in the urethra.
Sometimes on passing a catheter a calculus may be felt in the
bladder, or the filling up of one part of the bladder with a growth;
or fragments of a growth may be caught in the eye of the catheter
on withdrawing the instrument.

Catheters.—Three varieties of catheter are in use—the metal
catheter, the flexible catheter, and the rubber catheter.

x

Metal catheters have a curve corresponding to that of the urethra, a blunt conical end, and two small metal loops at the proximal end to assist in fixing the instrument in the urethra should it be desired to drain the bladder continuously. A " prostatic " catheter has a large curve and a much longer beak.

Flexible catheters have a basis of finely woven silk, which is coated without and within with a flexible preparation. They may be straight and taper to a point which has a bulb or olive tip, or they may be of the same calibre throughout and have a blunt rounded end, or the end may be bent upwards (coudé catheter), or there may be a double bend (bicoudé catheter). (Fig. 98.) The tip of the catheter beyond the eye should be solid. The proximal end of these catheters should be trumpet-shaped so as to admit the nozzle of a syringe or a glass nozzle. There should be no ornamental bone attachment.

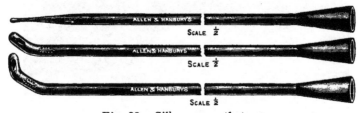

Fig. 98.—Silk-wove catheters.
From above downwards : Olivary, coudé, and bicoudé varieties.

Gum-elastic catheters are less flexible than those just described, and can be bent into the required shape for use. They have a mandarin.

Rubber catheters are soft and very supple. The tip of the catheter beyond the eye should be solid, and the proximal end should be trumpet-shaped.

Cleansing and sterilization of catheters.—*Metal* catheters are boiled before use. After use they should be syringed through with antiseptic fluid or attached to an apparatus which is fixed to the water-tap. The grease is removed from the surface, and the instruments are boiled, dried, and laid aside.

Well-made *flexible* catheters can be boiled in water. Additions to the water have been suggested, such as chloride of soda (40 per cent.) and ammonium sulphate (10–12 per cent.), with the view of preserving the surface of the catheter. They should be boiled from two to five minutes and then carefully placed in cold sterile water, or 1-in-80 carbolic, or 1-in-4,000 biniodide of mercury, or after removal from the sterilizer they may be placed upon a dry sterile towel and allowed to cool. They must not be grasped with forceps in removing them from the sterilizer.

A convenient form of *sterilizer* is that introduced by Zuckerkandl (Fig. 99). This compact apparatus is portable and durable. Another sterilizer for flexible catheters has been introduced by Herring. In this the catheter is boiled in liquid paraffin in a straight tube, which is then detached and the ends closed, so that the tube acts as a carrier.

After use, flexible catheters should be washed inside and out to remove grease, blood-clot, etc., then boiled for two minutes, and carefully dried and put away dry.

It is better to leave catheters exposed on a tray until they are thoroughly dry than to store them at once.

Glass tubes for storing and carrying catheters should' be open

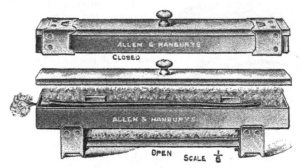

Fig. 99.—Zuckerkandl's catheter sterilizer.

at both ends, to facilitate cleaning and drying. Flexible catheters should be wiped with a little oil or dusted with lycopodium powder before being put away.

Formalin vapour is employed for the sterilization òf flexible catheters, and is especially useful when a large number of instruments must be sterilized. At St. Peter's Hospital a large oblong copper box is used. This contains perforated trays which hold several hundred catheters. On the floor of the box is a cup-shaped depression in which fluid formalin is placed. The box is closed and a lamp burns under the cup until the formalin has evaporated. The box is kept closed for two hours, and then air, filtered through cotton-wool, is pumped through to remove the irritating fumes. Boxes on a smaller scale can be obtained for formalin sterilization. For single catheters, a glass-stoppered tube, within which is a box perforated on the inside and containing a granular preparation of formalin, may be used. The efficiency of these tubes as sterilizers is very doubtful, and moisture tends to collect on the catheter and destroys its surface.

Rubber catheters can be boiled, and should be stored dry after carefully removing any oil or grease. For the convenience of patients who are compelled to pass a catheter upon themselves, small round sterilizable metal boxes with a receptacle for oil or vaseline are constructed. (Fig. 100.)

Lubricants should be sterile and non-irritating. Liquid paraffin, sterilized olive oil, and vaseline are the best.

Impregnation with powerful antiseptics should be avoided. Many elegant preparations are manufactured. In using metal bougies, especially those of large size, vaseline is the best lubricant. The following formula may be employed : Cocainæ hydrochloridi 5 gr., olei eucalypti 10 minims, adrenalin (1 in 1,000) 20 minims, olei ricini ½ oz., olei olivæ ½ oz.

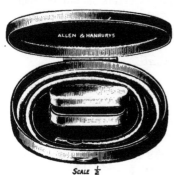

Fig. 100.—Sterilizable catheter box.

Method of passing catheters.—The passage of a catheter must be regarded as an operation of the first magnitude. The danger to the patient of infection introduced by the catheter is as great as that incurred by the infection of the peritoneum in an abdominal operation. The disastrous effects may not have their full fruition at once, but the ultimate result is none the less certain. It is true that a healthy bladder is able to deal with bacteria introduced in large numbers by a dirty catheter, no harm ensuing, or only a transient cystitis; it is also true that some patients with enlarged prostate use no antiseptic precautions and go for many years unscathed—most rural practitioners are able to relate such a case from experience or hearsay. These facts give a sense of false security, and are the cause of many surgical disasters. In the bladder obstructed by an enlarged prostate, or the seat of tuberculosis or other disease, bacteria find a ready soil, and the prognosis in these cases becomes immeasurably graver if sepsis is introduced.

It is impossible to ascertain the remote mortality of septic catheterization ; but the rate is very high.

Passage of a metal instrument.—The patient is recumbent in bed or on a couch, with the abdomen and thighs well exposed and sterilized towels placed across the knees and thorax. The surgeon stands on his left side. The penis is washed with antiseptic solution and the meatus carefully cleansed. An instrument is selected and well lubricated. The penis is grasped behind the glans with the forefinger and thumb of the left hand, and the tip of the instrument inserted into the meatus. The shaft of the instrument lies transversely across the patient's left Scarpa's triangle. The handle of the instrument is now carried gently towards the patient's abdomen and onwards to the middle line so that the point drops downwards and backwards. (Fig. 101.) During this manœuvre the left forefinger and thumb draw the penis on to the instrument like a glove. The handle is lightly held between the right forefinger and thumb and gently raised, and the slightest hitch receives instant attention. (Fig. 102.) As the point passes down the bulbous urethra the left hand leaves the penis and the fingers are used to support the perineum. The point passes into the membranous urethra as the handle becomes vertical (Fig. 103) and swings downwards, and the left forefinger and thumb replace the right while the handle is gently depressed between the thighs and pushed onwards (Fig. 104). The point of the instrument should move freely from side to side if it is in the bladder. Instead of swinging the handle of the catheter to the middle line, it is sometimes easier to carry it in the opposite direction so that it crosses the middle line below the scrotum, and then to carry it across the right Scarpa's triangle to the middle line of the abdomen, gradually raising it so that the point drops downwards along the urethra.

Passage of a flexible catheter.—In passing flexible catheters it must be remembered that the surgeon has little power of changing the direction of the point of the instrument, and the passage of a straight instrument into the membranous urethra depends upon its pliability. The penis is grasped behind the glans by the thumb and forefinger of the left hand, and kept on the stretch to render the urethra straight and obliterate the folds in its walls. The instrument is introduced vertically, and lightly held by the corresponding digits of the right hand and pushed carefully onwards until it reaches the bladder, which is recognized by the escape of urine.

Sounding the bladder.—Six ounces of sterile fluid are introduced into the bladder through a catheter. The instrument is passed in vertically until the beak reaches the membranous urethra, when the handle is slowly lowered in the middle line until it drops between the thighs, and then pushed onwards. It may assist the passage of the instrument to raise the patient's

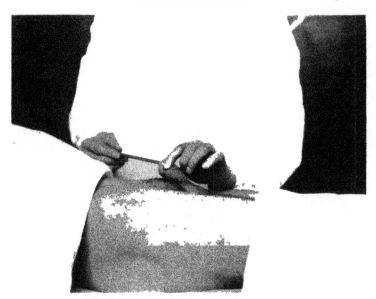

Fig. 101.—Passing metal instrument.

Position 1: Beak in anterior urethra, shaft lying parallel to left Poupart's ligament.

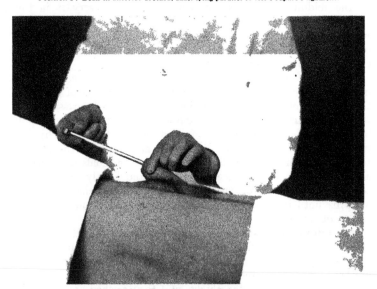

Fig. 102.—Passing metal instrument.

Position 2: Shaft swung to middle line, beak in bulbous urethra.

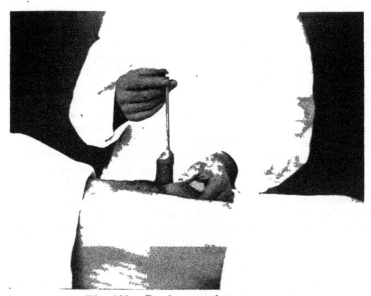

Fig. 103.—Passing metal instrument.

Position 3 : Shaft vertical, fingers of left hand on perineum, beak engaged in membranous urethra.

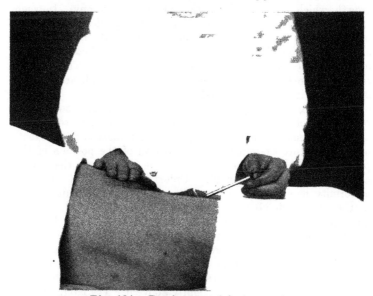

Fig. 104.—Passing metal instrument.

Position 4 : Shaft depressed between thighs by left hand, beak in bladder, right hand pressing on pubes to relax suspensory ligament.

pelvis on a sand pillow. The sound should be passed as far as possible in the middle line, and the handle, held lightly in the right thumb and forefinger, turned on one side and again upwards; and this is repeated, gradually drawing the instrument out until it reaches the internal urethral orifice, on which it hitches. It is now passed in again in the middle line, and the other side of the bladder searched in the same way. Finally, the beak is turned downwards and the post-trigonal or post-prostatic area searched. In manipulating the instrument the grating or click of a stone in the urethra or projecting from the prostate may be felt.

6. **Exploration.**—Exploration of the female bladder with the finger after dilatation of the urethra is an unsatisfactory method of examination. Only the terminal phalanx of the finger can be introduced, and by pushing the bladder down from above the pubes with the other hand a part of the superior wall can be palpated. Permanent incontinence of urine has frequently followed this procedure, which has now been entirely superseded by cystoscopic examination.

It is sometimes necessary, when the bladder has become filled with blood clot and cystoscopy has been found impossible, to explore the bladder by a cutting operation. In growths of the bladder information is also gained respecting the base of the growth which may not be obtainable by cystoscopy. In such cases the bladder should be opened suprapubically and the patient placed in the Trendelenburg position. By means of full exposure, by bladder retractors and the use of a head-lamp, the interior of the bladder can be thoroughly searched. The perineal route in the male and the vaginal route in the female are unsatisfactory and inadequate methods of exploration.

7. **Radiography.**—For the radiographic examination of the bladder, as of the kidneys and ureters, it is necessary to employ a fixed position which can be repeated with mathematical exactness at a future examination. Estimation of the position of the pelvic organs depends entirely upon the relation to the pelvis, a bony ring tilted at an angle. Unless some means of obtaining uniformity be employed the variation in different individuals, and in the same individual in different examinations, will be very great (see pp. 37, 305). In the radiographic plate the brim of the bony pelvis should be shown.

A normal bladder and prostate sometimes throw a shadow in a good plate. The prostatic shadow lies behind the pubic symphysis and the pubic bones. It does not project below the symphysis, but may rise very slightly above it. The lateral extent of the prostatic shadow varies, but it seldom extends laterally

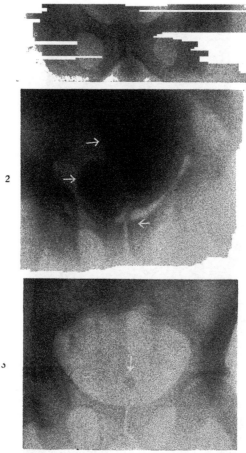

Fig. 1.—Shadow thrown by partly distended healthy bladder.
(P. 361.)

Fig. 2.—Shadow of greatly distended bladder (uppermost arrow)
and of diverticulum (middle arrow); catheter lying in urethra
(lowest arrow). (P. 361.)

Fig. 3.—Shadow of ureteral calculus in middle line of bladder. (P. 361.)

PLATE 27.

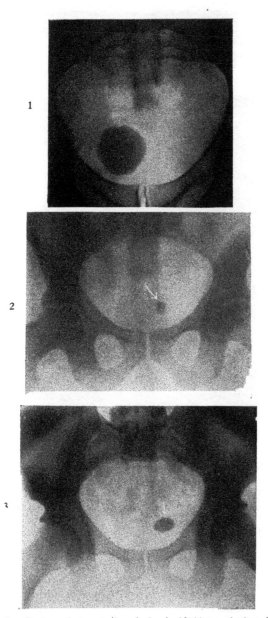

Fig. 1.—Shadow of phosphatic calculus in bladder pushed to right of
middle line by large growth on left side of bladder. (P. 361.)

Figs. 2, 3.—Calculus in bladder which has moved to the left of
middle line from patient lying on left side. (P. 361.)

PLATE 28.

beyond the middle of the pubic bones. The shape of the shadow thrown by the bladder varies according to its distension. The lower border of the shadow nearly corresponds to the upper margin of the pubic portion of the pelvic girdle. In moderate distension the bladder has an oval shape with the long axis placed transversely. (Plate 27, Fig. 1.) In full distension the shadow is more rounded and extends farther back towards the promontory of the sacrum. The lateral limits of the bladder in moderate distension do not pass beyond a vertical line drawn through the middle of the obturator foramen, and the posterior limit rather more than half-way to the promontory. If the bladder is distended with air a clear area appears on the plate.

Radiographic examination of the bladder is chiefly useful in stone and in diverticula of the bladder. A stone shadow in the bladder area may be thrown by a stone in the bladder, a stone in a diverticulum (Plate 29, Fig. 2), or a stone in the lower ureter. It is seldom possible by a radiographic examination alone to distinguish between these conditions. In Plate 27, Fig. 3, the round shadow in the middle line was thrown by a calculus which the cystoscope showed lay in the lower end of a solitary ureter opening in the middle of the distorted trigone. At a later date a radiogram showed the shadow in the middle line, and after water had been passed another radiogram showed that the shadow had moved considerably to the left, demonstrating that the calculus was free in the bladder. (Plate 28, Figs. 2, 3.)

In another case (Plate 29, Fig. 1) the shadow appears in the bladder area, but the calculus lay in a large diverticulum that opened into the bladder by an aperture which would admit a lead pencil. In a third case a large shadow lay on the left side of the bladder area, and on cystoscopy there was a stone on the left and a papillomatous growth on the right side of the bladder. (Plate 28, Fig. 1.)

A stone shadow constantly found in one position, not in the middle line, on several examinations, with varying distension of the bladder, is more likely to be thrown by a stone in the ureter or in a diverticulum than in the bladder, or the stone may be pushed to one side by a growth. Even when the shadow lies in the middle line it is not certain that the stone lies within the bladder, as the cases quoted above show.

Diverticula are demonstrated by filling the bladder with an emulsion of oxychloride of bismuth. The catheter, filled with the bismuth emulsion, should be left in the urethra during the radiographic examination to act as a guide, as the bladder is frequently distorted in these cases. (Plate 27, Fig. 2, and Plate 29, Fig. 3.)

8. **Cystoscopy.**—There are two methods of cystoscopy—(1) indirect, (2) direct.

1. **Indirect cystoscopy.**—The indirect method is carried out by means of a cystoscope after distension of the bladder with fluid.

(a) *Simple cystoscope.*—The simplest form of cystoscope, of which Nitze's was the original model, consists of a telescope and a lighting apparatus combined.

The instrument is 20 cm. long and has a calibre of 21 Charrière. At the distal end there is a short beak formed by a small detachable electric lamp which may have a metal or carbon filament. The shaft of the instrument consists of a double tube, between the layers of which is an insulated wire carrying the current and returned along the body of the instrument. At the proximal end is a double slot for the movable attachment which carries the

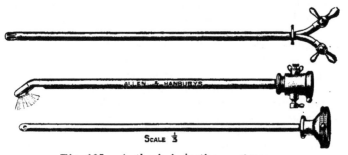

Fig. 105.—Author's irrigation cystoscope.

current and on which is the switch. The ocular apparatus consists of a prism window and a mirror that reflects the image along the tube, in which is a series of lenses. The proximal end is expanded, and on to this may be screwed an eye-piece. For use in children a small-calibre (15 Fr.) cystoscope is used. The current is supplied by a small accumulator or a dry cell giving about 4½ volts. The image is inverted.

(b) *Irrigation cystoscope.*—In the irrigation cystoscope the outer tube acts as a catheter and carries the lighting apparatus. At the proximal end of this there is a valve to prevent the fluid escaping. The telescope is separate, and is pushed along the lumen of the catheter. In the author's pattern (Fig. 105) the outer catheter and lighting tube can be boiled. At the proximal end of this is a valve which acts by a spring placed outside the lumen and may also be used as a turncock. The telescope, which is made by Zeiss, gives an erect image. The advantages of an irrigating

3

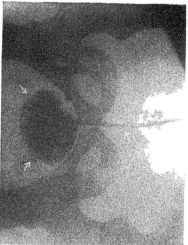

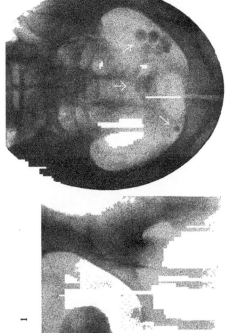

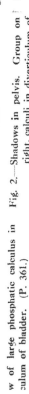

w of large phosphatic calculus in
culum of bladder. (P. 361.)

Fig. 2.—Shadows in pelvis. Group on
right, calculi in diverticulum of
bladder; middle shadow, calculus in bladder; shadow on left,
phlebolith. (P. 361.)

Fig. 3.—Diverticulum of bladder. Bladder is filled
with bismuth emulsion, and catheter is
seen in urethra. Arrow on right points
to diverticulum, that on left to dilated
ureter containing bismuth emulsion, and
that below to the opaque catheter.
(Pp. 361, 413.)

PLATE 29.

cystoscope are that only one introduction of the instrument is necessary, and that the bladder can be washed repeatedly by withdrawing the telescope and without removing the outer tube from the urethra.

(c) In the *catheter cystoscope* provision is made for catheterizing the ureters. In the simplest form a tunnel is placed on the upper surface of the simple cystoscope. This opens just short of the window, and at the end is provided with a small movable gutter which can be raised by turning a screw at the proximal end of the cystoscope and serves to project the point of the ureteric catheter away from the line of the cystoscope, facilitating its introduction into the ureter. Either one channel or two are provided, for single or double catheterization of the ureters.

The more recent models combine the catheterizing and irrigating cystoscope, and a very useful instrument is thus obtained.

Method of performing indirect cystoscopy.—The cystoscope is cleansed with ether soap and carbolic lotion, or, if the author's pattern is used, it is boiled. The patient either lies on a couch with a sand pillow beneath the hips, or sits in a special chair with the knees and hips flexed and the thighs widely apart. The urethra is anæsthetized by instilling 15 minims of a 4 per cent. solution of novocaine into the prostatic urethra by means of a Guyon's syringe, or by a combination of alypin with suprarenin —tablets of alypin 0·02 grm. ($\frac{1}{3}$ gr.), suprarenin boric 2 minims of solution in 1,000.

A catheter, or the catheter portion of the irrigation cystoscope, is lubricated with glycerine and introduced, and the bladder filled with 10 or 12 oz. of warm boric solution or sterile water. The " telescope " is now introduced, the light switched on, and the window turned to the base of the bladder. Air or oxygen has been used instead of water, but both have many disadvantages.

There may be difficulty in obtaining a clear medium owing to hæmorrhage from the bladder or the prostate. Careful washing with sterile water or very weak nitrate of silver solution (1 in 10,000) will usually overcome this. In persistent bleeding adrenalin may be used. I inject $\frac{1}{2}$ drachm of quarter-strength 1-in-1,000 solution of adrenalin, and leave it in for a half to one minute, and then wash it out. If the urine be purulent, prolonged washing may be necessary before a clear medium is obtained. Spasm of the bladder may prevent a full distension ; this may be due to using cold solution or injecting it too rapidly, or to cystitis. If it be due to cystitis, local anæsthesia may be obtained by washing the bladder with a 5 per cent. solution of antipyrin. A general anæsthetic may be necessary.

2. Direct cystoscopy (the open method).—This method was perfected by Kelly, and has been modified by Luys and others.

Kelly's specula (Fig. 106) are plated metal cylinders, 3½ in. long, and of the same diameter throughout. There is a funnel-shaped expansion at the outer end of the speculum, and a handle 3 in. long is attached to the funnel. The specula are made in various sizes, from 5 to 20, each number representing the diameter in millimetres. Each instrument has an obturator, which is used during introduction. A dilator is used to enlarge the orifice of the urethra (Fig. 107), and an evacuator to remove the urine which accumulates in the bladder during a prolonged examination. It consists of a rubber exhausting bulb and 14 in. of fine

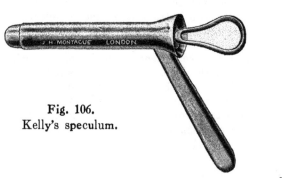

Fig. 106.
Kelly's speculum.

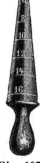

Fig. 107.
Kelly's dilator.

rubber tubing, and at the bladder end a small hollow perforated metal ball.

The lower bowel is emptied, and immediately before the examination the bladder is emptied in a sitting or standing position. General anæsthesia is necessary in nervous individuals. Local anæsthesia is obtained by cocaine introduced on pledgets of wool.

Two positions are used—(a) the elevated dorsal, (b) the knee-chest. (a) The *dorsal position* is the less trying to the patient, but it is only of service in thin patients, and the atmospheric expansion of the bladder is not so good. The bladder of stout patients will rarely distend at all in this position. The buttocks are raised 8 or 12 in. above the table level, the speculum is introduced, the obturator is withdrawn, and the atmospheric pressure distends the bladder. (b) In the *knee-chest position* the patient kneels, with the knees slightly separated, close to the end of the table, and lets the back curve in with the buttocks well raised.

If an anæsthetic is required the patient may be held by assistants, or a slinging apparatus may be used.

The speculum is introduced, the obturator withdrawn, and light projected through it from a forehead mirror reflecting lamp, or from an electric lamp held over the sacrum. After an examination the bladder is emptied by introducing a catheter and gently lowering the patient to the horizontal.

Kelly's method is only applicable to the female, and the position is an exhausting and embarrassing one.

Luys has modified this method, and uses it in the male also. His instrument consists of a metal tube of 10 cm. for the female and 18 cm. for the male. On the floor of the tube is a fine tunnel leading to a small tube to which a rubber tube and aspirator bottle are attached, and which prevents the accumulation of urine in the bladder. The plunger that closes the tube during introduction is straight in the instrument for the female, and angled in that for the male.

The patient is placed in the Trendelenburg position, with local or, preferably, general anæsthesia.

It is not always possible to obtain complete distension of the bladder, and there are folds and depressions in the mucous membrane. An area at the apex, the anterior and part of the lateral walls, are inaccessible to examination.

As a method of examination, direct cystoscopy is inferior to indirect. With the tube a small area of the bladder wall is seen, and the instrument must approach it closely in order to get a good view. With the indirect cystoscope an extensive field is displayed and a broad bird's-eye view can be obtained. The advantage of the direct or open method is the facility it presents for topical applications in cystitis, for operations on small papillomas, and for the removal of foreign bodies from the bladder.

Cystoscopic appearance of the normal bladder.—When the cystoscope is introduced the beak is turned downwards and the trigone comes into view. This is examined, and the interureteric bar at the base of the trigone recognized and followed out on either side, and the ureteric orifices noted. Then the posterior wall and the lateral walls, and finally the anterior wall and the apex, are examined.

A portion of the posterior wall near the apex is difficult to see, and the ocular end of the instrument must be fully depressed so as to tilt the window upwards and bring it into view. The anterior wall rises almost vertically from the urethral orifice, and the window of the cystoscope looks along it.

The mucous membrane is smooth and sandy-yellow, and it

reflects the light so that the whole viscus is easily illuminated. Fine vascular twigs appear here and there, and branch freely. Their number varies greatly in different healthy individuals. Larger vessels of a blue colour are usually seen here and there shining through from the deeper layers of the mucosa. The mucous membrane of the trigone is coarser and darker in hue. The vessels are larger, and pass in a fan-shaped arrangement from the urethral orifice, overlapping the sides and the base of the trigone.

The ureteric orifices are seen as fine pink slits on the ridge at the base of the trigone, and are found by following this ridge (the bar of Mercier) outwards on either side. One or two small blood-vessels emerge from the ureteric orifice and pass outwards and backwards. At the apex of the bladder there is usually a small bubble of air which has been introduced during the washing of the bladder.

The urethral orifice is seen by withdrawing the window until it is partly in the prostatic urethra. It has a slightly concave, even contour all round.

CHAPTER XXVII

METHODS OF COLLECTING THE URINE AND EXAMINING THE FUNCTION OF EACH KIDNEY

At the present time two methods are available for collecting the urine of each kidney separately :

1. The use of separators.
2. Catheterization of the ureters.

1. **Intravesical separation of the urines.**—Two models of separator are in use, those of Luys and Cathelin.

Luys' separator (Fig. 108) consists of a shank and a handle. The shank has a central metal stem, with a metal catheter fitted on each side. The distal end of the shank is curved to the extent of about half a circle, the curve lying below the straight portion of the shank. Attached to the end of the central flattened stem is a fine chain, which, when loose, lies snugly in the concavity of the curve. When drawn tight by a screw in the handle this chain bridges across the half-circle curve like the string of a bow. A fine rubber tube fits over the whole of the median stem. With the chain slack the rubber-covered central stem retains its peculiar curve ; with the chain taut the half-circle curve is filled in by a rubber membrane, forming a septum which divides the bladder in two parts. The metal catheters fit on each side of the central stem, and open one on each side of the membrane at the depth of the curve. At the handle of the instrument they curve outwards as fine tubes over two movable glass receptacles.

In *Cathelin's separator* the shaft is straight with a small curved beak. Concealed within the shaft is a membrane stretched on a spring hasp. When the membrane is projected by pushing in the shank the spring frame expands and a membranous division is formed. On each side small catheters project and drain each compartment of the bladder thus produced.

Method of using separators.—The instrument is prepared by adjusting the membrane and lubricating it. The patient lies on the back on an operating chair. The bladder is washed until the fluid returned into a glass vessel is clear. From 6–8 oz. of

fluid are allowed to remain in the bladder. A 1 per cent. solution
of cocaine hydrochlorate, 15 or 20 minims, is injected into the
urethra. In the female the instrument is readily passed into
the bladder; in the male the Luys separator passes easily until the

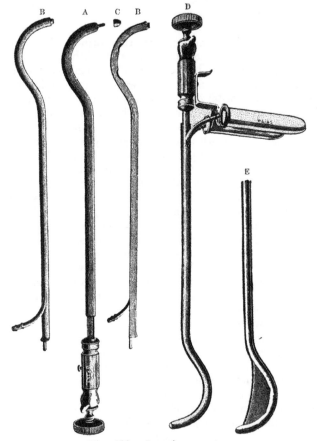

Fig. 108.—Luys' separator.

A, Shank and handle ; the rubber membrane has been drawn over the curve and shank, concealing the chain in the concavity of the curve. B, B, Metal catheters. C, Cap to unite shank with
catheters. D, Component parts adjusted ready for introduction. E, Curve of instrument with
chain drawn taut and separating membrane expanded.

curve lies in the prostatic urethra. The handle is now depressed
deeply between the thighs and pushed gently onwards. The
patient is gently raised into a sitting posture, and the instrument
is drawn towards the surgeon and held in the median line of the

body with a slight upward inclination. The screw is now turned and the chain rendered taut, forming the membranous septum in the bladder. A rectal or vaginal examination is made, to ensure that the instrument is in position. The first fluid is discarded, the tubes are placed in position, and the examination is continued

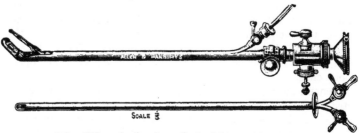

Fig. 109.—Author's catheterizing cystoscope.

for twenty-five minutes. In the case of Cathelin's instrument the introduction is easier, and the instrument is pulled towards the operator until the beak fits against the pubes. The membranous septum is then projected.

2. Catheterization of the ureters.—Many catheter cystoscopes are in use. Those of Nitze, Casper, Albarran, Freudenberg, Ringleb, and Israel are well known and reliable. The instruments have already been described. My pattern (Fig. 109) has the same valve as my irrigation cystoscope. Ureteral catheters are 30 in. long, and are of different sizes, varying from No. 5 to No. 8 Charrière. The end may be blunt or conical, or may have a fine

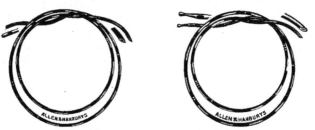

Fig. 110.—Author's ureteral catheters.

olivary bulb. There are two lateral eyes, or the eye may be terminal. Albarran's catheter has a slightly thicker part proximal to the second eye, to prevent the escape of urine alongside the catheter. My own catheters (Fig. 110) are graduated in divisions of black and brown of ½ in. each, and a narrow red band marks each 6 in. The end is blunt or olivary, the eyes are lateral.

Y

There is a slight thickening proximal to the second eye. The proximal end is obliquely cut, but is not trumpet-shaped, as it must pass through the tunnel of the cystoscope.

The catheters are sterilized by cleaning them with biniodide of mercury solution (1 in 1,000) and thoroughly syringing with the same solution before and after use with a special fine nozzle syringe which fits the catheter (Fig. 111). Before laying the catheter aside it is rubbed with a trace of sterile oil, and a little oil is injected through it to prevent cracking. The catheters should be kept in enamelled tin trays or in long glass tubes open at both ends.

A general anæsthetic is unnecessary unless in the case of a contracted tender bladder, such as may be met with in tuberculous disease. Local anæsthesia and the preparation of the bladder are the same as for cystoscopy. The amount of distension of the bladder for catheterization of the ureters is the same. It is sometimes necessary in an irritable contracted bladder to catheterize

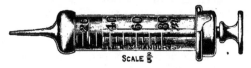

SCALE $\frac{2}{5}$

Fig. 111.—Author's syringe for washing out ureteral catheters.

the ureters with a small quantity of fluid in the bladder. I have occasionally had to be content with between 2 and 3 oz. of fluid.

The cystoscope should be loaded with a catheter before it is introduced, but the point of the catheter must not project from the tunnel. On the bladder being reached, the beak is turned downwards, the light switched on, and the interureteric bar comes into view. This is followed outwards on one or the other side by rotating the instrument, when the slit-like opening of the ureter comes into view. The ocular end of the instrument is now carried towards the opposite thigh, and the window and catheter opening travels towards the ureteric orifice. (Fig. 112.)

The catheter is projected so that the point lies about the middle of the field of vision. The catheter is then manœuvred as close to the orifice as possible, and finally the elevating gutter raised by a touch of the screw, the point of the catheter sinking between the lips of the opening and being slowly and gently pushed on. (Fig. 113.) When the catheter has passed a few inches up the ureter the elevator is lowered, and the catheter glides more easily. The catheter should be passed into the renal pelvis, which is reached when the double red band indicating 12 in. lies at the ureteric orifice. If it is intended to catheterize both ureters and a double-barrelled cystoscope is being used, the second catheter is now introduced; or if a single-barrelled cystoscope is being used, this is withdrawn—leaving the first catheter in position—reloaded, and introduced, and the second ureter catheterized. Each catheter is fixed with a piece of adhesive plaster to the thigh of the side to which it belongs, and it drains into a sterilized bottle labelled " right " or " left."

By Kelly's open method the ureteric catheters are introduced direct through the large tube.

The ureter may also be sounded by passing a catheter to ascertain if any obstruction exists; or a solid opaque bougie may be

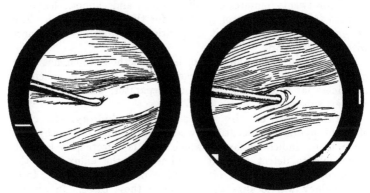

Fig. 112.—Catheter approaching ureteric orifice.   Fig. 113.—Catheter lying in ureter.

passed up the ureter in order to differentiate by means of the X-rays between stone in the ureter and extra-ureteral shadows.

Kelly has suggested the passage of a bougie tipped with wax which will receive scratches apparent to the naked eye from the rough surface of a calculus. This method cannot be used with the indirect method of catheterization of the ureters, as the wax would be scratched in the tunnel of the cystoscope.

Difficulties, such as temporary cessation of function of the kidney due to the catheterization, blocking of the catheter with blood clot, thick pus, or even gravel, inaccessibility of the ureter, smallness of the ureteric orifice, or enlarged or tuberculous prostate, may be met with, but are less formidable as greater expericuce is gained. With proper precautions there is no danger of infecting the ureter and kidney.

Choice of an instrument for separation of the urines.

1. *Ease of application.*—The separator is more easily introduced than the ureteral catheter. It is imperative, however, to make a cystoscopic examination before using the separator, so as to ascertain that the bladder is healthy.

2. *Danger of infecting the kidneys.*—In proper hands there is no danger of infection of the renal pelvis and kidney by a catheter.

3. *Accuracy of separation.*—The ureteral catheter is more accurate than the separator in obtaining the uncontaminated urine from one kidney. The results of the examination are so important that the surgeon cannot accept any report on which a doubt can be cast.

4. *Duration of the examination.*—The separation can only be borne for twenty minutes or half an hour, and cannot, therefore, be used for the majority of the tests for the renal function. The ureteric catheter can be left in position for four or five hours without discomfort.

Catheterization of the ureters is the method which has been most widely adopted. Its accuracy is greater and its sphere of usefulness far wider than that of the separator, which it has now entirely superseded.

Examination of the urine of each kidney.—In cases of slight pyuria or hæmaturia, where the bladder is healthy and there is no indication as to which side is affected, it is often impossible to detect a slight cloudiness of the efflux with the cystoscope. Examination of the urine drawn by catheter from each kidney will localize the disease in these cases. In disease of one kidney, when nephrectomy is proposed, the presence of a second kidney and its health and functional power are ascertained by the same method.

In examining the urines of the two kidneys, one may be normal and act as a standard of comparison for the other, or there may be signs of disease in each.

The quantity of urine is occasionally reduced by the presence of the catheter in the ureter. This is usually temporary, and can be avoided by giving a diuretic before the examination. The quantity may be reduced or the urine be absent on one side from blocking of the ureter or advanced disease of the kidney. There may be polyuria on the diseased side in conditions of cystitis such as early renal tuberculosis.

The urine should be examined for blood, pus, epithelial elements, and crystals, and also for bacteria.

The renal function is tested by the methods already described. Those suitable for the examination of one kidney are the quantitative estimation of urea, Casper's phloridzin test, Albarran's experimental polyuria test, and the phenol-sulphone-phthalein test. I use the phloridzin and phenol-sulphone-phthalein tests, and retain the catheters for two or three hours.

The details of the tests of the renal function have been already described (p. 20).

The following table gives the results of the examination of the urine of each kidney in a case in which nephrectomy was performed for advanced calculous disease of the right kidney:—

	RIGHT KIDNEY	LEFT KIDNEY
Quantity	206·5 c.c.	107 c.c.
Specific gravity ..	1004.	1011.
Freezing-point (Δ) ..	−0·18 C.	−0·76 C.
Colour	Pale, limpid.	Fairly coloured.
Urea	0·4 per cent.	1·3 per cent.
Uric acid	0·0067 per cent.	0·0150 per cent.
Chlorides as chlorine ..	0·09777 per cent.	0·1112 per cent.
Phosphates as P_2O_5 ..	0·08 per cent.	0·034 per cent.
Methylene blue.. ..	No change in colour.	Appeared in 1 hour 50 minutes, green colour, duration 18 hours.
Chromogen	Appeared in 25 minutes, faint green.	Appeared in 25 minutes, deep green.
Phloridzin glycosuria ..	0·395 grm.	1·623 grm.

The following is a report on a case in which nephrectomy was performed for tuberculosis of the left kidney:—

	RIGHT KIDNEY	LEFT KIDNEY
Total quantity	3 oz.	8 oz.
Specific gravity ..	1018.	1006.
Urea	1·4 per cent.	0·3 per cent.
Phloridzin glycosuria ..	2·81 grm.	Absent.
	No tubercle bacilli.	Tubercle bacilli.

LITERATURE

Albarran, *Exploration des Fonctions Rénales.* 1905.
Casper und **Richter,** *Functionelle Nierendiagnostik.* 1901.
Kapsammer, *Nierendiagnostik und Nierenchirurgie.* 1907.
Walker, Thomson, *Renal Function in Urinary Surgery.* 1908.

CHAPTER XXVIII

VESICAL SYMPTOMS OF DISEASE

HÆMATURIA and pyuria have already been discussed (*see* pp. 55, 62).

FREQUENT MICTURITION

Increased frequency of micturition may be a symptom in almost any disease of the bladder, and is observed also in many extravesical diseases.

The normal frequency of micturition varies in different individuals, and in the same individual under varying conditions.

The female bladder, by habit, is emptied less frequently than the male. The average number of micturitions during the day is three or four in the female and four to six in the male. During the night there is no call to micturate, partly from training and partly from the smaller quantity of urine secreted. Some healthy individuals, however, rise once during the night to pass water. This may be the continuation of a habit acquired in early life, or it may be the functional sequence of some pathological condition of the bladder, the organic disease having long passed off. The senile bladder is less sensitive, and micturition is usually performed less frequently than in earlier life. In old men increased diurnal frequency and the necessity for nocturnal micturition are signs of disease. In the tropics urine is passed less frequently than in cold climates, owing to the smaller quantity secreted. On returning from the tropics to the temperate zone, frequent micturition is usually observed. It may be distressing, and occasionally persists for some years. An Indian civil servant has told me that for over two years after returning to England from India he and his wife were unable to accept an invitation to dinner on account of frequent micturition. For convenience of description, frequency of micturition will be considered under four headings :

1. **Frequency of polyuria.**—In diabetes mellitus, diabetes insipidus, chronic Bright's disease, chronic interstitial nephritis from obstructive disease, nervous polyuria, and in the transient forms of polyuria such as those due to diuretics (tea, etc.), there

is increased frequency of micturition. The increased frequency is nocturnal as well as diurnal. In nephritis from obstructive disease the nocturnal frequency is especially marked. The quantity of the urine and the presence of abnormalities such as sugar or albumin render the diagnosis obvious.

2. **Frequency with normal urine and bladder.**—The mental state may affect the frequency of micturition. Fear and excitement may, apart from the production of polyuria, cause frequency. Prolonged intense concentration may reduce frequency. When disease of the bladder is present mental influences still affect the frequency of micturition. A patient with frequent micturition due to disease may have prolonged intervals when his attention is fully occupied, and shorter intervals when there is nothing to distract his attention from the calls to micturate.

Reflex frequency may be caused by disease of the kidneys. It is difficult to dissociate this from irritation of the bladder by descending ureteritis or by irritating urine. In early tuberculosis of the kidney, as well as in some cases of movable kidney and calculus, there is ground for believing that an increased frequency of micturition may be reflex, for the cystoscopic appearance of the bladder and ureteric orifices is normal. In other and advanced diseases of the kidney and ureter, such as pyelonephritis, stone, tuberculosis of the kidney and ureter, inflammation of the bladder base is present and is the cause of the frequency. In such cases the diagnosis as to the presence or absence of bladder disease is made by means of the cystoscope.

Reflex frequency of micturition may have its source in rectal irritation caused by worms, a condition which is often the cause of enuresis in children. In cases of rectal, anal, or vulvar irritation increased frequency of micturition is often due, not to reflex influences, but to a mild form of cystitis, with or without bacilluria, or there may be some disease such as diabetes.

Pressure on a normal bladder from without causes frequent micturition by reducing its capacity. Frequency is sometimes a marked and distressing symptom in the later months of pregnancy, and is generally associated with an abnormal position of the fœtus (retroversion). I have been consulted in regard to persistent frequency in a young lady which I found was due to the pressure of a large ovarian cyst.

3. **Frequency due to irritating urine.**—Apart from other causes the urine may cause irritability in a healthy bladder.

Blood poured out suddenly and in quantity may cause frequent micturition; usually, however, no change is caused by hæmaturia in the frequency of micturition. Where clots are formed they may act as foreign bodies and give rise to frequency. It is more usual to find that, beyond a temporary difficulty during the passage of the clot along the urethra, the patient is unaware of any irritation.

When the urine is highly acid, when it contains abundance of oxalate-of-lime crystals, or is milky with phosphates, extreme irritability of the bladder is present. In any of these states of the urine, but especially in phosphaturia, the irritability of the bladder is intermittent. It is more pronounced at certain times of the day ; in phosphaturia it is often worse after dinner. Bacilluria may be the cause of persistent frequency without other symptoms.

4. Frequency from disease of bladder, prostate, or urethra. —The frequency in mild cystitis is diurnal, but in severe cystitis it is also nocturnal, and the patient passes water at regularly spaced intervals of half to one or two hours day and night, accord‑ ing to the intensity of the inflammation and its distribution in the bladder. The frequency is unaffected by movement, but the intervals may be longer when the attention of the patient is held by other matters. In new growth frequent micturition, if present, is due to cystitis and has the characters already described.

The frequency due to stone in the bladder is characteristic. It is present during the day and disappears at night or on resting. Movements and exercise, or travelling by train or motor-car, increase the frequency. If there be severe cystitis the frequency is present at night as well as during the day.

In enlarged prostate there is an increase in the diurnal frequency, and the patient rises once or several times during the night. The first four or five hours of the night are usually undisturbed, and then the patient wakes at three or four o'clock and passes water, and this is repeated several times at short intervals. Movement and exercise have no effect upon prostatic frequency.

The frequency which results from urethritis of the prostatic urethra usually accompanies a urethral discharge. It is diurnal, and occasionally nocturnal, in character.

Frequent micturition due to nervous disease will be considered later.

Treatment.—The treatment of frequent micturition depends upon the cause, and the reader is referred to the various diseases which produce increased frequency of micturition for the lines along which treatment should be conducted. When the frequency is unconnected with any pathological condition of the urine or bladder, the prognosis for complete recovery is good only in mild cases. Washing the bladder with weak nitrate of silver solution

(1 in 10,000) or with a 5 per cent. solution of antipyrin, or gradual dilatation by the injection of progressively increasing quantities of fluid, may be tried, or instillations of silver nitrate solution (1 or 2 per cent.) into the deeper part of the urethra, or of cocaine (1 per cent.) or other local anæsthetic, may be given at intervals of a week. Gomenol may be instilled in small quantities (1 or 2 drachms of 5 or 10 per cent.) once or twice a week.

Electricity in the form of X-rays or high-frequency currents or radiant heat has been employed, but is rarely successful. Treatment by suggestion may be tried in severe cases.

The following drugs, which should be given with caution when urethral or prostatic obstruction is present, are valuable in reducing frequency, viz. camphor (2 gr. in pill) or camphor monobromide (2–4 gr. in suppository), cannabis indica (tincture in doses of 5–10 minims, or extract in doses of $\frac{1}{4}$ gr. in pill), belladonna (tincture, 5–10 minims, extract, $\frac{1}{4}$ gr., in suppository), collinsonia canadensis (tincture, $\frac{1}{2}$–1 drachm, liquid extract, 1–2 drachms, or as suppository 20 gr.), sandal-wood oil (10 minims in capsule), oil of copaiba (5–15 minims in capsule), hydrastis canadensis (tincture, 30–60 minims), kava-kava (liquid extract, 30–60 minims), argopyrum (decoction, $\frac{1}{2}$–1 oz., or liquid extract, 1–2 drachms), hyoscyamus (tincture, 10–15 minims), lupulin (pill containing 2–5 gr., or suppository 5 gr.), lycopodium (tincture, 15–60 minims).

When the urine is highly acid, diuretics and alkalis should be administered, such as Contrexéville, Vittel, or Evian waters, acetate or citrate of potash (15–20 gr.), liquor potassæ (5–10 minims), and sodium bicarbonate (5–30 gr.).

If phosphaturia is present, sodium acid phosphate (20 gr.) and mineral acids should be prescribed (*see* p. 49).

INCONTINENCE OF URINE

Incontinence consists in the involuntary escape of urine from the bladder, and is due to very widely differing causes.

The urine is retained in the bladder by the combined action of the involuntary sphincter at the outlet of the bladder and the voluntary compressor urethræ or external sphincter.

In infancy the bladder acts in an automatic reflex manner. After a certain quantity of urine has accumulated it is expelled. Towards the end of the first year mental control by inhibition is becoming established, and at the end of the second year the child has learned to intimate the desire to micturate and to exert an inhibiting influence for a certain time during the waking hours. Inhibition of micturition during sleep becomes gradually established, and under normal conditions and surroundings is complete, except for an occasional accident, at the end of the second year. During adult life the voluntary power of inhibiting micturition during waking hours and the unconscious inhibition exercised during sleep are much more powerful and less easily disturbed.

Incontinence of urine may be (1) false, (2) true.

(1) **False incontinence.**—Here the bladder is full of urine, and the escape is the overflow from the over-distended organ. This is observed in cases of chronic retention due to prostatic or urethral obstruction.

(2) In **true incontinence** the urine which escapes is the entire content of the bladder. Two types can be distinguished:

(a) A *passive* type, in which the urine dribbles away without distending the bladder and without contraction of the bladder assisting the expulsion. Here the sphincter is paralysed, and to this type belong cases of paralysis of the bladder involving the sphincter, or paralysis of the sphincter by mechanical means.

(b) An *active* type, in which the urine is expelled by contraction of the bladder. Here there is sphincter action, but it is either too weak to resist the normal contractions of the bladder or the contractions are so strong as to overcome a normal sphincter.

1. Incontinence due to mechanical causes.—This occurs more frequently in women than in men. A slight occasional escape of urine on coughing, sneezing, or lifting weights, or on exertion of any kind such as playing golf, is sometimes observed in women. In slight cases it may be difficult to assign a cause, but it is probably traumatic, for it frequently follows parturition. In older women more serious incontinence occurs in combination with cystocele.

When the now obsolete method of examination of the female bladder by dilatation of the urethra and introduction of the finger was in vogue, incontinence of urine from overstretching of the sphincter was commonly observed. Injury sustained during childbirth may cause incontinence.

In men perineal prostatectomy may produce incontinence of urine. I have also known it follow perineal drainage of the prostatic cavity after suprapubic prostatectomy, being caused by cutting through the compressor urethræ muscle, which acts as the vesical sphincter in these cases.

In a few cases (5 per cent.) of malignant disease of the prostate there is incontinence of urine without distension of the bladder. In these cases there is extensive infiltration of the bladder base, and the prostatic urethra is open and rigid.

Treatment.—In slight cases in women medicine may suffice. Strychnine (liquor, 5 minims) and ergot (liquid extract, 10–20 minims) are the best drugs. The introduction of a pessary may control the escape by pressure upon the urethra. In some severe cases operation is necessary. When cystocele is present an elliptical portion with the long axis vertical should be removed from the anterior vaginal wall and the edges united.

Duret has freed the urethra and excised the mucous membrane around its orifice, and transplanted the urethra forwards to the neighbourhood of the clitoris.

Gersuny dissects the female urethra with as much surrounding tissue as possible, twists it on its own axis for a complete turn, and fixes it in this position. The urethra is thrown into spiral folds in its whole length. This surgeon has also injected paraffin around the urethra and bladder orifice in incontinence of urine in the female, but the method has not been widely adopted.

Where incontinence in the male follows prostatectomy, recovery or improvement may take place by the perineal muscles assuming control. If not, the patient will have to wear a urinal.

2. **Incontinence due to nervous disease.**—This form of incontinence is considered at p. 532.

3. **Incontinence due to bladder spasm.**—The somewhat rare form of uncontrollable bladder spasm met with in disease of the spinal cord has already been mentioned.

In acute inflammation of the bladder uncontrollable spasm may give rise to active incontinence. This is usually nocturnal, as the patient, worn out by frequent micturition, sleeps heavily and the urine is passed involuntarily. Tuberculosis of the bladder in its advanced stage is the most frequent cause, but other forms of cystitis which persist in a subacute condition may also cause incontinence of this type.

Diurnal incontinence from uncontrollable spasm is also met with in the acute stages of cystitis and in acute inflammation of the prostate and prostatic urethra.

Treatment.—Means of soothing the bladder should be adopted. In acute cases hot fomentations should be applied suprapubically and on the perineum, and morphia and belladonna suppositories given. The rectum may be washed out with hot water, followed by a small enema of hot water containing antipyrin (30 gr.) to be retained. The urine should be diluted and rendered less irritating by large draughts of Contrexéville or Vittel water, and by the administration of sandal-wood oil (10 minims in capsule). Hot sitz-baths (106°–108° F.) are sometimes useful.

In chronic cases diuretics and sandal-wood oil should be administered and belladonna and hyoscyamus with small doses of opium given in mixture. Gomenol (5 per cent.) may be used as an instillation (30 to 60 minims) in the bladder and given by mouth in capsules. The treatment of the cystitis is carried out simultaneously with these measures. In tuberculous cystitis the bladder should not be washed.

4. Incontinence of childhood (nocturnal enuresis, essential enuresis).—Up to the end of the first year the bladder acts automatically. About that time, as mentioned above, mental control of the act of micturition begins, and by the age of 18 months or at most 2 years it is fairly established. At first the control is feeble and the inhibition can only be exercised for a very short time, and during sleep the automatic action continues. Gradually the control grows stronger and becomes a habit, so that it is exercised during the hours of sleep, although there may still be occasional lapses up to the age of 3 years. After that, constant or frequent bed-wetting must be regarded as abnormal. The period during which the incontinence of childhood occurs extends from the age of 3 to puberty. In 60 per cent. of Still's cases the onset was observed between the ages of 5 and 8 years, when the second dentition commences.

Enuresis is usually nocturnal, sometimes it is diurnal as well, rarely it is diurnal only.

There may have been a period of a year or more of complete control before the enuresis develops, or the nocturnal control may never have become established.

In 142 cases examined by Still, 67 had been incontinent since birth, and in 75 the incontinence began some time after infancy.

Boys and girls are about equally affected.

Etiology.—i. The cases first to be considered are those in which a source of irritation is found, such as threadworms, anal fissure, vulvitis, phimosis, and balanitis. These cases are looked upon as due to reflex irritation. The relation of phimosis to enuresis is doubtful. The great majority of cases that have come under my notice have already been circumcised in the hope of curing the enuresis, but without any effect upon it.

In some cases there are enlarged tonsils and adenoids, and the enuresis is ascribed to partial asphyxia during sleep. The importance of this as a causal factor is disputed, but most authorities are agreed that where enlarged tonsils and adenoids are present their removal, or, if small, the use of breathing exercises, should form an adjunct to the treatment of the enuresis.

ii. The next group of cases are those in which there is some abnormality in the urine or disease of the bladder. In young children the urine may be highly acid and contain large quantities of uric acid. Phosphaturia also occurs at this age. Bacilluria due to the bacillus coli is a common disease of childhood, and explains a small number of cases. Cystitis, stone in the bladder, and tuberculous cystitis may be found.

iii. Finally, there are cases in which no source of irritation and no alteration in the urine or disease of the bladder can be found. These form a class that has been named *essential enuresis*. There is frequently an heredity of nervous disease which may take the form of epilepsy, neurasthenia, alcoholism, insanity, or other disease. The child may be nervous, quiet, sensitive, and furtive. This is largely, however, due to a feeling of shame, and sometimes to the well-meaning but cruel and utterly futile attempts of parents or guardians to bring about a cure by chastisement. Stuttering and habit spasms are frequently observed, and betray a lack of co-ordination in the nerve centres. In some children there is a slight escape of urine on coughing or exertion, together with nocturnal enuresis.

The enuresis is always worse after excitement. It may occur when the child is at school and cease during holidays.

In a small number of cases the enuresis occurs during a minor epileptic seizure; and the possibility of the patient suffering from *petit mal* must always be remembered. Thursfield points out that in these cases the interval between the bed-wettings is much greater, and may be one or two months, and then several wettings occur in succession.

Prognosis.—In cases where an abnormality is found which is amenable to treatment the prognosis for immediate recovery is good.

In the great majority of cases of essential enuresis, continence becomes complete with or before the advent of puberty. Most cases get well after two or three months' treatment, but sometimes treatment for a year or even longer is required. In a small percentage enuresis persists into adult life.

Treatment.—In cases where some reflex influence, such as threadworms, is a factor, this should be treated. The prognosis should, however, be guarded, for the removal of a source of irritation may not be attended by the disappearance of the enuresis. Circumcision is often disappointing in this respect. This operation, and also that for the removal of enlarged tonsils and adenoids, should, nevertheless, always be done as a preliminary to other treatment.

Hyperacid urine with uric-acid or oxalate crystals should be treated with alkalis (potass. citrate, 5 or 10 gr. for a child of 3 or 5 years), and the intake of carbohydrates should be cut down. Sugar, starch, green vegetables, potatoes, and fruits should be restricted. This is more important than interdicting nitrogenous foods.

Phosphaturia is treated with acids and sodium acid phosphate, and attention to the diet and bowels. Bacilluria, cystitis, and stone should receive appropriate treatment.

In cases where all such causes of irritation are absent, treatment along the following lines should be adopted : All sources of mental excitement should be excluded. Late hours, theatres, parties, entertainments of all kinds, should be interdicted. The effect of removing the child from school and reducing, or for a time intermitting, book-work should be tried.

If, as sometimes happens, the enuresis ceases when the child is withdrawn from school, a three or six months' holiday should be prescribed. Country life in the open air is to be preferred to town life.

The principal meal should be taken in the middle of the day, and no fluids should be allowed after five o'clock. Tea and coffee, ginger beer and ginger ale should be interdicted. Meat may be taken, but in moderate quantities. All highly seasoned foods, with sugars and pastry, should be avoided. The nurse should train the child to hold water at longer periods during the day, and the child should be made to pass water before going to rest. He should be wakened for the same purpose once during the night. The enuresis usually occurs during the first two hours of sleep, and the nocturnal micturition should be arranged to take place after about one and a half hours' sleep, shortly before it is due. The mattress should be firm, and the clothing light but warm. The air of the bedroom should not be too cold.

Belladonna is largely used in the form of the tincture. The dose varies with the age and idiosyncrasy of the patient. It should commence with 3 minims of the tincture thrice daily for a child of 5 years or over, and slowly increase up to 30 or 40 minims, or even 1 drachm, three times a day, unless symptoms of dryness of the throat, flushing, dim vision, and commencing delirium appear. During the period in which this drug is being administered the child should be under daily medical supervision. Symptoms of poisoning with these large doses may set in rapidly. If the enuresis is controlled the dose should be kept a little beyond this point for a fortnight and then very gradually reduced.

Tincture of lycopodium is also useful and may be combined with belladonna. The dosage should commence with 5 or 10 minims thrice daily, and may rise to 20 minims. The tincture of nux vomica in doses of 3 or 4 minims thrice daily for a child of 5, and the liquid extract of ergot in doses of 10–20 minims thrice daily, are sometimes successful. I have found them most useful in cases where an occasional leak on laughing, sneezing, or other muscular effort shows weakness of the sphincter.

Potassium bromide and antipyrin have been found useful, and the fluid extract of rhus aromatica in doses similar to belladonna is recommended (Still). Hyoscine hydrobromide has also been used.

Leonard Williams and Firth have used thyroid extract. The latter observer found that of 28 cases 16 showed a marked improvement or were cured, and 12 showed no improvement. The initial dose was ¼ gr., and this was cautiously increased to 1 gr. or even 4½ gr. in twenty-four hours. The treatment was most successful when the child was backward, slow at school, lethargic, and under weight.

Local treatment should, if possible, be avoided, but in some cases it may be used and be successful.

Instillation of 10 or 15 minims of silver nitrate solution (1 per cent.) into the prostatic urethra once a week for three or four weeks may be followed by cessation of the enuresis. I have, however, known relapses occur after this treatment when it was completely successful for a time.

Treatment by the continuous current is applied by means of a urethral electrode introduced into the prostatic urethra and a pad applied over the suprapubic region. Two or three séances are given for five or ten minutes, with a week's interval between.

Cathelin has suggested the injection of fluid into the sacral canal with the object of causing pressure upon the sacral nerves. The method, which is employed also for adults, is carried out in the following manner: The patient is placed upon the side with the back bent and the thighs well flexed upon the abdomen. With the tip of the forefinger the opening at the lower end of the sacral canal is defined. This opening is covered with a membrane and lies a short distance above the lower end of the sacrum. On each side of it is a tubercle, and the bony arch surrounding the small opening can be felt. The skin is carefully cleaned and a hypodermic syringe sterilized and filled with 30 minims of saline solution. The needle is passed through the membrane and easily introduced into the sacral canal. The fluid is slowly injected and the needle removed. The procedure is painless. Cathelin claims 80 per cent. of cures by this method. I have used it in a few obstinate cases, but have had no success with it.

· Care should be devoted to training the child, and when the confidence is once gained much may be done by persuasion. Good results have been claimed for control by suggestion, employed during waking hours and also during sleep.

LITERATURE

Dudgeon, *Lancet,* 1908, i. 616.
Firth, *Lancet,* 1911, ii. 1619.
Still, *Diseases of Children.*
Williams, *Lancet,* 1909, i. 1245.

DIFFICULT MICTURITION

Difficult micturition results from obstruction to the outflow of urine, or from reduced power of expulsion.

In difficult micturition there is delay in the commencement of the act amounting to from a few seconds' hesitation to a wait of two minutes or more. The stream is feebly projected, and may drop vertically from the end of the penis. It may commence feebly, and gain in power, and then fall away again, or it may dribble throughout. The stream may be intermittent, one or several pauses occurring during the act. Occasionally the flow ceases, and only recommences after a pause of several minutes, or even a quarter of an hour. The abdominal muscles are brought forcibly into action to assist the expulsion of the urine. After-dribbling is usually observed.

The most frequent cause of difficult micturition is stricture of the urethra. Here the obstruction usually commences in young men, or below the age of 45. The onset is insidious, and the increase is gradual and persistent. Attacks of retention of urine following alcoholic excess or exposure to cold or wet supervene when the stricture has become narrow. Eventually there may be chronic retention with overflow.

Diseases of the prostate frequently cause difficult micturition. The commonest of these is simple enlargement of the gland. Here the symptoms commence at or after the age of 50 years. The difficulty is combined with frequency of micturition, which is most troublesome at night and especially during the early hours of the morning. Complete retention may occur without the patient being aware of previous difficulty in micturition. Malignant disease of the prostate causes difficult micturition which closely resembles that of stricture; it is insidious and persistent and is not combined with frequent micturition unless cystitis is present, but it appears in middle or late life. Tuberculous disease and calculi of the prostate, subacute chronic inflammation of the prostatic urethra, post-gonorrhœal or due to bacillus coli, may cause difficulty of micturition. Acute urethritis, prostatic abscess, impaction of a stone in the prostatic urethra, may cause difficulty and even retention.

Atony of the bladder, apart from obstruction, is usually due to disease of the spinal cord. The patient complains of increasing difficulty of micturition, or sometimes there is sudden complete retention. Tabes and Erb's "syphilitic spinal paralysis" are the most frequent causes of this form of atony. The symptom is often combined with nocturnal incontinence without over-distension of the bladder. I have described a form of atony of the bladder without obstruction and without signs of nervous disease ; it occurs at any age, but most frequently in young men ; the cases do not at a later date develop symptoms of spinal disease.

Functional difficulty of micturition. Stammering bladder.—It is well known that micturition may be difficult or impossible when there is urgent necessity that it should be quickly performed, or when it is attempted in the presence of others. There are many patients who pass water after considerable hesitation, or are unable to pass it at all, when called upon to do so in the surgeon's consulting-room. These are the minor phases of the condition described by Sir James Paget as the "stammering bladder." In its more severe forms it is found that otherwise healthy individuals cannot pass water in a public urinal, and may get complete retention of urine (hysterical retention). Complete retention from this cause occurs more frequently in women.

Treatment.—The treatment of difficult micturition can only be initiated after the cause has been ascertained. Urethral obstruction due to stricture is treated by dilatation or operation, enlarged prostate by operation. The obstruction of malignant disease of the prostate is much benefited by the careful passage of metal instruments at regular intervals. The treatment of atony of the bladder due to nervous disease will be discussed later (p. 538).

In any case of difficult micturition where obstruction has been relieved, or where a paralysed bladder is being emptied by catheter, the administration of small doses of ergot (liquid extract, 15–20 minims) and strychnine (liquor, 5 minims) is beneficial.

In "stammering bladder" ergot and strychnine are the most useful drugs, and they may be combined with bromides.

RETENTION OF URINE

Etiology.—The causes of retention of urine may be classified in the following manner :—

1. **Retention with obstruction.**
    (a) *Prostate.*
        (1) Simple enlargement.
        (2) Malignant disease.

z

(3) Stone.

(4) Acute prostatitis and prostatic abscess.

(b) *Urethra.*

(1) Rupture of urethra.

(2) Acute urethritis.

(3) Stricture.

(4) Stone and foreign bodies.

(5) Pressure from without, pelvic tumours, etc.

2. **Retention due to atony.**

(a) *With symptoms of nervous disease.*

Tabes, etc.

(b) *Without symptoms of nervous disease.*

Idiopathic atony.

3. **Retention in acute or chronic intoxications,** such as appendicitis, typhoid, salpingitis, or arsenical, mercurial, belladonna, or lead poisoning, or syphilis.

4. **Retention from inhibition or spasm.**

(1) Hysterical retention.

(2) Retention after anal and rectal operations.

Diagnosis.—It is necessary to distinguish between anuria and retention, and between retention due to atony and that due to obstruction, and, in the latter, to ascertain the form of obstruction.

A patient with anuria refers to previous attacks of renal colic, hæmaturia, or other signs pointing to progressive renal disease, and the cessation of periodic micturition may have followed immediately upon such an attack. Symptoms of bladder trouble are absent, and have been absent or insignificant during the course of the disease. The patient is in no pain, there is no distension of the bladder, and an instrument passes readily along the urethra into the bladder but draws no urine. In retention of urine there is usually a history of gradually increasing difficulty in micturition, the stream has become progressively smaller and more feeble, and there may be some involuntary dribbling of urine. The bladder is distended and appears as a smooth, rounded swelling above the pubes, firm on pressure and dull on percussion.

In retention from atony of the bladder muscle there is no pain and no desire to empty the distended viscus. In acute retention due to obstruction, recurrent spasmodic attempts of the bladder to overcome the obstruction usually double the patient up with cramp-like pain. In some patients, however, pain is remarkably absent, and this is especially the case in old men when the obstruction results from enlargement of the prostate. Here the retention is chronic and slowly progressive, and some urine is passed, voluntarily or involuntarily. The patient may be unaware that the bladder is distended even when the organ reaches above the umbilicus.

Diagnosis is made by the passage of a large-sized instrument, which enters the bladder easily if retention is due to atony, but is arrested if obstruction is present. The presence of signs of spinal disease clinches the diagnosis. In young men the most frequent cause of acute retention is gonorrhœa, and there will be a history of an acute discharge. In adult life retention is usually due to stricture, and there is a history of gradually increasing difficulty of micturition, culminating in retention after alcoholic excess or exposure to cold. The passage of an instrument confirms the diagnosis. In old men enlargement of the prostate is the most frequent cause of retention of urine. There is a history of nocturnal frequency and increasing difficulty, and rectal examination shows that the prostate is enlarged.

Treatment.—The following is the treatment suited to the chief types of cases met with in practice :—

1. *Acute inflammation of the urethra (gonorrhœa, etc.).*—Every means should be tried to relieve the retention without the passage of a catheter. Suprapubic puncture should not be performed. It has been recommended with the view of avoiding infection of the bladder by the catheter passing along the urethra. Retention does not, however, take place unless there is posterior urethritis or prostatitis, and in such cases the base of the bladder is already infected. The patient should be placed in a hot bath or made to sit in a hot sitz-bath and directed to pass his water in it. A large hot-water injection should be introduced into the rectum ; should this fail, a suppository containing extract of belladonna ($\frac{1}{4}$ gr.) and aqueous extract of opium ($\frac{1}{2}$ gr.) should be given. If relief is not obtained in half to three-quarters of an hour a catheter must be passed and the urine withdrawn. An anæsthetic will usually be necessary, for the urethra is intensely sensitive. The canal is first thoroughly washed with a solution of permanganate of potash (1 in 5,000) or protargol (1 in 10,000) from a douche can, a glass nozzle and bell shield being used to allow the fluid to rush in and out of the canal without splashing. To this 20 or 30 minims of cocaine solution (2 per cent.) may be added and may suffice to numb the urethra for the passage of the instrument. A soft rubber catheter is passed very gently and the urine withdrawn. The bladder should be washed out with protargol solution before the catheter is removed. If a morphia and belladonna suppository has not already been given, it should now be inserted into the rectum and the patient returned to bed. If

acute prostatitis and a prostatic abscess be present, operation as soon as possible is indicated.

2. *Blocking the urethra by stone, foreign bodies, pedunculated bladder growths, blood clot, etc.*—The diagnosis is made by the history, and relief by catheter should be given without delay. There is sometimes difficulty in introducing a catheter, due to intense spasm of the compressor urethræ muscle caused by impaction of the stone or foreign body. A metal catheter passes most readily. It may be necessary to pass several metal sounds before the catheter can be introduced.

The distension of the bladder with blood clot from a sudden copious hæmorrhage in a case of bladder growth will cause retention of urine. The condition is serious on account of the grave danger of septic infection of the clot. An attempt may be made with a large metal catheter to break up the clot and wash it out; or a lithotrite may be used, and an evacuating cannula. Very little time should be spent in these attempts, and the bladder should be opened suprapubically without further delay, the masses of clot removed, and a large rubber drain placed in the bladder. Treatment of the growth or other cause of bleeding will have to be postponed until a more convenient time.

3. *The distended atonic bladder of spinal disease.*—This should be relieved by catheter with the same precautions as are adopted in enlarged prostate. The introduction to regular catheterization is similar to that in enlarged prostate.

4. *Retention from reflex spasm in disease of or after operation on the rectum, anus, testicles, etc., and hysterical retention.*—In operation cases the catheter is passed without delay, to avoid distress. In other cases hot baths and other means of relieving spasm, such as are used in retention due to acute inflammation, should be tried before resorting to the catheter. A metal catheter is the best form of instrument in these cases. After relief of the retention the cause of the spasm should be treated.

5. *Retention with enlarged prostate.*—The diagnosis is made by the history of the case, by the age at which the symptoms commenced, and by rectal examination. The preliminary measures which are detailed above may be tried, but recourse to the catheter will nearly always be necessary. Three points must be insisted upon: (i) The most rigid asepsis; (ii) the delicate handling of instruments; and (iii) all the urine of the over-distended bladder must not be withdrawn at once, or it must be drawn off very slowly.

The catheters, whether gum-elastic or metal, must be boiled, the hands carefully cleansed, the penis washed with antiseptic, and the urethra with solution of oxycyanide of mercury (1 in 5,000) or permanganate of potash (1 in 4,000).

The instrument should be of gum-elastic or metal. Coudé and bicoudé catheters are useful, and may pass easily. Where a difficulty is encountered it may be due to the distorted shape of the prostatic urethra, and the greatest gentleness should be exercised in pushing the instrument onwards. Sometimes twisting it gently one way or another during the passage will make it ride over an obstacle. Occasionally false passages have been made by previous instrumentation. It may be necessary to withdraw the instrument one or two inches, and then push it on, so as to avoid being caught in the cul-de-sac. When the prostate is very large the urethra is greatly elongated, and it is necessary to push the catheter very deeply before the urine begins to flow. Bicoudé catheters are made specially long to allow for the additional length of the urethra in these cases. A very frequent cause of failure is the use of a catheter which is too small or too pointed. The obstruction to the catheter is not due to narrowing of the canal but to distortion of its lumen. A No. 18 or No. 20 Fr. is the best size for routine use.

If the coudé and bicoudé catheters fail, a metal instrument may be tried. Special prostatic catheters which possess a very long curve are found in every set of metal catheters. A method that may be adopted when other methods have failed is to bend an English gum-elastic catheter containing its stilet into a very complete curve which commences by dropping down from the plane of the shaft. If this does not pass, it has been recommended to pull the stilet out while holding the catheter in the urethra, so that the beak of the instrument bores forwards and enters the bladder.

These manœuvres failing, it may be necessary to puncture the bladder suprapubically with an aspirator needle.

Three dangers attend the rapid emptying of an over-distended bladder—hæmorrhage from the vessels of the bladder or kidney; acute urinary infection, either autogenous or introduced with the catheter; and suppression of urine. In order to avoid these the following procedure is adopted: The patient is in bed and in a warm atmosphere. Only 10–15 oz. should be drawn off, and an interval of half an hour or one hour should elapse before a similar amount is again withdrawn, and so on until the bladder is empty, the catheter being retained in the urethra meanwhile.

Another method is to withdraw a pint of urine and substitute half a pint of warm boric solution, and repeat this at intervals until only boric solution is left.

Or, again, a catheter of very small calibre is introduced and the urine allowed to dribble slowly away.

When the bladder is empty a few syringefuls of silver nitrate solution (1 in 10,000) should be injected and allowed to escape. The catheter should be tied in.

Stimulants are usually necessary in these cases. A mixture containing urotropine 10 gr., liquor strychninæ 5 minims, liquid extract of ergot 5 minims, citrate of potash 20 gr., and infusion of buchu 1 oz. should be given every four hours.

After several days' continuous bladder drainage, the decision will have to be made whether " catheter life " is to be commenced or an operation performed.

6. *Retention with stricture.*—A hot sitz-bath and hot rectal injection followed by a suppository of morphia ($\frac{1}{4}$ gr.) may be tried, but recourse to instruments will in most cases be necessary.

The method of passing instruments through a narrow stricture is described elsewhere (p. 631).

In cases where a No. 7 or No. 8 Fr. bougie can be passed it should be withdrawn and a catheter of this size introduced.

If only a filiform bougie will pass, it should be tied in place with a piece of silk, the ends of which are carried along the sides of the penis and fixed by means of strapping. After half an hour the urine begins to trickle alongside the bougie, a few hours later the stricture will allow of a larger instrument being passed, and eventually a catheter is introduced.

A more rapid method is to use a special instrument consisting of a metal catheter with a conical end which screws on to a filiform bougie. The bougie acts as a guide, and the catheter is forced through the stricture. Harrison's whip bougies are sometimes useful. They consist of a gradually tapering gum-elastic bougie 20 in. in length, the end of which is filiform, while the shaft rises to the size of 18–20 Fr. These may be made with a groove along one side, by which the urine trickles away. Another special instrument is a tunnelled catheter which can be threaded upon the filiform bougie and pushed through the stricture.

There is less danger in completely emptying a distended bladder in a case of stricture than in enlarged prostate, for the age of the patient is less, and the kidneys are usually not so extensively diseased as the result of obstruction and arteriosclerosis. At the same time diuretics and stimulants should be administered to guard against suppression of urine.

If instrumentation fail, the bladder should be emptied with an aspirator needle. The most suitable point for the puncture is an inch above the upper margin of the pubic symphysis in the middle line. The percussion note should be dull. The skin is cleansed, and incised with a sharp scalpel, and the aspirator needle introduced. The urine will flow from the cannula without a negative pressure being produced. The dangers connected with aspiration of the bladder are puncture of the peritoneum with subsequent peritonitis, leaking of the wound in the bladder, and the formation of a prevesical abscess, or in more virulent infections a spreading pelvic cellulitis. There is little risk of wounding the peritoneum when the bladder is distended and the percussion note dull. The aspirating needle should not be a large one, lest leakage at the point of puncture of the bladder take place.

Usually, after a single aspiration an instrument can be introduced through the stricture and tied in, but rarely the puncture must be repeated several times. In such a case operation for the relief of the stricture should be performed as soon as possible. The operation will take the form of a Wheelhouse operation.

CHAPTER XXIX

CONGENITAL MALFORMATIONS

Development of the bladder and urethra.—In order to explain malformations of the bladder and urethra it is necessary to make a brief note in regard to the development of this part of the urinary tract.

The allantois, a hollow tube of hypoderm with a covering of mesoderm, opens posteriorly into the hindgut. A septum develops between the allantois and the hindgut, and both come to open into a common cloaca. As the septum descends, the cloaca is divided into a dorsal or anal portion and a genital or urogenital sinus. The sinus and allantois form a tube on which a dilatation (the bladder) appears at the second month, implicating the portion belonging to the sinus, and probably also a part of the allantois. The remainder of the allantois is obliterated and forms the urachus. The Wolffian ducts, the progenitors of the vasa deferentia and ejaculatory ducts in the male, open into the sinus by a common opening with the ureters. Further growth leads to separation of these ducts from the ureters, so that the ureters come to open into the bladder dilatation and the Wolffian ducts into the urogenital sinus. The sinus eventually comes to form the prostatic and membranous urethra in the male, and the whole of the urethra and the vestibule in the female. The Wolffian ducts open on an eminence, and between them the fused Müllerian ducts end. This eminence persists as the crista urethræ in the male, and when the ureters become separated by elongation of this portion and diverge from each other the upper part forms the trigone of the bladder. It can thus be realized how malposition of the ureteric orifice in the prostatic urethra or into the seminal vesicle may take place by persistence of the fœtal condition.

The cloaca at first extends from the umbilicus to the root of the tail, and is covered by the cloacal membrane. On either side the mesoderm encroaches upon this until it meets in the median line from the umbilicus backwards for some distance. This union ends behind in an eminence, the genital tubercle, which lies at the anterior end of the reduced cloaca, and is at first contained in it. On each side of the cloaca ridges appear, forming the outer genital folds, which eventually form the labia majora or the scrotum. A groove forms on the under or posterior surface of the genital tubercle, the urethral groove. The edges of this groove constitute the inner genital folds, which form the labia minora in the female, and in the male unite to form the floor of the bulbous and penile urethra. At the surface the septum which divides the cloaca into anal and urogenital segments forms the perineum.

In the female the urogenital sinus becomes the vestibule, the inner genital folds form the labia minora, and the outer genital folds the labia majora. The genital tubercle forms the clitoris.

In the male the inner genital folds unite from behind forwards in the middle line, and as the penis becomes extruded from the cloaca this union passes forwards so as to close in the groove on the under surface of the genital tubercle, and the bulbous and penile parts of the urethra are formed. The orifice of the urethra is now on the under surface of the penis at the base of the glans penis, and this opening represents the orifice of the urogenital sinus. The end of the tubercle forms the glans penis, and the portion of the urethra which traverses this is formed separately by folding over the edges of the groove on its under surface. Berry Hart believes that this part of the urethra is formed by the ingrowth and hollowing of a rod of epithelium, but the above description is generally accepted.

The last part to be completed is the junction of this part of the urethra with the rest of the penile urethra. It is interesting to note how closely the various forms of hypospadias correspond to the stages of development of the urethra. The prepuce is formed by an ingrowth of solid ectoderm. The outer genital folds unite in the middle line to form the scrotum, and the median scrotal raphe represents their line of union.

ABSENCE OF THE BLADDER

The bladder is rarely absent, except in cases where there are extensive congenital deformities of the pelvic organs which are incompatible with life. A few cases have been observed clinically (Fleury, Benninger) in which the bladder was the only organ affected, and the ureters opened into the urethra. The bladder was represented by a small pocket, the size of a bean. Incontinence of urine is present, and ascending pyelonephritis occurs.

CONGENITAL DILATATION

The dilated bladder may be a cause of difficulty in labour. Urethral obstruction may be present in the form of atresia, folds or valves or cysts of the urethra, or torsion of the penis. Rarely, no obstruction of the urethra is present, and the condition is probably due to changes in the sympathetic ganglia. The ureters are usually dilated, and the kidneys greatly distended, and there is also congenital dilatation of the colon. The bladder may be greatly thickened and hypertrophied in congenital hydronephrosis.

FISTULA OF THE URACHUS

When the whole of the lumen of the allantois remains patent a urachal fistula results. Urethral obstruction is frequently the cause of the persistence of the lumen. In these cases the bladder is often dilated. In infants a membrane or fold in the urethra may cause the condition. The allantois may close and the fistula appear in adult life, when it may be due to urethral stricture or enlargement of the prostate. In some cases no urethral obstruction is present and it is supposed that a temporary obstruction has been present in fœtal life and has disappeared.

The fistula opens at the umbilicus, sometimes on a small, raspberry-like tumour. It is usually narrow, but it may admit a filiform bougie. The opening into the bladder may be minute, or it may be so large as to admit three fingers (Marshall). Urine escapes from the opening during micturition or constantly. There may be a leakage in drops, or a tiny jet may escape. Any doubt as to the nature of the fistula is settled by examination of the fluid for urea, or by injecting methylene blue into the bladder, when the fluid discharged from the fistula becomes coloured. A malignant growth may develop at the umbilical orifice. A portion of the urachus at the vesical end may remain unobliterated and form a diverticulum at the apex of the bladder. Dykes reports a case in which there was a calculus in such a diverticulum.

Pressure and cauterization are uncertain methods of treatment: The track of the fistula should be excised from the umbilicus to the bladder, and the bladder wall repaired. It may be necessary to open the peritoneum, but this should be avoided if possible.

URACHAL CYSTS

The majority of these cysts are found in women in adult life. They vary in size from a chestnut to large cysts occupying a large part of the abdominal cavity and containing many pints of serous or blood-stained fluid.

The cysts are thin-walled and lined with mucous membrane, and the wall contains non-striped muscle. In large cysts the wall is thin and the layers are indistinguishable. There may be a fine communication with the bladder or with the exterior at the umbilicus. Frequent micturition or incontinence of urine may be present. Infection of the cyst has been observed. In small cysts the position, and sometimes adhesions to the umbilicus, are relied upon for diagnosis. In large cysts diagnosis may be impossible.

Excision of the cyst is the proper treatment, but in some cases dense adhesions have prevented this being done and the cyst was drained.

MEMBRANES AND DOUBLE BLADDER

There may be incomplete division of the bladder cavity with a membrane or fold. This may be longitudinal and sickle-shaped, or transverse, and the bladder is partly divided into two unequal compartments, an hour-glass bladder being formed. Cathelin and Sempé collected 32 cases of double bladder. The bladder is divided by a vertical septum into two compartments which open into the urethra. Abnormalities in the ureters or other congenital malformations are sometimes present.

Von Frisch describes a case of double bladder in a man of 34 years. On cystoscopy there was a high septum in the middle line with transverse folds and covered with reddened œdematous mucous membrane. The patient had complained since childhood of delayed and difficult micturition, and eventually suffered from complete retention. The double bladder was demonstrated by the X-rays after collargol injection. Primrose records a case of a man aged 50 with the following malformations, viz. patent pericardium, solitary kidney, and septum in the urinary bladder. The septum was incomplete and formed two partly separated compartments, into one of which the ureter opened.

LITERATURE

Cathelin et **Sempé,** *Ann. d. Mal. d. Org. Gén.-Urin.,* 1903, p. 339.
Delbet, *Ann. d. Mal. d. Org. Gén.-Urin.,* 1907, p. 641.
Doran, *Lancet,* May 8, 1909.
Dykes, *Lancet,* 1910, i. 566.
Fortescue-Brickdale, *Rept. Soc. Dis. Child.,* 1904, p. 94.
von Frisch, *Verhandl. d. deuts. Gesell. f. Urol., III. Kongress,* 1912.
Hart, Berry, *Journ. Anat. and Phys.,* 1903, p. 330.
Holt, *Diseases of Infancy and Childhood.*
Marshall, *Journ. Obstet. and Gyn.,* 1907.
Pommer, *Wien. klin. Woch.,* 1904, Bd. xvii.
Primrose, *Glasg. Med. Journ.,* Sept., 1909.
Schlagenhaufer, *Wien. klin. Woch.,* 1896.
Schytzer, *Arch. f. Gyn.,* Bd. xliii.
Vaughan, *Trans. Amer. Surg. Assoc.,* 1905.
Weiser, *Ann. Surg.,* 1906, p. 529.
White, Hale, *Guy's Hosp. Repts.,* lv. 17.

EXTROVERSION OF THE BLADDER (ECTOPIA VESICÆ)

There is congenital absence of the anterior wall of the bladder, so that the mucous membrane is exposed and the urine is discharged on the surface. The condition is rare, and male infants are more often affected than female.

Hoenow found that one-quarter of the cases were female, two-thirds male, and in the rest the sex was uncertain. Wood found that only 2 out of 20 cases were females. The condition appears at birth as a dark-red swelling the size of a plum at the lower part of the abdomen. It is pear-shaped with the narrow end downwards. The eversion of the bladder wall is due to the intra-abdominal pressure. The upper, broader part of the mucous membrane is folded, irregular, and excoriated, bleeding readily when touched, while the lower part, which is somewhat triangular in shape and corresponds to the trigone, is smooth and partly hidden. At the margin of the mucous membrane there is a zone of scar tissue which forms a rigid border at the upper margin, the "hypogastric fold," and from the skin there are irregular ingrowths of epithelium into the mucosa. The epithelium of the mucous membrane is transitional in character with islands of squamous epithelium near the cutaneous margin. Columnar epithelium is frequently observed.

The umbilicus may be normal or displaced downwards and containing a hernial sac; it is separated from the extroverted bladder by healthy skin, or the bladder may fill the entire space from the umbilicus to the root of the penis.

On raising the prominent swelling a moister area of mucous membrane is seen, with two nipples on which the ureters open. These are closer together than in the normal condition, and the trigone is undeveloped. The ureters are frequently dilated. The muscular wall of the ectopic bladder is thicker than that of the normal bladder. The penis is a tubercle 1–1½ in. long, with undeveloped corpora cavernosa and glans. Along the dorsum there runs a median groove which represents the urethra (epispadias). At the base of the penis in a small pocket are the sinus pocularis and ejaculatory ducts. The foreskin is well developed in the form of an apron. The scrotum is split or rudimentary, and rarely contains the testicles, which are usually found in the inguinal canals. The prostate is absent or rudimentary. The pubic bones do not unite in the middle line, and are sometimes separated as much as 3 in. or more; a fibrous band has been stated to pass across the middle line, uniting the pubic bones, but this is now disputed. The ureters, owing to the absence of the bladder from the abdominal cavity, have a longer course than normal; they descend into the deep pocket between the rectum and the bladder, and then ascend to the bladder. Associated deformities, such as harelip, cleft palate, and spina bifida, are sometimes observed. The perineal muscles may be defective and the anal sphincter ill developed —an important point when the operation of transplantation of the ureters into the rectum is proposed.

The condition described above is the most common form, but other less extensive lesions are occasionally found. There may be scarring of the suprapubic region without separation of the pubic bones or defect of the abdominal wall or bladder. In other cases the pubic bones are separated, and there is scarring of the skin. In a still more advanced form there is a defect of the abdominal wall with exposure and thinning, but without perforation of the bladder wall. In a further stage a fistula of the bladder above or below the pubic symphysis exists. Finally, a more extensive congenital defect than the common variety of extroversion described above may rarely be observed: in this the bowel below the lower ileum or the cæcum is wanting, and the ileum opens behind the ureters in a common cloaca.

Etiology.—The cause of the malformation is unknown. Two theories have been advanced to explain the anatomical conditions present. According to one, there is an arrest at an early period of development. It has been pointed out, however, that at no period of development is the bladder open on its anterior wall. This, with the frequent coincidence of dilated ureters and kidneys, has led to the second suggestion, that there is an intra-uterine rupture of the bladder following obstruction and back pressure.

More recent work on embryology shows that the cloaca extends at first from the umbilicus to the base of the tail, and that the bladder is largely, if not entirely, formed from the cloaca. Ingrowths from mesoderm on each side reduce the size of the cloaca from before backwards (*see* p. 392). It is evident, then, that a failure of these lateral folds to meet on each side at the lower part of the abdomen, and the destruction of the cloacal membrane, sufficiently explain the anatomical conditions found in extroversion of the bladder.

There is a difficulty in accounting for the presence of the urethra as a gutter on the dorsum of the penis.

Symptoms and prognosis.—The thighs are widely separated owing to the cleft symphysis, and the body is bent forwards so as to protect the sensitive mucous surface. A peculiar waddling gait and bent attitude are thus developed.

The conditions of existence are extremely miserable. There is the constant escape of urine, saturating the clothes and leading to inflammation and excoriation of the skin. The child lives in the pungent atmosphere arising from decomposing urine, and his life is a burden to himself and to those around him. Progressive dilatation of the ureters and kidneys occurs. The mortality from ascending pyelonephritis is very high, but occasionally the patients attain adult life and even old age.

A malignant growth may develop in the exposed bladder. and may take the form of an adeno-carcinoma.

Treatment.—Many operations have been suggested and practised for ectopia vesicæ. The following are the chief types :—

I. **Formation of a reservoir in the body.**
    A. *From the bladder.*
        1. Closure of the defect by osteoplastic operations.
        2. Closure of defect by flaps.
            (*a*) Autoplastic methods.
                (i.) Of skin.
                (ii.) Of intestine.
            (*b*) Heteroplastic methods.
    B. *From the rectum.*
        1. By transplantation of the ureters.
        2. By vesico-rectal fistula.
    C. *From the sigmoid flexure.*
    D. *From the vagina.*
II. **No reservoir formed in the body.**
        1. *Implantation of the ureters.*
            (*a*) In urethra.
            (*b*) In skin.
        2. *Nephrostomy.*

A few of the more important of these operations will be described.

Trendelenburg's operation (osteoplastic operation).—This consists in opening the sacro-iliac synchondrosis, which allows of the approximation of the separated pubic bones and subsequent closing of the defect in the bladder wall.

The patient is placed in the prone position, and a longitudinal incision made over one sacro-iliac synchondrosis. Its posterior ligaments are cut through and lateral pressure is applied to the iliac bones, so that the pubic bone on the operated side swings towards the middle line. A similar operation is performed on the opposite side. The patient is placed on a special couch. Round the pelvis is passed a leather girdle, the ends of which cross in front and are attached to cords and weights acting over pulleys on each side. The pelvic bones are fixed in position for some weeks. Three or four months later an attempt to close the bladder is made by separating the bladder wall and uniting it, and bringing the component parts of the abdominal wall together in front of it. A later attempt may be made to reconstruct the urethra.

Results.—Katz collected 23 cases, with a mortality of 21·7 per cent. Improvement in rectal incontinence has been noted after these operations, and three patients were stated to have gained control of the urine. This must be exceptional, however, for no provision is made for sphincteric control, and an apparatus must be worn in almost all cases. The opened synchondrosis fills with clot and granulation tissue, and fibrous tissue is formed which contracts and drags the bones into their original position. Wiring the pubic bones together does not prevent this, for the wire cuts through the cartilage. There is some danger of injuring the sacral nerves and causing paralysis of the rectal sphincters.

Wood's operation (autoplastic skin method).—The defect is closed by skin flaps (Fig. 114), and the operation should be done about the age of 4 or 5 years. Several operations are usually required, and they should be completed before puberty, when hairs grow upon the skin flap and erections of the penis interfere with the success of the operation. If puberty be already passed some method should be adopted to remove the pubic hairs. Three flaps are used—a median superior flap from the abdominal wall above the bladder, broad above and narrow below, which is turned down over the defect skin inwards; and two lateral flaps from the abdominal wall on each side, which remain attached at their lower ends, are swung inwards to meet in the middle line, and are stitched in this position with the skin outwards. The trefoil surface thus laid bare is either covered at once with skin grafts or allowed to granulate and grafted later. The objections to this method are that there is no control and a urinal must be worn, and phosphatic deposit takes place on the skin surface which forms the anterior wall of the bladder.

Segond's operation.—The bladder is dissected from the abdominal wall and turned downwards so that the upper portion forms a roof for the urethra. The ample prepuce is now unfolded so that the upper surface is raw, and this is reflected backwards on the surface of the bladder flap, a hole being made through which the penis projects.

Implantation of the ureters into the rectum. — The dangers of implantation of the ureters into the bowel are sloughing of the wound and ascending pyelonephritis.

Fowler endeavoured to protect the implanted ureters from contact with the fæces. He cut the ureters obliquely and formed a flap valve of mucous membrane from the anterior wall of the rectum. To the under surface of this he attached the cut ends of the ureters in the hope that the descending fæces would press upon the valve and close the ureteric orifices.

Gersuny made an artificial anus at the sigmoid flexure and

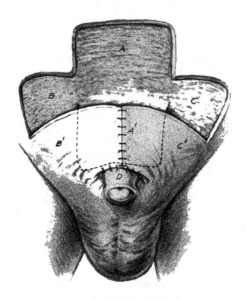

Fig. 114.—Wood's operation for extroversion ot bladder.

A, B, C, Raw surface left after cutting skin flaps. A', Central flap turned downwards (dotted line) with skin surface inwards. B', C', Lateral flaps swung inwards and stitched across back of A'. D Covering for urethral gutter formed from foreskin.

closed the upper end of the rectum. He then transplanted the ureters into the rectum.

Peters introduced catheters into the ureters, which he dissected from the wall of the bladder, leaving a collar of bladder mucous membrane round each. The catheters and ureters were passed through two small openings in the anterior rectal wall, each ureter projecting about 3 cm. into the cavity. The catheters were removed after three days.

Soubottine's operation (Fig. 115).—The coccyx is excised and the posterior rectal wall slit up longitudinally, cutting through the anal sphincter. A fistula is now made between the rectum and the bladder. A horseshoe incision is made with the convexity upwards round the recto-vesical fistula, including one-third of the rectal wall, the limbs of the horseshoe passing down to the skin at the anus. The edges of the portion of rectal wall included within this horseshoe are now united, and a reservoir formed. Finally, the rectal wall is united over this and the pos-

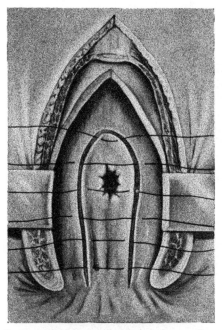

Fig. 115.—Soubottine's operation for extroversion of bladder.

The posterior wall of the rectum has been slit, a vesico-rectal fistula formed, the incision for the rectal pouch made, and the stitches introduced.

terior rectal wall repaired. The neck of this urinary receptacle is within the grasp of the anal sphincter.

The suprapubic gap in the bladder wall is closed by a skin-flap operation. One patient operated on in this manner obtained complete continence and held urine for four hours.

Maydl's operation (Figs. 116, 117).—The trigone of the bladder, together with the ureteric orifices, is transplanted into the sigmoid flexure of the colon. A catheter is introduced into

2 A

each ureter, and the bladder separated completely from the abdominal wall. The bladder wall is cut away, leaving an oval area on which the ureters open. Care is taken not to injure the vesical arteries. A knuckle of sigmoid flexure is isolated and incised longitudinally, and the bladder base is implanted into it and carefully sutured. Maydl fixes the bowel in the abdominal

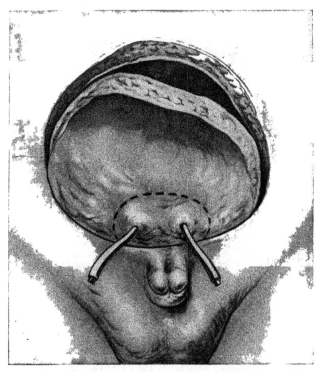

Fig. 116.—Maydl's operation for extroversion of bladder.

Stage 1. The bladder is being separated from the abdominal wall. Catheters are lying in the ureters, and the dotted line shows the portion of the bladder base that will be transplanted into the intestine.

wound on account of the danger of peritonitis from the line of suture giving way.

This method has proved the most successful of the bowel-implantation methods owing to the retention of the sphincter action of the lower end of the ureters.

Moynihan dissected up the whole bladder and implanted it into the colon. Kocher brings out a knuckle of sigmoid, implants the bladder base at the apex of the loop, and short-circuits the bowel at the base of the loop.

The immediate mortality of Maydl's operation varies from 5·5 per cent. (Josserand, 18 cases) to 26·7 per cent. (Katz, 57 cases). In Petersen's collection 31 patients recovered from the operation ; of these 2 died of pyelitis within a year. In the

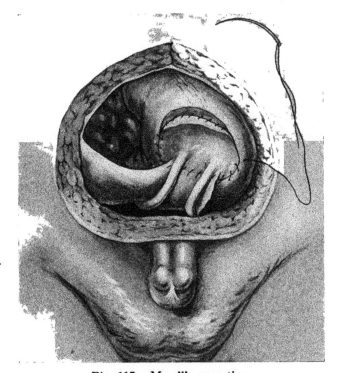

Fig. 117.—Maydl's operation.

Stage 2. The portion of the bladder base surrounding the ureteric orifices is implanted into the sigmoid flexure of the colon. The double row of stitching is seen.

other cases the control of the anal sphincter was good in every case but one. In 6 cases the operation was followed by fistula, which in every instance subsequently closed. Before embarking on this most satisfactory operation, the surgeon should ascertain if the anal sphincter retains fluid motions.

In **Sonnenberg's operation** the bladder is excised and the ureters implanted in the urethra. This allows of the fitting of a receptacle which will collect the urine.

LITERATURE

Connell, *Journ. Amer. Med. Assoc.,* 1901, p. 637.
Fowler, *Amer. Journ. Med. Sci.,* 1898, p. 270.
Frank, *Ann. Surg.,* 1903, p. 291.
Gersuny, *Wien. klin. Woch.,* 1898, No. 43.
Hager, *Münch. med. Woch.,* 1910, p. 2301.
Hoenow, Inaugural Dissertation, Berlin, 1884.
Josséraud, *Gaz. Hebdom. de Méd. et de Chir.,* 1895, p. 117.
Katz, Thèse de Paris, 1903.
Keith, *Brit. Med. Journ.,* 1908, ii. 1858.
Lendon, *Brit. Med. Journ.,* 1906, i. 961.
Maydl, *Wien. med. Woch.,* 1894, 1896, 1899.
Moynihan, *Ann. Surg.,* 1906, p. 237.
Newland, *Brit. Med. Journ.,* 1906, p. 964.
Peters, *Brit. Med. Journ.,* June 22, 1901 ; 1902, ii. 1538.
Petersen, *Med. News,* Aug. 11, 1911.
Segond, *Ann. d. Mal. d. Org. Gén.-Urin.,* 1890, p. 193.
Soubottine, *Wratsch,* 1901.
Trendelenburg, *Centralbl. f. Chir.,* Dec., 1885 ; *Ann. Surg.,* 1906, p. 281.
Watson, *Ann. Surg.,* 1905, p. 813.
Wood, *Brit. Med. Journ.,* 1880.
Zuckerkandl, *Handbuch der Urologie* (von Frisch und Zuckerkandl), 1905.

CHAPTER XXX

CYSTOCELE—PROLAPSE—DIVERTICULA

HERNIA OF THE BLADDER (CYSTOCELE)

HERNIA of the bladder is comparatively rare. Moynihan found 23 bladder hernias in 2,543 collected cases of hernia operations, or about 1 per cent. It is much more frequent in men than in women (115 in 144—Alessandri), and is most common in advanced life, although cases occurring in children have been described. The average age in males is 51 and in females 44 (Moynihan). The great majority of bladder hernias are inguinal; femoral are much less common, but are more frequent in women than in men (27 to 2). A few rare records of obturator, sciatic, and perineal hernia and of hernia in the linea alba exist.

Etiology.—A thin-walled bladder placed in close relation to a weak inguinal or femoral ring is either drawn through or forced into it. The following are recognized causes :—

1. Urethral obstruction with distension of the bladder (stricture, enlarged prostate, pelvic growths). The wall is usually thinned and its muscular power weak, but in a few cases there has been hypertrophy with thickening of the wall.

2. Weakness of the abdominal wall, such as is found in old age and other contributory causes of hernia.

3. Intermittent increase in intra-abdominal pressure, which may be caused by coughing, straining to pass water, etc.

4. Traction upon the bladder drawing it through the weak abdominal wall. This may be the traction (a) of an extraperitoneal lipoma, (b) of extraperitoneal fat on the sac of a hernia upon adherent perivesical fat, (c) of the peritoneum of a large hernial sac on the peritoneum covering the bladder, or (d) adhesions between the omentum or intestine and the intraperitoneal portion of the bladder dragging this into the hernial sac. A number of these factors unite to produce a bladder hernia. Bland-Sutton relates a case in which there was an enlarged prostate and distended thinned bladder and the inguinal canal contained a fibro-fatty tumour of the spermatic cord, a fat-covered " diverticulum " of the bladder, and a hernial sac in which there was omentum.

Varieties.—Three varieties are found (Fig. 118):

1. *Paraperitoneal*, in which a sac of peritoneum is present, and adherent to this is the bladder. The large majority of vesical herniæ are of this variety. Usually only a small portion of the bladder is involved, but a large part of the viscus, together with the ureters and even the prostate, has been found in the hernia.

2. *Extraperitoneal*, in which there is prolapse of the bladder without a hernial sac of peritoneum.

3. *Intraperitoneal*, in which the peritoneum-covered portion of the bladder is drawn into a hernial sac together with bowel and omentum.

Intraperitoneal cystocele lies outside the deep epigastric artery (oblique hernia). Extraperitoneal cystocele lies internally to this vessel (direct hernia), while paraperitoneal cystocele may

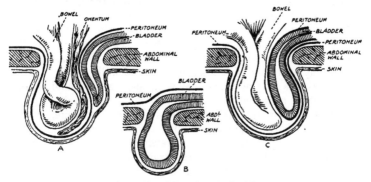

Fig. 118.—Hernia of bladder.

A, Paraperitoneal variety. B Extraperitoneal variety. C, Intraperitoneal variety.

be oblique or direct. The communication between the prolapsed portion of the bladder and the main cavity may be temporarily narrowed, but there is never a diverticulum in the true sense, and after the prolapsed portion is returned to the pelvis no change can be found with the cystoscope. Hernia of the bladder occurs most frequently in an inguinal hernia which has recurred after operation. One of Gifford's two cases of extraperitoneal bladder hernia was that of a child aged 5, on whom a previous operation had been performed. Cystitis may be present, and a phosphatic stone has been known to form in the prolapsed portion of the bladder.

Symptoms.—There is an inguinal or femoral swelling having the characteristics of an ordinary hernia. The swelling increases in size in the erect posture. It has the following characteristics:

(1) It is irreducible. (2) When the bladder is distended it is large, and when the bladder is emptied it subsides and only an indefinite thickening is left, or an ordinary hernia may persist. (3) Pressure upon the swelling causes a desire to micturate. (4) Fluctuation may be detected if the hernia is large. (5) The swelling is dull on percussion.

Symptoms pointing to implication of the bladder in the hernia may be present, but, as the prostate is enlarged or other urethral obstruction is present in many of these cases, the significance of the symptoms may be overlooked.

Micturition in two parts is a common symptom. Urine is passed, and then after a pause a second quantity is passed, sometimes after pressure upon the hernia or by assuming some particular position. There is difficulty in micturition, and sometimes complete retention, and the patient may only be able to pass water by pressing on the swelling or in a certain posture. Cystitis may complicate the condition. Urinary symptoms may be completely absent.

In a case under my care there were no urinary symptoms, but only constant deep-seated pelvic pain, which was unrelieved by operation. Cystoscopy after operation showed no abnormality of the bladder.

On introduction of a catheter it may pass into the hernial sac and be felt through the skin. Injection of fluid into the bladder distends the hernial swelling. Strangulation of a bladder hernia has occurred in several cases. The symptoms are those of strangulation of an intestinal hernia, but constipation is absent. Bladder symptoms are frequently wanting, but there may be strangury. Hiccough is sometimes a prominent symptom.

Diagnosis.—The diagnosis is usually made for the first time at operation, for there are frequently no symptoms to point to the presence of the bladder in the hernia. If suspicion of the nature of the swelling is aroused, some of the characteristic symptoms may lead to a diagnosis, and cystoscopy will help.

The diagnosis of the condition is made at operation on hernia in 67 per cent. of cases, and unintentional wounds of the bladder or inclusion in the ligature of the hernial sac seldom occur if due care be taken in clearing and inspecting the neck of the sac in a radical cure of hernia. The discovery is made when the sac is being freed, and the bladder in the most frequent form of vesical hernia (paraperitoneal) is found adherent to the median aspect of the surface of the sac. It is covered by perivesical fat, and when this is removed the muscular wall, on which veins course, is exposed. When the perivèsical fat is wanting and the bladder wall is thinned by distension, it may not be possible to recognize the organ until its cavity is opened. When this has occurred the nature of the case is demonstrated by the escape of urine, the appearance of the mucous membrane, and the freedom with which a probe passes behind the pubes, and, if necessary, the passage of a metal instrument through the urethra into the bladder can be felt from the inguinal cystotomy wound.

When the bladder alone forms the hernia (extraperitoneal) the same features assist in the diagnosis. If the bladder has passed unnoticed at a hernia operation, and has been included in or pierced by a ligature, hæmaturia and strangury follow the operation, and sometimes the escape of urine from the hernia wound. Fatal peritonitis usually supervenes. The significance of these symptoms is frequently overlooked. I have made an autopsy on a child who died of peritonitis following operation on an inguinal hernia. The bladder had been mistaken for the muscles of the abdominal wall and sutured to Poupart's ligament.

Prognosis.—There is danger that the surgeon may not recognize the bladder at the operation, may puncture it, or include it in a ligature, and fail to appreciate the significance of the symptoms which follow. If the bladder be recognized and treated at the operation the danger is not great. Hermes found the mortality of hernia operations involving the bladder to be 19·5 per cent. ; when the bladder was uninjured it was 6·5 per cent., and when it was injured 26·5 per cent.

Treatment. — When urethral obstruction is present this should be removed, and in some cases when the cystocele is intraperitoneal it may be controlled by a truss. In the great majority of cases, however, the hernia is irreducible and an operation is necessary. When the bladder is found within the hernial sac it is reduced with the other contents, adhesions to bowel or omentum being first separated, and the radical cure of the hernia carried out in the usual manner. If the prolapsed bladder is recognized outside the. sac it should be dissected off and returned to the abdomen without being opened. If a considerable portion of the bladder is covered by peritoneum, this may be left adherent to the bladder and excised from the sac. Great care is necessary to avoid tearing the bladder wall during the dissection.

After radical cure of the hernia, care should be taken to remove urethral obstruction, if such exists.

If the bladder be opened during the operation, it should be carefully dissected off the sac and the opening closed by a double layer of catgut sutures. The bladder is then returned to the pelvis, the hernia operation completed, and a catheter tied in

the urethra for a week. Should any sign of pericystitis supervene, a median suprapubic incision should be made and the
perivesical extraperitoneal space drained through this.

LITERATURE

Alessandri, *Ann. d. Mal. d. Org. Gén.-Urin.*, 1901.
Bland-Sutton, *Arch. Middx. Hosp.*, 1910, p. 10.
Brunner, *Deuts. Zeits. f. Chir.*, Bd. xlvii.
Curtis, *Brit. Med. Journ.*, 1903, ii. 69.
Foy, *Brit. Med. Journ.*, 1897.
Hamilton-Whiteford, *Lancet*, 1900.
Hermes, *Deuts. Zeits. f. Chir.*, Bd. xlv.
Malcolm, *Trans. Med. Soc. Lond.*, 1908, p. 26.
Martin, *Deuts. Zeits. f. Chir.*, Bd. liv.
Monod et Delagenière, *Rec. de Chir.*, 1889, p. 701.
Moynihan, *Brit. Med. Journ.*, 1900, i. 503.
Noall, *Pract.*, 1910, lxxxiv. 842.
Zuckerkandl, *Handbuch der Urologie* (von Frisch und Zuckerkandl), 1905, ii. 589.

INVERSION AND PROLAPSE OF THE BLADDER
(URETHRAL CYSTOCELE)

There are two forms of urethral cystocele. In one, inversion
of the bladder, the whole thickness of the bladder wall, including
the peritoneal investment, is inverted through the urethra, while
in the second the mucous membrane is prolapsed through the
urethra. The condition occurs in women and female children.
(Gross collected 7 cases of complete inversion, 5 in girls between
14 months and 4 years, and 2 in adult women.)

Etiology.—Except in one or two cases in which the urethra
was destroyed, little is known in regard to the causation. But
the exciting causes are straining from crying, coughing, sneezing,
constipation, and diarrhœa. Hirokawa has described a case
following pertussis.

Varieties and diagnosis.—Inversion of the bladder, which
is very rare, varies in degree. (i) The whole bladder may be
inverted into the urethra and appear at the external meatus
as a round swelling, the size of a walnut or an orange, covered
with reddened, easily bleeding mucous membrane. The tumour
is tender, elastic, increases in size on crying or straining, and is
felt to consist of several layers. It is reducible with difficulty or
not at all. If it project well beyond the urethral orifice it appears
to be pedunculated, and a probe passed along the urethra beside
the pedicle enters the bladder and can be swept round the
pedicle on all sides. Rarely the ureteric orifices are carried down
with the prolapsed bladder, and can be recognized emitting drops
of urine on the surface of the tumour. The patient complains of
incontinence of urine.

(ii) In an incomplete form of inversion the bladder wall is folded inwards into the cavity of the viscus, but is not prolapsed through the urethra. This variety is said to occur in men as well as in women. The diagnosis is only made by cystoscopy. Symptoms resembling those of stone in the bladder are usually present. There are increased frequency, pain on micturition and tenesmus, intermittent micturition, and the stream may only be initiated or recommenced by lying on the back. Hæmaturia is rare.

Prolapse of the vesical mucous membrane is more frequent than inversion. An area of mucous membrane is prolapsed through the urethra. According to Malherbe a glandular cul-de-sac in the neighbourhood of the internal meatus becomes distended with urine so that a ridge of mucous membrane is raised, and this becomes pedunculated. A small tumour of mucous membrane appears at the external meatus. It has a translucent appearance and is compressible.

The diagnosis from inversion of the bladder wall is made by the sensation of greater thickness and the presence of the ureteric orifices on the surface of the tumour in the inversion. A tumour of the bladder which has prolapsed through the urethra is firmer, does not vary in size, and is not compressible.

. In prolapse an instrument passes alongside the tumour into the bladder, and can be swept round it, but is not free in the cavity when it has passed the urethra. When it has been reduced, cystoscopy shows that there is no growth or prolapse of the ureter. Polypi of the urethra may protrude from the meatus, but they are small, and the attachment of the base to the urethral mucous membrane can be demonstrated by a speculum or urethroscope tube. Prolapse of the ureter has appeared at the external meatus in the female subject, but the thin, transparent appearance of the tumour and cystoscopic examination will make the diagnosis plain.

Treatment.—There are few cases recorded on which to base statements in regard to treatment. The tumour has been reduced and has not recurred (Leech). Leedham-Green reduced the inversion in his case and injected melted paraffin in a ring around the urethra; the hardened paraffin gave support to the urethra, and recurrence did not take place.

Cysto-uteropexy has been performed, the upper part of the bladder being fixed to the anterior surface of the uterus. This was successful in a case recorded by Peigné. Plastic operations on the urethra are necessary when prolapse has recurred.

When the mucous membrane is prolapsed the polypoid portion should be removed by suprapubic cystotomy.

LITERATURE

Carrel, *Ann. d. Mal. d. Org. Gén.-Urin.,* 1900, p. 299.
Hirokawa, *Deuts. Zeits. f. Chir.,* 1911, p. 575.
Leech, *Brit. Med. Journ.,* 1896, ii. 1128.
Leedham-Green, *Brit. Med. Journ.,* 1908, i. 976.
Lowe, *Arch. f. klin. Chir.,* v. 365.

DIVERTICULA OF THE BLADDER

A diverticulum is a pouch lined by vesical mucous membrane which communicates with the bladder by a narrow opening.

Diverticula should be distinguished from the pouches or saccules of a sacculated bladder, which is commonly seen in prostatic obstruction, where there is widespread or universal trabeculation, and between the trabeculæ are innumerable shallow and deep depressions, open, without contraction of the orifice, to the bladder cavity.

Pathological anatomy.—Diverticula may be single or multiple, small as a pea or as large as the bladder cavity, or even larger. Small diverticula may be solitary, but they are frequently multiple, and when multiple are frequently arranged in groups of two or three, or even six or seven sometimes, symmetrically arranged on each side of the bladder.

The orifice is small. It may barely admit a crow-quill, but more frequently will pass a pencil, or even the forefinger. The size of the orifice has no relation to the capacity of the diverticulum. The edges are sharply defined. The opening frequently appears as a round hole punched out in an absolutely healthy bladder wall. An oval or slit-like orifice is sometimes found, but is rare.

General trabeculation of the bladder wall is seldom if ever present. Trabeculation limited to an area around the orifice of the diverticulum is frequently found, and may be confined to the wall at one part of the circumference of the orifice.

The mucous membrane frequently shows puckerings and ridges which radiate from the orifice at one part of the circumference or all round. They resemble the puckering of the peritoneum at the neck of a hernia when viewed from within the abdomen, and give the impression that the mucous membrane is being dragged upon from without the bladder. (Plate 30, Figs. 1, 2.) When situated in the neighbourhood of the ureter the interureteric bar is usually hypertrophied on that side.

The ureteric orifice may open in the wall of the diverticulum or on the margin of the mouth of the diverticulum. In the former case the ureter has probably become dragged into the cavity in the process of development of the sac.

Diverticula may be found at any part of the bladder. They are most frequently found on the lateral walls, in the neighbourhood of the ureteric orifice, and next on the posterior wall. Less frequently they are found at the apex. Rarely they open on the trigone. I have seen the opening of a very large diverticulum in the middle line near the posterior part of the trigone.

The structure of the wall varies. The cavity is lined by mucous membrane continuous with and similar to that of the bladder, and is surrounded by fibrous tissue and usually by a considerable quantity of coarse fat. In some diverticula there is a layer of non-striped muscle, while in others this is wanting.

Virchow, Englisch, and others hold that when the muscle is present the diverticulum is congenital, and when absent the diverticulum is acquired. Young was always able to find muscle in the walls of diverticula, although the layer might be very thin.

Diverticula may have secondary pockets, and they are usually extensively adherent to the pelvic viscera.

Etiology.—The great majority of diverticula are found in men, but they sometimes occur in infants. They are frequently met with in young adults or in middle age.

While many of the diverticula are congenital, some are apparently due to urethral obstruction, and are met with in cases of stricture and enlarged prostate. In some cases I have found a history of pelvic cellulitis (from appendicitis, salpingitis, etc.), and traction from without by adhesions may have been a factor. Diverticula at the apex of the bladder result from incomplete obliteration of the urachus.

Symptoms.—These, apart from the symptoms of obstruction due to stricture or enlarged prostate which are present in some cases, and the symptoms of such complications as cystitis or new growth, are usually puzzling and irregular.

In a young man with clear urine there may be attacks of frequent micturition at varying intervals, or continuously. In other cases there are attacks of complete retention, relieved by catheter, or there may be gradually increasing difficulty in micturition, culminating in complete retention. In these cases I have usually found spasmodic contraction of the compressor urethræ.

In many cases there are no symptoms which can be ascribed to the diverticulum, and it is discovered accidentally during examination of the bladder for some other disease.

Micturition in two parts is a symptom which has been described, but is rarely seen except in very large diverticula. Sometimes the second supply is purulent when the first was clear.

On passing a catheter a somewhat similar phenomenon is

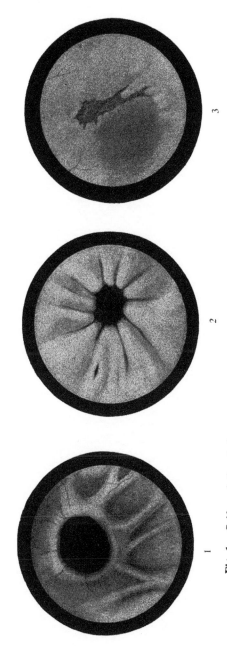

Fig. 1.—Orifice of diverticulum and trabeculation on posterior wall of bladder. (Pp. 411, 413.)

Fig. 2.—Orifice of large diverticulum of bladder close to right ureteral orifice. (Pp. 411, 413.)

Fig. 3.—Partial rupture of bladder; appearance of mucous membrane six days after accident. (P. 418.)

PLATE 30.

observed. The bladder is apparently emptied, when the point of the catheter slips onwards and a large quantity of urine, sometimes purulent, is passed. With a sound it is sometimes possible to feel the edge of the aperture with the beak.

One or several ounces of residual urine may be drawn off by catheter after the patient has passed all he can.

Small diverticula cannot be felt on abdominal or rectal palpation. A large diverticulum can be felt as a tumour in the lower part of the abdomen. In an extensive diverticulum on the right side of the bladder I could feel a large fluctuating mass in the right iliac fossa when the bladder was distended with fluid, and this almost disappeared when the bladder was emptied. The diverticulum was apparently adherent to the cæcum. Eventually a malignant growth developed in the diverticulum, and the patient died of pyelonephritis.

Diagnosis.—The symptoms are frequently those of cystitis with residual urine which is purulent. The only certain method of diagnosis is cystoscopy. The extent of the diverticulum cannot be gauged by the cystoscope. A stone lying in a diverticulum is sometimes seen cystoscopically. Usually, however, the orifice is so small that even a large stone cannot be seen. Drawings of the orifices of diverticula are seen in Plate 30. Figs. 1, 27, and the skiagram of a large stone which one contained is shown in Plate 29, Fig. 1. The stone could not be seen by cystoscopy.

To demonstrate the dimensions and position of a diverticulum, the bladder should be distended with an emulsion of bismuth and a skiagram obtained. (Plate 27, Fig. 2, and Plate 29, Fig. 3.)

Complications.—1. By pressure or dragging upon the ureter dilatation of the kidney may be produced. Both kidneys may be affected.

2. Infection is a common and very serious complication, and is usually due to septic catheterization. There may be acute general cystitis lasting for many weeks and finally subsiding, but recurring from time to time, or there is continuous subacute cystitis with recurrent exacerbations.

A collection of purulent urine, sometimes decomposing, is lodged in the diverticulum and pours out into the bladder from time to time. Pericystitis and peritonitis may occur. Ascending pyelonephritis is the usual termination in these cases.

3. A calculus may form in the diverticulum, and may follow long-standing infection of the diverticulum, but it also forms where a very mild infection is present.

4. A malignant growth may develop on the edge or in the neighbourhood of the orifice, or may arise within the diverticulum.

I have seen instances of each of these, and operated upon three cases of the former.

Prognosis.—The presence of a diverticulum is not in itself dangerous, but when infection has taken place the prognosis is extremely grave. Ascending pyelonephritis supervenes in these cases. Malignant growth occurs in a small percentage of cases.

Treatment.—The great danger of infection should render the

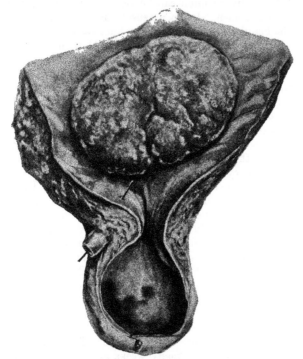

Fig. 119.—Operation specimen of resection of bladder wall.

The upper portion shows the excised part of the bladder wall, on which is set a malignant growth. Below this is the orifice of a diverticulum with the diverticulum itself. To the left is the lower end of the ureter, in which lies a bristle. The ureter was transplanted; perineal prostatectomy three weeks later; recovery.

surgeon doubly careful in regard to asepsis. Where infection has occurred, washing the bladder has little effect upon the contents of the diverticulum. In the female subject a Kelly's tube may be passed and a catheter introduced through this into the orifice and the diverticulum washed out.

A number of operations have been performed:

1. **Drainage outside the bladder.**—This may be tried in

large diverticula, but is impossible in small pockets and in those at the base of the bladder. This method leads to a permanent urinary fistula. It may, however, be combined with the next method.

2. **Closure of the orifice.**—After suprapubic cystotomy the edges of the orifice are cut away and the raw surfaces brought together. The diverticulum must previously have been aseptic.

3. **Drainage into the bladder.**—The walls of the bladder and diverticulum are split upwards or downwards and the edges stitched together so that the cavity of the diverticulum is thrown into that of the bladder. This permits of free drainage of the diverticulum into the bladder, and the cavity is more readily cleaned by washing the bladder.

4. **Excision of the sac and repair of the bladder wall.**— This has been performed by several surgeons, and I have carried it out in six cases. In the upper part of the bladder the operation does not present great difficulties, but it may be extremely difficult, owing to extensive adhesions, in diverticula deeply situated in the pelvis. A urinary fistula has persisted in some recorded cases and necessitated secondary operations. In one of my cases a small pocket deeply placed in the pelvis had been left and caused a purulent discharge for some time, but the communication with the bladder closed at once. In another case (Fig. 119) I removed a large malignant growth by resection of the bladder wall, and with it a diverticulum full of stones, and the lower part of the ureter, transplanting the ureter into the wound. A fortnight later an enlarged prostate was removed from the perineum. The patient, aged 73, made an uneventful recovery.

In order to facilitate removal of the sac, Lerche introduced a small collapsed rubber bag on the end of a fine catheter into the diverticulum, and then distended it with fluid.

LITERATURE

Berry, *Proc. Roy. Soc. Med.*, Surgical Section, 1911, p. 158.
Chute, *Boston Med. and Surg. Journ.*, Sept., 1912, p. 316.
Durrieux, Thèse de Paris, 1901.
Englisch, *Wien. klin. Woch.*, 1894, p. 91.
Lerche, *Ann. Surg.*, Nov., 1911, p. 593; Feb., 1912, p. 285.
Pagenstecher, *Arch. f. klin. Chir.*, 1904, p. 186.
Targett, *Trans. Path. Soc.*, 1896, p. 155.
Young, *Johns Hopkins Hosp. Repts.*, 1906, p. 401.

CHAPTER XXXI

INJURIES OF THE BLADDER

RUPTURE

In rupture of the bladder the outer coat may remain intact, or more commonly the whole thickness of the vesical wall is torn. The great majority of cases (90 per cent.) take place in male subjects, and usually during the most active period of life (20 to 40 years). The injury is said to occur more frequently in England and America, owing to the greater prevalence of field sports and boxing.

The bladder is invariably full at the time of rupture, sometimes it is over-distended. A considerable proportion of cases (35 per cent.—Bartels) occur during alcoholic intoxication.

The injury is usually direct, as from kicks, blows with the fist or knee, falls upon furniture or boulders, crushes between buffers or from machinery. In fracture of the pelvis a splinter of bone may penetrate the bladder. The injury may also be due to indirect violence, such as falls from a height or being thrown from a vehicle. The bladder may be ruptured by the muscular effort of lifting heavy weights, or by straining under an anæsthetic. Rupture has taken place from the effort of blowing a trumpet (Fenwick), and from leaning over the edge of a barrel (Zuckerkandl).

Over-distension of the bladder has caused rupture from great intravesical pressure. This usually occurs from the forcible injection of fluid by the surgeon into the bladder. It has been known to occur from the action of the evacuating bulb after the operation of litholapaxy. It is very doubtful if the bladder can be ruptured by intravesical tension from the collection of urine when the organ is healthy. Cases have, however, been described to show the possibility of such an occurrence.

In a bladder the seat of malignant or other ulceration rupture may take place spontaneously.

Pathology.—A few cases of incomplete rupture have been recorded, but they are very rare. In a case described later, only the mucous membrane was torn. The rupture is most frequently on the postero-superior wall, and opens the peritoneal cavity.

Extraperitoneal rupture occurs exceptionally, and affects the anterior wall. Rupture of the base and lateral walls is usually the result of fracture of the pelvis. The rupture is vertical, and in or near the middle line; it is single, and is usually small in size, with clean-cut or bruised edges. Later, inflammatory reaction is found around the wound. Rarely the tear is transverse or irregular.

When the peritoneal cavity is opened, coils of intestine may exceptionally become adherent and limit the extravasation of urine and peritonitis. Usually, urine escapes into the peritoneal cavity, and general peritonitis supervenes. When the urine is already septic this appears rapidly. Aseptic urine does not cause peritonitis, but it is toxic when absorbed, and even if aseptic at the time of the accident it very readily becomes infected. In extraperitoneal rupture the urine infiltrates the pelvic cellular planes, and inflammation and suppuration follow.

Fracture of the pelvis is present in 38 per cent. of cases (Bartels), the pubic bones being the most frequent seat of fracture, then the ischium, ilium, and sacrum. The mechanism by which the rupture is produced is open to discussion. It is stated that contact of the distended bladder with the pubic bone or with the promontory of the sacrum is the cause, and that the greater liability of the posterior wall to rupture is due to its being unsupported when compared with the anterior wall, and to the more frequent occurrence on it of saccules and diverticula.

When the bladder is fully distended above the pubes the danger from an antero-posterior blow is rupture of the postero-superior wall, while a partly distended bladder is more likely to be driven down into the pelvis and sustain injury to the base. The slower forms of violence are said to be more likely to produce a partial rupture.

Symptoms.—Shock is present as in other abdominal injuries, and is pronounced and frequently prolonged, but it may be absent, and when the rupture is uncomplicated by other injuries some time may elapse before other symptoms appear. These are pain, great desire to micturate, and straining, but inability to pass water. The spasms come on at intervals, and may be very severe. The abdomen is rigid, and tender on palpation. There is no dullness corresponding to a distended bladder, and the patient has not passed water for several hours. Per rectum there is bulging in the pouch of Douglas.

On a catheter being introduced a little bloody urine is with-

2 B

drawn. Rarely the catheter passes through the rent in the bladder wall into the peritoneal cavity, and a very large quantity of urine can be drawn off. If a catheter is passed several times within a short space it is found that the quantity of urine in the bladder is always the same, for any excess of fluid escapes into the peritoneum. If, after emptying the bladder, the patient be set upright for a very short time, a quantity of urine will be found to have filled the bladder again, having passed in from the peritoneal cavity (Morel).

When the rupture is extraperitoneal, dullness appears above the pubes, and there are tenderness and rigidity. The infiltration spreads in the pelvis and escapes by the sciatic notch into the buttock, by the obturator foramen, into the upper part of the thigh, or along the inguinal canal into the scrotum. Abscess formation and the development of fistulæ follow, and then thrombosis of veins and septicæmia.

In intraperitoneal rupture, peritonitis appears within the first twelve hours, the abdomen becomes distended, there are vomiting, hiccough, a rapid pulse, and other signs of severe peritoneal infection. Death may rarely take place without signs of peritonitis, and is then probably due to the toxic effect of the urine.

In a case of partial rupture of the bladder which I was asked to see by my colleague Mr. Jackson Clarke, a boy aged 5 was knocked down by a motor car, but it was doubtful if the wheels had passed over him. Soon after the accident he passed urine containing bright blood. Seven hours after the accident he was suffering from shock, there was a hæmatoma over the left iliac crest, left loin, and left inguinal region. The abdomen was slightly rigid, and there was tenderness to the right of the umbilicus and in the hypogastrium. The pelvic girdle was intact. On passing the catheter, clear urine flowed at first and was followed by bright blood. The blood disappeared from the urine in twenty-four hours. Cystoscopy six days after the accident showed the whole mucous membrane of the bladder dotted with tiny petechiæ like a rash ; in some places they were grouped. On the right side of the bladder near the apex there was a gutter-like tear of the mucous membrane about ¾ in. in length. The edges were sharp, raised, and slightly everted. The base was red and granular. (Plate 30, Fig. 3.) Convalescence was uneventful.

Diagnosis.—The diagnosis depends upon the history of an injury and the feeling of something having given way, followed by strangury and the inability to pass urine, and by the bladder being found empty with the catheter, or only a small quantity of blood-stained urine being withdrawn.

From rupture of the urethra the diagnosis is made by the absence of blood at the meatus and of perineal swelling, both of which are characteristic of injuries to the urethra.

In rupture of the kidney there may be symptoms similar to those of rupture of the bladder. The history of the blow in the lumbar region, the comparative absence of bladder irritation, and the absence of pain in passing water, together with tenderness in the loin, are characteristic features of renal injury.

In cases of fracture of the pelvis it is often doubtful if the bladder is ruptured, and the more so that retention of urine is frequently present. In these cases the bladder will be found distended. On rectal examination the pouch of Douglas is not filled with fluid. On passing a catheter the urine is drawn off, while in rupture of the bladder a small quantity of blood-stained urine dribbles feebly away.

The injection of fluids into the bladder in order to ascertain if a smaller quantity is returned, and thus assist in the diagnosis of rupture, is to be deprecated, for there is very grave danger of carrying infection and increasing the extravasation of fluid. The inflation of the bladder with air, which will escape into the peritoneal cavity and obliterate the liver dullness, is equally dangerous. Cystoscopy is only of service in partial rupture; in complete rupture it is not of diagnostic value, as distension of the viscus cannot be obtained.

When there is a fracture of the pelvis the rupture is more likely to be extraperitoneal. Here also there are no signs of peritonitis and no rigidity of the abdominal muscles. In the rectum the finger can feel a tender swelling, and there may be ecchymoses around the anus. Exploration of the bladder by suprapubic cystotomy is the most satisfactory method of making an exact diagnosis, and is a preliminary to treatment.

Treatment.—In complete rupture operation should be performed as soon as the diagnosis is made, unless the shock is very profound, when a few hours' delay is permissible in order to allow the patient to rally.

When the diagnosis of *intraperitoneal* rupture is clearly established, the abdomen is opened in the middle line below the umbilicus, and the urine and blood mopped up. The patient is then raised into the Trendelenburg position, the intestines packed aside, and the peritoneal surface of the bladder carefully examined. If the opening is within reach its extent is examined and brought up as near the surface as possible, and sutured in two layers, and Lembert's sutures added. A catheter should be tied in the urethra and a drain placed in the peritoneum. If the wound, from its position, is inaccessible, it will only be possible to drain the peritoneum and to tie a catheter in the urethra.

When the rupture is *extraperitoneal* a suprapubic incision is made down to the bladder and the anterior face examined. If the rupture is easily accessible it is sutured and a suprapubic drain inserted in the bladder. If the rupture is inaccessible—a very rare condition when the Trendelenburg position, good retraction, and proper lighting are used—the bladder is drained suprapubically, and if necessary a counter-drain is inserted in the perineum.

Results.—Dambrin and Papin found that the mortality of operations in intraperitoneal rupture was 43·5 per cent. in 78 cases, and when only the last six years were taken the mortality fell to 20·5 per cent. Death, when it occurred, was due to peritonitis, shock, urinary toxæmia, and hæmorrhage. The earlier operation is performed in intraperitoneal rupture the better the prognosis. Of 13 cases operated on within the first twelve hours after the injury, 8 recovered ; while of 21 cases operated on after this limit, 15 died (Zuckerkandl). At the same time it is never too late for operation, for recoveries have been recorded when six days have elapsed (Blumer), and Quick successfully operated on a case ten days fourteen hours after the injury.

In non-operated cases of extraperitoneal rupture Zuckerkandl gives a mortality of 27 per cent. Collected cases in which there was urinary extravasation show a high operative mortality. Mitchell collected 90 cases with a mortality of 83 per cent. in 1898.

Of 49 collected cases of extraperitoneal rupture, Wolfer found that 6 were fatal, and of 18 cases of intraperitoneal rupture 9 were fatal.

WOUNDS

Bullet wounds of the bladder are not common, but Bartels could collect 285 cases from the literature. Both in civil and in military practice they are usually incurred when the bladder is distended. Stab wounds of the bladder from a bayonet or dagger are rare. Accidental wounds during surgical operations are met with when the bladder is drawn into a hernial sac, in operations on the uterus, and in symphysiotomy. Falls upon sharp objects on which the patient is impaled are not infrequent. Puncture of the bladder base during attempts at abortion has been recorded. The wound is almost invariably complete, and frequently double. It may be intra- or extraperitoneal.

Bladder wounds are usually complicated by injury to the

bony pelvis, rectum, uterus, vagina, or urethra. Foreign bodies are frequently carried into the wound, with consequent infection. In intraperitoneal wounds a small opening may rarely be plugged by omentum or adherent bowel. Usually there is extravasation of urine, followed by acute peritonitis. In extraperitoneal wounds there are extravasation and suppuration, leading to urinary fistulæ.

Symptoms.—Shock is usually present, and may be profound. There are pain, tenesmus, and frequent desire to pass water, with inability to do so; often a few drops of blood are passed after much straining. Rectal spasm may also be present. Urine mixed with blood may escape by the wound, especially when it is extensive. The escape of urine may be prevented by plugging of the wound with bowel, or by the urine escaping into the peritoneal cavity through a second wound. In other cases, in which•the wound is small and the track oblique, urine may only escape during attempts at micturition. Occasionally there is profuse hæmorrhage from the external wound. Fæces and flatus may escape from the wound with the urine when the rectum is wounded. Spontaneous closure of a small intraperitoneal wound has been observed (Makins), but this is rare, and peritonitis almost invariably supervenes. The peritonitis may be delayed until the separation of sloughs on the seventh or eighth day. In small, oblique extraperitoneal wounds there is perivesical and periurethral extravasation of urine which becomes infected. This is followed by thrombosis in the vesical and prostatic veins.

Fistulæ are very common, especially after bullet wounds. Recto-vesical and vesico-vaginal fistulæ, and surface fistulæ on the abdomen, scrotum, perineum, thighs, and buttocks, result from suppuration and urinary infiltration. Bartels found that 23 cases out of 67 had a fistula for from six to twelve months, and in 5 the fistula was permanent. In many cases foreign bodies, such as bullets, fragments of bone, etc., are found in the bladder, and phosphatic calculi containing foreign bodies are frequent.

Diagnosis.—The escape of urine from the wound and the presence of blood in the urine passed or drawn by a catheter, and tenesmus of the bladder, are sufficient to establish the diagnosis. Examination of a perineal wound with a metal instrument in the bladder will assist. The diagnosis as to whether the wound is extra- or intraperitoneal may be impossible at first, and it is important not to wait until symptoms of peritonitis appear before operating.

Prognosis.—Intraperitoneal wounds are grave from the certainty of infection and the frequency of injury to other organs, such as the bowel. Extraperitoneal wounds have a much better prognosis.

Treatment.—The treatment is that of penetrating wounds of the lower abdomen. Laparotomy should be performed as early as possible, and the peritoneal surface of the bladder examined and any wound closed. Wounds of the intestine are searched for and sutured. If the bladder wound is not found on the peritoneal surface the peritoneum is closed and the anterior surface of the bladder examined. If a wound is found it may, if the position·is suitable, be used to drain the bladder, or the wound may be closed and a catheter tied in the urethra.

When the bladder has been wounded from the perineum the wound should be carefully examined and free drainage provided.

If symptoms of peritonitis supervene the abdomen should be opened.

The treatment of fistulæ is described later (p. 523).

LITERATURE

Ashurst, *Amer. Journ. Med. Sci.,* July, 1906.
Bartels, *Arch. f. klin. Chir.,* 1878, p. 519.
Berndt, *Arch. f. klin. Chir.,* 1899.
Blumer, *Brit. Med. Journ.,* Dec. 22, 1900.
Dambrin et **Papin,** *Ann. d. Mal. d. Org. Gén.-Urin.,* 1904, p. 641.
Goldenberg, *Beitr. z. klin. Chir.,* 1909, p. 356.
Makins, *Surgical Experiences in South Africa.*
Mitchell, *Ann. Surg.,* 1898, p. 157.
Morel, *Ann. d. Mal. d. Org. Gén.-Urin.,* 1906, p. 801.
Murray, *Liverpool Med.-Chir. Journ.,* 1906, p. 159.
Quick, *Ann. Surg.,* 1907, p. 94.
Seldowitsch, *Arch. f. klin. Chir.,* 1904, p. 859.
Treves, *Brit. Med. Journ.,* 1900.
Wolfer, *Therap. Gaz.,* Dec. 15, 1910

CHAPTER XXXII

CYSTITIS

Etiology.—Inflammation of the bladder is due to the combination of a bacterial infection with some factor which produces lowered resistance.

An injury will cause cystitis, and repeated injuries, such as are produced by the presence of a stone in the bladder, will lead to the persistence of the cystitis; but if the injury is not repeated the inflammation is transient, and if the cause of repeated injuries (such as the stone) is removed the cystitis spontaneously disappears. In some cases the presence of bacteria of most virulent type in the urine without any known local cause of diminished resistance gives rise to cystitis. On the other hand, if bacteria reach the healthy bladder by the urethra or through the kidneys, cystitis is not produced in the majority of cases. Urine which is swarming with bacteria may be passed through the bladder for years without producing cystitis. Pure cultures of bacillus coli and other bacteria have been injected in experimental work on animals, without producing cystitis. When, however, the penis has been ligatured, in addition to the injection of bacteria, cystitis is produced.

The predisposing causes of cystitis, such as masturbation, affections of the female genital organs, pregnancy, stricture, enlarged prostate, calculus, foreign bodies, malignant growths, operations upon the bladder, atony from nervous disease, etc., may act by producing congestion or injury to the bladder wall or stagnation of the urine. They vary at different ages and under different conditions. In childhood and infancy cystitis is the frequent complication of vulvo-vaginitis, enteritis, and stone. In young men gonorrhœal urethritis and stricture, in adult men stricture and atony of the bladder from nervous disease, in old men enlarged prostate, in women pregnancy and diseases of the uterus and ovaries, are the usual predisposing causes.

Bacteriology.—A large variety of bacteria are found in the urine in cystitis, and a mixed infection is frequent. Cystitis due to the tubercle bacillus will be discussed separately. The bacillus coli communis occurs more frequently than other bacteria, and is often found in pure culture. Other bacteria that occur alone, or in mixed infections, are the staphylococcus, streptococcus, proteus, gonococcus, the pneumococcus of Fraenkel and of Friedlaender, the bacillus pyocyaneus, and the typhoid bacillus. In chronic cystitis anaerobic bacteria are frequently found. The streptobacillus fusiformis, bacillus ramosus, micrococcus fœtidus, and others may be found alone or with aerobic bacteria.

The bacteriology of cystitis varies during the course of an attack, whether acute or chronic. At one time there may be a mixed infection, at another a pure culture. There is a tendency for certain bacteria to predominate, while others may be found in small numbers and have a feeble culture growth. When a dominant bacterium has been reduced in virulence or destroyed by vaccines, by bladder-washing, or by other means, other bacteria may be found to increase in numbers. Thus, in a case of almost pure bacillus coli cystitis the decline of this bacillus is not infrequently marked by the appearance or increase of staphylococcus.

The bacillus coli has a tendency to persist and to dominate the bacteriology of a. mixed infection ; the strepto- and staphylococci are readily displaced by other bacteria, while the pyocyaneus tends to persist.

The urine remains acid in cystitis due to the bacillus coli and the gonococcus, and also in about half the cases of cystitis due to bacteria which decompose urea.

Method of infection.—The bladder may be infected from the kidney, the bacteria being borne by the urine. The kidney may or may not participate in the inflammation, and the bacteria are usually blood-borne, and in the majority of cases bacillus coli is the infecting agent. Infection may be introduced by way of the urethra either by continuity of inflammation as in gonorrhœa or by the passage of an instrument. Bacteria may also reach the bladder through a cystotomy wound or a fistula, or from the rupture of an abscess or the formation of a fistula with the bowel.

Pathological anatomy and cystoscopic appearances.—Except in the most severe varieties of cystitis, little or no change is found post mortem. It is, therefore, necessary to take advantage of the cystoscope in studying the appearances presented in cystitis.

In the majority of cases of cystitis the inflammation does not affect the whole surface of the bladder mucous membrane. The base is most frequently involved, while the rest of the bladder may escape ; less frequently there is an area of cystitis at some part of the organ, sometimes at the apex, while the base is slightly affected. Occasionally there are patches of cystitis distributed over the bladder. In the more severe varieties of acute cystitis, and also in chronic cystitis, the whole of the mucous surface is usually inflamed. The earliest appearance of inflammation is engorgement of the capillary vessels, which appear as a fine intricate network. The mucous membrane becomes reddened and spongy or woolly, and the outline of the vessels grows less and less distinct until they are completely obscured. The surface is now bright red, and the mucous membrane thrown into stiff folds and ridges, with shreds of muco-pus or desquamated epithelium adhering to it. (Plate 31, Fig. 1.) Hæmorrhages may occur into the subepithelial tissues and appear as dark-red or black spots or blotches surrounded by a halo of intense inflammation. If there are numerous hæmorrhages the condition is known as hæmorrhagic cystitis.

In bullous cystitis the surface is covered with closely-set yellow semitransparent bullæ. This appearance is usually confined to some part of the bladder, such as the orifice of a diverticulum, the neighbourhood of the ureter in a virulent descending inflammation, or the area around a malignant growth, or it may extend over the whole base. It may be quite evanescent. Small, closely grouped granules in the inflamed mucous membrane are characteristic of follicular cystitis.

In cystic cystitis there are yellow sago-grain-like follicles which may be scattered or grouped together, and may be surrounded by a halo of inflammation, or by only a few injected vessels. (Plate 31, Fig. 2.) Groups of small cysts may form in inflamed areas and project from the surface in masses like bunches of grapes, or there may be solid projecting masses. In these cases there may be cysts in the ureter and renal pelvis. Stoerk and Zuckerkandl have found that the cysts result from the closure of the orifices of small invaginations of epithelium, or by the fusion of papillary excrescences on the surface. Adeno-carcinoma may take origin in these cysts.

Extensive deposit of phosphatic salts may take place in patches, along the ridges of inflamed mucous membrane or over large areas of the bladder. This may be heaped up into irregular projecting masses.

Necrosis of the superficial layers of mucous membrane mixed with fibrin forms a membrane which is cast off, and the condition is named croupous or diphtheritic cystitis. The infection in these cases is usually streptococcal.

In very virulent infections exfoliation of the bladder mucous membrane may take place, and the. necrosed membrane is passed as a cast of the bladder. Emphysema of the mucous. membrane has been described.

Ulceration is usually confined to the superficial layers. It is frequently found along the summit of ridges and folds, and may extend more widely. Less frequently there is a circumscribed deep round or oval ulcer, with a heaped-up, sharply. defined edge. (Plate 31, Fig. 3.) I have also seen a spreading ring-like ulcer commencing at the apex and advancing to the base.

Leucoplakia is found in stone and other conditions of. chronic irritation, and there may be a single patch or several patches. The surface is dry, greyish or yellowish white, and parchment-like. The edges are irregular, and the surrounding mucous membrane is deep red and intensely inflamed.

The epithelium becomes transformed into squamous epithelium, which is heaped up in thick masses. In chronic cystitis there are infiltration and sclerosis of the submucous tissue and muscular layer, and a great increase in the perivascular fat, which becomes fibrous and adherent. The bladder becomes contracted and the cavity permanently diminished.

When cystitis complicates urethral obstruction there is thickening of the bladder wall from hypertrophy of the muscle.

In stricture, trabeculation is always less marked and sacculation less pronounced than in enlarged prostate. In the latter, sacculation with thinning and atrophy of the muscular layer is frequently present. Calculi often form in the bladder in chronic cystitis, especially when there are sacculi or residual urine. .

Symptoms.—The symptoms of cystitis are frequent micturition, pain, and changes in the urine.

Increased frequency of micturition usually draws attention to the condition. The frequency varies with the intensity of the cystitis. In slight cases the urine may be passed every two hours, and there is some urgency when the call to micturate is felt. In severe cases a few drops of urine are passed every few minutes, and necessity to pass water is uncontrollable, so that a form of active incontinence is produced. In the lesser grades the patient sleeps throughout the night, but in severe cystitis the call to micturate is powerful and frequent during the night as well as the day. The bladder may be so sensitive that spasm is induced by jarring the bed, or a breath of cold air, or a hot or cold drink. Polyuria frequently accompanies the frequent micturition, and is said to be due to a reflex influence on the kidney. It diminishes as the frequency subsides.

Pain is present to a varying degree. There is scalding pain

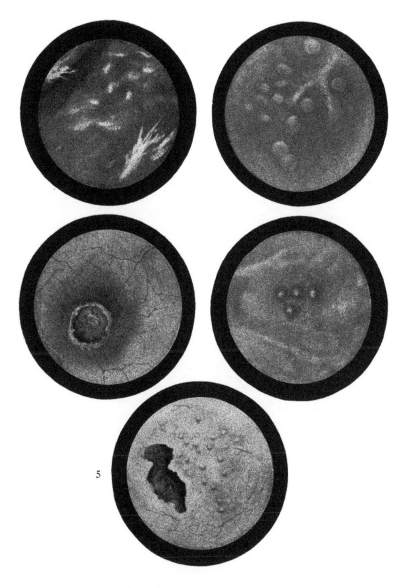

5

Fig. 1.—Acute cystitis. (P. 425.)

Fig. 2.—Cystic cystitis. (P. 425.)

Fig. 3.—Ulcer of bladder in cystitis due to Bacillus coli
communis. (P. 426.)

Fig. 4.—Tuberculosis of bladder; group of caseous
tubercles. (P. 439.)

along the urethra on passing water, and intense desire and pain when an attempt is made to hold the urine. In moderately severe cases there is discomfort at the end of micturition, and a feeling that the bladder has not been emptied; and in severe cases a cramping pain at the neck of the bladder, in the rectum, along the urethra to the end of the penis, and sometimes radiating down the thighs.

Pyuria is always present, but varies greatly in amount. The pus is mixed with mucus in varying proportion. It may form a haze which settles to the bottom of a glass as a billowy semitranslucent mass, or in more severe or chronic cases it forms a slimy tenacious deposit which clings to the bottom of the receptacle. The quantity of mucus and pus is not subject to sudden variation unless the cystitis is complicated by sacculation or diverticula of the bladder, pyelitis, or some other disease which permits of accumulation and sudden discharge of pus. The urine is mixed with blood in severe cases; in less severe cases there may be terminal hæmaturia. In most cases no blood is seen with the naked eye, but very frequently blood corpuscles are found with the microscope in the acute stage.

Fever is not present unless cystitis is complicated by renal, prostatic, or some extravesical inflammation. There is tenderness on pressure above the pubes and on rectal and vaginal examination. The bladder wall can be felt from the rectum thickened and contracted. The capacity of the bladder is reduced to a degree corresponding to the intensity of the inflammation. In acute cystitis the bladder may not retain more than ½ oz. of fluid ; in less acute cystitis the organ may hold 1 oz. or several ounces.

Cystoscopy is difficult and may be impossible in acute cystitis, and it is advisable to wait until the acute stage has passed before using the cystoscope. There is difficulty in obtaining adequate distension of the organ or a medium clear of pus and blood. Cystoscopy shows that in a large proportion of cases of cystitis the inflammation affects a small area of the bladder, usually at the base. When the inflammation is descending and mild, an area surrounding one ureter and involving the trigone is alone affected ; when inflammation has reached the bladder by extension from the urethra (urethro-cystitis) the trigone is most acutely inflamed. In other cases cystitis consists of scattered patches of inflammation over the mucous surface or of an inflamed area at the apex or elsewhere.

The illumination is more difficult in cystitis than in a normal bladder, for the reflecting property of the mucous membrane is diminished by desquamation of the surface epithelium.

The appearances seen on cystoscopy have already been described (p. 424).

Complications.—Retention of urine may occur as a compli-' cation of cystitis, usually in cases of stricture of the urethra or of enlarged prostate, but also in atony of the bladder from nervous disease. Ascending infection of the kidneys is a constant danger, especially when obstruction is present, and is the cause of death in most of the fatal cases of cystitis.

Abscess of the wall of the bladder, or surrounding a saccule, or in the perivesical tissue, may complicate chronic cystitis.

Diagnosis.—The diagnosis of cystitis involves a number of questions :

1. **Are the symptoms due to cystitis or to some condition outside the bladder?** (a) *Extra-urinary causes of vesical symptoms.*—Pain in the bladder of a dull constant aching character, sometimes also in acute attacks, may occur in tabes, and reflex pain is observed in cases of hæmorrhoids and anal fissure, and there is a condition known as " neuralgia " of the bladder in which pain is present without recognizable cause. In these conditions there is pain but no pyuria.

Frequent micturition may also be caused by extravesical conditions, such as pregnancy, ovarian or fibroid tumours, prolapse of the uterus. Here also pyuria is absent.

(b) *Urinary causes of vesical symptoms without cystitis.*—Frequent micturition may be due to the passage of large quantities of urine in diabetes mellitus, diabetes insipidus, hysterical polyuria, etc. In such cases pain is usually absent, but there may be dull aching vesical pain.

In highly acid urines and urines containing oxalate crystals, and in phosphaturia, frequent and urgent micturition with pain is often present. The condition of the urine, the absence of pus, and the effect of treatment distinguish these cases.

Occasionally frequent micturition due to urethral obstruction in stricture may be ascribed to the effect of the obstruction on a sensitive bladder, apart from cystitis.

In enlarged prostate frequent micturition is an early and prominent symptom when no cystitis is present. This is due partly to the pressure of the enlarging prostate on the base and sphincter of the bladder, and partly to the exposure to the urine in the bladder of the sensitive mucous membrane of the prostatic urethra, which is dragged up through the vesical sphincter by the intravesical projection of the prostate.

Urethral polypi in the male or female urethra may cause frequent painful micturition. Reflex bladder pain and frequency of micturition are common in certain diseases of the kidney, notably in tuberculous disease, calculus, and pyelitis. In these cases the ureter of one side may show congestion and other slight changes, and the trigone be infected, but usually no changes referable to cystitis can be found in the bladder. In pyelitis the frequency is principally nocturnal. The diagnosis is made by the discovery of pus and bacteria in the urine and by the use of the cystoscope.

2. **Is the cystitis primary or secondary ?**—This question only applies to the condition at the time of the examination, for the bladder is an internal organ at which bacteria arrive by the urethra, the ureter, or the blood stream, or from the bursting of an abscess through the bladder wall; and primary infection in the strict sense only occurs in cystotomy or other wounds of the bladder.

In a secondary cystitis the removal of the primary extravesical focus is followed by disappearance of the cystitis.

The bladder may be infected from the kidney in cases of renal calculus, pyonephrosis, pyelonephritis, renal tuberculosis, etc., or there may be infection from the urethra (urethro-cystitis) in acute, subacute, or chronic urethritis. The source of infection in subacute and chronic cases is the prostatic urethra, and there is usually chronic prostatitis as well.

In renal suppuration there may be symptoms of disease of the kidney, such as pain, tenderness, enlargement of the kidney; and if no cystitis is present, tenderness of the bladder and pain on distension with fluid are absent. The urine sometimes contains cells from the renal pelvis, and tubules, and occasionally tube casts, while vesical epithelium is absent. The reaction of the urine in renal affections is usually acid from the blending of acid urine from the second kidney; but this is not a reliable point in diagnosis, for the urine may be alkaline in renal disease and acid in some forms of cystitis. The pus in pyelitis or pyelonephritis, and especially in pyonephrosis, is greater in quantity than in cystitis, and forms a heavy, flat layer at the bottom of the glass; and it is liable to sudden and marked variations in quantity. In cystitis the pus is mixed with mucus, and forms an irregular deposit which is slimy and tenacious. Variations in quantity do not occur. When cystitis complicates suppurative renal disease, the combination of a heavy substratum of pus with an upper layer of muco-pus is observed.

The diagnosis of cystitis secondary to renal disease is made by the cystoscopic inspection of the ureteric orifices. The inflammatory area may surround one ureter, or it may affect the whole bladder surface. The orifice shows inflammatory changes, and the efflux is purulent. In slight cases the ureteral catheter may be necessary to ascertain the origin of the infection.

In urethro-cystitis there are signs of urethral inflammation, and the use of the urethroscope and cystoscope confirms the diagnosis. Entero-vesical fistula may be the cause of acute cystitis, and of chronic cystitis with acute exacerbations. The diagnosis is made by examination of the urine and by cystoscopy.

3. **In primary cystitis, what is the cause ?**—Acute spontaneous cystitis is most frequently due to the bacillus coli, but also to other bacteria. Subacute and chronic cystitis may be purely bacterial, or there may be a diverticulum, stone, or growth of the bladder with secondary infection. Of cases of malignant growth of the bladder, 40 per cent. come under observation as cases of chronic spontaneous cystitis. The urine in all subacute chronic cases should be carefully examined bacteriologically and histologically, and the bladder inspected with the cystoscope.

Prognosis.—In acute cystitis without complications the prognosis is good. The attack lasts from two to four or five weeks, and, if there is no focus of recurrent infection inside the bladder, recovery is usually complete. When a diverticulum or sacculi of the bladder are present, recurrent attacks, and eventually chronic cystitis, may be expected.

Cystitis complicated by urethral obstruction rarely disappears unless the obstruction is completely removed. Cystitis in an atonic bladder in nervous disease usually becomes permanently established, and the chronic inflammation is subject to acute exacerbations from time to time, usually as the result of infection from outside sources. When suppuration in the kidney is the primary disease and cystitis is secondary, the latter will not be relieved until the renal infection is removed.

Ascending pyelonephritis is the final stage of most of the fatal cases of cystitis. The infection may ascend spontaneously or may follow upon bladder-washing.

Treatment. Acute cystitis.—In acute cystitis the patient should be confined to bed and treatment chiefly directed to soothing the inflamed bladder. The diet should consist mainly of milk, eggs, custards, soups, and light farinaceous foods. Alcohol should be interdicted. Diuretics such as Contrexéville, Vittel, Vichy, and Evian waters, barley water, buchu and parsley tea are administered to render the urine less irritating. When the urine is acid the administration of alkalis is of great value. Citrate of potash 20 gr., pot. bicarb. 20 gr., magnesium sulphate 30–60 gr., and liquor potassæ 5 minims, may be given, and sandalwood oil has a soothing effect (10 minims in capsule or emulsion). To reduce the painful spasm of the bladder the following are useful, viz. : tincture of belladonna 5 or 10 minims, tincture of hyoscyamus 15 minims, tincture of opium 5–15 minims, and bromide of camphor 5 gr., by the mouth; and lupulin 4 gr., extract of belladonna ¼ gr., and morphia ⅛–¼ gr., given singly or in combination as suppository, and repeated twice or thrice in the twenty-four hours provided morphia and belladonna are not being administered by the mouth. Hot sitz-baths are given twice or thrice a day, the patient being well covered up during the bath, which lasts for ten or twenty minutes, and thoroughly rubbed down afterwards. Hot fomentations, to which laudanum may be added, are applied to the lower abdomen and perineum, and when intense strangury is present a small enema of hot water containing antipyrin 20–30 gr., or a vaginal douche of similar composition, may be given. Two teaspoonfuls of starch and 15 or 30 minims of tincture of opium may be added to the enema.

Occasionally a hypodermic injection of morphia ¼ gr. with atropine $\frac{1}{120}$ gr. may be necessary.

The bowels should be freely opened by a smart saline purge, and a daily aperient such as Apenta, Hunyadi János, or cascara given. No attempt should be made to wash the bladder at this stage. In very painful cystitis an instillation of a few drachms or ounces of distilled water containing antipyrin 2 per cent., and laudanum ½ to 1 per cent., or of orthoform 5 to 10 per cent., in oil, may be cautiously introduced.

Subacute cystitis.—The acute stage lasts from three to ten days, and is followed by a subacute stage. In subacute cystitis the patient may be allowed up and a less restricted diet permitted, but all highly spiced foods, curries, much meat, coffee, and all alcoholic drinks are forbidden.

Urinary antiseptics should be administered by the mouth, such as urotropine, hetralin, or helmitol 10 gr. of each, urodonal 1 drachm, and salol 5–15 gr. ; and sometimes benzoate of soda or ammonia 10 gr., and boric acid 15 gr., will be found valuable.

If the cystitis is due to the bacillus coli or to other bacteria which flourish in an acid urine, alkalis should be given. If, on the other hand, the urine becomes alkaline from ammoniacal decomposition owing to the presence of the bacillus ureæ liquefaciens in mixed infections, alkalis should be withheld, and dilute mineral acids, benzoate of soda and ammonia, and boric acid given. Sodium acid phosphate 20–30 gr. is especially useful, together with large doses of urotropine or other urinary antiseptics. Bladder-washing should be commenced when the acute symptoms have passed off. Vaccine treatment with an autogenous vaccine will be found of use in this stage.

Chronic cystitis.—In chronic cystitis a very careful examination with the cystoscope is necessary to ascertain whether there is some factor such as renal suppuration, stone, enlarged prostate, or diverticula which may act as a contributory cause and prevent resolution of the cystitis. Should any such complication be present it must be dealt with before the cystitis can be cured.

The treatment is similar to that of subacute cystitis. The only restrictions of diet that are necessary are the avoidance of articles such as curries and all highly spiced foods and alcohol. Alkalis or acids and urinary antiseptics are administered as in subacute cystitis.

Bladder-washing plays a prominent part in the treatment ; a visit to one of the Continental spas, such as Wildungen, Contrexéville, or Vittel, is frequently of great service. Vaccine treatment is occasionally beneficial, while drainage of the bladder with daily flushing or continuous irrigation may become necessary.

Bladder-washing.—This is suitable for subacute or chronic cystitis. A large rubber or silk-wove coudé catheter with a trumpet-shaped outer end is sterilized and carefully passed into the bladder. An irrigating can hung 2 or 3 ft. above the level of the recumbent patient contains the solution selected, the temperature of which is about 100° F. A glass bladder syringe with metal fittings and asbestos plunger may be used to replace the irrigator. The fluid is allowed to flow through the catheter slowly until the patient begins to feel slight discomfort, when the nozzle is removed and the fluid run off. Several pints of solution are used in this way, and the mechanical action of free washing with large volumes of fluid plays an important part.

A double-way catheter does not wash the bladder so thoroughly as a single-bore instrument.

In some cases masses of tenacious muco-pus adhere to the bladder wall or obstruct the lumen of the catheter. In acid cystitis a preliminary washing with a weak alkali such as bicarbonate of soda, 1 or 2 per cent., is useful, while in very alkaline cystitis with deposit of phosphates I have found much benefit from the use of a weak solution of acetic acid, $\frac{1}{2}$ per cent. Solutions that may be used for washing the bladder are potassium permanganate 1 in 5,000 or 10,000, oxycyanide of mercury 1 in 1,000 or 5,000, biniodide of mercury 1 in 10,000 or 20,000, tincture of iodine $\frac{1}{2}$-1 drachm to the pint, nitrate of silver 1 in 10,000 or 20,000, peroxide of hydrogen 1 in 10 or 1 in 20 of the twenty volumes, lysol $\frac{1}{2}$-1 per cent., protargol $\frac{1}{2}$ per cent.

Instillations. — The instillation of small quantities ($\frac{1}{2}$–2 drachms) of more powerful solutions is sometimes useful. These are introduced by means of a small syringe and catheter such as Guyon's syringe. Iodoform in sterilized liquid paraffin (5 per cent.) is a useful solution; the oil floats in the urine, and, if the patient is careful to stop micturition before he has completely emptied his bladder, some of the solution may be retained in the bladder for several days. Gomenol is analgesic as well as antiseptic; it is used in oil solutions of 5 to 20 per cent., and may also be given internally in capsule. Silver nitrate 2 per cent., protargol 2 per cent., and acid picric $\frac{1}{2}$–1 per cent., may also be used. In chronic alkaline cystitis instillations of lactic acid bacillus in the form of trilactine may be beneficial. I have instilled $\frac{1}{2}$–1 drachm of freshly prepared trilactine daily after washing the bladder with sterile water, with marked improvement in the condition of the urine.

Bladder drainage.—Drainage of the bladder is very exceptionally required in acute cystitis, and then only in the rare cases of fulminating cystitis with sloughing of the mucous membrane. It is chiefly of use in intractable subacute or chronic cystitis, and may be carried out through the urethra, or by the perineal or the suprapubic route.

In *urethral drainage* a catheter is " tied in." A silk-wove coudé catheter (No. 10 Fr.), a Jacques rubber catheter, or a Pezzer's self-retaining rubber catheter is used. In the female subject the last is most suitable, and is introduced with a stilette.

In the male subject the catheter is passed until the eye is just within the internal meatus, and its position is tested by injecting a little fluid with a syringe and allowing it to flow off, gradually withdrawing the catheter until the flow becomes arrested, and then pushing the catheter in again until the flow is re-established. Two strands of silk or two short strips of narrow tape are tied firmly around the catheter, without constricting its lumen, $\frac{1}{2}$ in. beyond the external meatus, and if there is any tendency for them to slip a small safety-pin is oiled and passed through the tape and catheter at this point.

The four tails of silk or tape are laid along the penis, and a strip of adhesive plaster 1 in. broad is wound round the penis over these, just behind the corona glandis, care being taken not to apply it so tight as to cause constriction. The ends of the tape may be turned back under a second round of plaster. The adhesive plaster may be applied longitudinally to avoid causing oedema of the foreskin. A short length of rubber tubing is attached

2 c

to the end of the catheter and carried into a bottle between the patient's thighs. If the catheter becomes blocked, this may be due to tenacious mucus or blood clot, or to gravel, or there may be a kink of a silk-wove catheter, or the instrument may have slipped so that the eye is in the urethra.

Perineal drainage is carried out by opening the membranous urethra on a staff by a median incision and introducing a rubber perineal drainage tube through the prostatic portion of the urethra into the bladder. A stitch through the edges of the wound fixes the tube, and a length of tubing carries the urine into a vessel.

When a stiff gum-elastic tube is used, metal loops are provided for perineal tapes passing anteriorly in the fold of the groin and posteriorly in the fold of the buttock to a waist-band. The mortality of this operation is high—25 per cent.—as it is frequently practised in severe cases, and often at a late stage.

Suprapubic drainage is carried out by distending the bladder with fluid and opening it by a vertical median suprapubic incision. The bladder should be thoroughly explored, and any cause for the persistence of the cystitis ascertained and, if possible, removed. In the case of a middle-aged woman whose bladder was encrusted with phosphatic deposit heaped up in parts so as to resemble a large phosphate-covered growth, I applied pure acetic acid to the interior, and afterwards washed the bladder with a weak solution of acetic acid for a fortnight. The recovery from a long-standing and intractable cystitis was rapid and uninterrupted.

A large rubber drainage tube ($\frac{3}{4}$–1 in. diameter) is introduced, and the bladder wound closed around this with catgut stitches. A smaller tube is placed in the prevesical space. Both tubes are removed on the fourth day, and a smaller tube is introduced into the bladder. An alternative method.is to stitch the edge of the bladder wound to the skin, but there is often difficulty in obtaining healing later and a fistula persists.

The mortality of suprapubic drainage is 10 per cent. (Joubert). In the female subject a fistula may be created between the bladder and the vagina for the purpose of draining the bladder. This is frequently successful in curing cystitis, but a fistula remains in 50 per cent. of cases.

Comparative value ·of methods.—Urethral bladder drainage may suffice, but it is less thorough than either of the other methods.

Suprapubic drainage is preferable to perineal unless there is a stricture of the urethra, when perineal drainage can be combined with external urethrotomy. In other cases the bladder can be more thoroughly explored by the suprapubic route, and drainage and washing can be more easily carried out. The perineal tube does not drain the lowest part of the bladder, since the end of the tube projects into the bladder at the internal meatus, which is the highest part of the fixed portion of the bladder when the patient lies on his back. The suprapubic drainage tube passes to the bottom of the bladder, and this part is more readily drained and washed.

Continuous irrigation.—This is carried out by the suprapubic route, and can conveniently be arranged by using an Irving suprapubic drainage apparatus. Through the small hole in the lid of the apparatus a rubber catheter passes, and descends through the rubber tube in the suprapubic wound to the lowest part of the bladder. To the outer end of this catheter rubber tubing is attached, and leads from a reservoir placed above the level of the patient. The flow is regulated by screw clips so as to allow of a gentle continuous stream, and arrangements must be made for keeping the fluid in the reservoir warm.

Serum and vaccine treatment.—*Serum-therapy* consists in supplying the patient with antibodies contained in the serum of an animal artificially immunized by inoculation with bacteria. In acute cystitis this method may be useful. Antistreptococcic serum is obtained from animals inoculated either with one strain of streptococcus or with several strains from different sources (polyvalent). Anti-colon-bacillus serum has not yet been widely used. The serum is injected subcutaneously, and a large initial dose (20 c.c.) is given, followed by smaller doses (10 c.c.). Calcium lactate should be given at the same time as the serum in order to prevent serum rashes and joint troubles. Care must be taken not to continue the treatment too long, lest the state of hypersensitiveness to the serum, known as anaphylaxis, be produced.

Vaccine treatment is most suitable for cases of subacute and chronic cystitis. It consists in the inoculation of the patient with graduated doses of vaccine with the object of increasing the resistance to the special bacteria by the production of antibodies. The vaccine should be prepared from cultures of the patient's urine. Stock vaccines are of much less value. The bacteriology of the urine is investigated, and if the infection is by a pure culture a vaccine from that strain is obtained. If several varieties of bacteria are present the dominant species is selected, or if more than one grows luxuriantly a mixed vaccine is prepared. The vaccine consists of a measured number of the bacteria sterilized.

For a period of forty-eight hours after the inoculation the resistance of the patient is lowered (negative phase), and then it rises, and remains high for several days, falling again to its previous level or a little above it. For the earlier inoculation it is often necessary to examine the opsonic index, so that too large a dose may not be given and a second dose may not encroach upon the negative phase of a previous inoculation. In the majority of cases, however, it is possible to dispense entirely with this examination, and to rely upon experience and clinical observation as guides to dosage. The inoculations should begin with small doses at intervals of three or four days, the doses rising continuously, and the interval being extended to a week or longer. The more acute the disease the smaller the dose of vaccine. If possible, a reaction should be avoided. It is shown by a feeling of malaise, pains in the back and head, and a slight rise of temperature, with increased irritability of the bladder. The most frequently used vaccine is that of the bacillus coli, and this may be employed alone when the culture is pure, or in combination with other vaccines when it is mixed. The inoculations can usually . be commenced with a dose of 3 millions given every three or four days, the dose being raised to 4 and 5 millions with extension of the interval to a week, and then to 10, 15, 20, 30, 40, 50, 60, 80, 100, 150, and eventually to 200 millions, and even higher. The staphylococcus is given in doses commencing at 100 to 250 millions, and rising to 500 or 1,000 millions; the streptococcus in increasing doses of 2, 3, 5, 10, 20 millions, and more. The treatment may extend over several months.

Vaccine treatment is frequently successful in reducing and causing the disappearance of cystitis, but in many cases bacilluria remains and resists all treatment, and at a later date relapses of the cystitis occur.

LITERATURE

Brown, *Johns Hopkins Hosp. Repts.*, 1901, p. 1.
Faltin, *Ann. d. Mal. d. Org. Gén.- Urin.*, 1902, p. 176.
Hallé et **Motz,** *Ann. d. Mal. d. Org. Gén.- Urin.*, 1902, p. 17.
Joubert, VIIe Sess. de l'Assoc. franç. d'Urol., Paris, 1903, p. 7.
Lichtenstein, *Wien. klin. Woch.*, 1904; *ibid.*, 1907, Nr. 40.
Melchior, *Monats. f. d. Krankh. d. Harn- u. Sex.-Apparat.*, 1898, p. 581.
Motz et **Denis,** *Ann. d. Mal. d Org. Gén.- Urin.*, 1903, p. 898.
Motz et **Montfort,** *Ann. d. Mal. d. Org. Gén.- Urin.*, 1903, p. 1211.
Newman, *Lancet*, 1912, i. 490, 570.
Raskai, *Monats. f. Urol.*, 1905, p. 1.
Stoerk, *Zieglers Beitr. z. path. Anat.*, 1911, l. 361.
Stoerk und **Zuckerkandl,** *Zeits. f. Urol.*, 1907, p. 3.
Suter, *Zeits. f. Urol.*, 1907, p. 97.
Zuckerkandl, *Monats. f. Urol.*, Bd. vii.

CHAPTER XXXIII
TUBERCULOUS CYSTITIS

TUBERCULOUS cystitis is said to be primary or secondary, according to whether it is the original focus in the genito-urinary organs, or is dependent upon a tuberculous focus in the kidney or the male genital system.

Primary tuberculosis in the strict sense that the vesical tuberculosis is the primary focus in the body does not exist.

Etiology.—Vesical tuberculosis occurs in youth and early adult life, and is more common in men than in women. Cases of senile vesical tuberculosis are occasionally observed.

Primary tuberculosis invades the mucous membrane of the bladder by the blood stream. At the present time there is considerable doubt as to whether this form of tuberculosis ever occurs. The evidence for it is clinical and cystoscopic. The clinician finds that symptoms of vesical tuberculosis are present without symptoms of renal or genital infection, and the cystoscopist sees tuberculosis of the bladder mucous membrane while the orifices of the ureters are healthy. Neither of these observations is reliable, for it can be proved by catheterization of the ureters that under these conditions tuberculosis of the kidney may exist. Since I have relied upon the ureteral catheter in every case for a decision on this point, I have not met with a single case of primary tuberculosis of the bladder.

In cystitis secondary to renal tuberculosis there is either direct spread by continuity along the ureter to the bladder, or the deposit of tubercle from the infected urine. In cystitis secondary to genital tuberculosis the tuberculous process either passes directly through the bladder wall from the seminal vesicles or prostate, or spreads from a dilated and tuberculous prostatic urethra into the bladder. In cases in which the bladder and kidneys are tuberculous, much discussion has arisen as to whether the tuberculous process is primary in the kidney and the infection of the bladder a descending one, or the tuberculosis of the bladder is primary and the infection of the kidney ascending and secondary.

At one time the ascending theory was universally held, and

was based upon (1) the early appearance of vesical symptoms in urinary tuberculosis, (2) some post-mortem records, and (3) experimental work.

Cystoscopy has proved that the early symptoms of cystitis in urinary tuberculosis are, in the majority of cases, reflex; that the bladder is healthy, or at least non-tuberculous; and that the kidney may be totally destroyed by tuberculosis without giving rise to renal symptoms. Post-mortem records which are quoted in support of the ascending view show the tuberculous process surrounding the ureteric orifice of the affected kidney, and might equally be quoted in proof of secondary descending infection of the bladder. Apart from cases of genital tuberculosis, tuberculosis of the bladder is almost without exception accompanied by tuberculosis of the kidney; whereas tuberculosis of the kidney, or kidney and ureter, is frequently present without tuberculosis of the bladder. The experimental production of ascending tuberculosis of the kidney in animals by Albarran, Wildbolz, and others has proved that by injecting tubercle bacilli into the bladder and ligaturing the urethra, or into the ureter and ligaturing the ureter, a tuberculous infection of the kidney can be produced. In all these experiments the element of obstruction, temporary or permanent, is superadded to the introduction of the tubercle bacillus, a condition not found in tuberculosis in the human subject.

Baumgarten has demonstrated that the tuberculous infection cannot spread against the stream of the secretion in which the bacilli are suspended. Not only does he deny the possibility of ascending infection of the kidney, but he holds that tuberculosis of the prostatic urethra cannot affect the epididymis by spreading back along the vas deferens.

In the female the combination of urinary tuberculosis with genital tuberculosis is very rare, and the infection of the urinary from the genital tract does not occur.

Pathology.—The distribution of the tuberculous process is frequently significant of its origin. It surrounds one ureter in cases in which the infection has spread along the ureter from the kidney. When the process has commenced in the seminal vesicle it is found immediately behind the trigone; when a tuberculous collection has ruptured through the bladder wall from the prostate a crater-like ulcer is found on one side of the trigone. In tuberculosis of the prostate tubercles may be found in the prostatic urethra, and tuberculous ulceration extending from this part of the urethra into the bladder. A tuberculous collection of the prostate may rupture into the prostatic urethra and spread thence into the bladder, the outlet of the bladder and the prostatic urethra being sometimes indistinguishable.

The tuberculous process commences in the mucous membrane as greyish tubercles surrounded by inflammation. (Plate 31, Fig. 4.) These become yellow from caseation and break down, forming a tiny superficial ulcer, the size of a pin's head, with sharply cut edges, and sometimes covered with blood clot. Several of these fuse and form larger ulcers.

Very extensive superficial ulceration may be present, covering a large area of the bladder wall. The exposed surface is pinkish-red and granular, and to it adhere numerous small white flakes. Deep ulcers may also be found. (Plate 31, Fig. 5.) They are round, oval, or serpiginous. The base is greyish-red and granular, the edge deeply undermined, and often with a thin, frayed margin of necrosing mucous membrane. The edge is not heaped up above the mucous membrane, and, where the condition is chronic, yellow tubercles are dotted around with little surrounding inflammation. Evidence of healing may be found at one part of the ulcer, and of spreading at another. In chronic tuberculous cystitis where there is no infection by other bacteria the lesions are discrete, the intervening mucous membrane being healthy. If infection with other bacteria is superadded these characteristics are lost, but the serpiginous outline is retained. Irregular masses of graunlation tissue may be found. Widespread infiltration of the submucous tissue and of the muscular coat takes place. In long-standing tuberculosis the bladder becomes contracted and fibrous. The perivesical fat is thickened and fibrous, and the bladder becomes adherent to the rectum and intestine and, in the female, to the genital organs. The pelvic lymphatic glands are tuberculous, but the formation of a tuberculous abscess is very rare. In a few cases the bladder cavity remains large and the wall is transformed into a thin fibrous layer, the contractile power of which is lost.

Together with these changes there is tuberculosis of the kidney on one or both sides, or tuberculosis of the seminal vesicles or prostate. Genital tuberculosis in the female is rarely found combined with vesical tuberculosis.

Symptoms.—The symptoms are those of spontaneous cystitis in a young man or woman. The onset is insidious, and the progress gradual but persistent. Variations in intensity of the symptoms frequently follow dietetic indiscretions and climatic changes. Frequent micturition is the earliest symptom. At first this is diurnal and moderate, the call coming every two or three hours, but it is progressive and becomes nocturnal and sleep is disturbed.

Small quantities of urine are passed every quarter- or half-hour during the day, and slightly less frequently at night. Micturition is urgent, and if the patient sleeps heavily the urine is passed involuntarily. Pain and intense desire are felt at the neck of the bladder when the patient attempts to hold water too long. There is scalding along the urethra during micturition, and cramp-like pain in the bladder and pain at the end of the penis, or at the external meatus in the female.

Hæmaturia is a frequent symptom, a few drops of bright blood passing at the end of micturition. In some cases there are occasional attacks of more severe hæmaturia at long intervals.

The urine is pale, faintly acid, of low specific gravity, and contains numerous fine dots and shreds, and a small quantity of pus well mixed, which gives it an opalescent appearance. Polyuria is present, and may be ascribed to the reflex effect of the frequent contractions of the bladder, but is probably the result of tuberculous changes in the kidneys. The quantity of pus is small, but it is constant. The symptoms are unaffected by movement, but are influenced by dietetic indiscretions and cold damp weather.

Complications.—Severe hæmaturia is rare. Retention of urine is an unusual complication. It may occur when there is tuberculosis of the prostate, and I have met with it twice as a post-operative complication lasting several days after nephrectomy for renal tuberculosis in women. The most serious complication is septic infection. The bacillus coli, staphylococcus, and streptococcus are the bacteria most frequently present, and are almost invariably introduced by the passage of instruments or by washing the bladder. With the advent of a mixed infection the symptoms increase in intensity. The cystitis, which may have been localized to one part of the bladder, becomes general, and septic pyelonephritis may be superadded to the tuberculous process in the kidney.

Course and prognosis.—The course of tuberculous cystitis when instrumental interference is withheld is slowly progressive, with periods of improvement and periods of relapse, dependent partly upon changes of diet and climate. There may be a period of acute cystitis at the commencement, which subsides, a slight subacute cystitis persisting. More frequently, however, the onset is insidious and the progress very gradual. After some years the nocturnal calls to micturate become very distressing, and the patient is worn out with loss of sleep. If septic complications are avoided, death takes place after some years from renal failure due to bilateral renal tuberculosis. More often there are septic complications, occasionally with secondary stone formation and subacute or chronic septic pyelonephritis. Where vesical tuberculosis is secondary to renal tuberculosis which is unilateral, and nephrectomy is performed, the tuberculous disease of the bladder may entirely disappear without further treatment. The same may occur when the lumen of the ureter becomes permanently obliterated without operation (*closed renal tuberculosis*). When the tuberculous process is secondary to disease of the prostate or seminal vesicle the prognosis is less favourable, owing to the difficulty of eradicating the primary focus.

Diagnosis.—The spontaneous development of slight persistent and progressive vesical irritation in youth or early adult life, when venereal disease can be excluded, should raise the suspicion of tuberculosis of the bladder.

On cystoscopy the presence or absence of cystitis is definitely ascertained. If it is present, the following questions must be answered :—

1. **Is the cystitis tuberculous ?**—(*a*) Examination of the urine. The urine is pale, faintly acid, opalescent, with a small quantity of suspended pus, and contains small white dots and shreds. The discovery of the tubercle bacillus in the urine is conclusive. The bacilli are more easily found when slight hæmorrhage is in progress. Failure to discover the tubercle bacillus on one occasion should not be accepted as final, and repeated examinations may be necessary. Inoculation of animals with the suspected urine should, if necessary, be carried out.

(*b*) Tuberculous disease may be found in the epididymis, seminal vesicles, or prostate, or in the lungs or elsewhere in the body.

(*c*) The cystoscope shows characteristic appearances. There are greyish-yellow opaque tubercles distinguished by being small, discrete, opaque, and having the appearance of pushing through the inflamed mucous membrane, which distinguishes them from the small cysts of cystic cystitis—semitransparent, often closely grouped, and set upon the surface of the mucous membrane, which is seldom much inflamed.

Chronic deep ulceration with undermined edges, healing at one part and spreading at another, is characteristic of tuberculosis. There may be general acute cystitis, or extensive superficial ulceration, or heaping-up of granulation tissue, none of which is characteristic of tuberculosis.

2. **Is the tuberculous cystitis secondary to renal or to genital tuberculosis ?**—Basal grouping of the tuberculous cystitis behind or on one side of the trigone, together with nodules

in the seminal vesicles or prostate, shows that the primary focus
is in these organs.

The presence of tuberculosis of the kidney is ascertained by

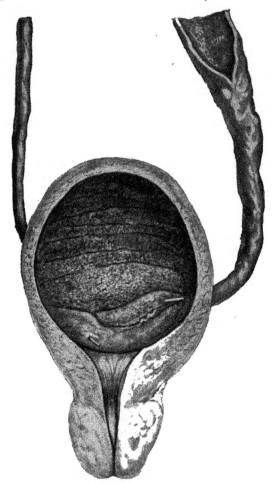

Fig. 120.—Specimen of bladder, ureters, and prostate in
case of urinary tuberculosis.

Universal tuberculous ulceration of bladder, the wall of which is much thickened ; right ureter
normal, left ureteric orifice dragged upwards and outwards and ureter thickened and dilated.
There was advanced tuberculosis of the left kidney.

examining the orifice of the ureter. Changes at the orifice and
grouping of tuberculous inflammation round it show disease of

the corresponding kidney. (Fig. 120.) The absence of changes at the second ureteral orifice does not exclude tuberculous disease of that kidney, and when both ureteric orifices are healthy renal tuberculosis may still be present. · The only reliable test is the passage of the ureteric catheter and examination of the urine withdrawn by it for pus and the tubercle bacillus.

Treatment.—When tuberculous cystitis is secondary to renal tuberculosis, the kidney, if one only is affected, should be removed, and in the majority of cases the cystitis diminishes and completely disappears. When bilateral renal tuberculosis is present, when the cystitis is secondary to tubercle of the prostate or seminal vesicle, when an active focus of tubercle exists elsewhere in the body, when no renal or genital tuberculosis can be demonstrated, or when the cystitis does not disappear after nephrectomy, other treatment is necessary.

General treatment.—Residence in a warm, dry climate, such as Egypt and Algiers, has a very beneficial influence. Arcachon, Biarritz, and the French or Italian Riviera are also suitable resorts for these tuberculous patients. The food should be plain and nourishing. Articles known to irritate the urinary tract, such as curries and highly spiced foods, and all alcoholic drinks, should be avoided. Plenty of milk and eggs and cod-liver oil in suitable quantity should be taken.

If the infection is mixed, urinary antiseptics should be used, but in pure tubercle they have no effect.

Guaiacol, 5 minims in capsule, thrice daily, has been recommended, and cacodylate of soda, $\frac{1}{2}$–1 gr. hypodermically, or guaiaco-cacodylate, $\frac{1}{2}$–2 gr. hypodermically, and disodium methylarsenate, $\frac{2}{5}$–3 gr. hypodermically, have also been used. Sandalwood oil, 10 minims in capsule, should be given for its soothing effect on the bladder, and belladonna and hyoscyamus to reduce the spasm of the bladder.

Tuberculin should be given in all cases, and very striking results are frequently obtained. The pain, frequency, and irritability diminish, the blood disappears from the urine, and the patient increases in body weight. When the cystitis is secondary to renal tuberculosis marked improvement is observed in early cases, sometimes with the disappearance of pus and tubercle bacilli for varying periods. The tuberculous disease of the bladder may completely disappear, and the ureter of the diseased kidney is found to be occluded. Relapses, however. occur, and observations extending over a few months are worthless in regard to the permanence of the cure. In genito-urinary tuberculosis the results are less favourable, but amelioration of the symptoms may be anticipated, and occasionally the genital tuberculosis heals under the treatment. The method of administration has been described elsewhere (p. 238).

Local treatment.—I am opposed to the local treatment by means of bladder-washing and instillations. Temporary improvement is observed in many cases, but septic complications almost invariably supervene and the patient is placed in a much worse condition. As, however, this view is not universally held, the following details of these methods are given: The bladder has been washed with boric acid and other solutions containing antipyrin or opium to soothe the pain. Instillations of ½–1 drachm of various drugs have also been given with a small syringe under strict aseptic precautions. Corrosive sublimate is used in strengths of 1 in 10,000 up to 1 in 5,000, the injections being repeated every two or three days and continued for a long time. With iodoform in liquid paraffin, 5 per cent., may be combined guaiacol, 5 per cent., which has the advantage of being analgesic. Gomenol, 10 or 20 per cent., in oil, has been instilled daily, or given in alternation with the corrosive sublimate instillations. Picric acid, ½–1 per cent., and carbolic acid, 5 per cent., have also been used.

Treatment by direct applications may be made in either sex through Luys' direct cystoscope. In this way ulcers may be scraped or cauterized with the electric cautery, with nitrate of silver, or lactic acid. Cystotomy may be performed either for drainage alone or for drainage after treatment of the tuberculous ulcers.

In the extremely rare cases where a single ulcer is present it is excised. In other cases the ulcers are curetted, cauterized, or treated with silver nitrate, chloride of zinc, or other caustics, and the bladder is drained. Suprapubic cystotomy is preferable to perineal cystotomy, for it permits of local applications.

Temporary relief may be obtained by these methods, but in a few months the condition relapses, and sepsis is invariably superadded, so that the condition of the patient is worse than before the operation.

LITERATURE

Casper, *Deuts med. Woch.*, 1900, p. 661.
Fenwick, *Trans. Med. Soc.*, 1905, xxvii. 242.
Hallé et Motz, *Ann. d. Mal. d. Org. Gén.-Urin.*, 1904, p. 161.
Karo, *Med. Rec.*, Oct. 2, 1909.
de Keersmackers, *Centralbl. f. d. Krankh. d. Harn- u. Sex.-Org.*, 1906, p. 413.
Pardoe, *Lancet*, 1905, ii. 1766.
Rovsing, *Arch. f. klin. Chir.*, 1907, p. 1.
Suter, *Centralbl. f. d. Krankh. d. Harn- u. Sex.-Org.*, 1901, p. 657.
Walker, Thomson, *Pract.*, May, 1908.

CHAPTER XXXIV

OTHER INFECTIONS OF THE BLADDER

BILHARZIOSIS

Etiology.—Bilharziosis is caused by a trematode worm named the *Bilharzia hæmatobia* or *Schistosomum hæmatobium.*

The disease is endemic in certain countries. In Africa, including Egypt, it is most prevalent, especially in Lower Egypt, where it is found in about one-third of the autopsies. Ferguson states that about one-half of the agricultural population of Egypt are shedding blood and bilharzia ova in their urine and fæces daily—a very serious drain on themselves, and a constant menace to their neighbours as a source of infection and re-infection. He found the disease present post mortem in 40 per cent. of 600 male subjects from 5 years of age upwards. Madden found that 10 per cent. of 11,698 patients had bilharziosis. It occurs also in Tunis, Algiers, on the west coast of Africa (Nigeria, etc.), and on the east coast (Abyssinia, Zanzibar, Madagascar). In South Africa it is common in Delagoa Bay, Natal, the Eastern Province of Cape Colony, and the Transvaal. The disease has been met with in Japan and China. In England a large number of cases were imported after the South African War. Major Smith, R.A.M.C., reports: "In ordinary times soldiers serving in South Africa were little subject to the disease, and it seems to have been of very minor importance as a cause of ill-health in former campaigns in that country. The Army Medical Department Reports for the period 1890 to 1898, when the garrison had an average numerical strength of 4,164, made no mention of bilharzia, while the reports dealing with the sick statistics of the Zulu and first Boer Wars contain no reference to it." The actual number admitted to hospital during the South African campaign (1899–1902) was 187, but the slighter cases were probably unnoticed or disregarded. All the cases that came under observation were mild (Simpson).

Mode of infection.—Infection takes place after bathing or prolonged immersion in infected rivers or pools, and, it is also stated, from the constant soaking of the bare feet in the rice fields. The incubation period is about three to six months. Males are much more frequently affected than females in the proportion of 93·2 males to 6·8 females (Madden). The disease is very common in boys; Kautsky found that 79 per cent. of boys in a school near Cairo had bilharziosis. Agricultural labourers and dwellers in the country are more frequently affected than town dwellers. Looss found that 30·5 per cent. of boys in a school in Cairo, and 80 per cent. in a school in the outskirts of the same town, had hæmaturia. The path by which invasion takes place is disputed.

(a) *The stomach.*—The embryo is supposed to be swallowed in the water during bathing or in drinking water. Against this theory is the fact that the embryo is killed by a much weaker solution of hydrochloric acid than is present in the normal stomach.

(b) *Through the urethra or anus.*—Allen holds that the parasite enters the urethra during prolonged immersion in infected water, and that it is more likely to do so if there is a long prepuce and care is not taken to dry the parts thoroughly after bathing. Circumcision he regards as a valuable preventive measure.

(c) *Penetration of the skin.*—This is held by most authorities to be the probable path of invasion. It is chiefly male earth-workers in country districts and their children who are affected.

Life-history of the trematode.—The male worm is 1 cm. long, flat, and with the lateral margins incurved to form a canal, and the female 2 cm. long; they are thread-like, and possess two suckers. The sexes are separate in the early stage, and at this time they occupy the portal vein. With sexual maturity they unite and find their way against the blood-stream to the veins of the submucous tissue of the bladder and rectum. (Fig. 121.) The eggs deposited by the female penetrate the mucous membrane, and are shed and appear in the urine and fæces. The ova are elliptical, and are contained in a thin yellow envelope which has a spine at the posterior end. Larger ova with a lateral spine are also found, most frequently in the liver or the rectum, and are probably deformed. If the ovum is placed in fresh water a ciliated embryo (Miracidium) escapes from the envelope and swims vigorously, and can be kept alive for twenty-four to forty-eight hours. The length of life of the worms is unknown. When they die the supply of ova ceases and the symptoms subside and disappear. The severe cases met with in Egypt are probably the result of often-repeated infection.

Pathology.—The disease affects the ureter (Fig. 121), bladder (Figs. 122, 123), urethra, and rectum, and rarely other parts of the body. Only urinary bilharziosis will be considered here.

1

2

3

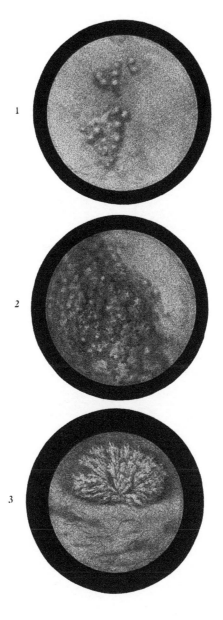

Fig. 1.—Bilharzial nodules in bladder. (P. 447.)

Fig. 2.—Bilharzial granulations in bladder. (P. 447.)

Fig. 3.—Villous papilloma of bladder. (P. 461.)

The mucous membrane becomes red and injected, and then inflamed and œdematous in patches. In these areas small yellowish-grey nodules the size of a millet-seed appear, and these rupture and leave ulcers, sometimes of considerable extent, which become covered with granulation tissue. (Plate 32, Fig. 1.) The mucous membrane has a brownish, sandy appearance in patches. Irregular excrescences of granulation tissue spread from the surface, forming

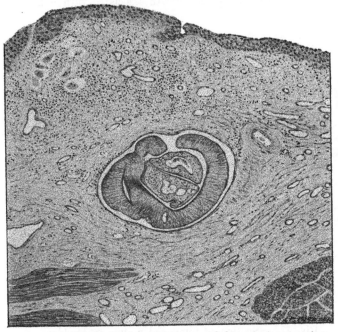

Fig. 121.—Wall of ureter in case of bilharziosis, showing male and female worms in vein.

The worms are cut transversely. The outer body with radiating structure is the male worm, while the female lies enfolded in the genital groove. A fold of the female worm has been cut so that it appears as two bodies. (*Section presented by Professor A. R. Ferguson, Cairo.*)

papilloma-like masses, or in ridges like the comb of a cock. These patches are adherent to the submucous tissue. (Plate 32, Fig. 2.)

Microscopically there is proliferation of the epithelium, which may grow downwards in glandular and cystic forms. (Fig. 123.) The submucous tissue is infiltrated and adherent. Ova are found in the mucous membrane, especially in the epithelial layer. They are perivascular in their grouping, suggesting a position in the lymphatics. They increase in numbers with the duration of the infection, few being seen in children and large numbers in adults. Stained with hæmatoxylin, the living ova are blue, and dead ova violet. (Fig. 122.) Old dead ova may become calcified. The granular masses consist of thickened inflamed mucous membrane with granulation tissue and numerous ova. True papillomatous tumours may develop, and malignant growths (carcinoma and sarcoma) are very frequently observed. Ferguson has described 40 cases of malignant growth associated with bilharziosis

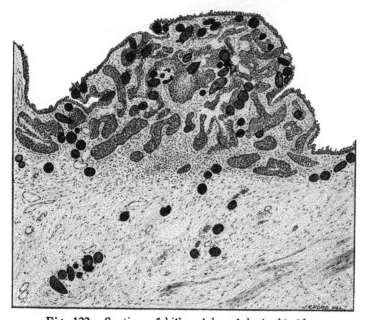

Fig. 122.—Section of bilharzial nodule in bladder.

There is a heaped-up mass of tubes of epithelium, in which are embedded numerous bilharzial ova.
(*Section presented by Professor A. R. Ferguson, Cairo.*)

of the bladder. The posterior wall was most frequently affected, but in many cases the whole bladder was a rigid spherical mass. In 34 cases the growth was carcinomatous—usually squamous epithelioma; in 6 it was sarcomatous. Lymph-glands were frequently affected.

In severe cases sepsis is almost invariably superadded, the urine becomes alkaline, there is widespread ulceration and sloughing of the epithelium and granulation tissue.

The interior of the bladder becomes encrusted with phosphatic material, from which portions may be detached, forming the nucleus of larger calculi. The bladder is contracted, and ascending pyelonephritis combined with dilatation of the ureters and the pelvis of the kidneys is common, and leads to a fatal termination. In a number of cases the urethra also becomes involved ; ulceration of the mucous membrane follows, and a deep crater coated with phosphates is formed. Around this an abscess usually develops, which ruptures in the perineum, and sinuses form. Madden, who has described this condition, points out that the bulbous urethra is the part affected, and that the sinuses start

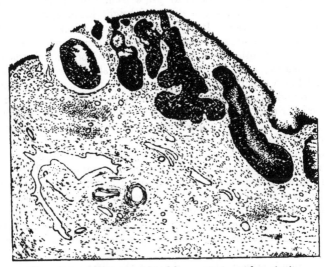

Fig. 123.—Section of bladder wall in bilharziosis.
Down-growths of epithelium into submucous layer.
(*Section presented by Professor A. R. Ferguson, Cairo.*)

from the urethra either laterally or even from the roof and track round between the corpus cavernosum and corpus spongiosum, opening to one side of the middle of the perineum and sometimes tracking round the anus on to the buttocks, scrotum, or pubes. A characteristic false elephantiasis of the scrotum and perineum may be produced by multiple fistulæ. The penile urethra may also be affected, and when the lesions are confined to the terminal one or two inches there is solid œdema of the glans and prepuce, sometimes accompanied by purulent urethral discharge. The whole penis may be involved, and there may be numerous fistulæ communicating with the urethra. Ulceration of the glans may lead to epithelioma. There may be nodules in the subcutaneous

2 D

and erectile tissues of the penis. The latter lead to extensive infiltration of the erectile tissue and great distortion of the organ and the urethra. The prostate and seminal vesicles are less frequently affected.

Symptoms.—Bilharziosis may exist without giving rise to symptoms. Milton found that of 35 cases in which bilharzia ova were found in the urine, in only 2 were symptoms of bilharziosis complained of. In bilharzial cystitis the chief symptom is hæmaturia. This appears spontaneously, and is persistent, although there may be intervals of clear urine from time to time. The hæmaturia is terminal, a few drops of bright blood appearing at the end of micturition. It is unaffected by movement. Rarely more severe hæmorrhage occurs. The hæmaturia may be unaccompanied by other symptoms. The urine contains shreds of various shapes, and frequently there are shreds with a small terminal blood clot in which an ovum can be found. The ova are readily found on microscopical examination of the urine. Frequent micturition and slight pain at the end of the penis are early symptoms in most cases. The irritability gradually increases and becomes distressing day and night.

On cystoscopy small yellow bodies about the size of a canary-seed are found projecting from the mucous membrane. They are usually grouped together in colonies, and a colony may have little or no surrounding inflammation. These bodies may closely resemble tubercles in tuberculous cystitis, but are larger, more prominent, more numerous, and more distinctly grouped. The formation of ridges of infiltrated mucous membrane on which are excrescences of granulation tissue, often with the bilharzial bodies dotted around, is very characteristic of the disease. Larger areas may be raised, and granular and papillomatous new growths may develop. As the disease advances the bladder becomes intensely irritable and cystoscopy becomes more and more difficult.

Complications.—In the later stages complications occur. Sepsis is the most constant of these, and leads to an intensely painful form of cystitis with alkaline urine and phosphatic encrustation. Madden describes a peculiar grey-green urine characteristic of the advanced stages of the disease.

Stone is a frequent complication. Of 65 cases, Goebel found stone in 34, and probable stone in 10 others. When the urine is still acid the stones may be composed of uric acid and oxalate of lime, sometimes with alternating layers of phosphates. They have as a nucleus bilharzia ova or portions of papillomas. When the urine has become alkaline they are invariably phosphatic, and may originate in detached portions of the phosphatic encrustations of the bilharzial ulcers. Papillomatous tumours develop late and may fill the whole of the bladder. Fistulæ appear in the perineum and suprapubically, and track in various directions. Malignant growth in the papillomatous tumours is not uncommon (p. 448).

Prognosis.—The type of bilharzial disease met with in South Africa and imported into this country is benign compared with the bilharziosis of Egypt. Colonel Simpson, R.A.M.C., states, in reference to the cases which occurred in the South African campaign, that " secondary changes involving the bladder and other parts of the urinary tract have not come under observation."

The virulence and malignancy of the Egyptian form appears to some extent to depend upon the prevalence of the disease and the habits of the agricultural population, which give opportunity for repeated re-infection. In ordinary cases, if the patient leaves the bilharzial country the symptoms disappear in about four years. I have re-examined the bladder in a case of vesical bilharziosis after an interval of four and a half years, and found the mucous membrane quite healthy.

The mortality of Egyptian bilharziosis or its immediate complications is just over 10 per cent. (Madden).

Treatment.—The treatment is prophylactic and symptomatic. No method of destroying the schistosomum is known. Preventive measures consist in forbidding bathing in infected rivers or pools, in thorough drying where a risk of infection has been taken, in circumcision of boys, and in boiling drinking-water. Removal of the patient from the bilharzial country is usually followed by recovery.

In the early stages Madden recommends 15 minims of the liquid extract of male fern thrice daily. The treatment of the cystitis is similar to that already described. Urotropine, methylene blue, and other urinary antiseptics are usually administered. Washing the bladder with weak solutions of silver nitrate, 1 in 10,000, or quinine, 4 per cent., or other antiseptics, or instillation of stronger solutions, may be carried out, especially where cystitis is present. Treatment of the bladder is, however, unsatisfactory, for the ova in the mucous membrane are constantly being renewed. When stone complicates the disease litholapaxy is to be preferred to cystotomy, and when in advanced disease bladder drainage is necessary the suprapubic route is more suitable than the perineal.

Day and Richards have tried salvarsan in the treatment of bilharziosis and found that it was worthless.

LITERATURE

Allen, *Lancet,* May 8, 1909, and Aug. 6, 1910.
Day and **Richards,** *Lancet,* 1912, i. 1126.
Elgood, *Brit. Med. Journ.,* Oct. 31, 1908.
Ferguson, *Journ. of Path. and Bact.,* 1911, p. 76.
Goebel, *Deuts. Zeits. f. Chir.,* 1906, p. 288.
Kautsky, *Wien. klin. Runds.,* No. 36.
Looss, *Menses Handbuch der Tropenkrankheiten.*
Madden, *Bilharziosis,* 1907; *Lancet,* Oct. 23, 1909; *Journ. of Trop. Med.,*
    Dec. 1, 1909; *Brit. Med. Journ.,* Oct. 1, 1910.
Simpson, *Journ. of R. A.M.C.,* 1910, p. 653.
Wilson, *St. Bart.'s Hosp. Repts.,* xlv.

SYPHILIS OF THE BLADDER

Scattered through the literature there are descriptions of syphilitic affections of the bladder. In the majority of cases proof of the syphilitic nature of the affections has been confined to the history of a syphilitic infection and the effect of treatment; cystoscopic and bacteriological examinations have been wanting. Recently, however, the writings of Frank, von Englemann, Pereschiwkin, and especially an exhaustive article by Asch, have placed the subject on firmer ground.

In secondary syphilis symptoms of an acute or chronic cystitis develop, frequent micturition and the presence of pus being most prominent. On cystoscopic examination there is congestion and swelling of the mucous membrane, and multiple small superficial ulcers with indurated edges may be present. Multiple (twelve) superficial round or oval ulcers with undermined edges and whitish base, resembling syphilitic plaques, have also been described.

In tertiary syphilis there may be gummata or ulcers, or both may be combined. The gummata may form papillomas which are indistinguishable from other forms of papilloma, except that they disappear under antisyphilitic treatment. In other cases a gumma has formed a round, circumscribed, nodular swelling, the size of a walnut, and covered with ulcerated mucous membrane. The ulcers have high infiltrated edges and a grey base. The symptoms resemble those of a new growth. There is hæmaturia, sometimes severe and terminal, and uninfluenced by rest. There are also frequency of micturition and pyuria.

Diagnosis.—The urine must be examined for the bacillus coli, tubercle bacillus, and other bacterial causes of cystitis and ulceration. The history, the presence of signs of active syphilis or the scars of postsyphilitic affections, and the effect of antisyphilitic treatment without local treatment are important in diagnosis.

. · Syphilitic papilloma and gumma disappear rapidly under treatment.

LITERATURE

Asch, *Zeits. f. Urol.*, 1911, p. 504.
von Englemann, *Folia Urol.*, 1911, p. 472.
Frank, *Verhandl. d. II. deuts. urol. Kongress*, Berlin, 1909, p. 356.
Heberern, *Centralbl. f. Chir.*, 1911, p. 663.
Hinder, *Austral. Med. Gaz.*, 1901, p. 92.
Lefur, VIᵉ Sess. de l'Assoc. franç. d'Urol., 1902, p. 524.
MacGowan, *Journ. Cutan. and Gen.-Urin. Dis.*, 1901, p. 642.
Margoulies, *Ann. d. Mal. d. Org. Gén.-Urin.*, 1902, p. 384.

ACTINOMYCOSIS OF THE BLADDER

Actinomycosis very rarely affects the bladder, and is always secondary to intestinal actinomycosis. The disease reaches the bladder by direct continuity, taking origin either in the appendix or in the rectum.

Extensive perivesical inflammation is present and there is usually a perivesical abscess.

The symptoms are those of cystitis, and on examination there is an indurated mass in the perivesical tissue and in the region of the appendix or round the rectum. Malignant growth or chronic appendicitis may be diagnosed. The diagnosis can only be made by the discovery of the yellow actinomycotic granules in the urine. The treatment consists in administering large doses of iodide of potash and in opening collections of pus if they exist. Iodides have not proved so successful as was at one time anticipated. If the bladder is invaded the cystitis is treated by urinary antiseptics and washing.

LITERATURE

Ruhrah, *Ann. Surg.*, 1899, p. 417.
Stanton, *Amer. Med.*, 1906, p. 401.

CHAPTER XXXV
TUMOURS OF THE BLADDER

TUMOURS of the bladder form about 3 per cent. of diseases of the urinary organs (Küster). Men are much more frequently affected (78 per cent.—Albarran) than women. In children vesical growths are rare, and are usually of the connective-tissue varieties. The age most frequently affected is from 40 to 60 years. Secondary growths of the bladder are uncommon, and result from the spread of malignant growths from the prostate, urethra, or rectum in the male, and from the uterus in the female. In the rare papillomatous tumours of the renal pelvis or ureter papillomatous new growths may become implanted on the bladder mucous membrane or spread from the ureteric orifice.

Etiology.—There is little exact knowledge of the origin of vesical neoplasms. The frequent situation of papillomatous growths in the immediate vicinity of the ureteric orifices has led to the view that some irritant in the urine may be the cause of the growth. The usual position is, however, above and to the outside of the ureteric orifice, while the stream of urine is directed downwards and inwards, the current passing just below the orifice of the opposite ureter.

Workers in aniline dyes (fuchsin, etc.) are stated (Wendel, Lichtenstein) to be especially liable to the development of papilloma of the bladder, and this is ascribed to some irritating effect these dyes exert upon the bladder mucous membrane. Malignant growths have been found to develop in a bladder the seat. of long-standing cystitis, but in the majority of cases where malignant disease and cystitis are combined the cystitis occurs as a complication of the growth. In 40 per cent. of malignant growths spontaneous cystitis is the first sign of disease. A malignant growth may develop in a patch of leucoplakia caused by chronic cystitis. In some cases of chronic cystitis papillomatous masses develop. These are cystic or solid (cystitis cystica, cystitis glandularis). Stoerk and Zuckerkandl have traced the development of glandular carcinoma of the bladder from cystitis glandularis. In bilharzial cystitis the development of papillomâtous and malignant new growths is so frequent as to indicate an etiological relationship.

Classification.—New growths of the bladder are conveniently divided into the following groups and subgroups :—

1. **Epithelial growths.**
    (1) *Benign.*
        (*a*) Papilloma.   Villous tumour.
        (*b*) Adenoma.
        (*c*) Cholesteatoma.
    (2) *Malignant.*
        (*a*) *Papillomatous.*
            Malignant villous growth.
            Nodular growths.
        (*b*) *Infiltrating.*
            Epithelioma.
            Adeno-carcinoma.
            Alveolar carcinoma.
2. **Connective-tissue new growths.**
    (1) *Simple.*
        (*a*) Fibroma.
        (*b*) Myoma.
        (*c*) Angioma.
    (2) *Malignant.*

    Sarcoma $\begin{cases} \text{Spindle-celled.} \\ \text{Round-celled.} \\ \text{Melanotic.} \\ \text{Rhabdo-myoma.} \\ \text{Chondro-sarcoma.} \end{cases}$

3. **Dermoid cysts.**

1. EPITHELIAL GROWTHS

PAPILLOMA—VILLOUS TUMOUR

Pathology.—These tumours are covered with villi or tendrils, and are either spread out over the surface of the mucous membrane (sessile) or set on a stalk (pedunculated). They vary in size from a split pea to a Tangerine orange, and may be single or multiple (30 to 40 per cent.—Albarran). The great majority are situated at the base, in the neighbourhood of the ureteric orifices, usually behind and to the outer side of these orifices, and frequently concealing them. They are rarely situated on the trigone, but frequently around it, and they may surround the urethral orifice. Other parts of the bladder are also affected, especially the posterior wall.

On section (Fig. 124) a papilloma shows a central fibrous trunk with branches subdividing in all directions. Microscopically the trunk consists of fibrous tissue containing elastic and plain muscle fibres, and supporting numerous large blood-vessels. Each branch and twig has a fibrous core containing blood-vessels, and is covered by a thick layer of epithelium (Fig. 125). This consists of layers of cells of the transitional epithelium type. The deeper cylindrical cells radiate from the core in characteristic manner, and are regular in arrangement and size. (Fig. 126.) Where the villi are closely

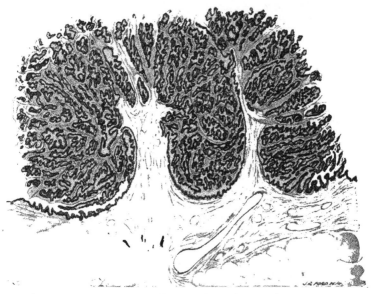

Fig. 124.—Slightly magnified section of operation specimen of papilloma of bladder.

Two papillomas are seen with villi closely packed together. The relation to the mucosa and muscular wall of the bladder is shown.

pressed together the superficial flat cells disappear and the cylindrical cell layers unite. The nuclei show karyokinetic figures in abundance. Vacuolation of the cells and the formation of spaces containing colloid material or epithelial débris are frequently observed. Œdema of the stroma of a branch may result from kinking. The tumour may consist of closely set, short finger-like processes (Fig. 127), looking, on surface and section, not unlike a cauliflower. A papilloma may remain solitary and increase to the size of a Tangerine orange ; more frequently small villous tumours appear around the parent growth, and others are dotted over the bladder, and finally the cavity may be filled with masses of papillomatous growth.

Dilatation of the ureter and kidney on the side corresponding to the growth is not infrequent.

The histological appearance of these growths is benign, but they possess certain characters by which they differ from other benign tumours.

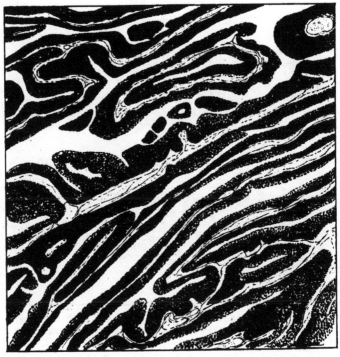

Fig. 125.—Microscopical section of papilloma of bladder.

i. They may spread by implantation. A portion of a papilloma of the kidney may be detached and implanted at the lower end of the ureter or in the bladder. Small buds of papilloma appear on normal mucous membrane around the parent tumour. Recurrence after an operation shows signs of implantation of papillomas in the track leading from the site of the original growth to the cystotomy scar, and the frequency with which a papilloma, usually the largest of the recurrent growths, is situated at the cystotomy wound.

ii. Recurrence very frequently takes place after removal, and the recurrent growth is multiple although the primary growth may have been single.

iii. The recurrent growths after operation or the multiple papillomas in a non-operated bladder become sessile and irregular in growth, and in a large number of cases eventually infiltrate the bladder wall

Symptoms.—Hæmaturia is the characteristic, and usually the

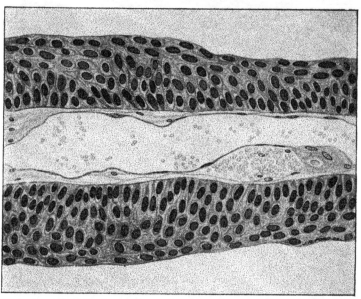

Fig. 126.—Highly magnified villus of papilloma of bladder with central capillary blood-vessel and covering of transitional epithelium.

only, symptom of papilloma of the bladder. It appears suddenly without ascertainable cause, continues for one or two micturitions or for a day or a week, and suddenly ceases. Rest has little effect on the hæmorrhage. The blood is copious, and mixed throughout the urine. Occasionally the first part of the urine is blood-stained, and a few drops of pure blood are expelled at the end of micturition. Flat or irregular clots may be present. After an interval of a few weeks, but more often of several months, and occasionally of one or two years, another attack of hæmorrhage occurs similar in character and duration to the first; and this recurs with diminishing intervals, and often with increasing duration of the hæmorrhage. The hæmorrhage comes from a ruptured vessel in a villus, and clot may be seen adhering when the hæmaturia has ceased.

Slight aching pain in one kidney is frequently present if the papilloma is situated in the neighbourhood of one ureter. Occasionally other symptoms are added. A patient under my care had an attack of intense pain and strangury, with the discharge of a few drops of bright blood from the urethra every few minutes. A pedunculated papilloma had engaged in the prostatic urethra and caused spasm of the bladder. Another patient with a pedunculated papilloma had five attacks of retention of urine from plugging of the internal meatus.

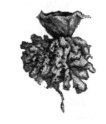

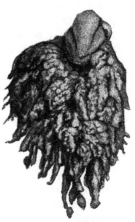

Complications.—Profound anæmia from recurrent hæmorrhages is not infrequent. Spontaneous cystitis is very rare, but cystitis very often follows the introduction of instruments, especially in cases of pedunculated papilloma, where some degree of urethral obstruction from plugging is usually present.

Cystitis leads to sloughing of portions of the growth, to the deposit of phosphates on the growth, and occasionally to the formation of stone.

Retention of clot from excessive hæmorrhage is rare. Retention of urine may occur from a pedunculated papilloma obstructing the internal meatus.

Fig. 127.—Papillomas of bladder, removed by operation.

At the upper part of each drawing is a portion of the mucous membrane and muscle of the bladder wall, removed with the tumour.

Course and prognosis.—The duration of papilloma of the bladder may extend over many years (ten to fifteen, even twenty-five); meanwhile the growth increases in size and forms a large single tumour, or multiplies and covers large areas of mucous membrane. It may very rarely remain quite stationary for many years, and I have seen a case of multiple recurrent papillomas in which the growths slowly diminished in size during seven years and have almost disappeared.

The average duration of life after the appearance of symptoms is stated to be about three years. In my experience it is much longer. Recurrence of growth after operation is very common, and is due to (a) new development of papilloma from the original cause, (b) incomplete operation, (c) implantation of fragments in the bladder wall during removal.

Malignant transformation is frequent, and may occur in un-operated or in recurrent growths. However benign the histo-logical characters of the original papilloma may be, clinical experience shows that recurrence after removal is very common, and that infiltration of the bladder wall occurs eventually in a large proportion of cases. Papilloma of the bladder cannot, there-fore, be looked upon as a benign tumour, and it is better to regard it as a precancerous condition in all cases.

Diagnosis.—" Symptomless " hæmaturia in a young or middle-aged adult is usually due to papilloma of the bladder, to " essen-tial renal hæmaturia," or to early renal growth. If tube casts are present the condition is renal. The quantity and appearance of the blood may be the same in all three conditions. The passage of fragments of papillomatous growth in the urine is important but rare. It is impossible to distinguish by the microscope be-tween fragments from papilloma of the bladder and from similar tumours in the renal pelvis or ureter, but the passage of papillo-matous masses from the kidney almost invariably gives rise to ureteral colic, and these papillomas are very rare. Evidence may also be obtained by the removal of portions of growth in the eye of a catheter.

Histologically there may be nothing to show whether the portion of papilloma has been detached from a benign papilloma or from the surface of a malignant growth.

Palpation of the bladder from the rectum and bimanually gives negative results in the great majority of papillomas, but when the growth is large and firm it can be felt in bimanual palpation in favourable cases. The diagnosis can only be certain when the cystoscope is used.

Cystoscopy.—Cystoscopy for symptomless hæmaturia should be made during an attack of bleeding, for should the hæmorrhage prove to be renal it will be seen from which ureter the blood is issuing. When the hæmorrhage arises from a vesical papilloma there is seldom difficulty in obtaining a clear medium.

A papilloma is seen as a round or irregular tumour with tendrils of varying length which float in the fluid and are stirred by every current or eddy. (Plate 32, Fig. 3.) They may resemble the fronds of a luxuriant fern or ostrich feathers, or they may be short and leaf-like and the tumour may be like a coarse bath sponge.

Each villus has a fine central vessel with lateral branches. The majority of papillomas have a short pedicle (subsessile), some have a long delicate stalk (pedunculated), and others are sessile. The tumour is most frequently situated on the upper and outer aspect of the ureteral orifice, which may be hidden by its branches. Usually a leash of vessels passes up to the growth from the trigone. Small buds of papilloma may be found on the mucous membrane in the neighbourhood, and other papillomas may be scattered about the bladder. Adherent clots appear as dark-red or black masses, and the tumour may be powdered with phosphates.

When the growth is very large the beak of the cystoscope may plunge into it, and the light is obscured so that no view is obtained.

Treatment. Non-operative.—Prolonged treatment by washing the bladder with solutions of nitrate of silver and resorcin with the object of causing necrosis of the tumours has been advocated by Casper, Herring, and others. Daily instillations of 2 oz. of nitrate of silver solution (1 in 3,500 at 100° F.) are made by means of a catheter and retained for a few seconds, and then repeated once. The instillations are best made at night, and the patient feels only a slight warmth for half an hour. The strength of the solution is gradually increased to 1 in 1,000, and the treatment continues for six months.

Solutions of resorcin (2 per cent. up to 10 per cent.) have also been used bi-weekly. This method has apparently met with an occasional success or partial success. It may be useful in cases which are unsuitable for operation, or which have recurred and are still small.

Radium and the high-frequency current (fulguration) are under trial. Radium is inserted in a catheter into the bladder and a radium plate applied suprapubically, or radium may be suspended in the rubber drainage tube after suprapubic operation as a prophylactic measure. For high-frequency treatment an electrode is applied to the growth through a catheterizing cystoscope, a flat electrode being applied suprapubically.

Operative treatment. (a) *Removal through the urethra.* "*Intravesical operations.*"—This is carried out by means of the Nitze operating cystoscope (or some modification of it), or by Luys' direct cystoscope, or in the female through Luys' or Kelly's cystoscope. A fine platinum wire is projected from a tunnel in view of the cystoscope window and is passed over the tumour, which is snared and left in the bladder to be expelled in the urine. If the papilloma is very large, portions of it are removed at several sittings. Hæmorrhage is sometimes severe after these operations. The growths must be favourably situated. Tumours near the neck of the bladder are unsuitable. Those at the base and on the posterior wall are most suitably placed.

With the direct cystoscope the growth can be touched with the electric cautery, or removed with forceps or a snare and the base cauterized.

Malignant growths should not be operated on by this method. The advantages claimed for it are the small mortality, the avoidance of complications such as sepsis, fistula, phlebitis, or pneumonia, the ability of the patient to continue work, the avoidance of danger of implanting tumour cells, and its greater applicability to recurrent tumours. The open operation applied to cases suitable for intravesical removal should, however, have no mortality; complications such as those mentioned should not occur with thorough aseptic operation, and the after-treatment of the bladder (see p. 465) should prevent any possibility of implantation. Very small recurrent growths may be treated by intravesical removal, but the tendency of recurrent growths to become malignant must be remembered.

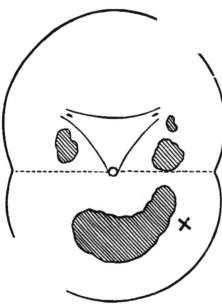

Fig. 128.—Cystoscopic chart of multiple papilloma of bladder.

The trigone with ureteric and urethral orifices is shown, and the number and position of the growths. At X a small papilloma was concealed from the view of the cystoscope behind the larger growth.

Good results in small growths have been obtained by some surgeons. Weinrich found that 71 cases out of 101 operated before 1902 had no recurrence. There were 18 cases of recurrence, and 12 cases were untraced. The mortality was 1 in 150.

(b) *Removal by open operation.*—This is the most radical form of treatment, and, in view of the pathology, should be adopted in all cases when no contra-indication to an operation exists. If multiple papillomas are present a chart showing their number and position must be drawn at a preliminary cystoscopy. (Figs. 128, 129.)

Suprapubic cystotomy is performed by a vertical median incision 3 in. in length, the peritoneum being pushed aside. The edges of the bladder wound are held by two catgut traction sutures, and the patient is placed in the Trendelenburg position. Suitable bladder retractors (Fig. 130) are introduced, a small retractor being placed on the side of the growth and a large one on the opposite side. With a powerful head-lamp the interior of the bladder is thoroughly examined. A solitary pedunculated papilloma (Fig. 131) is picked up with forceps, the pedicle put on the stretch, and a double catgut suture passed through it and tied. The pedicle is then cut through, and with it an area of bladder mucous membrane which was raised by the traction. In sessile papilloma (Fig. 132) the mucous membrane is raised and cut through half an inch from the tumour, and the incision carried round it at this distance, so that a good margin of healthy mucous membrane is removed with the growth (Fig. 133). The mucous membrane is then

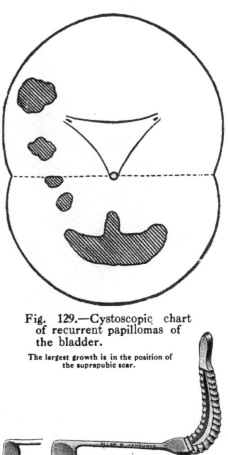

Fig. 129.—Cystoscopic chart of recurrent papillomas of the bladder.

The largest growth is in the position of the suprapubic scar.

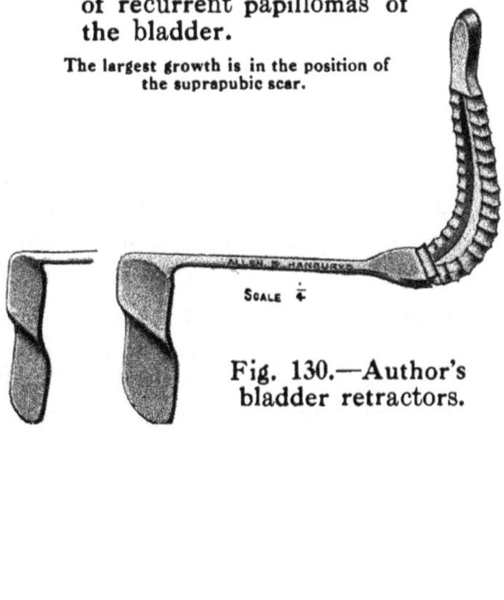

Fig. 130.—Author's bladder retractors.

brought together and bleeding controlled by catgut stitches. I use special needles on pliable handles (Fig. 134), long fine forceps (Fig. 135), and curved scissors (Fig. 136) for these operations. If a number of papillomas are situated close together the whole area of mucous membrane bearing them is removed

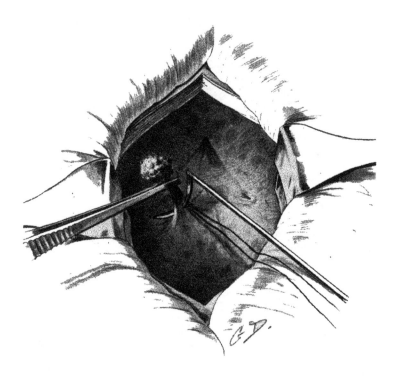

Fig. 131.—Removal of pedunculated papilloma of bladder.

The patient is in the Trendelenburg position, and the edges of the suprapubic cystotomy wound are widely retracted. The papilloma is grasped with long forceps, and the base of the pedicle is transfixed by a needle with catgut.

in one strip (Fig. 137). I have removed an area as large as the palm of the hand, and in one case half the mucous membrane of the bladder was stripped off. When the papilloma lies near the orifice of the ureter a catheter should be passed up the duct in case it may be included in the stitches. Great care is taken not to soil the mucous membrane by contact with the papilloma during removal. At the end of the operation I treat

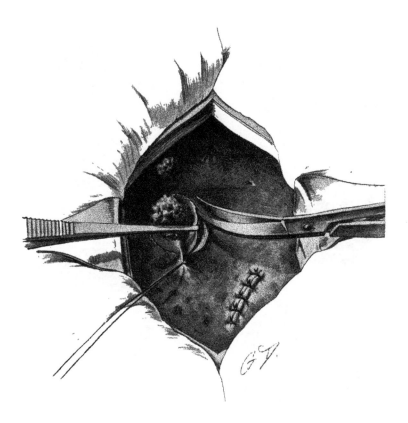

Fig. 132.—Removal of multiple sessile papilloma of bladder.

A traction suture steadies and raises the mucous membrane on the near side of the papilloma. The mucous membrane is cut round the base of the growth with long curved scissors and dissected up, carrying with it the growth. The cut edges of mucous membrane are united with catgut. On the right is a wound already closed.

the bladder with silver nitrate solution 5 or 6 per cent., formalin 1 in 300, resorcin 10 per cent., or other albumin coagulant, with the object of destroying stray cells or microscopic papillomas.

2 E

The bladder is drained through a large suprapubic tube, and washed daily with weaker solutions of these drugs.

The suprapubic wound may be closed at the end of the operation with catgut sutures and a catheter placed in the urethra, but

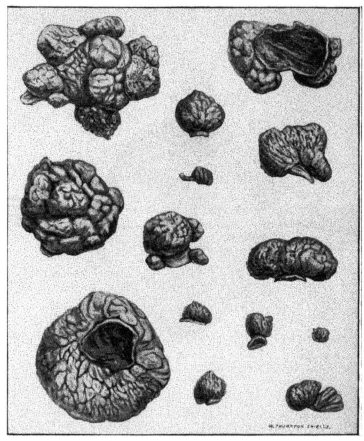

Fig. 133.—Group of papillomas removed from bladder.

The tumours are removed with an area of mucous membrane, which shrinks after removal. In two the under surface is shown. An area of mucous membrane bearing eight separate tumours is seen at the upper left-hand corner.

if this is done the treatment of the bladder with strong solutions must be omitted. Complete immediate suture of the bladder with catheter drainage may even in the simplest operation for papilloma lead to hæmorrhage which necessitates opening up the suprapubic wound, and I have now abandoned it and drain every case supra-pubically.

In removing the papillomas a Guyon's clamp may be used,

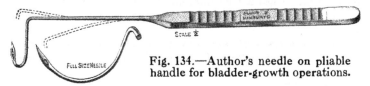

Fig. 134.—Author's needle on pliable handle for bladder-growth operations.

but it is rarely necessary, and may injure the ureteric orifice. After convalescence the bladder should be examined at regular intervals with the cystoscope for recurrence.

In its earliest stage a recurrent bud of papilloma should be treated by a fine electric cautery applied through a Luys' cysto-

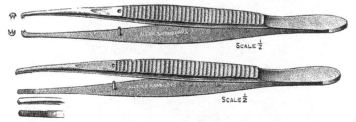

Fig. 135.—Long toothed and serrated forceps for bladder-growth operations.

scope, or instillation of nitrate of silver may be tried. If the recurrent tumour is large or multiple a second suprapubic operation is necessary.

When the bladder cavity is filled with large numbers of papillomatous growths the operations described are inapplicable. The

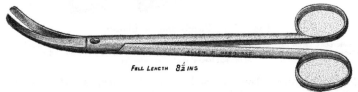

Fig. 136.—Long curved scissors for bladder-growth operations.

choice then lies between palliative, non-operative treatment, and operative treatment. Operative treatment consists in (1) opening the bladder and clearing out the contents, and stopping the bleeding by means of the cautery, hot douche, nitrate of silver, adrenalin, or, better, packing the bladder with gauze round a large rubber tube which leads down to the ureters ; or (2) the total removal of the bladder (cystectomy) after ureterostomy. The latter operation has a high immediate and remote mortality, but it is the only method by which cure can be obtained in these cases.

Transperitoneal cystotomy has been advocated (Harrington, Mayo) as an easier method of approach in operating on papilloma

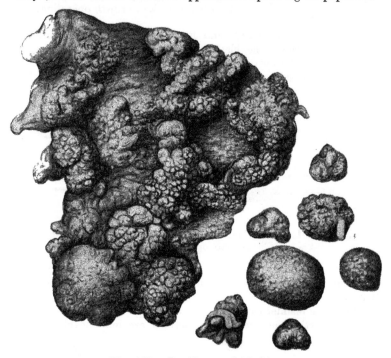

Fig. 137.—Papilloma of bladder.

Numerous discrete papillomas, and one large area of mucous membrane covered with papillomatous masses. The extent of this portion of mucous membrane was half the posterior and the whole of the left lateral wall of the bladder.

of the bladder. This method is unnecessary, as there is no difficulty in obtaining full exposure and room for manipulation by the ordinary extraperitoneal route.

Palliative treatment.—In cases in which radical operation is abandoned, certain complications and symptoms may arise which require treatment.

Hæmorrhage.—Unless the case is acknowledged to be inoperable, the proper treatment for hæmorrhage is early removal of the growth, and the less the bladder is interfered with before the operation the better. Hæmorrhage so severe as to cause acute anæmia seldom occurs. The patient is kept in bed and a morphia suppository ($\frac{1}{4}$ gr.) or a hypodermic injection of morphia ($\frac{1}{6}$–$\frac{1}{4}$ gr.) given. Calcium lactate in doses of 10 or 15 gr. every four hours is given for two days, but if hæmorrhage persists beyond this time it is then omitted. Ergot, iron salts, tannin, acetate of lead, and suprarenal extract given internally have all been used, but in my experience they are worthless. Washing the bladder should be avoided if possible, as there is a very serious risk of introducing sepsis. Should it become necessary, a large coudé catheter (10 or 12 Fr.) should be passed under the strictest aseptic precautions and the bladder washed out by means of an irrigator. About 4 or 6 oz. are allowed to run in and to escape, and this is repeated until several pints have been used. The best solution is silver nitrate, 1 in 10,000, and it should be used hot (110° to 120° F.).

Another method is to pass a double-way catheter and run a continuous stream of hot silver nitrate solution through the bladder. A weak solution of adrenalin (1 in 100,000) may be used, but it is not so efficacious.

Instillations of stronger solutions may be used, such as silver nitrate solution (3 oz. of 1-in-1,000 or 1-in-500 solution) or adrenalin (1 oz. of 1-in-2,000 solution). These are allowed to remain in the bladder for a few minutes and then run off. The following may also be used, viz. 3 oz. of a sterilized solution of gelatin (2 per cent.), or 2 oz. of creolin solution ($\frac{1}{2}$–1 per cent.) at a temperature of 105° F., retained for twenty or thirty minutes.

If clotting has occurred in the bladder the clots are extracted with a large evacuating cannula with rubber bulb, such as is used in litholapaxy. This method should be employed with the utmost caution and under strict aseptic conditions, and should not be persisted in if it is not at once successful. After removal of the clots a large catheter should be fixed in the urethra and the bladder washed frequently with normal saline solution to prevent recurrence of clotting, or a double-way catheter and continuous irrigation with normal saline solution should be installed. Finally, should these methods fail, the bladder should be opened suprapubically, the clots cleared out, and a large rubber tube inserted.

Bladder spasm.—In the later stages of recurrent and inoperable papilloma and in infected cases there may be distressing frequency of micturition and painful spasm of the bladder. The general and local treatment for cystitis should be carried out.

Instillations into the bladder of a few ounces of distilled water containing antipyrin (2 per cent.) and laudanum (1 per cent.), or of orthoform (5 to 10 per cent.), or the use of suppositories containing belladonna ($\frac{1}{4}$ gr.) and morphia ($\frac{1}{8}$-$\frac{1}{4}$ gr.) or lupulin (4 gr.), may give temporary relief.

The injection of 20 or 30 minims of sterilized water, or eucaine (2 per cent.) or cocaine (1 per cent.), into the sacral canal may also assist (see p. 383).

Permanent suprapubic drainage may become necessary, and the opportunity may be taken to clear out the papillomatous material and apply nitrate of silver solution.

In some cases the pain and spasm continue in spite of this, and nephrostomy or permanent drainage of the kidneys, or ureterostomy, by bringing the ureters to the surface in the loin or groin, may be necessary in order to direct the urine from the hypersensitive organ.

Results.—The mortality of open radical operations on papilloma of the bladder is very small under modern conditions. Rafin found a mortality of 3·8 per cent. in 156 cases operated on in recent years. Recurrence of papilloma after operation is frequent. In Rafin's collection there were 33 cases of recurrence out of 115 cases traced (28 per cent.). In 18 cases there was no recurrence for over three years, and non-recurrence was reported in periods as long as fourteen and twenty years. Recurrence four and eight years after operation has been recorded. The recurrent tumours are usually multiple, and may have the same characters as the primary growth. There is a marked tendency, however, for the type to change. The tumour becomes more and more sessile, the villi shorter, and the surface smoother, and finally infiltration of the submucous and muscular coats takes place.

Watson found that about 60 per cent. of pedunculated papillomas were cured by operation, but only 2 per cent. of sessile and multiple papillomas. The number of cases of recurrence will, I hold, be greatly reduced by careful preoperative charting of multiple growths, by thorough operation, and by treatment of the bladder with strong solutions after the operation.

ADENOMA

Adenoma is a rare tumour so far as the bladder is concerned. It arises in the glands in the region of the base of the bladder, and is found in two forms, a diffuse and a circumscribed (Rochet and Martel). The tumours have a smooth or villous surface. Rafin collected 11 operated cases.

CHOLESTEATOMA

This rare condition was described by Rokitansky, and 10 cases were collected from the literature by Rafin. There is great thickening of the epithelium, which becomes squamous and presents a pearly appearance. Masses of epithelial débris are thrown off and collect on the surface. The whole urinary tract may be affected.

CARCINOMA

A number of malignant growths differing widely in their gross and microscopic characters are grouped under this heading.

The following grouping of varieties is clinical, and will be of greater use to the surgeon than a strictly pathological classification:

(1) *Malignant Papilloma*

However benign the macroscopic appearances of a villous growth of the bladder may be, the majority, as already stated, eventually become malignant if untreated. Some papillomas are malignant from their earliest stage of development. Macroscopically, malignant papillomas may be similar in appearance to those of benign form, but certain characters can usually be detected. The villi are more stunted and less regular in size and shape, the tumour is sessile and irregular in contour. Infiltration of the bladder wall commences, and the mucous membrane at the base is thickened and adherent to the submucous tissue. Microscopically the epithelial cells show rapid and very irregular proliferation. The base shows the invasion of lymphatic spaces and veins by irregular masses of cells. Another type of malignant papilloma is malignant from its earliest appearance. The growth is very rapid and irregular, and luxuriant on the surface, so that the bladder is rapidly filled with a friable mass from which portions slough off and are discharged in the urine.

(2) *Nodular Growths*

These are sessile, or rarely have a short pedicle, and vary in size from a hazel-nut to a chestnut or a Tangerine orange. The surface may be irregular with nodules varying in size, or there may be a large single mass with a regular nodular surface. Occasionally there is a round tumour with flat surface, the centre of which is depressed and shows short villi, with sometimes a hard, brown, pigmented, calcareous mass adherent to it. The margin is rounded and vertically ridged. (Plate 33, Figs. 1, 2, 3.)

These tumours belong to the papillomatous group. (Fig. 138.) The surface consists of a dense mass of irregular villi closely welted together, and sometimes necrotic on the surface about the centre. In the deeper part there is a fine stroma of fibrous tissue supporting irregular spaces filled with cells. In these spaces papillary

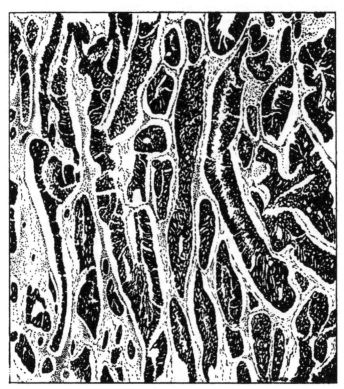

Fig. 138.—Microscopical section of a nodular malignant growth (papillomatous variety).

formations are frequently seen. Masses of cells infiltrate the muscular planes passing along the lymphatic vessels.

(3) *Infiltrating Growths*

The growth forms flat nodules on the surface of the mucosa, but its most extensive growth is intramural. Not infrequently it takes the form of a hard, depressed ulcer surrounded by nodules or by a raised, hard ring of growth. (Plate 34.) The histological structure varies.

(a) *Squamous epithelioma (chancroid)*.—This takes origin in a patch of leucoplakia (Fig. 139). The greatly thickened and heaped.

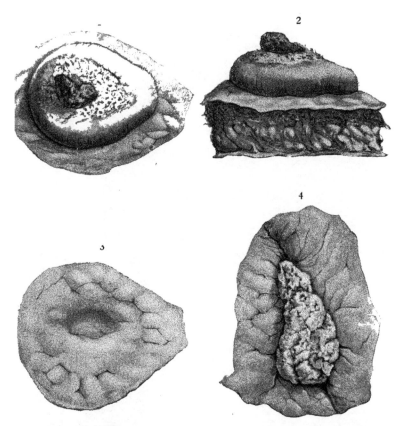

Figs. 1, 2, 3.—Views of operation specimen of malignant growth of bladder (nodular papilloma). On surface is a mass of clot encrusted with phosphates. The third figure shows peritoneal surface. (Pp. 473–8.)

Fig. 4.—Recurrence of malignant growth of bladder in scar of resection wound. Operation specimen of second operation. Patient well three and a half years later. Primary tumour, *see* Plate 35, Fig. 3. (P. 485.)

PLATE 33.

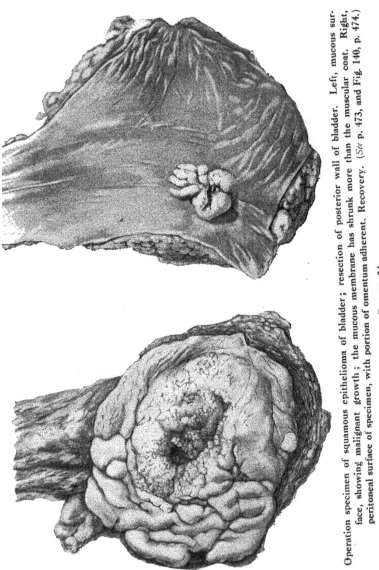

Operation specimen of squamous epithelioma of bladder; resection of posterior wall of bladder. Left, mucous surface. Right, the mucous membrane has shrunk more than the muscular coat. Right, face, showing malignant growth; the mucous membrane has shrunk more than the muscular coat. Right, peritoneal surface of specimen, with portion of omentum adherent. Recovery. (*See* p. 473, and Fig. 140, p. 474.)

PLATE 34.

up epithelium infiltrates the submucous tissue and a depressed
ulcer is formed. The growth has the structure of a squamous
epithelioma with cell nests. (Figs. 140, 141, and Plate 34.)

(b) *Cylindrical epithelioma* or adeno-carcinoma consists of round
or oval spaces lined with one or two layers of cylindrical epithelium.
These tumours develop at the base of the bladder, and are comparatively rare. Stoerk and Zuckerkandl have shown the close
relation between this form of growth and cystitis glandularis.

(c) *Alveolar carcinoma.*—Alveoli of varying sizes, branching and

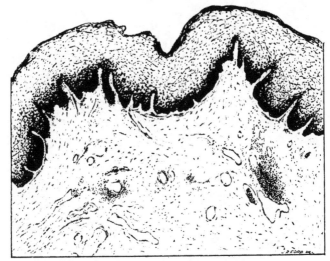

Fig. 139.—Leucoplakia of mucous membrane in neighbourhood
of large squamous epithelioma of bladder.

Note the presence of papillæ and the large, clear, flat nucleated cells.

tubular, filled with cells of varying shape and size, many of which
are cylindrical and others spheroidal, are set in a stroma of connective tissue. The proportion of the cellular elements to the
stroma varies. With an excessive development of the former
a soft tumour is formed, while a highly developed stroma forms
a scirrhus. When stroma and cellular elements are equally
balanced it is customary in German literature to term the growth
" carcinoma simplex."

Spread of growths of the bladder.—Growths remain for a
long time localized in the bladder. The spread is intravesical,
intramural, perivesical, glandular, and metastatic.

The intravesical spread of papillomatous growths may be

rapid and extensive. It appears to take place by implantation, small papillomas occurring on the mucous membrane around the original tumour. After removal of a papilloma recurrence takes place in a form which also suggests implantation. A track of papillomas is seen from the site of the original growth to the suprapubic scar, and the largest, and occasionally the only, recurrent tumour is situated on the vesical aspect of the cystotomy scar.

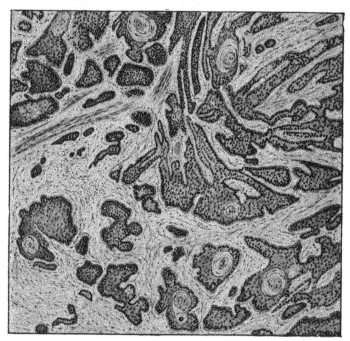

Fig. 140.—Section of squamous epithelioma of bladder showing cell nests. (*See* Plate 34.)

Propagation by contact is occasionally seen in malignant growths of the bladder. A small secondary growth develops on the portion of the bladder wall which comes in contact with the parent tumour when the viscus is empty. The anterior and superior walls are those affected in this manner. (Fig. 141.)

Owing to the peculiar distribution of the lymphatic vessels (*see* p. 348) malignant growths may spread widely in the muscular coat while their extent is still limited in the mucous and submucous layers. Rapid penetration of the growth through all the coats of the bladder wall is a feature in some tumours which do not spread laterally.

The perivesical spread is sometimes as extensive as the intra-vesical growth, and this part of the growth is surrounded by dense fibrous fat. Adhesions to the vagina, uterus, rectum, and intestines take place in the later stages, and perforation may occur. The spread along the lymphatics follows the large trunks (*see* p. 348). The first glands are a few small lymph nodules in the outer coat of the bladder, and then the larger lymph-glands serving the different regions of the bladder are affected. Pasteau states that the glands along the internal iliac arteries are affected

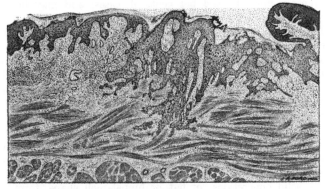

Fig. 141.—Small epitheliomatous ulcer (contact growth) on anterior wall of bladder.

There was an extensive nodular malignant growth at the base.

in 79 per cent. and the lumbar glands in 26 per cent. of cases. This refers to the advanced stage found post mortem.

In the latest stages secondary deposits may be found in the lung, pleura, liver, spleen, or kidney.

Symptoms.—The onset of symptoms is usually insidious; occasionally there is a sudden severe attack of hæmaturia with-out previous symptoms.

Hæmaturia is the most frequent (90·2 per cent. of cases) and the earliest (61·7 per cent.) symptom. The bleeding usually com-mences gradually. A little blood appears at the end of micturi-tion. This passes off, and reappears and increases till the whole urine is stained. Clots are frequently present (34 per cent.). Persistent slight terminal hæmaturia may be observed, with occasional attacks of severe hæmorrhage.

Frequent micturition occurs in 68 per cent. of cases, and may be the first symptom (14·7 per cent.). It is nocturnal as well as diurnal, and may increase until urine is passed every ten or fifteen minutes during the day, and every half-hour at night. There is urgency, and sometimes the necessity to empty the bladder is uncontrollable. These symptoms are usually due to cystitis, but may occur without cystitis and with a clear urine.

Pain may be due to cystitis, to obstruction by blood clot, or to pressure upon nerves. It is felt along the urethra, at the end of the penis, in the suprapubic region and groin, in the perineum, anus, and down the thighs or along the sciatic nerve. Posterior renal pain may be unilateral or bilateral, and is due to obstruction of the ureters or to ascending pyelonephritis. Although pain is frequently present (63·4 per cent. of cases) and may be the first symptom (8·8 per cent.), it is never severe.

The urine may be clear in the intervals of hæmaturia, and contain no abnormal elements. Occasionally a persistent excess of epithelial cells from the bladder may be found. Portions of growth may be passed. These are villi from the surface of the growth, and their structure may be that of a benign papilloma. In some cases the irregularity of cell growth and rapidity of proliferation suggest malignancy.

When cystitis is present the urine contains pus, mucus, and blood. The urine may be alkaline and stinking. It contains greyish or brownish shreds, which may be blood clot, muco-pus, or necrotic portions of growth. Masses of mucus and phosphatic or more solid concretions, of flat or limpet-shell shape, form on ulcerated patches and are discharged with the urine. Difficult micturition (12 per cent. of cases) is due to large luxuriant growths, or to smaller growths situated near the urethral orifice.

Emaciation is present in advanced cases. It is not a reliable sign of malignancy, for it may be caused by chronic septic pyelonephritis.

Diagnosis.—Cases of malignant growth of the bladder present two chief types, a cystitis and a hæmaturia type.

(1) **Cystitis type** (40 per cent.).—The onset may be sudden or gradual, and occurs without the passage of an instrument.

The following conditions may also give rise to spontaneous cystitis in a man of 50 years or over :—

(a) *Stone.*—Here the onset is less acute. Pain is a much more prominent symptom ; it is sharp, is felt at the end of the penis and at the close of micturition. Hæmaturia, if present, is terminal and moderate, and the blood is bright. Frequent micturition only appears during the day ; the patient sleeps throughout the night without waking. All the symptoms of stone are greatly increased by movement and shaking.

(b) *Simple enlargement of the prostate.*—The onset of frequent micturition is gradual. Nocturnal frequency is pronounced and commences in the early morning after a rest of five or six hours. Hæmaturia may be absent, and there is no pain.

(c) *Malignant disease of the prostate.*—In this condition there is gradually increasing difficulty in micturition, pain is a prominent and persistent symptom (72·5 per cent. of cases), hæmaturia is rare, and movement has no influence on the symptoms.

(2) **Hæmaturia type** (60 per cent.).—These cases are most likely to be confused with simple papilloma or with tuberculous disease of the bladder. In simple papilloma the patient is usually younger (under 45) than in malignant growth (average, 57 years). The hæmaturia is sudden, copious, and intermittent in papilloma; it is insidious, terminal, persistent, and increasing in malignant growth. The hæmaturia of papilloma is usually the only symptom, while frequent micturition and other symptoms are present in malignant growth. There is no change in symptoms to show when a simple papilloma takes on malignant characters.

Tuberculous disease usually occurs in younger patients. It can frequently be detected in the genital system (epididymis, prostate, seminal vesicle), or there are tuberculous lesions elsewhere in the body. The tubercle bacillus is found in the urine.

Examination.—Discrete, shotty enlargement of the groin glands is occasionally present (12 per cent. of cases). Enlarged lymphatic glands can be detected in the pelvis on rectal examination in the advanced cases. These are found in a band of tissue at the upper and outer angle of the prostate on each side, and are the lowest glands of the lymphatic chain.

Palpation of the base of the bladder from the rectum or vagina, and especially by bimanual examination, may detect a thickening of the wall.

Cystoscopy.—Hæmorrhage and spasm of the bladder may render cystoscopy difficult.

The following are the chief types of malignant growth as seen with the cystoscope :—

(a) **Villous growth.**—In some cases there is nothing to distinguish simple from malignant papillomas. Usually, however, the latter are sessile, the villi are stunted, more closely packed, and less regular. In the same bladder there are pedunculated and sessile growths. Signs of infiltration of the bladder wall may be present. The pedicle is thickened and more fleshy, the surrounding mucous membrane is ridged and puckered, and may have an infiltrated, velvety appearance. Small œdematous tags may project from the mucous membrane, and separate nodules may be seen.

(b) **Nodular sessile or pedunculated growths.**—These vary in size from a large pea to a Tangerine orange. The surface is smooth, and may be firmly or coarsely nodular, opaque, and pink or yellowish-pink in colour. (Plate 35.) The surrounding mucous membrane may show signs of infiltration. The centre of the growth is sometimes depressed and covered with a gritty mixture of blood clot and phosphates (Plate 33), or may be necrotic (Plate 35).

(c) **Infiltrating nodular growths and depressed ulcers.**—The appearances have already been described. (Plate 34.) The unaffected portion of the mucous membrane is usually the seat of subacute or chronic cystitis. Phosphatic deposit may take place on the growth.

Course and complications.—The average duration of life after the first appearance of symptoms is said to be under three years, but this estimate requires qualification. The duration of symptoms in papilloma of the bladder which eventually becomes malignant may be ten or fifteen years. Hard infiltrating growths forming a depressed ulcer are very chronic, although the duration is shorter than that of papilloma. Those of the rapidly growing papillomatous variety have a very short history, death taking place frequently under a year and always under two years.

Septic complications usually result from the passage of instruments, and if untreated ascending pyelonephritis eventually follows.

Obstruction of the ureters is a frequent complication of bladder growths. If one ureter is involved and the obstruction is gradual an intermittent hydronephrosis results. If both ureters are occluded, obstructive anuria supervenes. Anuria may come on suddenly with no previous symptoms, or after symptoms lasting a few hours. Lymphatic glands are involved late, and metastatic deposits in the lungs and liver are rare.

Treatment.—The treatment is operative or non-operative, and the operative treatment is radical or palliative.

Selection of cases for radical operation.—Of 41 consecutive cases under my observation, only 15 (36·5 per cent.) were fit for the operation when first submitted for examination.

Cases suitable for a radical operation must fulfil the following conditions : (1) The growth must be confined to the bladder. (2) The patient must be sufficiently robust to undergo a severe operation.

Evidence of disease of the kidneys or of renal failure, of bronchitis or emphysema, of a weak or failing circulation, must be held as a contra-indication to radical operation.

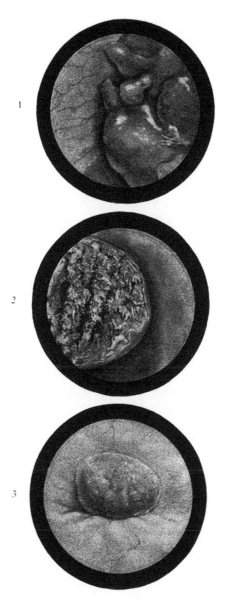

Fig. 1.—Nodular malignant growth of bladder.

Fig. 2.— Nodular malignant growth of bladder with necrotic surface.

Fig. 3.—Small nodular malignant growth of bladder. Recurrent growth after removal. (*See* Plate 33, Fig. 4.)

The radical operations that may be performed in suitable cases are (1) resection of the bladder wall and (2) cystectomy.

Choice of radical operation.—Wherever possible, resection of the bladder wall should be performed in preference to total cystectomy, because the mortality of resection varies from 10 per cent. (Thomson Walker, in 30 cases) to 22 per cent. (Enderlein and Walbaum), while cystectomy has an operation mortality of from 46·1 per cent. (Thomson Walker, collected cases) to 61·5 per cent. (Goldenberg).

The cases unsuitable for resection are—
(1) Growths covering a very large area of the bladder wall.
(2) Rapidly growing malignant papillomas.
(3) Growths involving both ureters, or the trigone or urethra.
(4) Intractable cystitis.

None of these is a contra-indication to cystectomy provided the conditions previously stated are fulfilled.

Resection of the bladder wall.—Before operation the position and intravesical extent of the growth are ascertained by cystoscopy. At the operation the perivesical extent is examined before commencing to resect the bladder wall. Tumours of the lateral wall should be examined from the outer aspect of the bladder. In all tumours of the posterior wall the peritoneum should be opened and the peritoneal surface of the bladder examined. Tumours at the base are examined by palpation after cystotomy.

A vertical median suprapubic incision of 3½ in. with undercutting of the rectus muscle on the side of the growth and subsequent repair suffices for the majority of resections.

In stout patients a transverse curved suprapubic incision may be necessary.

The bladder is opened and the patient placed in the Trendelenburg position, illumination being obtained from a powerful headlamp. In tumours of the anterior wall and apex of the bladder the cystotomy wound should be placed well away from the growth. An area of bladder wall extending for at least an inch on all sides of the growth is removed, and the edges of the bladder wall are brought together by catgut stitches round a rubber tube, which is retained for four days.

In tumours situated on the posterior wall (Figs. 142, 143, 144) cystotomy is first performed, and then the peritoneal cavity is opened and the peritoneal aspect examined. An area of peritoneum is marked out behind the growth with scissors, and the edges are stripped off, leaving this portion adherent to the bladder. The peritoneal cavity is now closed. The cystotomy wound is

carried back and surrounds the growth, which is removed with
the area of bladder wall and peritoneum on which it is set. When
the growth lies in the neighbourhood of the ureters a second wound
is made from within the cavity of the bladder. A catgut suture
is passed through the bladder wall 1½ in. on the near side of the

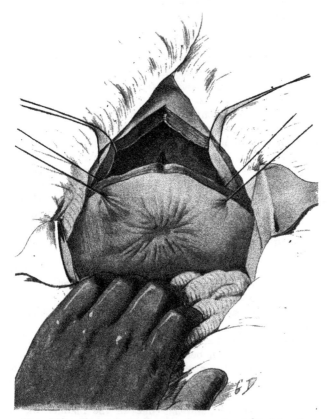

Fig. 142.—Resection of posterior wall of bladder for
malignant growth.

The bladder has been opened by suprapubic cystotomy, the peritoneum opened, and the
intestines packed off, exposing the puckered peritoneal surface of the growth.

growth. By traction on this the bladder wall is steadied, and
with a long, curved pair of scissors a transverse incision is made
through the whole thickness of the bladder wall an inch from
the growth. This is carried round the growth, leaving an inch

margin of healthy bladder wall. As the section proceeds catgut traction sutures are inserted every half-inch through the edge of the bladder wound, while traction on the growth is made by a stitch passed through it. Any spouting vessels are readily controlled.

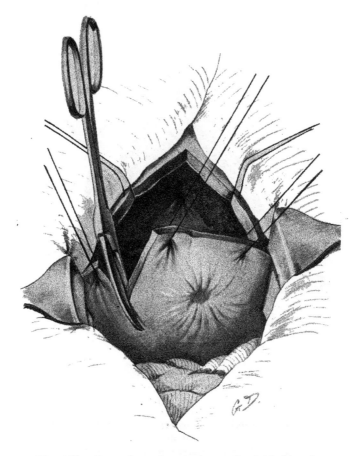

Fig. 143.—Resection of posterior wall of bladder for malignant growth.

The portion of wall bearing the growth is being removed.

If the ureteric orifice comes within the area of the resection the lower end of the ureter must be excised. This is done by continuing the wound down on each side of the growth and raising

2 F

the flap thus made. The ureter is exposed on the extravesical aspect of this flap, secured by toothed forceps, and cut across. The resection having been finished, the cut end of the ureter is raised to the bladder edge of the growth wound at the nearest point, and a catgut stitch passed through the wall of the ureter, and then through the bladder wall, and tied. Bleeding-points having

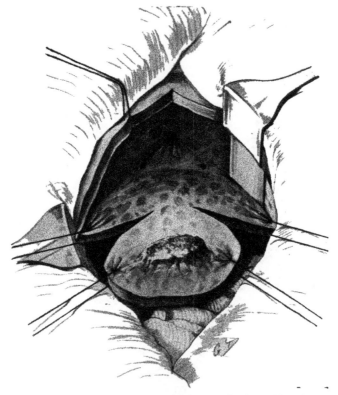

Fig. 144.—Resection of posterior wall of bladder for malignant growth.

Bladder surface of growth shown ; resection nearly completed.

been ligatured, the growth wound is stitched with catgut sutures from below upwards, using the traction sutures as stitches. When the level of the ureter is reached a second stitch is passed through its wall and through the opposite edge of the growth wound, to which it is already fixed. I then place a rubber drainage tube with a lateral perforation near the terminal opening alongside the ureter in the extravesical space, and this passes through the growth wound across the bladder and out of the cystotomy wound. It is fixed in the growth wound by a catgut stitch. The remaining portion of the growth wound is now closed, the bladder mucous membrane treated with nitrate of silver as in papilloma (p. 465), and a large drain placed in the cystotomy wound, which is then closed around the two tubes. The abdominal wall is now repaired.

The catgut stitch holds the tube alongside the ureter for seven days. It drains the extravesical space and leaves a weak spot in the bladder wall which prevents constriction of the ureter. I have used this simple method of ureteral transplantation successfully in ten cases, and prefer it to more elaborate methods. In none of my cases has there been any postoperative pyelonephritis after resection and implantation of the ureter.

Cystectomy: treatment of the ureters.—Some method of derivation of the urine must be adopted, and a large part of the high operative mortality of cystectomy is due to the operation for derivation of the urine being performed at the same time as the removal of the bladder. The two operations should be performed at an interval of some weeks.

The ureters have been implanted into the rectum, large intestine, urethra, vagina, or on to the skin in the loin or at the suprapubic wound, or bilateral nephrostomy may be performed.

Maydl's operation of transplanting the trigone of the bladder with the ureters cannot be done in growths of the bladder.

Implantation of the ureters into the rectum is seldom successful, and in the majority of cases in which the patient has survived operation a fistula has formed on the surface. In cases of implantation into the large bowel there is a grave danger of ascending septic inflammation. Implantation of ureters into the urethra has not given good results. Fixation of the ureters in the suprapubic wound has been successful in several cases. After ureterostomy there is considerable danger of stenosis and of ascending inflammation. In one case I implanted the appendix into the dilated right ureter (*uretero-appendicostomy*, see p. 342).

The most successful operation is one done in two stages, of which the first stage consists in derivation of the urine by vaginal implantation in the female, and nephrostomy or ureterostomy in the male subject.

Cystectomy in the male: the combined perineo-abdominal method.—The bladder is distended with fluid and the patient placed in the lithotomy position. A curved transverse prerectal incision, concave forwards, is made, and the posterior surface of the prostate and seminal vesicles is exposed.

The patient is now placed horizontally, and then raised into the Trendelenburg position, and a transverse suprapubic incision made down to the bladder. The peritoneum is then stripped by blunt dissection from the apex and posterior wall until it meets the dissection made from the peritoneum. The vas deferens is separated, the seminal vesicles are detached and pushed backwards, the bladder is pulled to one side, and the ureter and large vessels on the opposite side are isolated and clamped; and the same is done on the other side. The bladder is emptied and pulled up, and dissection carried transversely between the front of the base of the prostate and the bladder, and the prostatic urethra is clamped and cut arcoss. The trigone is dissected off the upper surface of the prostate and the bladder removed. The lateral pedicles are now ligatured. The peritoneum may be opened, and, instead of being stripped off, the adherent portion is excised (intraperitoneal method).

Cystoprostatectomy.—The preliminaries are the same as already described, but the prostate is completely separated from the perineum, the membranous urethra is cut across, and the anterior surface of the prostate separated from the back of the pubic bones. The patient is placed in the Trendelenburg position and the bladder exposed, the peritoneum stripped off, and the lateral pedicles clamped as before. The bladder is drawn upwards and backwards, the pubo-vesical ligaments are cut across, and the bladder, prostate, and seminal vesicles removed.

Cystectomy in the female (Pawlik's operation).—The ureters are exposed from the vagina, cut across, and implanted into the vaginal wall. After some weeks the bladder is exposed and separated from the peritoneum by a vertical suprapubic incision. A vaginal incision is made immediately above the urethra, and the bladder delivered into the vagina and removed after cutting across the urethra. The urethra is then implanted into the vagina and the outlet of the vagina closed by a second operation later, so that the vagina forms a reservoir for the urine.

Results. *Partial resection.*—In 96 collected cases of partial resection of the bladder for carcinoma there were 21 deaths (21·8 per cent.—Watson). The author has performed (March, · 1911) resection of the bladder in 30 cases of malignant growth, with 3 deaths (10 per cent.). In 10 of these cases one ureter was transplanted.

Late results.—Of 50 cases of partial resection collected by Watson there was recurrence in 58 per cent. within three years, and in 10 per cent. there was no recurrence. Kümmel reports that of 47 cases of bladder resection for malignant growth 10 are well after sixteen, fifteen, eight, and six and a half years, and 1 died of recurrence ten years after the operation.

In 25 cases of resection by the author in which late information was obtained there were 3 deaths from ascending pyelonephritis and 6 recurrences, 1 of which was re-operated (Plate 33, Fig. 4) ; in 17 cases the patients were alive and without recurrence (1) six months after the operation in 6 cases, (2) twelve months in 3 cases, (3) eighteen months in 6 cases, (4) two years in 1 case, and (5) four and a half years in 1 case (statistics in March, 1911).

Cystectomy.—Of 39 cases collected from the literature, death occurred after the operation in 18, a mortality of 46·1 per cent. Only 10 cases could be traced, and in only 2 of these was the period after the operation longer than fifteen months. One was well five years afterwards (Hogge) and one sixteen years (Pawlik).

Later statistics give an even higher mortality. Verhoogen and de Graeuwé collected 59 cases of total cystectomy, with an operative mortality of 52·7 per cent. Of the 27 cases that survived the operation, 6 died in the first year, 7 died before the third year, and only 2 survived more than three years. In 12 cases the result was unknown.

Watson, basing his statistics on collected cases, holds that the only operation that offers reasonable hope of success in carcinoma of the bladder is total extirpation of the organ, and that this operation should be done in every case that is suitable for operative interference. He also holds that cystectomy should be performed for benign growths whenever recurrence takes place, " or at least if there is more than one recurrence." With the high operative mortality of cystectomy and the lack of encouraging statistics of the after-results, the views of Watson are not likely to be generally accepted, the more so that the results of partial cystectomy have greatly improved. Cystectomy must at the present time be looked upon as a desperate measure which holds out little, if any, prospect of cure.

Palliative treatment.—This is adopted when radical operation is contra-indicated, and consists in treating symptoms as they arise.

Hæmaturia.—In severe hæmaturia the patient is confined to bed, the lower end of the bed being raised. Opium and ergot are given hypodermically and calcium lactate by the mouth, the latter in doses of 10 gr. every four hours for forty-eight hours. The bladder should be washed with a large quantity (several quarts) of hot weak silver nitrate solution (1 in 10,000). Continuous irrigation may be arranged with a double-way catheter. This is followed by the instillation of a small quantity of adrenalin solution (1 in 1,000).

If the bladder becomes distended with clots, an attempt may be made to break them up and remove them by means of an evacuating cannula and bulb. If this is not quickly successful the bladder should be opened suprapubically, the clots cleared out, and a large drain inserted.

Partial operations involving the removal of the salient portion of a large growth by the suprapubic route and subsequent drainage are sometimes successful in relieving severe bleeding.

Pain.—Pain is frequently the result of chronic cystitis, and in such cases the urine is usually ammoniacal, and there may be phosphatic deposits on the bladder wall. Severe pain may, however, be present in infiltrating growths with little, if any, cystitis. Treatment consists in giving suppositories of extract of belladonna $\frac{1}{4}$ gr. and morphia $\frac{1}{4}$ gr., to which cocaine $\frac{1}{2}$–1 gr. may be added.

The injection of tincture of opium 20 minims, with antipyrin 30 gr., in a small enema of hot water, frequently gives relief.

Washing the bladder with silver nitrate solution (1 in 10,000) may be beneficial, and, if the urine is alkaline and phosphatic material is being deposited, washing with a very weak solution of acetic acid (1 in 5,000) and the administration by mouth of sodium acid phosphate, 20 gr. thrice daily, should be tried. Urinary antiseptics (urotropine, etc.) are also useful.

Suprapubic cystotomy may become necessary, and the cystitis should be treated by continuous irrigation. A permanent drain should be established, an apparatus being fitted, and the urine drained into a rubber urinal attached to the thigh (p. 549).

Partial operations upon the growth give relief from pain and from serious hæmorrhage. They are attended with some danger of septic pyelonephritis where cystitis is present. Nephrostomy, or permanent drainage of the kidney with ligature of the ureter just below the renal pelvis, may be done. Each kidney is treated in this way, and an apparatus applied to the loin to collect the urine (Watson). Harrison suggested the implantation of one ureter on the skin of the loin and the removal of the second kidney. Fenwick has adopted this method, applying it to both sides without nephrectomy.

2. CONNECTIVE-TISSUE NEW GROWTHS

FIBROMA

These rare tumours are small, round, pedunculated, covered with smooth mucous membrane, and of a yellowish-white colour. They consist of somewhat loosely-set fibrous tissue containing few blood-vessels. They are likely to be confused with malignant growths. Clado collected 25 recorded cases. The author removed a fibroma the size of a hazel-nut from the neighbourhood of the right ureter in a man aged 30.

Myoma, Fibro-Myoma

These tumours, of which about 20 examples are on record, form single, very rarely multiple, round nodules, which project from the outer surface of the bladder (extravesical), or into the interior of the viscus (intravesical or submucous), or are buried in the wall (interstitial). The submucous variety are pedunculated or sessile, firm, round, or oval tumours found at the base of the bladder. The growth consists of closely-set non-striped muscle fibres in whorls or irregularly interlacing. The vascular supply is peripheral and abundant.

Sarcomatous, rarely epitheliomatous, degeneration of these tumours has been described.

Myxoma

Pure myxoma of the bladder is rare, and is found almost exclusively in children. The tumours are situated at the base of the bladder, are almost always multiple, and form polypi not unlike those of the nose, but of firmer consistence and darker-red colour. Growth is extremely rapid, and recurrence takes place in a short time after removal. Microscopically there is an abundant granular intercellular substance, in which are round cells and a few branching myxomatous cells. The vessels are large and numerous, and formed of a single layer of endothelium.

Sarcoma

Sarcoma of the bladder is found in infancy and late adult life, and, relatively to epithelial tumours, is a rare growth. Wilden states that in 50 cases of sarcoma 26 of the patients were over 40, and 14 were under 10 years.

Horder found 4 cases in 60 growths, and Targett described 4 in 36 specimens. The proportion is much higher in children. Phocus found that 7 in 15 bladder growths in children were sarcomas. Secondary sarcoma is rare. The sarcoma originates in the submucous areolar tissue, less frequently from the extra-muscular areolar tissue (Targett), and rarely from the connective tissue of the muscular layer (Bernstein).

The majority of these tumours arise from the posterior or lateral walls (57 per cent.—Albarran), and the trigone is seldom affected unless with other parts. The tumour may be pedunculated or sessile, and infiltrating. Not infrequently the bladder wall is widely infiltrated, and projecting into the interior are numerous polypoid bodies. The cavity of the bladder may be filled with masses of these polypi. The surface is smooth and pink, or deep red, and of the consistence of hail. The ureteric orifices may be surrounded without obliterating the lumen.

The urethra is sometimes blocked by polypoid bodies which may protrude from the external meatus in the female. The rectum, intestine, and vagina may be involved, and perforation of the bladder wall occasionally occurs.

The spindle-celled, round-celled, and rarely the melanotic varieties of sarcoma are found. Myxoma and myxo-sarcoma are also described.

Rhabdo-myoma is a very rare tumour, probably arising from the striped muscle of Henle which passes up the anterior surface of the prostate as far as the bladder. Chondro-sarcoma is another rare form. Angioma has been described by Albarran and others; it is a rare form of tumour, which may become sarcomatous. Two cases of chorion-epithelioma have been described.

3. DERMOID CYSTS

Dermoid cysts are occasionally found as pedunculated tumours the size of a pigeon's egg, or buried in the wall of the bladder. Occasionally a perivesical dermoid cyst ruptures into the bladder. Clado described 8 examples, 2 of which were pedunculated and 6 sessile tumours.

LITERATURE

Albarran, *Les Tumeurs de la Vessie.* 1891.
Bangs, *Med. Rec.,* 1911, i. 359.
Binney, *Boston Med. and Surg. Journ.,* 1911, p. 226.
Block and **Hall,** *Amer. Journ. of Med. Sci.,* 1905, p. 654.
Casper, *Berl. klin. Woch.,* 1908, Nr. 6; *Zeits. f. Urol.,* 1909, *Suppl.,* 441.
Cassanello, *Ann. d. Mal. d. Org. Gén.-Urin.,* 1908, i. 641.
Enderlein und **Walbaum,** *Festschr. z. 60 Geburtstage, O. Ballingers.* Wiesbaden, 1903.
Gredenberg, *Beitr. z. klin. Chir.,* 1904.
Harrington, *Ann. Surg.,* Oct., 1893.
Kümmel, IIe Congrès de l'Assoc. Internat. d'Urol., London, 1911.
Lichtenstein, *Deuts. med. Woch.,* 1898, p. 709.
Mayo, *Ann. Surg.,* 1908, p. 105.
Motz, IIIe Sess. de l'Assoc. Franç. d'Urol., Paris, 1898, p. 347.
Paschkis, *Folia Urol.,* 1908, ii. 450.
Pawlik, *Wien. med. Woch.,* Nov. 7, 1891.
Rafin, *Proc.-verb. Assoc. Franç. d' Urol.,* 1906, p. 1.
Rehn, *Centralbl. f. Chir.,* 1904, *Suppl.,* 122.
Rochet et **Martel,** *Gaz. Hebdom. de Méd. et de Chir.,* 1898, p. 337.
Rovsing, *Arch. f. klin. Chir.,* 1907, p. 1407.
Shattock, *Proc. Roy. Soc. Med.,* Pathological Section, 1909, p. 31.
Stoerk und **Zuckerkandl,** *Zeits. f. Urol.,* 1907, p. 1.

LITERATURE (*continued*)

Stumpf, *Zeiglers Beitr.*, 1911, p. 171.

Treplin, *Deuts. med. Woch.*, 1906, No. 19.

Verhoogen, de Graeuwé, and **von Rihmer,** XVIe Congrès Internat. de Méd., Budapest, 1909, p. 118.

Walker, Thomson, "Operations on the Bladder," in Burghard's *System of Operative Surgery,* 1909, vol. iii. ; *Lancet,* Nov. 12, 1910 ; II. Congrès de l'Assoc. Internat. d'Urol., London, 1911.

Watson, *Ann. Surg.,* Dec., 1905 ; *Diseases and Surgery of the Genito-Urinary System,* 1909.

Weinrich, *Arch. f. klin. Chir.,* 1906, p. 887.

Wendel, *Mitt. d. Grenzgeb. d. Med. u. d. Chir.,* 1900, p. 15.

Wilder, *Amer. Journ. Med. Sci.,* 1905, p. 63.

CHAPTER XXXVI

VESICAL CALCULUS

Etiology.—The etiology of stone formation in the urinary tract is discussed under Renal Calculus (p. 249).

Stone in the bladder is less frequent in children than in adults, and much more frequent in men—especially old men—than in women.

In children vesical calculus is more frequent in the lower class than in the well-to-do. When stone occurs in children it is found in the bladder in the great majority of cases. Bokay found that 1,150 out of 1,621 cases of urinary calculus in children were vesical.

Calculi are primary when they are formed in an aseptic urine, and secondary when they result from changes in the urine caused by bacteria. The nucleus of a vesical calculus may be formed by a small oxalate-of-lime or uric-acid calculus which has descended from the kidney, or the stone may form around a portion of blood clot or a foreign body such as a fragment of a catheter, a pin, a silk ligature from a previous operation on the bladder (Figs. 152, 153) or neighbouring organs, a fragment of necrosed bone, etc.

The two important predisposing factors in the production of secondary calculi are bacterial action and stagnation of urine. Of these bacterial action is the more important.

The following proof of the presence of bacteria in the interior of calculi is of interest. In a woman of 50 years I removed a large phosphatic vesical calculus by litholapaxy. Previous to the operation the urine had been aseptic. The centre of the stone was composed of soft, greyish, stinking material, and cultures made from this gave an abundant growth of bacillus coli. The operation was followed by a smart attack of cystitis due to the bacillus coli released from the interior of the stone at the litholapaxy. The patient gave a history of removal of a urethral caruncle, followed by an attack of cystitis, three years before.

Calculi are very frequently found in old men with enlarged prostate and infected urine, and they may form in the stagnant urine in a diverticulum of the bladder.

490

Chemical composition and physical characters.—Vesical calculi are composed of 'uric acid, phosphates, or oxalate of lime, in that order of frequency, and rarely of cystin, xanthin, indigo, or calcium carbonate.

Uric-acid calculi (Figs. 145, 146, 147) may be pure uric acid, or ammonium or sodium urate. They are single or multiple, varying from the size of a split pea to that of a hen's egg. They are rounded or oval and may be flat ; the surface is smooth, or very finely nodular, and easily polished. They are sandy yellow to a dark brown in colour, and on section show a regular concentric lamination. They are hard, but not so hard as oxalate-of-lime calculi. Calculi composed of urates are similar in contour, but lighter in colour and harder in consistence.

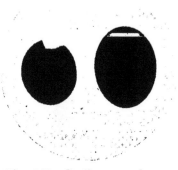

Fig. 145.—Radiogram of pure uric-acid calculi from bladder, taken after removal.

These calculi did not throw a shadow when in the bladder.

Oxalate-of-lime calculi (Fig. 148) are round and usually single. They vary from a pea to a chestnut in size and have a dark-brown colour. The surface is covered with closely-set conical bosses (mulberry calculus), or there may be a few sharp projecting spines (star form). The calculi are very hard. On section they are composed of closely set, irregularly disposed laminæ.

Phosphatic calculi (Figs. 149–53) may consist of basic calcium phosphate, either alone or mixed with ammonio-magnesium phosphate, and in addition there may be ammonium urate.

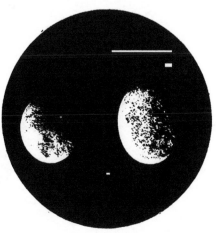

Fig. 146.—Uric-acid calculi removed from bladder.

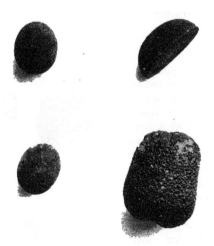

Fig. 147.—Uric-acid calculi removed from bladder.

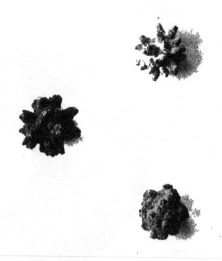

Fig. 148.—Oxalate-of-lime calculi (mulberry calculi)
removed from bladder.

These stones vary greatly in consistence. They may be soft and easily crumble, but when composed of crystalline phosphates they are very hard. Sometimes there is a hard outer shell and a soft interior. On section they are granular and rarely show lamination.

Cystin calculi are oval, granular, yellowish-brown, and have a soapy appearance. They turn a greenish-yellow when exposed to air. *Xanthin* stones are smooth and yellow, and *indigo* are blue, while *calcium-carbonate* calculi are greyish-white, earthy-looking, hard stones.

Calculi are rarely composed of a single ingredient, and are frequently named uric-acid, oxalate - of - lime, etc., only from their principal ingredient.

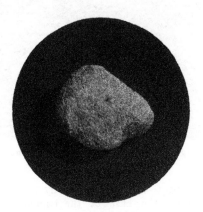

Fig. 149.—Phosphatic calculus of bladder.

The nucleus in primary stones is most frequently uric acid, less often oxalate of lime. Around the nucleus the laminæ of oxalate of lime or of uric acid are disposed. The layers may alternate. The surface is frequently covered with a smooth layer of phosphates. Large calculi are usually single, but there may be one large calculus and many small ones.

Multiple hard stones are rounded like peas, while the softer varieties (phosphates) are angular and faceted. As many as 400 or 500 may be present. Very large

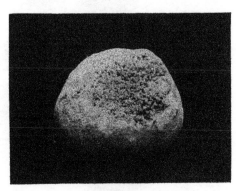

Fig. 150.—Phosphatic calculus removed from bladder.

stones have been recorded : Preston found one weighing 51 oz., and Earle another of 44 oz., at an autopsy ; and Milton removed one of 34 oz., and Clive another of 46 oz., by operation.

The average weight is 200 or 300 gr. Phosphatic stones develop
rapidly, and a large stone may form in a few weeks. Uric-acid
calculi form less ra-
pidly, and oxalate-of-
lime very slowly, some
years being usually
taken to form a cal-
culus of moderate size.

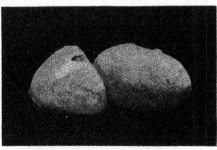

Fig. 151.—Phosphatic calculi removed
from bladder.

Vesical calculi are
either movable or fixed.
A *movable stone* rolls
about in the bladder,
and its position varies
according to the atti-
tude of the patient.
With the patient re-
cumbent the stone usually lies on the posterior wall, just
behind the base of the trigone. Large calculi in an inflamed,
sensitive bladder are occasionally found at the apex spasmodically

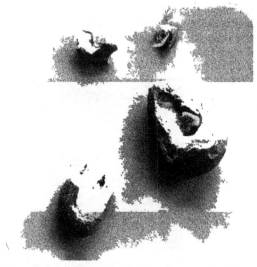

Fig. 152.—Phosphatic calculi formed around silk sutures
used in removal of bladder growth.

grasped in a partial contraction of the bladder. The lower part
of the bladder is not contracted, and contains fluid. Freely
movable stones take a rounded or flat oval form.

Ultzmann holds that the contour of the stone depends upon the crystals of which it is composed. Urates, uric acid, earthy phosphates, and cystin belong to the rhomboidal crystalline form, and produce flat ovoid stones varying in the three axes. Calcium oxalate belongs to the quadrate crystal form, and produces a rounded calculus. Secondary deposits change the contour of the stone: a rounded oxalate stone covered with uric acid becomes egg-shaped, while an ovoid uric-acid nucleus becomes rounded when oxalate of lime is deposited upon it.

When a number of calculi are closely packed together they

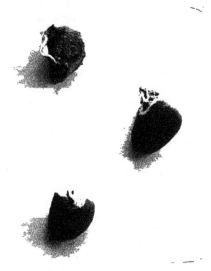

Fig. 153.—Phosphatic calculi formed around silk sutures used to close a cystotomy wound.

take a polygonal form with facet-like surfaces; when freely movable they take a rounded form.

A *fixed stone* is found in a diverticulum or saccule, or project-ing into the bladder from the lower end of the ureter or from the urethra, or in a diverticulum at the apex of the bladder, the patent lower end of the urachus (Dykes). When a stone lies within the cavity of a diverticulum it is rounded or oval, and it may be movable within the diverticulum or fixed. The opening of the diverticulum may be so small that the stone cannot be seen from the bladder. Stones which project from the prostatic urethra into the bladder increase rapidly in the shape of a mushroom or umbrella.

Spasmodic contraction of the bladder wall around a large stone may fix the stone in the upper or, in children, in the lower part of the bladder. Such contractions may give the bladder an hour-glass form, one part of the bladder being distended with fluid, while the other is firmly contracted round the stone.

In enlargement of the prostate, stones may be wedged in the deep pocket behind the intravesical projection so that they become fixed.

Pathology.—Cystitis may precede the formation of stone, or may result from its presence. The inflammation may be confined to the base of the bladder, or it may be universal. The bed on which the stone lies frequently consists of a thick, shaggy, greyish-white membrane formed of thickened and necrosed epithelium with muco-pus.

Papilloma or malignant growth is present in rare cases. Chronic pyelonephritis is found in cases of long-standing calculous cystitis, and is the cause of death in most fatal cases of stone.

Spontaneous fragmentation of a vesical calculus has been known to occur, and it has been most frequently observed in uric-acid calculi. Watson, Dabout d'Estrées, Kasarnowsky, and others have described such cases. The phenomenon is ascribed either to mechanical or to chemical action. Ord believed that it was due to the colloid cement substance of the calculus becoming saturated with urine of low specific gravity, such as is produced by diuretic waters. Leroy d'Etoilles regarded a drying and shrinking of the calculus as an essential factor. Heller explained the fracture by supposing that tension was produced within the calculus by decomposition of ammonium urate lying between layers of uric acid. Civiale, and later Kapsammer, held the view that the mechanical action of bladder contractions produced the fragmentation. If the mechanical view were correct, fracture would be expected to occur more frequently in multiple calculi and when the bladder was spasmodically contracted; but this is not the rule, and Zuckerkandl points out that fragmentation may occur in an atonic bladder. At the present time the factors which govern this rare phenomenon are unknown.

Symptoms.—A stone which descends from the kidney may give rise to a varying series of symptoms. There are one or several attacks of renal colic, which may be followed at once by symptoms of bladder irritation and the immediate discharge of the calculus with the urine. Frequently, however, a period of relief from symptoms follows the discharge of the calculus into the bladder, and this may last for some days, weeks, or even months. Symptoms commence again when the calculus is swept into the urethra to be impacted in that tube or passed through it, or when irritation of the bladder is produced by the continual movement of the stone, or finally when infection takes place.

Leguen states that calculi which form in infancy may remain quiescent for ten or even twenty years.

Fixed calculi give rise to no symptoms directly referable to stone, and very large calculi are frequently "latent."

Frequent micturition.—This is the most common and the earliest symptom. The increased frequency commences gradually and is progressive. There is urgency to pass water, and the desire, once felt, becomes an imperative necessity. After passing water there is discomfort, and a feeling that the bladder has not been emptied. These symptoms are aggravated, and may only be present, when the patient moves about or is subjected to the jarring of horse-riding, bicycling, or travelling in a railway carriage or a bus. In the recumbent position the stone falls away from the sensitive neck of the bladder, and the desire to pass water is no longer felt. The patient sleeps peacefully throughout the night.

Pain.—Pain is a prominent symptom. It is felt at the neck of the bladder and at the end of the penis, either at the external meatus, at the base of the glans on the dorsum, or most frequently beneath the frænum. The pain occurs at the end of micturition, is sharp and "cutting," and is increased by movement and jarring.

Hæmaturia.—Terminal hæmaturia is a frequent symptom. A few drops of blood are squeezed out at the end of micturition. The blood is bright, and the hæmorrhage not severe. Movement and rest influence this in the same manner as the other symptoms.

An intermittent stream may be observed. Arrest in the middle of the act, accompanied by severe pain, is due to impaction of the stone at the internal meatus. The arrest may be momentary, or it may be impossible to start the flow for some minutes, or even a quarter of an hour. If the patient lies down the stone rolls away from the internal meatus and water can be passed freely.

Continued retention of urine, necessitating the use of the catheter, is rare when the stone is still in the bladder. It may occur when the stone has become impacted in the prostatic urethra, and is usually accompanied by severe pain and strangury.

The urine contains crystals of oxalate of lime, uric acid, or phosphates. The urinary deposit for the time indicates the composition of the surface layer of the calculus.

Microscopic quantities of blood and an excess of leucocytes and epithelial cells are usually found in the urine.

In children, screaming on micturition and retention of urine are not infrequent. In other cases there is incontinence from

2 G

frequent involuntary expulsion of the urine caused by the irritation of a stone forced down into the neck of the bladder. In small boys ".milking" of the penis is an attempt to ease the pain, and leads to an enlarged, turgid, semi-erect condition of the penis which is very characteristic.

When cystitis complicates stone the symptoms are modified. The frequency is increased, and is continued at night as well as during the day; the pain grows more intense, and pus and mucus appear in the urine, which often becomes alkaline and stinking.

In old-standing cases symptoms of ascending pyolonephritis appear, and the patient rapidly loses weight, and eventually dies of " urinary septicaemia " (see p. 133). Pericystitis with perforation into the rectum or vagina is a rare complication.

Diagnosis.—Pain similar to that of calculus may occur in other diseases of the bladder, such as cystitis or malignant growth; but the pain in calculus is a prominent symptom, it is sharp, occurs at the end of micturition, and is markedly affected by movement and rest. The hæmaturia and frequent micturition are also increased by movement. The gradual onset of frequent micturition, diurnal in character, is very characteristic of stone. When cystitis is present a calculus may be suspected if the pain is unusually severe and all the symptoms are markedly increased by movement and jarring. The previous passage of a calculus is an important aid to diagnosis. Tuberculous cystitis in children or adults may give rise to difficulty in diagnosis. Pain is seldom so acute, and the frequency is continued at night as well as during the day, while movement has little effect upon the symptoms.

Malignant growth of the bladder may give rise to symptoms closely resembling stone. Here the pain is constant, is not so sharp, and movement has no effect upon the symptoms.

Calculus in combination with enlarged· prostate may be attended by no distinctive symptoms, and the stone is usually found during an examination of the bladder, or at the operation for enlarged prostate.

Has a stone which is known to have been descending the ureter been discharged into the bladder, or is it still in the lower end of the ureter ? The symptoms of stone in both these situations may be similar, but the effect of movement is seldom so marked in ureteral calculus, and symptoms of irritation of the genital system, such as erections and emissions, are frequently observed when the calculus is in the lower ureter. Usually, when the calculus passes into the bladder the symptoms suddenly cease, and they may not recur until the calculus is passed through the urethra or impacted in that tube.

The only certain method of distinguishing between stone in the lower ureter and stone in the bladder is by the use of the cystoscope.

Examination.—As a rule, it is not possible to detect a stone of moderate size by rectal or vaginal examination. Even large stones may not be palpable from the rectum, on account of the thickened bladder wall. They may, however, be felt on bimanual examination.

Sounding the bladder.—Before sounding a patient it is necessary to exclude urinary tuberculosis by bacteriological exam-. ination of the urine and other means. If tuberculosis is present the bladder should not be sounded.

The most stringent precautions in regard to asepsis must be exercised in this examination. The instruments are boiled, the hands rendered surgically clean, and the area of operation is surrounded by clean towels. The penis is washed with antiseptics. In children a general anæsthetic is usually necessary, but in adults none is required.

The patient lies on a high couch, and the surgeon stands on his right. Four or six ounces of fluid are introduced into the bladder through a catheter, which is then removed. The sound is introduced and pushed on until it is arrested at the apex of the bladder in the middle line. The beak is turned first to one side and then to the other, and the instrument drawn slowly out, tapping the bladder on each side of the middle line by turning the beak from side to side, until it is arrested at the internal meatus. Then the postprostatic area is examined by raising the handle of the sound until it is vertical, and finally by turning the beak down behind the prostate if it is enlarged. As the instrument is withdrawn the surgeon should pay particular attention to grating or impact with a stone in the prostatic urethra. When the beak of a sound comes in contact with a stone in the bladder a sharp metallic click is heard, and the impact can be felt with the thumb and forefinger lightly holding the instrument. An idea of the size of the stone may be gained by noting the distance to which the sound is withdrawn while the beak still rings upon the stone. Multiple calculi may be detected by the impact taking place when the beak is turned first on one side and then on the other.

In children the stone lies at the neck of the bladder, and the sound at once impinges upon it ; in adults in the dorsal decubitus the stone falls into the post-trigonal area, and in old men

the stones are usually found behind an intravesical projection of
the prostate (postprostatic pouch). A calculus may not be felt
with the sound when it is embedded in the folds of a partially
distended bladder, when it is grasped by a spasm of an irritable
bladder, when it lies behind an enlarged prostate or in a diverticulum, or when it is covered by a thick layer of mucus and pus.
The ridges of a trabeculated bladder, or phosphatic deposit on
the mucous membrane in chronic cystitis or on a new growth,
may give rise to difficulties in diagnosis with the sound; and the
operator should be careful that the handle of the instrument
does not come in contact with hard bodies such as a ring or a
button.

When a small stone cannot be felt with the sound the following method may detect it (Freyer): The cannula of a litholapaxy
evacuator is passed, a few ounces of fluid are introduced, and the
evacuating bulb is applied. At diastole of the bulb the small
calculus is sucked against the eye of the metal cannula with an
easily detected click.

Cystoscopy (Plate 36).—This is the most certain method of
detecting a calculus. Movable calculi are found just behind the interureteric bar. Large calculi in a contracted bladder may be difficult
to view, as they are pushed aside by the beak of the cystoscope.
Calculi lying behind the prostate or in a sacculus or at the mouth
of the ureter are readily seen with the cystoscope, while they may
escape detection with the sound. When a diverticulum has a
small opening it may contain a large calculus which cannot be
seen with the cystoscope. The number of calculi present in the
bladder and their position and appearance are readily ascertained.
I have seen a small spherical growth of the bladder entirely covered
with phosphates, which exactly resembled a phosphatic stone,
except that the position was constant to the outside of the right
ureter in different positions of the patient. In another case where
a stone shadow was shown by radiography the cystoscope revealed
in addition a large papillomatous growth, and litholapaxy was
abandoned for suprapubic cystotomy.

Radiography.—A shadow in the vesical area (*see* p. 360) may
be cast by a stone in the bladder, in the lower end of the ureter,
or in a diverticulum. A vesical stone shadow is usually in the
middle line, and it can be made to change its position by movements of the patient. The shadow thrown by a calculus in a
diverticulum is more likely to be to one side of the middle line,
and this position may also be taken by a shadow thrown by a
stone in the bladder pushed aside by a growth.

Treatment.—There is no means by which a stone in the

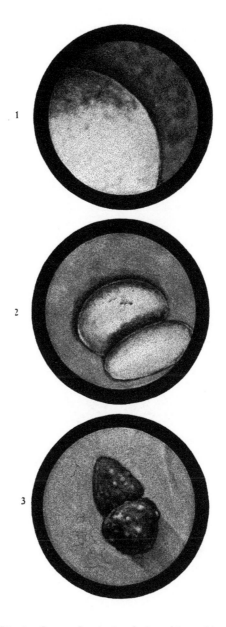

Fig. 1.– Large phosphatic calculus with cystitis.

Fig. 2.—Uric-acid calculi covered with thin layer
of phosphates.

Fig. 3.—Oxalate-of-lime calculi in bladder.

PLATE 36.   P 500

bladder can be dissolved, whether by medicines, or waters administered by mouth, or washes used locally.

When a stone has been passed in the urine a thorough examination with the cystoscope or X-rays should follow to make certain that no other calculi are present in the bladder, ureters, or kidney. When a stone has been passed down the ureter into the bladder and has not immediately been discharged through the urethra, its removal from the bladder should be proceeded with as soon as possible; for, although there is a fair probability of the stone passing through the urethra, there is also considerable danger that it may become impacted in that tube—an accident that may give rise to much pain and considerable difficulty in attempting to push the calculus back into the bladder, and may necessitate a perineal operation for its relief.

A small calculus may sometimes be removed by means of the cannula and aspirator (Fig. 154) used in litholapaxy. This should

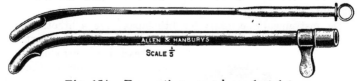

Fig. 154.—Evacuating cannula and stylet.

be performed under the same aseptic conditions that are necessary in a crushing or cutting operation. A general anæsthetic is preferable, although it may be dispensed with, or local anæsthesia used when the operator is skilful and the patient placid.

The largest cannula that the urethra will take is passed and the bladder emptied. Four or five ounces of warm boric lotion are introduced by means of a bladder syringe, and the aspirating bulb, filled with boric solution, is applied to the cannula. The bulb is raised so that the beak of the cannula lies at the lowest part of the bladder, and is compressed and relaxed. At diastole the calculus is felt to click at the eye of the cannula, and it drops into the glass bulb. The aspirating bulb is removed, the bladder emptied and then washed with a few syringefuls of silver nitrate solution (1 in 10,000).

This method is only applicable to small stones which have recently descended from the kidney, or to small fragments of phosphatic grit found in the course of chronic cystitis. It should not be attempted unless the surgeon is skilled in litholapaxy and is prepared at once to proceed to this operation if suction fails.

The operations which are performed for stone in the bladder are of two kinds—(1) crushing (litholapaxy or lithotrity), and (2) cutting (lithotomy).

1. Litholapaxy or lithotrity.—The modern operation of litholapaxy, which consists in crushing a stone and removing the fragments at one sitting, was introduced by Bigelow, of Boston, in

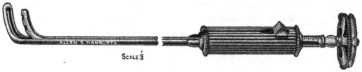

Fig. 155.—Thompson's lithotrite.

1878, and became firmly established as the operation of choice for vesical calculus through the work of Freyer, Keegan, and other officers of the Indian Medical Service. Previous to this date the operation consisted in crushing the stone and allowing the fragments to be swept out by the urine.

The instruments necessary for litholapaxy are a lithotrite and evacuating apparatus. Lithotrites of slightly varying construction have been introduced by Weir, Bigelow, Guyon, Thompson (Fig. 155), Freyer, and others.

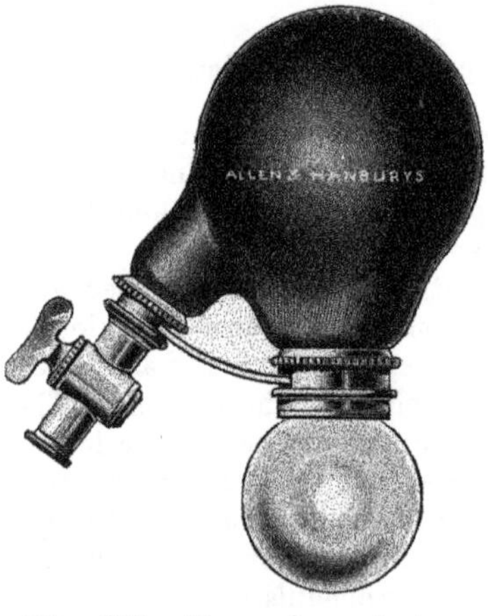

The lithotrite consists of two blades, one of which, the male blade, glides in a sunken groove in the other. The beak is set at an angle, and the female portion of it is concave and fenestrated, while the male is convex and toothed. The handle, by which the instrument is held in the left hand of the operator during the crushing, is attached to the female blade, and the screw, which is manipulated with the right hand, passes through this and belongs to the male blade. By a mechanical device, controlled either by a movable button on the handle (Thompson) or a screw cap attached to the male blade (Bigelow), the two blades can be locked, and can then only be approximated by means of a powerful screw worked on the male blade by a wheel (Thompson), or by

Fig. 156.—Freyer's aspirator.

a conical serrated handle (Bigelow). The cannula consists of a
straight metal tube with a short beak and a large eye, the proximal
end of which fits into the tube of the aspirator. The size of the
cannulæ varies from 12 to 18 English scale. There have been many
modifications of Bigelow's aspirator. That of Freyer (Fig. 156)
is the simplest and best. It consists of a bulb of thick rubber,
on the lower aspect of which is an opening to which a glass bulb
is attached; close to this, and steadied by a metal bridge, is a
metal tap and stopcock. This fits on to the proximal end of the

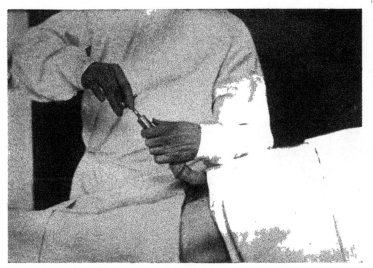

Fig. 157.—Litholapaxy: Grasping the stone and locking
the blades.

Note the angle of the instrument; the blades are in the most dependent part of the bladder.
The stone is grasped between the blades, and the thumb of the operator's left hand is pushing
up the locking button.

cannula. Pardoe has modified this by replacing the pressure
band of twisted wire which holds the rubber bulb and glass bulb
together by a metal band with a spring clip.

The operation of litholapaxy (Figs. 157, 158, 159, and Plate
37) is carried out as follows: The patient is prepared by the
administration for some days of 10 gr. of urotropine thrice daily,
the bowels are emptied by an aperient, and the rectum cleared
before the operation by an enema. A general anæsthetic is administered. The pelvis is slightly raised on a low, flat cushion. The
bladder is thoroughly washed with warm boric solution and the
catheter withdrawn, leaving 4 or 5 oz. of the solution in the bladder.

If the meatus is narrow it is slit downwards. The surgeon stands
on the right side of the patient, and the lithotrite, with the male
blade pushed home and well lubricated, is passed along the urethra
until the beak is inside the bladder. The handle is then raised
so that the beak descends to the lowest part of the bladder (the
post-trigonal area in this position), and the blades are separated.
The stone, which is lying at the lowest part of the bladder, rolls
in between the blades, and is caught when the male blade descends
upon it. Should the stone not be grasped by the manœuvre the

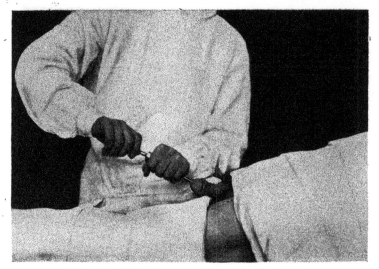

Fig. 158.—Litholapaxy : Crushing the stone.

The stone having been caught between the blades of the lithotrite and the blades locked, the
handle is firmly grasped in the left hand ; the right hand is turning the screw.

blades are separated and the instrument turned to the right or
left, or pushed well up into the apex of the bladder, or finally
turned downwards behind the prostate if this is enlarged. The
blades are now locked, the beak raised slightly from the bladder
wall, and the screw rapidly turned, the female blade being kept
absolutely steady by holding the handle rigid with the left hand.
When the blades have closed the screw is thrown out of gear and
the blades are separated, a fragment seized as before and crushed.
The crushing should proceed with the lithotrite in this position
until no more fragments are grasped, then it may be turned on one
side, opened, and a fragment (if any are left) grasped, the beak
again turned into the erect mid-line position, and the fragment

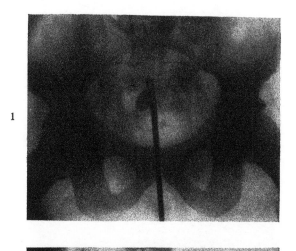

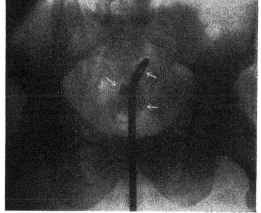

Fig. 1.—Shadow of calculus in grasp of lithotrite. (P. 504.)

Fig. 2.—Shadow of evacuating cannula, upper arrow on right; lower arrow on right points to small fragments of crushed calculus, arrow on left to large fragment that could not pass the eye of the cannula. (P. 503.)

PLATE 37.

crushed; and this manœuvre is repeated until no fragments are left. The beak is now turned to the other side, and the process repeated. All the fragments having been crushed, the blades are closed and the lithotrite withdrawn.

The largest cannula that the urethra will admit is now passed and the fluid in the bladder allowed to escape. Four or five ounces are again injected, the aspirator bulb is applied to the cannula, and the cock opened. . The bulb is now raised in the middle line, so that the beak of the cannula lies at the lowest part of the

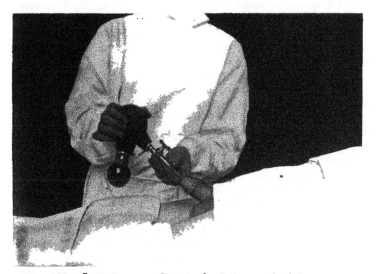

Fig. 159.—Litholapaxy: Removal of the crushed fragments
by evacuator.

The beak of the evacuating cannula is at the most dependent part of the bladder. It is supported by the left hand, and the eye has been turned towards the onlooker by pressing the thumb on the flange. The right hand is in the act of squeezing the bulb.

bladder, and the bulb is grasped in the right hand and compressed, the cannula being firmly held by the left hand. At diastole of the bulb the fragments of the stone are sucked into the rubber bulb, and, being heavier than water, they fall down into the glass bulb. The aspiration is continued until no further fragments fall, then the beak of the cannula is turned to the right and aspiration repeated, and then to the left, each new position being retained until the supply of fragments is exhausted at that spot. During diastole there may be " stammering " of the suction, which indicates that the beak of the cannula has been applied too close to the wall of the bladder and the loose mucous membrane sucked into the eye. This must be avoided, as it is tantamount to dry-cupping the wall of the bladder. If it should happen, the eye is set free by compressing the bulb, and is then turned away from the mucous membrane.

Two aspiration bulbs should be in use, to save time by changing them when one is filled or the fluid has become cloudy. The bulb may become fixed and fail to expand. This is due either to aspiration of the mucous membrane, and is freed by squeezing the bulb and turning the eye away from the mucous membrane, or to a fragment of stone too large to pass the cannula becoming fixed in the eye. This may be dislodged in the same way, but will probably necessitate the bulb being detached from the cannula and a stylet being pushed along the tube, after which the fluid comes away in a gush.

When removal of the stones is complete the fragments cease to fall into the glass bulb at diastole, and on listening carefully no click of a fragment against the eye of a cannula can be heard. Frequently at the end of the crushing several large greyish-white shreds of muco-pus and necrosed epithelium fall into the bulb. This is the bed on which the stone has been lying. If the clicking of fragments can still be heard the lithotrite is again introduced, and the fragments are crushed, and removed by the aspirator.

The type of fragment which is most difficult to pick up with the lithotrite is a thin shell from the outer part of the calculus.

The bladder is now washed out through the cannula with nitrate of silver solution (1 in 10,000), and the cannula removed. If the fluid returns clear on washing the bladder a cystoscope may be introduced and the bladder examined to see that it is clear of fragments. Usually, however, the cystoscopy may be deferred for a few days. The operation lasts from five or ten minutes to an hour or more, according to the size of the stone and the condition of the bladder.

If cystitis is present, or if the bladder is irritable or the prostate enlarged, the bladder should be drained by tying a catheter in the urethra for a few days, and should be washed daily with silver nitrate solution. The patient is kept in bed from two to fourteen days, according to the condition of the bladder and the temperature. Three to five days will suffice when the stone is small and the bladder aseptic.

Litholapaxy in children.—There are theoretical objections against the performance of litholapaxy in children. The urethra is very small and narrow, and its mucous membrane delicate and easily torn, and the bladder is small and pear-shaped, so that the space for manipulation is confined.

Keegan has shown, however, that litholapaxy in young children is not only possible, but is preferable to other methods. Freyer has further established this operation on a sound basis. The latter authority advises that the surgeon be provided with a series of small instruments similar to those used in adults, ranging from No. 4½ to 10. Boys aged from 13 to 16 take a lithotrite of No. 11 or 12 size; while the cannulæ suitable for children vary from No. 6 to 11 English scale. The small sizes of cannulæ should be short, as the suction power is diminished by the small lumen. The aspirator is used with the utmost gentleness, and only a small quantity of water is pressed into the bladder at each systole. The calibre of the urethra varies more in the child than in the adult. The meatus and first inch and a half are the narrowest part of the urethra in the child. Having passed this, the lithotrite enters the bladder without further difficulty, except a slight hitch at the internal meatus. The operation in children takes longer, and there is more danger of leaving fragments behind, but this can be avoided by care and experience.

If the lithotrite does not lie easily in the canal, there may be difficulty in withdrawing and reintroducing instruments. For this reason care should be taken to finish the crushing before withdrawing the lithotrite. The earliest age at which litholapaxy can be performed depends upon the calibre of the urethra. Freyer performed the operation on a male child aged 18 months. In January, 1912, the author performed litholapaxy on a boy aged 15 months. The stone consisted of calcium phosphate. Metal sounds up to 10 English gauge were passed before the urethra would accommodate the lithotrite. The difficulty lay in the first inch and a half of the urethra. After crushing the stone there was some difficulty in removing the lithotrite, as it was firmly gripped at the internal meatus. The size of the lithotrite and evacuating cannula was 11 Fr.

Litholapaxy in the female.—The operation presents no difficulty in the female subject. The shank of the instrument should be well lubricated, so that it does not drag on the labia majora, and if there is any tendency to incontinence an assistant presses the forefinger against the urethra from the vagina during the operation.

Difficulties and contra-indications of litholapaxy. i. *The urethra.*—The external meatus is frequently too narrow to admit a large lithotrite, and meatotomy should be performed before commencing the operation. Stricture of the urethra may prevent the introduction of the lithotrite. In all cases of vesical calculus the urethra should be examined before operation, and large sounds passed to estimate the calibre of the tube. The adult urethra should have a capacity of 16 or 18 English scale (28 to 30 Fr.) for large lithotrites, and 12 or 13 (21 to 23 Fr.) for small lithotrites. There may be difficulty in passing through the membranous urethra, from spasm of the compressor urethræ. A large metal instrument should first be passed, and the lithotrite will readily follow. Organic stricture must be treated before the lithotrite can be passed. This may be done at the time of the litholapaxy. Internal urethrotomy is performed and large metal instruments are passed, the bladder filled with fluid, and then the lithotrite used. I prefer to treat the two conditions separately, allowing a fortnight's interval to elapse between the internal urethrotomy and the litholapaxy, for the passage of large irregular instruments like the lithotrite and cannulæ several times through a urethra the seat of an internal urethrotomy wound causes unnecessary bruising and tearing of the incision, and may lead to recontraction of the stricture at a later date. The narrow urethra of the child in relation to litholapaxy has already been discussed.

ii. *Enlarged prostate.*—A moderate enlargement of the prostate is not a barrier to litholapaxy, but a large prostate causes considerable difficulty in the introduction of the lithotrite, and a well-developed intravesical projection hampers the movements of the lithotrite, so that stones wedged behind it are reached with difficulty by the lithotrite. Hæmorrhage may be severe. The best method of treatment of stone with enlarged prostate is suprapubic prostatectomy with removal of the stones. There is no difficulty in performing litholapaxy in cases of recurrent stone where prostatectomy has previously been done. When a stone forms in or passes into the cavity left after prostatectomy it may sometimes be manipulated back into the bladder by means of the lithotrite or a large metal sound, and it is sometimes possible to crush it in the prostatic cavity with a small lithotrite, but as a rule a median perineal incision will be necessary for the removal of the stone.

iii. *The bladder.*—In acute cystitis the bladder does not hold sufficient fluid to allow of litholapaxy being performed. The patient should be confined to bed, and treatment for acute cystitis adopted. Litholapaxy may be performed when the cystitis has subsided. If, however, improvement is tardy, suprapubic lithotomy and drainage of the bladder is preferable.

In chronic cystitis litholapaxy should be performed and the cystitis actively treated.

Advanced sacculation of the bladder should be looked upon as a contra-indication to litholapaxy. The fragments and powder fall into the saccules, and are not removed by the aspirator. A stone in a saccule is unsuitable for litholapaxy. Such stones have been crushed, but there is a danger of injury to the bladder wall and of rupture of the thin-walled saccules that should deter the surgeon from using this method.

Spasmodic contraction of the bladder around the stone at the upper part of the bladder, forming a species of hour-glass bladder, may develop; and a similar condition in children at the lower part of the bladder may interfere with the intravesical manipulation. This contraction may relax after a time, but in one case of an adult at the upper part of the bladder, and in two cases of children at the lower part, I have had to abandon litholapaxy and remove the tightly wedged stones by suprapubic lithotomy.

New growths of the bladder when combined with stone contra-indicate litholapaxy.

iv. *Size of the stone.*—No rule can be laid down as to the limits of size that are suitable for litholapaxy. Large stones which are egg-shaped may be crushed when grasped in the short axis, when the long axis is too great for the grasp of the lithotrite.

Very large stones are more quickly and safely removed by suprapubic cystotomy with drainage of the bladder than by litholapaxy. Stones that are too hard for crushing by a well-made lithotrite are very rare, if other conditions be favourable. When the lithotrite is fully screwed up on a very hard calculus, fracture may be delayed for quite an appreciable interval.

Perineal litholapaxy.—A median external urethrotomy is made on a grooved staff and the membranous urethra opened longitudinally. A large-sized Bigelow lithotrite is introduced, or a Harrison's lithoclast, and the stone crushed and removed by an evacuator or forceps. It is claimed that this operation is useful when it is desired to examine the prostatic urethra and remove the prostate by the perineum. There may be difficulty in grasping the stone. The operation is inferior to litholapaxy and to suprapubic lithotomy.

Dangers of litholapaxy.—Ascending pyelonephritis is a rare sequel in septic cases. These cases should be carefully prepared by washing and urinary antiseptics before the operation, and drainage of the bladder by catheter should be installed after the operation. When the urine is septic a sharp rise of temperature may follow the operation from absorption of septic material from the urethra, which may have suffered some slight mechanical injury during the operation. This can be prevented by thorough preparation of the bladder before, and by drainage with a catheter after the operation, and it is less likely to occur when skill and gentle manipulation have been exercised than when the urethra has been roughly handled. Hæmorrhage may result from enlargement of the prostate, from growth in the bladder, or from unskilful manipulation.

Perforation of the bladder wall has occurred, and has apparently been due to operating in a small contracted bladder containing an insufficient quantity of fluid. The perforation is situated immediately behind the trigone and is extraperitoneal, and allows fluid and fragments to escape into the pelvic cellular tissue. Pelvic cellulitis and peritonitis supervene, and unless promptly treated by free drainage are fatal.

2. **Suprapubic lithotomy.**—The bladder is exposed and opened by a vertical median suprapubic incision, and the left forefinger passed into the cavity. A pair of . lithotomy forceps is introduced, and, guided by the finger, grasps and removes the stone. A number of calculi may be removed in this way or by means of a scoop. When there are numerous small stones, or when a friable phosphatic stone is removed, great care must be exercised to avoid leaving small stones or fragments in the bladder or in the perivesical space in withdrawing them. A copious stream of fluid from a large reservoir is useful for removing débris and small stones. In dealing with large calculi the wound in the bladder should be sufficiently large to pass the stone without tearing or bruising. The bladder wall may have to be peeled off a large calculus. When the prostate is enlarged, prostatectomy should immediately follow removal of the calculi. The treatment of a calculus in a diverticulum depends upon whether the calculus is shut in a diverticulum which communicates with the bladder by a small opening, or whether the opening is large and the calculus easily accessible or projecting into the bladder cavity. In the former case the treatment is described under that of diverticula (p. 411). In the latter the calculus is grasped by lithotomy forceps guided by the forefinger, or, if the calculus is impacted or difficult to reach, the patient is placed in the Trendelenburg position and the operation conducted under the light of a head-lamp, the opening of the diverticulum being enlarged if necessary. A large calculus in a diverticulum has been broken up by a chisel and mallet, counterpressure being obtained by the finger of an assistant in the rectum. The fragments were then extracted. In such cases it is better to remove the diverticulum by dissection outside the bladder, and with it the stone.

After suprapubic lithotomy, drainage by means of a large rubber tube should be installed in cases where cystitis or a diverticulum or urethral obstruction is present, or where the kidneys are diseased by sepsis or back pressure. A smaller tube is placed in the prevesical space, and both are removed on the fourth day. The bladder is washed daily with solutions of nitrate of silver (1 in 10,000 to 1 in 5,000) or some other antiseptic.

When a small calculus is removed from an aseptic bladder the cystotomy wound may be completely closed and a catheter tied in the urethra.

Median perineal lithotomy.—A curved staff with median groove is introduced into the bladder and the patient placed in the lithotomy position. The handle of the staff is held vertically by an assistant, who grips the handle of the instrument with the right hand, and includes the lowest part of the scrotum in this grasp. An incision 2 in. in length is made from above downwards in the middle line of the perineum, ending $\frac{1}{2}$ in. in front of the anus. This is deepened to the membranous urethra, which is opened longitudinally on the staff, and the point of the knife is run longitudinally along the groove till it reaches the prostatic urethra. A probe-pointed gorget is introduced and pushed along the groove, and the surgeon draws the handle of the staff towards him and at the same time pushes the gorget on into the bladder, when a gush of urine escapes. The staff is withdrawn and the forefinger of the left hand introduced along the gorget into the bladder, and the gorget withdrawn. Forceps or a scoop is passed along the finger into the bladder, and the stone removed.

A rubber perineal drainage tube is tied in the bladder and kept there for a few days.

Lateral lithotomy is now abandoned in favour of one of the methods already described.

Vaginal lithotomy consists in opening the bladder on a sound from the anterior vaginal wall. The operation is inferior to those described, and vesico-vaginal fistula is a frequent sequel.

Choice of operation for vesical calculus.—Only two methods, litholapaxy and suprapubic lithotomy, need be discussed. The advantages of litholapaxy are that it is applicable to the great majority of calculi, and that in recurrent calculi it may be repeated time after time without increased difficulty. The death-rate in experienced hands is low and the convalescence rapid. This operation is unsuitable for very large stones, encysted stones, stones in a sacculated bladder, for cases of enlarged prostate, foul cystitis, or those in which advanced pyelonephritis is present.

Suprapubic lithotomy requires less manipulative skill and has the advantage of providing thorough postoperative drainage. It is thus especially useful in cases of foul cystitis and those in which there is urethral obstruction. It should be performed in cases of encysted stone, of very large calculi, where the kidneys are diseased, of enlarged prostate, and of bladder growths. In stone complicating bilharziosis or cystitis, lithotomy is preferable to litholapaxy, and the perineal operation is invariably performed. In other cases it has the disadvantage of a longer period of convalescence (fourteen to twenty-one days), the death-rate is higher, and in recurrent calculus the succeeding cystotomy becomes increasingly difficult.

Litholapaxy should be performed as the routine operation, and lithotomy reserved for cases that are unsuitable for crushing. The proportion in which a cutting operation is necessary is small. Of 66 cases of vesical calculus treated in St. Peter's Hospital during the year 1910, litholapaxy was performed in 56 with 1 death, suprapubic lithotomy was performed 3 times with 1 death, and prostatectomy with removal of calculi in 7 cases without a death. In children litholapaxy is a very successful operation, and cystotomy should be reserved for cases in which the urine is foul, or the calculus is very tightly wedged in the neck of the bladder, or the urethra is too small to admit a lithotrite.

Results.—The following are the results in 1,814 cases of stone in the bladder operated on at St. Peter's Hospital from 1864 to 1912 :—

Decade	Operations	Cured or relieved	Died	Death-rate (per cent.)
1864–73	.. 118	.. 100	.. 18	.. 15·25
1874–83	.. 196	.. 166	.. 30	.. 15·30
1884–93	.. 362	.. 332	.. 30	.. 8·29
1894–1903	.. 600	.. 571	.. 29	.. 4·83
1904–12	.. 538	.. 520	.. 18	.. 3·34

The proportion of the different operations has already been given. The decline of the death-rate under the aseptic performance of litholapaxy is very striking.

Sir Henry Thompson recorded 49 deaths in 850 cases of *lithotrity*, a mortality of 5·76 per cent. Only 372 of these operations were performed according to the modern Bigelow method at one sitting, and in these the mortality was 3·22 per cent.

The death-rate of *litholapaxy* in the hands of various surgeons is as follows :—

Guyon	..	..	..	..	..	2·7 per cent.
Zuckerkandl	..	..	..	..	..	3·6 ,,
v. Frisch	..	..	..	..	..	2·6 ,,
Legueu	..	..	..	..	..	2·0 ,,
Freyer	..	..	..	..	..	2·61 ,,

In 19 cases of *suprapubic lithotomy* Thompson had 5 deaths (26·3 per cent.), and in 149 cases Freyer had 19 deaths (12·75 per cent.).

The high death-rate of suprapubic lithotomy compared with litholapaxy is due to the fact that all the grave cases were treated by lithotomy. When the same cases are treated by the two operations the results are less disproportionate. Thus, Assenfeldt in 460 cases of suprapubic lithotomy found a death-rate of 3·6 per cent.

Late results.—Watson found 19 per cent. of recurrence in 902 cases of litholapaxy, and in more than two-thirds of these the patients were over 50 years of age. There is no difference in recurrence after the two operations of lithotomy and litholapaxy in the hands of an experienced surgeon. Recurrence takes place most frequently from new formation of phosphatic stones, usually in the subjects of enlarged prostate. Recurrence of oxalate-of-lime and uric-acid calculi is much less frequent, but may occur from the descent of calculi from the kidney or by new formation in the bladder. The latter is very rarely the result of fragments left behind at a crushing or cutting operation. The recurrent calculus after removal of a uric-acid or oxalate-of-lime calculus may be phosphatic, and is due to changes in the urine. The effect of removal of an enlarged prostate upon the recurrence of calculi varies according to their composition and the state of the urine. Uric-acid and oxalate-of-lime calculi rarely recur, phosphatic calculi frequently. In 7 out of 112 cases of prostatectomy in which the author removed calculi at the time of operation there was no recurrence in 4, and all these were cases of uric-acid or oxalate-of-lime calculi. In the remaining 3 cases the urine was alkaline and the stones were phosphatic, and there was recurrence in all.

LITERATURE

Assenfeldt, *Arch. f. klin. Chir.*, 1899, p. 669.
Civiale, *Traité de l'Affection Calculeuse.* Paris, 1838.
Dykes, *Lancet*, 1910, i. 566.
d'Étoilles, Leroy, *Union Méd.*, 1855.
Freyer, *Surgical Diseases of the Urinary Organs.* 1908.
Heller, *Die Harnkonkretionen.* Wien, 1860.
Histon, *Brit. Med. Journ.*, 1904, ii. 833.
Kapsammer, *Wien. klin. Woch.*, 1903.
Kasarnowsky, *Folia Urol.*, 1909, p. 469.
Keegan, *Ind. Med. Gaz.*, 1885.
Knorr, *Zeits. f. Geb. u. Gyn.*, 1911, Heft i.
Milton, *Lancet*, 1893, p. 687.
Ord, *Trans. Path. Soc. Lond.*, 1878.
Petit, *Ann. d. Mal. d. Org. Gén.-Urin.*, 1904, p. 1281.
Walker, Thomson, IIᵉ Congrès de l'Assoc. Internat. d'Urol., London, 1911.
Watson, *Boston Med. and Surg. Journ.*, Dec. 2, 1886
Wildt, Iᵉʳ Congrès Égyptien de Méd., Cairo, 1905.
Zuckerkandl, *Handbuch der Urologie* (von Frisch und Zuckerkandl), 1905, B. ii.

CHAPTER XXXVII

FOREIGN BODIES IN THE BLADDER

FOREIGN bodies reach the bladder by the urethra or through the bladder wall.

A silk suture placed in the bladder wall at an operation acts as a foreign body and forms the nucleus of a calculus. A number of such calculi may be found when silk has been used as suture material. (Figs. 152, 153.) Soft absorbable catgut should therefore be used in all bladder operations.

A silk ligature used in operations upon the pelvic viscera, such as ovariotomy or hysterectomy, may later penetrate the bladder wall and act as a foreign body. A mop or gauze roll may be accidentally left in the bladder at the time of an operation. The flexible guide of a urethrotome may become detached from the instrument by being imperfectly screwed on, or it may break across the junction of the flexible and metal portion. To avoid this the metal part should taper inside the flexible. Portions of rubber or gum-elastic catheters which are old and friable may break off and remain in the bladder.

Foreign bodies may be introduced by the patient along the urethra by design, either in innocence or to excite erotic sensations, and the bodies may slip into the bladder. This occurs more frequently in the short female urethra than in the long, tortuous male canal. I have seen in the female bladder a coiled piece of wire, a hairpin, a pin ; and in the male a collar-stud buttoner, a metal pencil-case, a cylindrical piece of hard wax. (Plate 38, Figs. 1, 2.)

The following are a few of the articles which have been found, viz. : needle, bone knitting-needle, rubber tube, thermometer, glass rod, nozzle of an irrigating apparatus, pessary, mouthpiece of a pipe. A splinter of bone from a bone abscess or after fracture of the pelvis has penetrated the bladder wall. A pair of artery forceps, left in the pelvis at a gynæcological operation, has been known to ulcerate through the bladder wall (Spencer Wells).

Effect upon the bladder.—Unless the body is sharp and irritating, it remains for a week or more without giving rise to

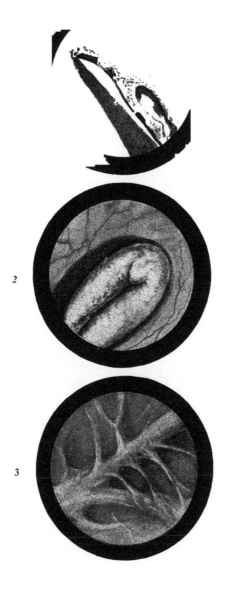

Fig. 1.—Stud-buttoner covered with phosphatic
deposit in male bladder. (P. 514.)

Fig. 2.—Doubled-up piece of wax in male bladder. (P. 514.)

Fig. 3.—Atrophy of bladder wall in tabes dorsalis.
(P. 534.)

PLATE 38.

irritation ; at the end of that time, or even sooner, the mucous
membrane becomes inflamed at the situation usually occupied by
the foreign body, and in patches elsewhere which come in contact with it. Ulceration and even penetration of the bladder
wall may follow. Penetration of the body into the bowel or
vagina may occur. The foreign body quickly becomes encrusted
with phosphatic deposit, and this occurs when the urine is still
clear. According to Zuckerkandl, wax does not become encrusted,
silver slowly, while iron, rubber, and vegetable materials are most
rapidly coated. A phosphatic stone forms, and may reach large
dimensions. A portion only of an elongated body may become
covered with phosphates—only the head of a pin, and in a needle
the sharp end, projects. Long flexible bodies, such as catheters
or urethrotome guides, may form knots. Finally, infection occurs,
and the urine becomes alkaline and offensive. Very rarely a
calculus forms in acid urine. Zuckerkandl describes a large uric-
acid calculus which formed around a fragment of iron.

Symptoms.—For some hours after the introduction of the
body there is vesical irritation, but this may subside, and for a
varying time symptoms may be absent. Smooth, regular bodies
may remain quiescent unless they are swept into the internal
meatus, when retention of urine results. Later there is increased
frequency of micturition, with pain, the urine becomes turbid,
and infection takes place. The symptoms are then similar to
those of stone in the bladder. Retention of urine is common
when the body has penetrated the bladder wall, pericystitis
results, and there is high fever with pelvic pain, and a swelling
can be detected.

When a mop or a gauze roll is left in the bladder after an
operation there is unusually severe and prolonged vesical spasm.
The urine may remain aseptic for several weeks, but afterwards
becomes infected. The suprapubic sinus remains open, and
eventually the body appears at the wound, or is removed at
an exploratory operation.

Diagnosis.—The history of the introduction of the foreign
body may be difficult to elicit, and the patient is examined for
spontaneous persistent cystitis. In the course of this examination
the foreign body is discovered with the cystoscope. Its usual
situation is on the posterior wall behind the trigone. In the case
of a long body, one end, when the bladder is distended, is near
the internal meatus, and the body lies obliquely towards one or
other side ; when the bladder is empty, the body lies transversely.
The gradual onset of cystitis some time after an operation on
the pelvic viscera, or the development of stone after an operation

in which silk is known to have been used as suture material, or the presence of an inflammatory mass alongside the bladder detected by rectal, vaginal, or bimanual examination, should arouse the suspicion that a foreign body may be present.

The X-rays may assist when the foreign body is opaque.

Treatment.—Urethral operations are most suitable for the female subject, but are also feasible in some cases in the male. In the female a large Kelly's tube should be used after dilatation of the urethral orifice, and the patient placed in the Trendelenburg position. When the bladder is distended with air the foreign body may be seized with fine forceps or with specially constructed instruments and removed. The manœuvres may be assisted by a finger in the vagina. There may be difficulty in obtaining inflation of the bladder or in seizing the foreign body. In the male, urethral operations are less likely to be successful. Luys' direct cystoscope should be used, and the patient placed in the Trendelenburg position. A catheter or urethrotome guide may be seized with a lithotrite and removed.

When these methods fail (50 per cent. of cases) the bladder should be opened suprapubically and the foreign body extracted. If a septic cystitis or ulceration is present and no penetration of the wall of the bladder has occurred the cystotomy wound should be sutured, but in the other cases a large suprapubic drain should be introduced.

When a foreign body such as a hair-pin forms the centre of a calculus the ends usually project, so that a diagnosis can be made. The calculus should be removed by suprapubic cystotomy. In other cases a foreign-body nucleus is entirely buried in a calculus, and is only revealed by the difficulty experienced in crushing this part of the calculus or by the peculiar sensation imparted on grasping it with the lithotrite. Such bodies are usually small, and may be broken up with the lithotrite. If this fails the bladder should be opened and the object removed.

LITERATURE

Grosglik, *Centralbl. f. d. Krankh. d. Harn- u. Sex.-Org.*, 1897, p. 641.
Heresco, *Ann. d. Mal. d. Org. Gén.-Urin.*, 1898, p. 802.
Hirsch, *Deuts. Zeits. f. Chir.*, 1903, p. 45.
Ravasini, *Wien. med. Presse*, 1902, p. 31.
Zuckerkandl, *Handbuch der Urologie* (von Frisch und Zuckerkandl),1905, B. ii.

CHAPTER XXXVIII

PERICYSTITIS AND PERIVESICAL ABSCESS

THE perivesical tissue consists of fatty and areolar tissue, and forms part of the freely intercommunicating areolar planes of the pelvis, which partly surround the bladder, rectum, uterus, and vagina, and lie between the layers of the broad ligament in the female. They communicate above with the areolar tissue of the iliac fossæ, closely related with the cæcum and appendix on the right and the sigmoid flexure on the left side. In front of the bladder there is a space (the space of Retzius), limited anteriorly by the pubic bones and filled with loose areolar tissue. A partial floor is formed by the anterior extremities of the visceral layers of pelvic fascia. These do not meet in the middle line, and the space is continued down the front of the prostate to the triangular ligament and membranous urethra.

Etiology.—Pericystitis may be secondary to disease of the bladder, or it may arise in neighbouring organs or structures; rarely it is idiopathic. The diseases and injuries of the bladder which most commonly give rise to it are chronic cystitis, tuberculous cystitis, malignant growth, diverticula, and perforation of the bladder wall, which may be caused by mechanical injury with a sound or lithotrite, stabs or bullet wounds, fracture of the pelvis, or by diseases such as stone, malignant or (rarely) simple ulcers. Men are more often affected than women, owing to the frequency of obstructive disease in the male.

Diseases of the pelvic organs frequently give rise to pericystitis. Of these the commonest are malignant disease or ulceration of the rectum, inflammation of the seminal vesicles, uterus, and Fallopian tubes. Appendical abscesses spread into the pelvic areolar tissue, and cause acute or chronic pericystitis.

Suppuration in the prevesical areolar tissue or abscess of the space of Retzius forms a special group of cases. The abscess may follow rupture of the membranous urethra, or tearing of the canal with septic instruments; infiltration behind a stricture; suprapubic puncture performed with a septic trocar, or followed

517

by leakage of septic urine from the bladder; or necrosis of the pubic bones.

Pathology.—Two forms are met with, similar to those which occur around the kidney, namely, (1) chronic fibro-lipomatous pericystitis, with or without points of suppuration, and (2) perivesical suppuration and abscess.

1. In the *fibro-lipomatous* type a mass gradually forms around the bladder, confining its movements and forming dense adhesions to the peritoneum and surrounding structures. This is usually most marked around the base of the bladder and around the lower ends of the ureters and the seminal vesicles. It may increase until the bladder forms a small cavity surrounded by a mass of fibrous tissue and coarse fat several inches in thickness. In this, small isolated collections of pus may be found. In such cases there is advanced disease of the bladder, the wall of which is thick, contracted, and fibrous. In cases of bygone appendicitis the perivesical areolar tissue may be dense and fibrous.

2. Perivesical *suppuration* is diffuse or circumscribed. In the diffuse form the areolar tissue is widely infiltrated. In the circumscribed form the pus is thick and foul, and it may be confined by adhesions to the anterior, lateral, or posterior aspect of the bladder.

The abscess may surround a diverticulum, or it may form in the outer layers of the bladder wall.

The abscess may rupture into the bladder and also into the rectum or peritoneum, or, after forming adhesions, into the bowel, and a recto- or entero-vesical fistula results.

Symptoms.—The varying etiology and position of the pericystitis give rise to a variety of symptoms. Clinically the cases may be divided into those in which the bladder is primarily diseased and those in which there is disease of other organs, while the prevesical abscess forms a special group.

1. **Pericystitis following disease of the bladder.** — In the course of chronic cystitis there is little to show that pericystitis is present. The capacity of the bladder is diminished, and distension becomes impossible.

On rectal examination, and especially on bimanual palpation, the greatly thickened ·bladder wall is recognized. When the upper part of the bladder is affected an abdominal tumour may be formed.

Great fibro-lipomatous thickening may develop around a large diverticulum, which can be felt as a hard mass resembling a malignant growth. In these cases it may be impossible to obtain a good cystoscopic view of the interior of the bladder. The presence and size of the diverticulum may be demonstrated by obtaining a radiogram after distension of the bladder with bismuth emulsion or collargol solution.

Localized perivesical suppuration may develop insidiously, so that it is not recognized during life.

The abscess may be more acute and may rupture into the bladder cavity, giving rise to an attack of acute cystitis superadded to the symptoms of subacute or chronic cystitis which already exist. There is intense pain and strangury, the urine is alkaline, purulent, and blood-stained. Suprapubic tenderness and sometimes distension of the bowel and obstinate constipation are present. The temperature is high, and there may be repeated rigors. The appetite is lost, the tongue dry and glazed, with intense thirst and occasional vomiting and rapid wasting.

The case may, however, pursue a much milder course. A tumour may be found on suprapubic or bimanual palpation, which may be mistaken for a malignant growth, or there is a boggy mass felt in the rectum at the bladder base or to one or other side of the pelvis.

Cystoscopy is often impossible owing to the spasm of the bladder. When a view is obtained the mucous membrane is seen to be intensely inflamed, and thrown into large, irregular, œdematous folds.

Finally, the abscess may rupture into the rectum or bowel, and urine is discharged with the fæces, and gas and fæculent urine are passed by the urethra. ˙

2. **Prevesical suppuration or abscess of the space of Retzius, acute or chronic.**—In acute cases there is a high, swinging temperature, often with repeated rigors, frequent micturition and strangury, suprapubic pain and tenderness, and dullness on percussion. A prominent rounded swelling appears above the pubes, which closely resembles the contour of the distended bladder. On the bladder being emptied the swelling remains unchanged. When there is previous disease of the bladder and urethra the urine is purulent, and may be alkaline and stinking.

The abscess may develop more slowly and insidiously. In a case under my care there was gradual onset of increased frequency and pain on micturition, with slightly purulent urine, and after some weeks cystoscopy showed a prominent patch of bullous cystitis on the anterior wall of the bladder closely resembling a growth. This rapidly subsided when the abscess was drained.

3. **Pericystitis following disease of other organs.**—An appendicular abscess may invade the areolar tissue of the pelvis and open into the bladder. During the course of an attack of

appendicitis bladder symptoms appear. Before any change is observed in the urine, there are increased frequency of micturition, spasm and pain on passing water, and the mucous membrane of the bladder is at first unchanged. This is followed by the discharge of a quantity of fetid pus in the urine and an attack of acute cystitis, and a fistula may form between the appendix or cæcum and the bladder.

General symptoms are prominent. There are pain in the lower part of the abdomen, high, swinging temperature, and rapid emaciation. There is suprapubic tenderness, and tenderness on rectal examination. The pain is not affected by micturition, but is increased by movement. The urine remains clear until the abscess has ruptured into the bladder, when it becomes purulent and fetid; if a fistula forms it contains fæcal material, and gas is passed with a peculiar sensation that attracts the notice of the patient. On examination there is a hard mass in the region of the bladder, which may fill up the pelvis and extend suprapubically, or there may be a circumscribed mass in the pelvis in close relation to the bladder. On rectal examination the bladder base is tender, thick, and boggy.

The cystoscope shows at first a patch of cystitis of varying size, and later œdema and intense cystitis, with hæmorrhages, and finally necrosis at some point of the wall, giving rise to a fistula. Similar symptoms are produced by pericystitis originating in the rectum, sigmoid flexure, or small intestine.

Pyosalpinx may rupture into the bladder, but this termination is less frequent than rupture into the rectum or vagina. Gras found that rupture into the bladder occurred in 11 out of 60 cases. The bladder may remain free from cystitis for a long period, even when pus is being discharged into it from such a collection. After rupture of the abscess the cavity may heal in a few days. The abscess may discharge intermittently, causing pain and fever in the intervals of retention of pus, or there may be prolonged discharge of pus without general symptoms.

The **diagnosis** is made by the intermittent discharge of large quantities of pus in the urine and the absence of pyonephrosis. Cystoscopy shows a patch of thickened inflamed mucous membrane, and a round or irregular opening may be seen in this area.

Pericystitis following surgical operations or resulting from rupture of pelvic organs from injury tends to spread widely and rapidly. There are repeated rigors and high, swinging temperature, and the patient sinks and dies.

Prognosis.—Spontaneous recovery after rupture of an abscess into the bladder not infrequently takes place. In cases of malignant disease or tuberculous cystitis the duration of life is shortened by the development of a perivesical abscess. Pericystitis following operations upon the bladder is rapidly fatal in many cases. The formation of a recto- or entero-vesical fistula is not infrequent.

Treatment.—No radical treatment is possible for chronic fibro-lipomatous cystitis. The application of heat by means of fomentations, Leiter's tubes, etc., has been followed by the disappearance of extensive inflammatory thickening of recent origin.

In acute cases the perivesical areolar planes should be freely drained. A prevesical abscess should be incised by a median suprapubic incision, large rubber drainage tubes introduced, and the cavity freely irrigated daily. In some cases when the diagnosis is obscure the perivesical or interstitial abscess is opened during an exploration of the bladder.

Chronic abscesses are surrounded by a thick wall of inflammatory tissue which mats the pelvic organs together so that it is impossible to distinguish anatomical structures. The incision should be suprapubic and vertical. Occasionally a transverse incision may be necessary, and rarely the abscess is drained from the perineum. Great care should be taken not to open the peritoneum. When pus is reached by careful blunt dissection, the finger is introduced and the opening enlarged, and large drainage tubes are inserted.

LITERATURE

Englisch, *Wien. klin. Woch.,* 1889, p. 25.
Gras, Thèse de Paris, 1905.
Müller et Petitjean, *Gaz. des Hôp.,* 1908, p. 819.
Schmidt, *Surg., Gyn., and Obst.,* 1911, p. 281.
Walko, *Münch. med. Woch.,* 1904.
Zuckerkandl, *Handbuch der Urologie* (von Frisch und Zuckerkandl), 1905, B. ii.

CHAPTER XXXIX

FISTULA OF THE BLADDER AND PERIVESICAL HYDATID CYSTS

SUPRAPUBIC VESICAL FISTULA

THE orifice of the fistula is usually situated at the lower end of a suprapubic operation scar. It is small, and a bud of granulation tissue may project from it, or it may lie at the bottom of a depressed scar. The surrounding skin is usually healthy, but if the urine is decomposing and constant cleanliness is not observed the scar is thick and red, and the skin inflamed and excoriated. The whole of the urine may pass this way, or the fistula may leak only when the bladder contracts, the urine being discharged partly by the urethra and partly by the fistula. Sometimes a tiny jet of urine is discharged from the fistula for some distance at each micturition. The fistula may close for a time and then leak again.

Etiology.—A permanent fistula may be intentionally formed by the surgeon for incurable urethral obstruction or other disease. Very rarely the fistula is the result of a wound of the bladder, unconnected with operation. A spontaneous fistula from extension of disease of the bladder, such as malignant growth or tuberculous disease, is rare. The scar of an old suprapubic cystotomy wound may break down and a fistula form some months or years after the operation.

The most frequent form of fistula results from the non-healing of a suprapubic cystotomy wound. The principal causes of its persistence are mistakes in technique and sepsis, but other factors may be present.

Too long retention of drainage tubes in a cystotomy wound causes a thick hard tube of fibrous tissue to form, which prevents healing by granulation. A cystotomy wound which lies low down in the anterior wall of the bladder near the urethra and behind the pubic symphysis heals less readily than a wound placed high up above the pubes. The bladder wall becomes adherent to the posterior surface of the symphysis, and this interferes with the healing of the fistula.

522

.Prolapse of a peritoneal sac between the muscles of the abdominal wall interferes with the healing of the suprapubic wound. This difficulty is most frequently encountered after the transverse incision from cystotomy, but it may also follow a vertical incision. In both it is due to breaking down of the wound from sepsis, or to imperfect technique in the repair of the abdominal wall.

The spread of a rapidly growing malignant growth of the bladder along the suprapubic tract and tuberculous infection of the wall are rare causes of fistula. Unrelieved urethral obstruction caused by simple or malignant enlargement of the prostate or stricture results in the formation of fistula after cystotomy. Cystitis resulting from recurring infection from a congenital diverticulum may cause a persistent fistula after cystotomy. After the operation of suprapubic prostatectomy, fistula may be due to sepsis or to obstruction resulting from incomplete removal of the enlarged prostate, stenosis at the vesical outlet, stone in the prostatic cavity, or the recurrence of carcinoma of the prostate. Delayed healing of suprapubic wounds is not infrequently observed in very old and feeble patients, and in patients suffering from nervous disease.

Treatment.—Sepsis must be energetically treated by the administration of urinary antiseptics and by daily washing the bladder, a catheter being tied in the urethra. The urine should be examined bacteriologically, and a vaccine prepared from the predominant organisms and given in increasing doses.

Should these measures fail, and should phosphatic débris or calculi or unrelieved urethral obstruction be present, operation is necessary. The track of the suprapubic fistula should be dissected out down to the bladder wall. Care is taken to avoid opening the peritoneum, which is frequently adherent to the scar or may form a pocket in it. If the peritoneal cavity is opened the forefinger should be introduced and used as a guide to dissect the peritoneum up, and the wound should then be closed with catgut and the operation continued. The thick mass of scar tissue should be removed, exposing the rectus muscle on each side, and dissection should be carried down behind the pubic symphysis so as to free the bladder wall. The fistulous track is removed and the bladder cavity explored with the finger. Phosphatic débris or stone is removed, stenosis at the neck of the bladder is treated by free cutting on a sound, and obstructing portions of an adenomatous prostate are shelled out. Should it be considered advisable, the wound in the bladder is closed with one or two rows of interrupted catgut sutures, a small drainage tube placed in the lower end of the abdominal wound, and the recti muscles and sheaths carefully united with interrupted catgut sutures. A catheter. is tied in the urethra for a week.

The septic state of the bladder, or the possibility of hæmorrhage, or the presence of symptoms of renal disease may render it unwise to close the wound after dissecting out the fistula. A rubber tube is inserted, and the bladder treated by constant irrigation or repeated washing. After a week the tube is removed and the wound allowed to heal.

VESICO-INTESTINAL FISTULA

Etiology.—The fistula may be spontaneous or traumatic. Spontaneous fistula may take origin in the bladder in chronic cystitis, malignant growth, or some other condition which will cause perivesical abscess (*see* p. 517). The abscess forms adhesions to the rectum or intestine, and ruptures both into this and the bladder.

Rarely, tuberculosis of the bladder or prostate or malignant growths of these organs is the cause of the fistula.

Simple, tuberculous, or malignant ulceration of the rectum or intestine may lead to adhesions to the bladder and the formation of a fistula. Pascal found the following order of frequency in collected cases: Malignant growth of the intestine 35 cases, tuberculosis 6, syphilis 3, actinomycosis 3. Of 13 cases of fæcal fistula of the bladder under my care only 3 were due to malignant growths, 1 at the ileo-cæcal valve and the other 2 in the sigmoid flexure and rectum. The remaining 10 cases were due to —abscess round the bowel of unknown origin 2, stricture and abscess of the wall of the sigmoid flexure following dysentery 2, diverticulitis and abscess round the sigmoid flexure 1, appendicitis 1, typhoid fever 1, perivesical abscess following cystitis 1, non-tuberculous prostatic abscess 1, diverticulum of the bladder 1.

Traumatic fistula follows wounds of the abdomen or perineum, the opening either resulting from a wound or from subsequent suppuration and sloughing.

Pathology.—The opening in the bladder is most frequently found on the posterior wall, high up, or it may be in the neighbourhood of the ureters. Fistulæ are less often found in other parts of the bladder, and are rarest on the anterior wall. A fistula on the right side of the bladder usually communicates with the cæcum or the appendix, and one on the left side with the sigmoid, but I have known a fistula due to abscess round the sigmoid open on the right side of the bladder. The opening may be so small that it will only admit a probe, or it may be the size of a sixpenny-piece. It is surrounded by an area of inflammation of varying intensity. The vesical opening may enter directly into the bowel, but there is usually either a tortuous track or an intermediate cavity. Rarely there are several openings into the bowel or into other organs, such as the uterus, and only one into the bladder. The following is the order in which, according to Pascal, the different parts of the bowel are affected : Rectum, 57·9 per cent. ; sigmoid flexure, 21·5 per cent. ; ileum, 13·3 per cent. ; cæcum, 1 per cent.

The coils of intestine are usually matted in a dense mass, adherent to the bladder and filling the pelvis, and there may be narrowing of the bowel and dilatation above the narrow part. There is cystitis to a varying degree, and ascending pyelonephritis is the cause of death in the majority of cases.

Symptoms.—When the fistula forms in a previously healthy bladder the onset is frequently insidious, and the cause of the symptoms at first obscure. Spontaneous cystitis gradually develops, and persists sometimes for some weeks before a fistula is actually formed. I have cystoscoped a patient at this stage, and found cystitis distributed over the posterior wall but not otherwise distinctive. Obscure abdominal or pelvic pain may be present, and occasionally there are rigors, high temperature, and other symptoms of deep-seated suppuration. A history of rectal or intestinal disease may be given, or there may have been long-standing disease of the bladder when the primary disease is in this organ. The preliminary stage may be rupture of an abscess into the bladder. A quantity of pus is discharged in the urine, and blood may also be present ; rarely there is a sharp attack of hæmaturia. These symptoms may, however, be absent.

Pneumaturia, or the escape of gas by the urethra, is a constant and characteristic sign, and is frequently the first intimation that perforation has occurred. The gas is usually discharged at the end of micturition with a bubbling sound and a peculiar sensation. It may appear during micturition, or may only be present when the bowels move. Distension of the bladder with gas has occurred.

The passage of fæcal material in the urine may be constant or intermittent. There are only a few brown shreds, or irregular masses of brown fæcal matter of considerable size may be passed. The condition of the urine is characteristic. When the quantity of fæcal matter is moderate, the urine is hazy with mucus and bacteria, and contains brown shreds, and irregular white flakes or semitransparent shreds of meat fibre. There may be a distinct fæcal odour or only a faint trace. When larger quantities are present the urine may resemble weak beef-tea ; fragments of undigested food, portions of grape-skin, grape-seeds, orange-pips, fish-bones or fins, etc., may be distinguished. When the fistula is connected with the small intestine the urine is yellow with bile. The reaction of the urine is acid, and it contains albumin and mucus and many varieties of bacteria, among which the bacillus coli predominates.

When the escape of bowel contents into the bladder is inter-mittent, the "attacks" occur after some dietetic indiscretion which induces diarrhœa.

Frequent micturition is present and is due to cystitis. There are acute exacerbations and periods of quiescence. Urine is often passed by the bowel, the quantity varying from some ounces to the entire urinary secretion. Frequent watery stools of urine and fæcal matter are passed, or if constipation is present the urine may be discharged from the rectum with little fæcal matter. The diarrhœa varies inversely with the quantity of urine passed by the urethra.

Cystoscopy may be very difficult owing to the irritable condi-tion of the bladder, but in some cases the capacity amounts to 8 or 12 oz., and the examination is easy. The opening of the fistula is frequently hidden behind a fold or ridge of mucous membrane, and cannot be seen. In an old-standing fistula the cystitis is often moderate, and may be confined to the immediate neighbourhood of the opening The orifice of the fistula may be a small round opening level with the general surface, with a plug of fæcal matter protruding from it, or it may be surrounded by a button of closely set œdematous "bullæ." There may be a malignant growth in the bladder, surrounding the orifice.

Course and prognosis.—The condition may continue for many years without affecting the health of the patient unless the original disease is fatal. I have seen patients in good health three, four, and twenty years after the fistula became established.

The complications which may supervene are recurrent retention of fæcal material and pus in an intermediate cavity, peritonitis, ascending pyelonephritis, and intestinal obstruction.

Diagnosis.—Pneumaturia and fæcal material in the urine are constant and characteristic. It may be impossible to distinguish between fistula resulting from malignant growth of the bowel and that produced by other causes. A history of typhoid fever, dys-entery, or other probable cause of ulceration of the bowel is against malignant growth, while the presence of a well-defined hard mass in the region of the cæcum or sigmoid and the history of hæmor-rhage from the bowel and of the early onset of obstruction are in favour of a malignant growth. A mass of inflammatory material with matted coils of intestine in a case of non-malignant disease may readily be mistaken for a malignant growth, even after opening the abdomen. The lower bowel should be examined with the proctoscope and sigmoidoscope. It may be very difficult to ascertain the position of the intestinal orifice. When the small intestine is affected, the yellow biliary colour of the urine is characteristic.

A mass · in the right iliac fossa, and the fistula seen by the cystoscope on this side of the bladder, will point to the cæcum or appendix, and these signs on the left side to the sigmoid. If the orifice is rectal, the diagnosis can usually be made with the finger and the proctoscope, aided by the injection of coloured fluids into the bladder.

Treatment.—In some cases washing the bladder and rectum and careful attention to diet may be followed by closure of the fistula.

Palliative surgery.—A short circuit may be made so that the portion of bowel is excluded, and fæcal material thus prevented from entering the fistula. When the fistula opens into the rectum colotomy may be performed. A patient under my care was well and comfortable after sixteen years, but the recto-vesical fistula persisted.

Radical treatment consists in attempting to close the fistula by operation. This has been performed through the rectum after dilatation of the anal sphincter, with some successes, and a few cases have been operated upon through a suprapubic cystotomy wound. These methods are, however, inferior to the perineal route practised by Zuckerkandl. A transverse pre-anal incision is made, the rectum separated from the prostate and bladder, the fistulous tract cut across, and the openings in the bladder and rectum are closed. The bladder and rectum are kept apart with a gauze plug. In fistula originating above the rectum the abdomen is opened and the adherent coils of intestine are separated until the portion from which the fistula arises is identified. A part of this is excised and the ends are anastomosed; or it may be possible to close the openings in the intestine and bladder without resection of the former.

VESICO-VAGINAL FISTULA

Etiology.—Traumatic vesico-vaginal fistula is rare apart from surgical operations and parturition. In operations upon the genital organs an accidental vesico-vaginal fistula may be produced. In order to drain the bladder in cystitis a temporary vaginal fistula is sometimes made, and this may resist attempts at closure; or the opening may have been made for the removal of a stone in the bladder. Injury to the vaginal wall and subsequent formation of a fistula may result from the pressure of the fœtal head or of instruments during parturition. Foreign bodies in the vagina, such as a pessary, may ulcerate into the bladder. Spontaneous fistula may form from the ulceration of malignant growths of the bladder or cervix uteri, or from ulceration due to tuberculosis or other infection.

Pathology.—The common form opens directly from the base of the bladder at or behind the trigone, in the upper part of the anterior vaginal wall. Less frequently the fistula opens into the cervix uteri. The ureter may be implicated when extensive destruction has occurred in prolonged labour, and a vesico-ureterovaginal fistula results.

In large fistulæ there is generally some prolapse of the vesical mucous membrane into the vagina.

There is usually much scarring around the fistula, and if the fistula has followed a vaginal hysterectomy the upper part of the vagina is rigid and fixed.

The vagina is irritated by the urine, especially when it is decomposing, and the vulva and upper part of the thighs are excoriated. There is cystitis, and frequently stone in the bladder.

Symptoms.—The escape of urine from the vagina is the only symptom. This will vary according to the size of the fistula. The whole of the urine may escape day and night, or only a part of it, and sometimes it only escapes when the patient walks and is retained when she is recumbent. The urine is alkaline and decomposing, and a urinary odour surrounds the patient.

Diagnosis.—Vesico-vaginal fistula is recognized by examination with a vaginal speculum. In vesico-uterine fistula urine can be seen trickling from the os uteri, and injection of coloured fluid into the bladder is followed by its appearance at the os.

In vesico-uretero-vaginal fistula there is widespread destruction, and the position of the ureteric orifices will be distinguished after careful examination aided by the intramuscular injection of methylene blue or indigo carmine.

Prognosis.—If the fistula does not close in a few weeks after the injury it is unlikely that it will heal spontaneously. The chief danger is ascending pyelonephritis, but, apart from this, unless the fistula is cured the patient must become a recluse, and sometimes is bedridden.

Treatment.—This consists in plastic operation, but before it is undertaken the urine must, if possible, be rendered aseptic by urinary antiseptics and by washing the bladder. Calculi must be searched for and removed, and inflammation of the vagina and vulva treated by soothing douches and lotions. Free drainage of the urine by suprapubic cystotomy should be established for at least a week before all these plastic operations. At the operation free access to the fistula must be obtained, and if the vagina is scarred and narrowed a preliminary plastic operation may be necessary. The ureters should be properly safeguarded by passing a catheter along each at the commencement of the operation.

There are three methods of approach—(1) vaginal, (2) vesical, (3) peritoneal. The *vaginal method* is that which is most frequently employed. A number of operations have been used, and for these special works should be consulted. The author makes use of Young's prostatic retractor, introduced from the vagina through the fistula, in order to pull down and steady the fistula during the operation, and dissects up large anterior and posterior flaps of the vaginal wall, which are brought together after excision of the track. Whatever method is used, the bladder and vagina should be dissected very freely from each other, and if the cervix of the uterus is involved this should be freed. The free edges of the bladder and then those of the vagina should be accurately sutured. A plug of antiseptic gauze should be placed in the vagina to keep the surfaces of the flaps in apposition, and should be changed daily. A White's suction apparatus is fitted to the suprapubic wound to keep the bladder dry. The vagina and bladder are flushed out daily. At the end of a week the tubes are removed and the suprapubic wound is allowed to heal.

I have found a *combined vesical and vaginal operation* useful. The bladder is opened suprapubically with the patient in the Trendelenburg position, and the bladder wall round the fistula freed and sutured. The patient is then placed in the lithotomy position and the vaginal aspect of the fistula treated in the same way. Postoperative suprapubic drainage is essential.

LITERATURE

Bishop, *Lancet,* 1897, i. 1675.
Legueu, *Traité Chirurgical d' Urologie.* 1910.
Pascal, Thèse de Paris, 1899.
Walker, Thomson, Burghard's *System of Operative Surgery,* iii. 481.

PERIVESICAL HYDATID CYSTS

These are situated in the subperitoneal tissue of the pelvis, and may be primary or secondary. The primary cysts are very rare, only a few examples having been recorded. Secondary cysts are more common, the primary hydatid cyst being in the liver or elsewhere in the abdominal cavity. It has been proved by experiment that when scolices are introduced into the peritoneal

2 I

cavity they may penetrate the peritoneum, and hydatid cysts develop in the subperitoneal tissue of the pelvis.

The cyst forms in the subperitoneal tissue of the recto-vesical pouch, and becomes adherent to the bladder, prostate, and rectum. As it develops it mounts above the brim of the pelvis and grows into a cyst the size of a child's head or larger. It is usually single. The peritoneum is stretched over it and adherent to the cyst wall. Pressure upon the ureters in the pelvis may cause obstruction and dilatation.

Symptoms.—Frequent micturition and pain in the pelvis and on micturition are the earliest symptoms. Sciatica has been observed. Retention of urine occurs later from prostatic obstruction. A swelling appears above the pubes, which is firm, rounded, and dull on percussion, and closely resembles a distended bladder. In a case that came under my observation there were difficult micturition and a large, globular suprapubic swelling in a young man. The swelling was looked upon as due to a distended bladder, but on passage of a catheter the tumour remained after the bladder was emptied.

On rectal examination a tense swelling is felt in the region of the recto-vesical pouch, and bimanually fluctuation can be detected between the rectal finger and the hand above the pubes.

Hydatid fremitus is rarely detected. Rectal obstruction may be produced by a large cyst, and the ureters become dilated by pressure in the pelvis.

Diagnosis.—The diagnosis is not likely to be made before a suprapubic swelling has appeared. Previous to this, malignant growth of the prostate or pericystitis is the condition for which it will probably be mistaken. The presence of a fluctuating cyst in the male, in close relation to the bladder and unaffected by distension of the bladder, with no opening of a diverticulum in the bladder, should raise a strong suspicion of hydatid cyst.

The reaction known as " fixation of the complement " has given important results, and a diagnosis of hydatid cyst can be made by this means.

Treatment.—The cyst is exposed by a vertical median suprapubic incision, and the contents removed. If the cavity is septic it should be drained by. large tubes or by stitching the edges of the sac to the skin. If sepsis is not present the cavity should be closed.

LITERATURE

Cranwell and Vegos, *Rev. de la Soc. Méd. Argentina*, 1904, xii. 215.
Frustemberg, *Ann. d. Mal. d. Org. Gén.-Urin.*, 1901, p. 1160.
Kaliontzis, *Ann. d. Mal. d. Org. Gén.-Urin.*, 1909, p. 397.
Legueu, III⁰ Sess. de l'Assoc. Franç. d'Urol., Paris, 1899, p. 312.

CHAPTER XL

NERVOUS DISEASES OF THE BLADDER

THE nervous diseases which affect the bladder are principally spinal lesions. Cerebral disease rarely affects the organ so long as consciousness is retained, and it is doubtful if it is affected by changes in the peripheral nerves.

Symptoms.—Nervous disease of the bladder gives rise to pain, increased desire, diminished desire, difficulty, retention, incontinence.

1. **Pain.**—There is occasionally aching pain in the bladder. This is constant, capricious, and unaffected by micturition. In tabes attacks of acute pain (vesical crises) are sometimes observed.

2. **Increased desire and bladder spasm (hypertonic bladder).**—Increased frequency may be the only symptom of nervous disease of the bladder, or it may be one of a group of symptoms. It is not seldom combined with partial retention. In rare cases bladder spasm is present. There is increase in frequency, and the bladder expels the urine forcibly when a small quantity has collected. On introduction of a catheter and injection of fluid into the bladder the fluid is expelled with force, and the catheter may also be ejected. This form of irritability leads to an active incontinence. I have met with the symptom in cases of multiple sclerosis.

Frankl-Hochwart and Zuckerkandl found the intravesical tension in such cases (hypertonic) excessively high (80 cm. water).

3. **Diminished desire.**—The patient may pass urine twice in twenty-four hours, and then only because he considers it necessary, not from the sensation of desire to micturate. With this there is residual urine in varying amount.

The absence of desire is usually combined with a diminished sensibility of the bladder which may affect the mucous membrane over the whole surface or sometimes over half of the organ. The prostatic urethra may retain its sensibility. The condition is most frequently observed in tabes, but may also occur in transverse myelitis, syringo-myelia, diseases of the cauda equina, spinal meningitis, etc.

531

4. Difficult micturition.—Micturition is difficult in almost all cases of nervous disease of the bladder from spinal lesions. There is delay in commencing, and the patient waits a few seconds to two or more minutes before the flow appears. The stream is poor, it drops vertically from the meatus, and may be merely a dribble. By straining with the abdominal muscles, and sometimes by pressure with the hand above the pubes, the stream increases, but falls away again into a final dribble. Intermission of the flow is frequently observed. Sometimes the patient can only pass urine when at stool, or by assuming some peculiar position.

An early symptom may be the inability to interrupt the stream during the flow. The patient is usually aware that the bladder has not been completely emptied. The cause of the difficult micturition is paresis of the bladder muscle. Frankl-Hochwart mentions spasm of the vesical sphincter as an additional cause occurring in multiple sclerosis and other spinal diseases, but he admits that it is often diagnosed in error. In paresis of the bladder there is a varying quantity of residual urine, of which the patient may be unconscious. Tabes is the most frequent cause, but other spinal diseases such as transverse myelitis, multiple sclerosis, and syringomyelia may produce it. In many of these cases the nerve symptoms are slight and are overlooked, and the patient is treated for stricture or other urethral obstruction—a diagnosis which may appear to be confirmed by some difficulty in entering the membranous urethra with a sound. The slack urethral muscles in these cases allow the bulbous urethra to sag downwards when the patient lies on his back, so that the point of the instrument drops past the opening. For some days after the passage of a large instrument micturition may be more easily performed, and this may further lead the surgeon astray. Paresis is said to result from prolonged active retention of urine in a normal individual. After forcibly retaining the urine for many hours the patient is unable to pass urine. Cases where permanent paresis has followed have been recorded.

5. Complete retention (atonic bladder).—Nervous retention is due to paralysis of the bladder muscle. There may be complete retention when the bladder is first affected, and, later, improvement takes place and urine is passed but the bladder is incompletely emptied. Periods of complete retention lasting several years may alternate with periods of partial retention (difficult micturition with residual urine).

6. Incontinence of urine.—The following varieties of incontinence are observed in nervous diseases :—

    i. Active incontinence.
        (a) Reflex micturition.
        (b) Incomplete reflex micturition.
    ii. Passive incontinence.
        (a) Distension with overflow.
        (b) Collapse with outflow.

When the bladder is cut off from the control of the cerebrum it acts automatically. A quantity of urine collects, the reflex of micturition is initiated, and the bladder empties itself. This is repeated at intervals. The bladder is here in the state which is normal in the infant. This is observed in lesions above the lumbar centre, and, as Müller has shown, in lesions involving the lumbar centre also. There is sometimes uncontrollable spasm of the bladder, which empties itself forcibly whenever a small quantity of urine collects (hypertonic).

In many cases, in addition to being cut off from control, the bladder muscle is partly paralysed, either temporarily from over-distension, or permanently from disease of the lumbar or sympathetic centres, and here the organ is distended and small quantities of urine are discharged involuntarily from time to time. This state is likely to be mistaken for distension with overflow unless careful observations are made.

The bladder may only be partly distended, and the reflex micturition leaves behind a residuum of 8 or 10 oz.

In passive incontinence the contraction of the bladder is abolished and the outflow is purely mechanical.

In one type of nervous incontinence the bladder is fully distended and the surplus urine dribbles away continuously. Here the vesical sphincter is still active. In a second form there is no distension of the bladder, both the detrusor and the sphincter being paralysed and the urine dribbling away. As Corner points out, the bladder is seldom if ever empty, even where both detrusor and sphincter are paralysed. A certain amount of urine collects before the pressure is sufficient to overcome the elastic resistance of the urethra.

Changes in the bladder in nervous disease.—Cystitis is the most frequent complication in paresis of the bladder. The infection is usually introduced by the catheter, but it occasionally occurs spontaneously, bacteria reaching the bladder either through the urethra or after excretion by the kidneys. With the advent of cystitis there is increased frequency of micturition and increased sensibility of the bladder mucous membrane in cases where anæsthesia of the bladder has been a prominent symptom. The quantity of residual urine is usually much reduced. Sometimes there is painful desire to micturate with inability to expel the urine.

Cystitis becomes chronic in the majority of cases, and the urine may be alkaline and ammoniacal. Phosphatic calculi form rapidly.

Trabeculation in the early stages of tabes dorsalis was first observed cystoscopically by Nitze, while Orth and others have described the conditions post mortem in old-standing cases of tabes. Böhme described 8 cases of tabes in the early stage when trabeculation was present, and he regards this condition of the bladder as a diagnostic sign of tabes in the earliest stage. I have examined (1911) the bladder cystoscopically in 31 cases of tabes in its early and irregular forms. (Plate 38, Fig. 3.) Trabeculation was generally present, but was occasionally absent. Trabeculation in nervous disease is most frequently found in tabes, but it is not confined to that disease. I have seen it in atony from postero-lateral sclerosis and from spina bifida. It was absent in cases of multiple sclerosis and supralumbar myelitis that I examined. I have also described trabeculation in atony without nervous disease or urethral obstruction.

The trabeculation found in obstruction differs in several particulars from that found in spinal disease.

The trabeculation of an obstructed bladder is coarse, the muscular ridges being thick and irregularly branching, the interspaces deeply pouched, and the openings of the saccules often narrow. In trabeculation without gross obstruction the muscle ridges are fine and evenly set, and the branching is regular and orderly. Very fine twigs can frequently be seen branching and interlacing. A solitary muscle band may stand up sharply for 2 or 3 in. on the bladder wall. The interspaces are not so deep and are saucer-shaped.

In the obstructed bladder the whole organ is affected, the trigone is broken up into hypertrophied ridges among which the ureteric bar is hidden, and the ureteric orifices are difficult to find. In the unobstructed trabeculated bladder the side walls and apex are affected while the trigone escapes.

Frankl-Hochwart and Böhme believe that the trabeculation is due to hypertrophy caused by obstruction, which they state results from inability of the sphincter to relax. I hold that the earliest change in these cases is atrophy, and that the prominence of some muscle bundles is largely due to atrophy of neighbouring bundles. There may be compensatory hypertrophy of some of the remaining bundles, but it is insufficient to replace those that have atrophied.

Rarely in spinal disease ulceration of the bladder may develop and rapidly perforate. Such cases have been described by Hertig, le Fur, Posner, and others.

Bladder symptoms in special nervous diseases.—The bladder is more often affected in **tabes dorsalis** than in other forms of nervous disease. The type which most frequently comes under the observation of the surgeon is an irregular form when the bladder is early affected while the symptoms of spinal disease are only partly developed.

There is gradually increasing difficulty in micturition, delay in commencing the act, a loss of power of projection so that the stream tends to fall more vertically, intermittent flow with pauses of varying length, and dribbling after the act appears to be completed. There is not infrequently a diminished desire, so that the patient passes water less often than usual, and this only from habit, not from a natural call to micturate. If the patient is examined at this time there will be found a varying quantity of residual urine (6–12 oz.), with widespread trabeculation of the bladder. The tabetic symptoms may be confined to "rheumatic" pains in the legs and modification of the patellar reflex, or the presence of Argyll-Robertson pupils. The atony of the bladder gradually increases until there is complete retention of urine, or a sudden attack of retention may be the first symptom of which the patient complains. The bladder is greatly distended, and there is incontinence from overflow, or the patient may be able to expel some urine voluntarily by contraction of the abdominal muscles or pressure with his hand. Nocturnal enuresis is usually present, and this may be the first symptom.

The patient may feel the urine escape, but frequently the urethra is anæsthetic and the first feeling is one of dampness of the linen.

After a period varying from weeks to months some improvement in the tone of the bladder may take place, the residual urine being reduced to from 8 to 10 or 12 oz. and the bladder remaining in this condition.

I have not met with a spasmodic bladder (hypertonic) in tabes. Vesical and urethral crises are rare. Sudden pain is felt at the neck of the bladder, or along the urethra, or at the external meatus, and this may be accompanied by intense and frequent desire to micturate when the bladder is empty. The attacks may recur several times in an hour, and last one or several days.

In acute and chronic **spinal meningitis,** and acute and chronic **myelitis,** and in **multiple sclerosis,** there may be initial increased frequency of micturition, but the characteristic change in the bladder is gradually increasing atony, and complete retention develops. There may be difficulty in passing a catheter, from spasm of the sphincter. Dribbling of urine from over-distension . follows. The complete retention may continue, but usually after a time the bladder is emptied automatically. Spasmodic contraction of the bladder (hypertonic) is occasionally observed. When this is present it usually subsides gradually, and is succeeded by reflex micturition or atony.

In acute and chronic **anterior poliomyelitis, Friedreich's disease,** and **amyotrophic sclerosis** the bladder is unaffected.

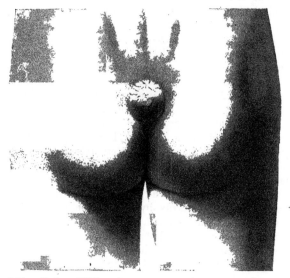

Fig. 160.—Spina bifida of sacrum, with atony of bladder.

In **cerebral disease** unassociated with loss of consciousness or spinal disease the bladder may be affected. These are cases of lesions of the corpus striatum or cortex, and possibly of the optic thalamus or cerebellum.

The bladder is rarely affected in **polyneuritis.**

In a case of **spina bifida** affecting the sacral canal in a man aged 38 (Fig. 160) there was difficult micturition and a poor stream from infancy. At the age of 19 complete retention developed, and the patient became dependent upon the catheter for ten or twelve years, with intervals of a few days at a time. After that he gave up using the catheter and passed water with difficulty for seven years. For three weeks he was again dependent on the catheter.

There was loss of desire and an absence of feeling of distension when the bladder was full. He also suffered from weakness of the anal sphincter, and a loose motion could not be retained.

Atony of the bladder without obstruction or signs of nervous disease.—I have described a series of cases under this title. The condition frequently occurred in patients under 30 years (22, 22, 23, 28, 30), and a history of syphilis could only be obtained in two cases. There were gradual onset and increase of difficulty in micturition, delay in initiation of the act, a feeble, often intermittent stream. Chronic distension of the bladder was present in four cases. The power of voluntary micturition remained, although greatly impaired. In the remaining cases there was residual urine varying from 4 to 10 oz. in amount.

Incontinence of urine was present in two cases, amounting in one to the escape of some urine on coughing or sneezing, and in another to nocturnal dribbling from an over-distended bladder.

There was loss of sensation in the bladder with reduced frequency of micturition in all but three cases, in which there was increased frequency without cystitis.

Well-marked trabeculation of the bladder wall was found in all.

In these cases there was atony of the bladder muscle to a varying degree, while the sphincter was weak but not paralysed in two cases, and active in all the others.

Urethral obstruction and spinal disease were eliminated. The lesion in these cases was probably in the lowest reflex centres of the bladder, namely, the hypogastric and hæmorrhoidal plexuses of the sympathetic.

In 9 cases there had been atony of the bladder for two, two and a half, four, five, six, eight, twelve, fourteen, and eighteen years respectively, without development of symptoms of spinal disease.

The absence of any evidence of spinal disease on examination of the cerebro-spinal fluid obtained by lumbar puncture (by Dr. Purves Stewart), and the long duration of the bladder atony without development of other symptoms, exclude the possibility of the atony being an early symptom of tabes.

It is possible that a lesion localized in the spinal reflex centre of the bladder might be the cause of this atony, but why such a lesion should remain .confined to the bladder centre in all these cases is difficult of explanation.

Blum and, later, Hahn have recorded cases of injury to the nervous system from falls or crushes, where permanent injury to the spinal bladder centre remained after the immediate results had passed off.

Injury to the nervous system.—Corner has investigated the state of the bladder in cases of injury to the nervous system. The following tables are extracted from his admirable article :—

Concussion of the brain.
1. Reflex or unconscious micturition.
2. Active retention.
    (a) Active overflow.
    (b) Passive overflow.
    (c) Absolute retention.

There is first retention of urine, which, if unrelieved, may proceed to active overflow (reflex contractions expel the surplus urine while the bladder remains distended), or to passive overflow (constant dribbling of overflow without reflex contractions), or, if urethral obstruction be present, absolute retention remains.

Compression.
1. Passive retention.
2. Active paralytic overflow. .
3. Passive paralytic overflow.

The symptoms differ from concussion in that they grow progressively more severe. In the later stages there is a paralytic condition of the bladder, in which a little urine collects, although the sphincter is also paralysed, and at first the escape is due to contractions of the bladder which are entirely local, but later these are lost and the urine dribbles away.

Spinal injuries.
1. Supralumbar lesions.
    (a) Active retention and its possible sequels.
    (b) Reflex micturition.
    (c) Exaggerated reflex micturition.
2. Lumbar lesion (the same as compression).
    (a) Passive retention and its possible sequels.
    (b) Active paralytic overflow.
    (c) Passive overflow.

Treatment of nervous diseases of the bladder. 1.—Relief of retention and residual urine.—The greatest care must be exercised in all instrumental interference to avoid introducing bacteria into the bladder. For complete retention catheter life is necessary. The catheter should be passed at regular intervals. It will usually suffice to pass it thrice in twenty-four hours—namely, in the morning, at night, and once during the day. With regular catheterization the tone of the bladder frequently improves, so that the number of times the catheter is passed may be reduced. When the residual urine does not exceed 8 or 10 oz. the catheter should be passed once a day, and if less than that once or twice a week will suffice. A soft rubber catheter of large calibre is most suitable for self-catheterization in these cases, as it is easily kept clean by boiling, and there is no urethral obstruction to overcome. Careful note should be kept of the quantity of residual urine as an indication of improvement or deterioration in the tone of the bladder.

When urethral obstruction is present it must be removed.

I have performed prostatectomy with success on a patient suffering from multiple sclerosis. Stricture of the urethra should be treated by urethrotomy.

2. **Prevention and treatment of cystitis.**— The measures which are elsewhere described of attaining asepsis in catheterization should be adopted. From the first, urinary antiseptics should be given (urotropine, hetralin, helmitol, etc.), and care should be taken to prevent constipation so as to avoid hæmatogenous infection. In women careful cleansing of the vulva is important as a safeguard against ascending infection.

If infection has occurred the bladder should be washed out with antiseptic solutions, of which silver nitrate (1 in 5,000 or 1 in 10,000), oxycyanide of mercury (1 in 5,000) and iodine (1 in 500 to 1 in 300 of the tincture) are the best. The patient can be instructed to do this by using an irrigator, or a trained nurse may be provided. Once a week will suffice in mild cystitis, but it is necessary to wash the bladder daily in more severe cases. When the urine is alkaline, sodium acid phosphate, 20 gr. thrice daily, should be administered with urotropine. The bladder should be examined from time to time with the cystoscope to ascertain if phosphatic calculi have formed, and if these are present they are removed by litholapaxy.

3. **Treatment of atony.**—With regular catheterization improvement in the tone of the bladder usually takes place. The patient should be encouraged to try to expel the urine. The liquid extract of ergot, 20–30 minims thrice daily, and liquor strychninæ, 5 minims, should be administered ; they are frequently of great service in increasing the contractile power of the bladder.

The administration of mercury and iodides has no beneficial effect on the bladder in these cases.

The electrical current may be used with advantage. One terminal is placed over the suprapubic region or over the sacrum and the other on the perineum, or a urethral electrode is introduced into the bladder or a rectal electrode into the rectum. A urethral electrode consists of a gum-elastic bougie enclosing a wire. At the proximal end is a connection for the wire, and at the distal end a small metal cone. A rectal electrode has a handle with a connection for the wire, and a metal cylinder which is oiled and introduced into the rectum.

The interrupted current is most frequently used, and the current should at first be weak and the sitting short. The galvanic current may also be used, commencing with 3 ma. and rising gradually to 5 ma. or more.

LITERATURE

Albarran, Noguès, and others, Ier Congrès de l'Assoc. Internat. d'Urol., 1908, p. 265.

Asch, *Münch. med. Woch.,* 1909, No. 7.

Bierhoff, *Derm. Zeits.,* 1904, Nr. 3.

Böhme, *Münch. med. Woch.,* Dec. 15, 1908.

Corner, *Ann. Surg.,* 1901, xxxiv. 456.

von Frankl-Hochwart und **Zuckerkandl,** *Die nervosen Erkrankungen der Blase.* 1898.

Goltz und **Ewald,** *Pflügers Arch.,* Bd. lxiii.

Goltz und **Treusberg,** *Pflügers Arch.,* Bd. viii., ix.

Hahn, XVIe Congrès Internat. de Méd., Budapest, 1909, xiv. 428.

Hertig, *Arch. f. Psychiatrie,* xxvii. 2.

Hirt, *Centralbl. f. d. Krank. d. Harn- u. Sex.-Org.,* 1902.

Le Fur, Thèse de Paris, 1901.

Müller, *Deuts. Zeits. f. Nervenheilk.,* 1901, p. 86.

Rinaldo, *Gaz. degli Osped.,* Jan. 18, 1910.

Walker, Thomson, *Ann. Surg.,* 1910, p. 577.

CHAPTER XLI

OPERATIONS UPON THE BLADDER

THE operations upon the bladder performed for growths, stone, and other diseases are described under the headings of these diseases. Preliminary to most of these operations are certain preparations and the operation of cystotomy, and these will be described here.

The **general preparation of the patient** differs in no way from that adopted for other surgical operations. In suprapubic operations the pubic region is shaved, in perineal operations the scrotum and perineum are shaved, and the whole region thoroughly washed with ether soap. The skin is prepared by painting with a solution of iodine in rectified spirit (2 per cent.) twelve hours previous to the operation, and again immediately before it.

When an operation for growth or prostatectomy is proposed, and cystitis is present, every endeavour should be made to render the bladder aseptic. This may be done by careful washing through a catheter in the urethra; or, if the cystitis persists, and especially where renal complications from sepsis and back pressure are present, a week or a fortnight of drainage by tying in a catheter or by suprapubic cystotomy should be allowed as a preliminary to the main operation.

The preliminary to most operations upon the bladder is cystotomy, and the postoperative treatment, in the majority, consists of temporary or permanent drainage. These two procedures will therefore be described.

Cystotomy.—The bladder may be opened above the pubes (suprapubic cystotomy) or from the perineum (perineal cystotomy).

Perineal cystotomy.—This may rarely be used for exploration, for the extraction of foreign bodies and calculi, or for drainage. For all of these objects suprapubic cystotomy is preferable Perineal cystotomy is seldom employed, except in cases of stricture of the urethra with severe cystitis, or of stone in the prostate or prostatic urethra complicated by stone in the bladder.

A curved staff with a deep groove on the convexity of the

curve is introduced into the bladder, and the patient placed in the lithotomy position. The staff is held vertically by an assistant, who holds up the scrotum. An incision 1½ in. in length is made in the middle line, ending ½ in. in front of the anus. The bulb is seen at the upper part of the wound, and the staff is made prominent in the membranous urethra. The point of the knife, guided by the left forefinger, enters the groove in the staff, and is pushed along horizontally into the prostatic urethra. The knife is withdrawn and a probe-pointed grooved director pushed along the groove while the handle of the staff is depressed towards the perineum. This is replaced by a gorget, which enters the bladder, and the staff is removed. The forefinger of the left hand is introduced along the gorget into the bladder, and the gorget then removed. If the object of the operation is exploration of the bladder, the right hand is placed above the pubes and pushes the bladder downwards.

If drainage is desired, the gorget is again slipped into the bladder, and a rubber tube along this.

Suprapubic cystotomy.—A catheter is passed and the bladder distended with 12 oz. of warm boric lotion by means of a bladder syringe. If the urine is foul the bladder is repeatedly washed before final distension. The catheter is left in the urethra and plugged. An incision 2½ in. long is made in the middle line, commencing just below the upper border of the symphysis (Fig. 161). In a stout individual this is prolonged. The anterior layer of the rectus sheath is exposed and cleanly cut in the middle line. The pyramidalis and recti muscles come into view, and are split in the middle line with the handle of a scalpel. The finger seeks the upper border of the symphysis pubis and tears through the transversalis fascia. The pocket of peritoneum which dips in front of the bladder is pushed upwards; the bladder wall is recognized by its coarse muscle fibres, and the large veins which course over it are exposed. The wall is picked up with two pairs of tissue forceps, and the knife plunged sharply through it (Fig. 162). As the fluid wells up, the forefinger is inserted into the cavity and hooks up the bladder wall (Fig. 163). The further procedure depends upon the object for which the cystotomy is performed.

Cystotomy with air instead of water distension has no advantage and many disadvantages. Cystotomy without distension is necessary in some cases, as in vesico-vaginal fistula.

If possible, a large metal sound is introduced along the urethra and acts as a guide. If no instrument can be passed the surgeon depends upon good illumination and careful dissection.

After-treatment of the wound.—When the object of cystotomy has been attained it is sometimes possible to close the wound by immediate suture; in other cases temporary drainage will be adopted; in yet others permanent drainage must be installed.

Immediate suture is contra-indicated when urethral obstruction or cystitis is present, when there is a danger of hæmorrhage,

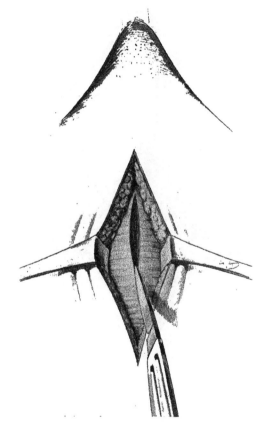

Fig. 161.—Suprapubic cystotomy.

A vertical median incision has been made through the skin, and the rectus sheath is being incised.

and in operations affecting the orifice of the ureter. The cases favourable to immediate closure are cystotomies for aseptic calculi or foreign bodies or small papilloma when there is no risk of hæmorrhage. The edges of the bladder wound are united by interrupted catgut sutures passed through the whole thickness of the wall, including the mucous membrane. Over these is placed a row of Lembert's sutures, and a drainage tube is inserted in the prevesical space, around which the abdominal wound is closed. A catheter is tied in the urethra.

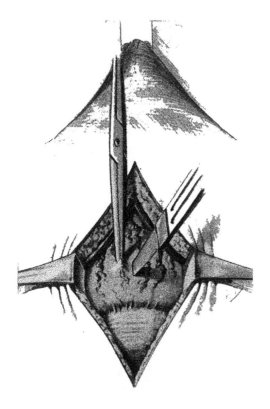

Fig. 162.—Suprapubic cystotomy.

The bladder, with its large, irregular veins, has been exposed and the peritoneum pushed upwards. The bladder wall is seized with forceps and the knife plunged vertically through it.

Measures for providing permanent drainage are described at page 549.

Dangers.—Wounds of the peritoneum should rarely occur if proper care is taken to push the peritoneal pouch out of the way.

If the peritoneum is opened the rent is at once repaired by means of a continuous catgut suture, and the operation continued. I have never seen ill effects follow when the wound has been recognized and immediately repaired.

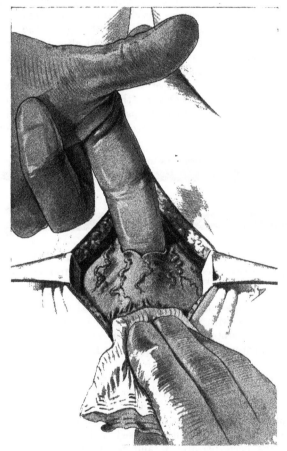

Fig. 163.—Suprapubic cystotomy.

The finger is introduced into the cystotomy wound, and the apex of the bladder hooked up while the peritoneum is brushed off it with a gauze swab.

Hæmorrhage may take place from the veins or an artery of the bladder wall. This is controlled by stitching the wound after the operation, either completely closing it or closing it around a drainage tube.

2 J

Modifications of suprapubic cystotomy. Transverse suprapubic cystotomy.—A transverse curved incision about 6 in. long is made across the lower part of the abdomen, 1 in. above the symphysis pubis and 2 in. above Poupart's ligament. The sheath of the recti muscles is cut through, and the recti and pyramidales muscles divided transversely, one or two sutures being placed through the upper cut edge of the muscles and assisting in repairing the abdominal wall after the operation. The fascia transversalis is incised and the peritoneum exposed and stripped off the bladder. A transverse incision is made through the bladder wall. After the operation careful repair of the abdominal wound is necessary; this is carried out by means of catgut sutures after lowering the patient to the horizontal from the Trendelenburg position. Free access is gained by this method,

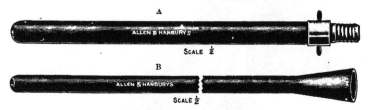

Fig. 164.—Perineal cystotomy drainage tubes.

A, Harrison's rigid tube with metal attachment for fixing tapes. B, Thick red rubber tube with terminal opening and a trumpet-shaped outer end.

but there is great weakening of the abdominal wall, and vertical median cystotomy with incision of the recti muscles is preferable.

Suprapubic cystotomy with resection of the pubic bones or with symphysiotomy has been performed, but is very rarely necessary.

Bladder drainage.—This may be required as a temporary measure after operation on the bladder or urethra, or as a means of treatment of cystitis. Permanent drainage may be necessary in cases of malignant disease of the prostate or bladder.

Perineal drainage.—This is used only when a perineal operation has been performed, and is unsuited for permanent drainage. The best form of drain is a flexible rubber tube with a terminal opening and lateral eyes (Fig. 164, B). The edges of the opening are smooth and rounded. The opening of the tube should lie just within the sphincter, and it is retained in position by a silkworm-gut suture passed through each lip of the perineal wound.

A stiff gum-elastic tube with a metal ring which has lateral eyes may be used (Fig. 164, A). The tube is held in position by passing a length of tape through each eye and carrying it along the fold of the groin in front and the fold of the buttocks behind. The tapes are knotted on each side above the great trochanter and attached to a waist-belt.

A short length of rubber tubing is attached to the tube and carried into a bottle containing antiseptic fluid.

Temporary suprapubic drainage.— This is practised after the majority of suprapubic operations on the bladder. The drainage must be free, and a rubber tube with a diameter of ¾–1 in. should be used. The tube is about 4 in. long—longer if there is a considerable development of fat —and it has a large lateral eye near the vesical end. The tube lies above the base of the bladder, but does not press on it. The part of the bladder wound unoccupied by this tube is stitched with catgut sutures. A small rubber tube is placed in front of the bladder behind the pubes. The tubes are held in position by silkworm-gut sutures passed through the skin after repair of the abdominal wound.

Stitching the edges of the bladder wound to the skin is to be avoided, as it is frequently followed by a urinary fistula. After four or five days the tubes should be removed and the wound allowed to granulate. It should close in fourteen to twenty-one days from the operation.

The skin should be protected by being smeared with an ointment containing lanoline, zinc oxide, and castor oil.

Methods of draining away the urine.—To avoid the discomfort of soaking the dressings with urine and to reduce the expense of dressings many methods have been adopted.

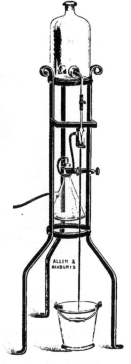

Fig. 165.—White's exhaust apparatus for bladder drainage.

1. *Exhaust methods.*—Cathcart's and White's apparatus may be used. White's (Fig. 165) consists of a water reservoir leading to a drop pump that sucks air out of a bottle, which again is connected with a double tube in the suprapubic wound. These evacuators can be applied only during the short period that a drainage tube is retained in the wound.

⌐.⌐ 2. *Siphonage.*—A small tube in the bladder may be connected with a length of rubber tubing and carried into a vessel below the bed. The siphon action is difficult to control, and, as a rule, acts too powerfully, sucking air, and eventually the bladder wall, into the tube.

I use a more satisfactory method, which is an overflow rather than a siphon method. To the top of the large bladder drainage tube a length of Paul's soft rubber colotomy tubing is attached by tying a ligature around it. This is brought over the side of the bed into a bottle. A little oil should be run through the tubing after boiling, in order to prevent the surfaces from adhering.

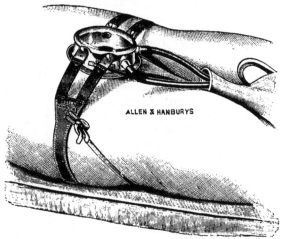

ALLEN & HANBURYS

Fig. 166.—Hamilton Irving's overflow apparatus for suprapubic cystotomy wounds.

3. *Overflow apparatus.*—Colt's and Hamilton Irving's are the methods in use, and of these Irving's apparatus (Fig. 166) is the more efficacious. It consists of a celluloid cap with a movable perforated lid. This is fastened over the wound by means of a rubber belt round the waist and two tapes which pass round the perineum to keep the cap from riding upwards. Two openings in the lower part of the circumference of the cap are provided with rubber tubes which conduct the overflow urine into a receptacle between the thighs. This is much the most satisfactory method. It can be applied at the time of the operation and used until the wound is healed. The pressure of the apparatus tends to cause eversion of the lips of the wound, and may slightly delay healing.

Permanent suprapubic drainage.—This may be required for malignant disease of the prostate or for other irremediable obstruction.

Having exposed and opened the bladder by the suprapubic route, the edges of the bladder wound are drawn into the suprapubic wound and stitched with catgut to the sheath of the rectus on each side. The upper part of the opening in the rectus sheath is closed with catgut, and the skin wound closed, leaving room for a rubber tube the size of the forefinger, which is passed into the bladder at the lower end of the wound. The wound is allowed to contract to the size of a No. 12 English rubber catheter. The catheter, which lies in the suprapubic fistula, is brought through a metal tube attached to a metal plate (Fig. 167) that is strapped to the abdomen. The catheter is carried into a rubber receptacle which is strapped to the patient's thigh. The patient can get about and pursue an active business life with this apparatus in place.

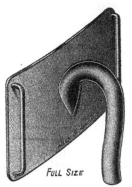

Full Size

Fig. 167.—Metal plate with tube for catheter, for permanent suprapubic drainage.

An ingenious method, and one which promises good results, has been introduced by Pardoe. The bladder is exposed by a vertical median suprapubic incision, and the peritoneum stripped off its posterior and lateral walls. The skin is undercut and retracted, exposing the sheath of the right or left rectus, in which a small vertical incision is made 2 in. from the middle line. The rectus is split from the mid-line cut to this opening, and a cone of bladder pulled through and out of the opening in the sheath, to the edges of which it is stitched. The cone is then brought through a small opening in the skin corresponding to that in the sheath. The cone is opened and a small self-retaining catheter inserted. The median wound is now closed. After a few days the catheter is removed, and a rubber catheter is passed at intervals through the fistulous opening. The bladder may be continent, or only a little urine may escape, which can be controlled by a light truss. The operation is not applicable to contracted or extensively adherent or infiltrated bladders.

PART IV.—THE URETHRA

CHAPTER XLII

SURGICAL ANATOMY

THE male urethra is about 8½ in. long, and is divided anatomically into three parts : the prostatic urethra (1¾ in.), the membranous urethra (¾ in.), and the spongy urethra (about 6 in.). A *pars intramurales*, where the canal passes through the base of the bladder, is also described (E. Zuckerkandl). Clinically, the canal is more conveniently divided into (1) the posterior urethra, which lies behind the compressor urethræ muscle and corresponds to the prostatic urethra, and (2) the anterior urethra, which lies in front of the compressor. The anterior urethra is divided into the bulbous or perineal urethra, and the penile, the names of which sufficiently explain their position and relation.

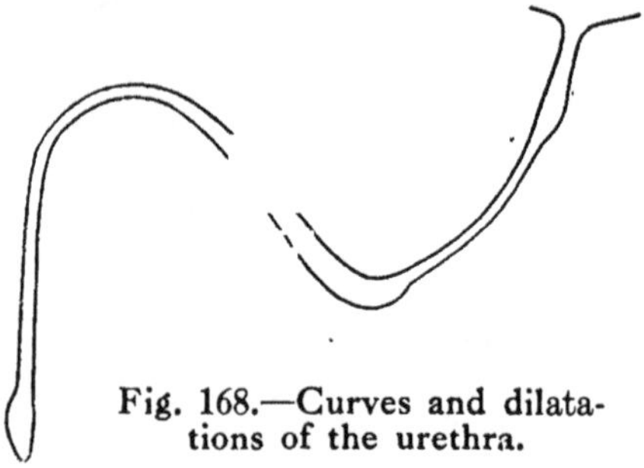

The urethra in the flaccid state of the penis has an S-shaped curve (Fig. 168). The internal meatus is on a level with the middle of the pubic symphysis and about 2 cm. behind it. From this the canal passes vertically downwards for about ½–¾ in. to the level of the verumontanum, and at this point it turns slightly forwards and maintains a forward and downward direction to the junction of the membranous and bulbous urethra. The canal now turns sharply upwards and forwards along the under-surface of the triangular ligament. At the peno-scrotal junction the urethra turns vertically downwards in the flaccid penis to the meatus.

The penile urethra is freely movable. At the base of the penis, the peno-scrotal junction, the canal becomes fixed, this part being slung up by a dense fibro-elastic band, the suspensory ligament

Fig. 168.—Curves and dilatations of the urethra.

of the penis, which has a vertical median attachment to the front of the pubic symphysis. (Fig. 169.)

Behind the peno-scrotal junction the urethra is fixed, the corpus spongio-sum being adhe-rent to the tri-angular ligament. Between the layers of the tri-angular ligament the membranous urethra is rigidly fixed, and the prostatic urethra is immobile, being surrounded by the prostate

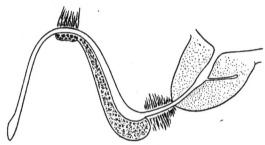

Fig. 169.—Relations of the prostate, compressor urethræ, bulb, and suspensory ligament to the urethra.

gland. The fixed curve of the urethra (Fig. 170) is 7 cm. long, and extends from the internal meatus to the peno-scrotal junction, the deepest part of the curve lying at the termination of the bulbous urethra, the *cul-de-sac du bulbe*. This is 4 cm. from the internal meatus, and 3 cm. from the peno-scrotal junction. The angle formed by these two segments is almost a right angle (93°). The most fixed part of the urethra corresponds to the triangular ligament.

A straight rigid instrument, such as a stone sound or cysto-scope, the beak of which is passed into the bladder, modifies the canal in the following man-ner: The penile urethra is first brought into line with the bulbous

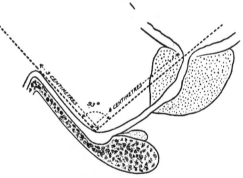

Fig. 170.—Fixed curve of the urethra.

urethra, and becomes vertical in the recumbent position. In order to pass the instrument into the membranous urethra the penile urethra is depressed and the suspensory ligament of the penis dragged upon. This, together with the elasticity of the wall of the bulbous urethra, allows the lumen to come into line with the membranous portion. If the recti abdominis muscles are contracted by the patient straining, or trying to raise his head and shoulders, the suspensory ligament is dragged upon and the straightening of the canal is considerably impeded. The elasticity of the prostatic urethra, combined with slight mobility of the prostate gland, allows these parts of the urethra to come into line, so that a straight line passes through the external meatus, the urethral opening in the triangular ligament, and the internal meatus; and the segment which remains fixed and immobile is the membranous urethra, in the grasp of the triangular ligament.

The walls of the urethra lie in contact. The external meatus is a vertical slit, the penile and bulbous urethra a transverse slit; the membranous urethra is star-shaped, and the prostatic urethra horseshoe-shaped with the convexity forwards, the internal meatus also having this form.

The **calibre** of the urethra varies at different parts. (Fig. 168.) The narrowest point is usually the external meatus; this part is more fibrous and has less elasticity than any other. The external meatus opens into the fossa navicularis, a dilatation of the canal situated in the glans penis, and formed by an arching of the roof, the floor being level with that of the penile urethra. At the junction of the fossa navicularis and the penile urethra the canal is again narrowed; and this part, the valve of Guérin, is not infrequently narrower than the external meatus. This valve is composed of a fold of mucous membrane, which usually takes the form of a transverse fold on the roof and two vertical folds at the lateral walls. In the fossa navicularis anterior to the roof fold is seen the opening of the lacuna magna, which passes backwards. The penile urethra is of even calibre. Across the roof of this, under full distension, fine transverse fibrous arches are seen. These supporting arches are frequently mistaken for strictures of wide calibre by the tyro in aero-urethroscopy. As the bulbous urethra passes backwards it gradually dilates until the opening of the membranous urethra is reached, when the floor rises sharply to this opening. The opening of the membranous urethra is thus on the roof of the bulbous urethra. In old men, and when the perineal muscles are slack, some sagging of this part is observed, so that a veritable *cul-de-sac du bulbe* is produced.

The membranous urethra is firmly closed by the tonic contraction of the compressor urethræ, but it offers no obstruction to the passage of large instruments. The normal prostatic urethra is elastic and capable of expansion; the internal meatus is more rigid.

The following are the **dimensions** of the anterior urethra, as given by Calle :—

Meatus, 25–30 mm.

Fossa navicularis, 30–35 mm.

Penile urethra, 35–37 mm.

Bulb, 35–38 mm.

Otis held that the calibre of the urethra had a constant relation to the circumference of the penis : when the circumference was 3 in. (75 mm.) the calibre was 30 mm. ; when the circumference was 3½ in. (87 mm.) the calibre was 34 mm., and so on. This rule is not generally accepted, and has certainly many exceptions.

Structure.—The urethra consists of a mucous, submucous, and muscular coat. The mucous membrane is lined with columnar epithelium, except at the fossa navicularis, where it is squamous. There is a basement membrane surrounded by a vascular layer, and this by a circular layer of non-striped muscle. In the penile urethra the circular muscle lies on the ventral surface of the urethra only. In the bulb the circular non-striped muscle is well developed ; on the dorsal wall it is wanting, but there is a layer of longitudinal fibres. In the prostatic urethra there is a well-developed internal longitudinal layer of non-striped muscle continued from the longitudinal muscle of the trigone, and outside this is a layer of circular fibres.

These layers are continued through the membranous urethra.

The anterior wall of the prostatic urethra is even and shows no openings. On the posterior wall is a vertical ridge commencing at the vesical orifice (uvula vesicæ) and rising gradually to the middle of the prostatic portion, where it culminates in an eminence, the verumontanum. Below this the ridge gradually sinks again. On each side of the ridge is a gutter, the prostatic sinus. The ducts of the prostatic glands open into the urethra in the prostatic sinuses in the immediate neighbourhood of the verumontanum and above this. No gland ducts open into the urethra between the part immediately adjacent to the verumontanum and the membranous urethra.

The sinus pocularis, a blind tube ¼–½ in. in length, opens on the verumontanum, and on each side of this are the slit-like openings of the ejaculatory ducts.

The mucous membrane of the membranous urethra shows the openings of numerous mucous glands. This portion of the urethra is surrounded by the compressor urethræ muscle, the external sphincter of the bladder, and on each side he Cowper's glands. The mucous membrane of the anterior urethra is thrown into longitudinal folds. In the mucous membrane there are numerous openings of small mucous glands, the glands of Littré, the ducts of which pass obliquely forward. There are also ten or twelve larger openings leading into lacunæ which pass obliquely backwards through the mucous membrane, and are found only on the roof of the bulbous and penile urethræ. (Plate 40, Fig. 1, facing p. 626.) Opening into the roof of the fossa navicularis is the largest and most constant of these, the lacuna magna, 6–8 mm. in length. The ducts of Cowper's glands converge and run for an inch or more in the wall of the bulbous urethra, opening separately on the floor about this distance from the membranous opening. Covering the under-surface of the bulb is the bulbo-cavernosus muscle, which acts powerfully in ejecting fluid from the bulbous urethra.

Lymphatics.—The lymphatics of the prostatic urethra join those of the prostate and pass to the chain along the internal iliac vessels. Those from the membranous and the bulbous urethra pierce the triangular ligament, and pass partly to the glands along the external iliac vessels, and partly to those in relation to the internal pudic vessels. The lymphatics of the spongy portion of the urethra pass round the sides of the penis or out at the frænum and join the lymphatics which accompany the dorsal vein. At the base of the penis these pass in a superficial set to join the superior group of inguinal glands, and in a deep set to the glands along the femoral vessels or along the inguinal canal to the external iliac artery. Other lymphatics pass beneath the pubic arch with the dorsal vein, and then join the glands along the external iliac vessels.

Female urethra.—The female urethra is 1½ in. in length, is almost straight, with a slight anterior concavity, and is intimately united with the anterior wall of the vagina. The internal meatus is situated at a lower level than in the male, being on the level of the lower border of the pubic symphysis, and is a little nearer to it.

The external meatus is a vertical slit immediately in front of the entrance of the vagina. It is the narrowest portion of the canal. The mucous membrane is thrown into longitudinal folds, the most marked of which is on the posterior wall. Numerous mucous glands and a few lacunæ open in the depression between these ridges. The epithelium is squamous at the external end and columnar near the bladder.

LITERATURE

Albarran, *Médecine Opératoire des Voies Urinaires.* 1909.
Walker, Thomson, *Med.-Chir. Trans.*, 1904, lxxxvii.
Zuckerkandl, E,. *Handbuch der Urologie* (von Frisch und O. Zuckerkandl), 1904, Bd. i.

CHAPTER XLIII

EXAMINATION OF THE URETHRA—URETHRAL SHOCK—URETHRAL FEVER

EXAMINATION

1. Inspection.—The size and appearance of the external meatus are examined. In acute and subacute urethritis the condition of the lips gives a fair indication of the state of the urethral mucous membrane. Congenital and acquired malformations are noted. A sinus or fistula may be found on one or on both sides of the frænum.

The swelling of a periurethral abscess may be seen in the penile or bulbar areas, or urinary fistulæ may be found. On examining a perineal urinary fistula I have found the rounded end of a large urethral calculus projecting through the opening.

When a sacculus of the urethra is present it will be seen to swell up during micturition and subside at the end of the act.

2. Palpation. — A small lacunar abscess of the penile urethra can be felt as a rounded body the size of small shot, and is made more evident on passing a bougie. Larger ab-

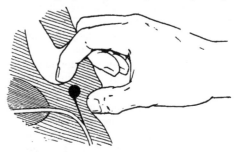

Fig. 171.—Palpation of Cowper's gland.

The forefinger is in the rectum and the thumb on the perineum, the patient being in the knee-elbow position.

scesses are less defined, and the skin over them is usually reddened. A cartilaginous stricture in the bulbous or penile urethra can frequently be felt when palpated with a bougie in the canal. A calculus or foreign body can be detected in the anterior urethra, but rarely in the prostatic portion unless it is of considerable size.

Cowper's glands, when inflamed, can be felt by introducing the forefinger into the rectum, sinking it alongside the membranous urethra, and placing the thumb upon the perineum (Fig. 171). The enlarged gland is felt as a hard pea-sized body between the finger and thumb. It cannot be felt in the normal state.

The membranous urethra is felt in the middle line below the prostate on rectal examination, and the prostatic urethra lies in the vertical sulcus between the lobes of the prostate.

3. Examination of the urethra with sounds.—An acorn-tipped bougie or *bougie à boule*, or a conical bougie (No. 18 Fr.), is used. The penis is raised with the left forefinger and thumb behind the corona glandis, and the instrument, well oiled, is passed gently along the anterior urethra, and any obstruction noted. If it is arrested, the distance from the meatus is noted and a smaller instrument tried.

There may be a creaking in passing through a cartilaginous stricture, grating in passing over a stone or a phosphatic deposit, or a tearing sensation when a false passage is made. These sensations are frequently confused, the most usual mistake being to make a diagnosis of calculus when a cartilaginous stricture is present or when the mucous membrane has been torn.

Slight resistance is felt, or the bougie is arrested, at 5½ or 6 in. from the meatus when it reaches the contracted membranous urethra. When the urethral muscles are atonic and a well-marked *cul-de-sac du bulbe* is present, the point of the bougie sinks past the opening. This is avoided by pressure upon the perineum with the disengaged hand, or by using a metal instrument and raising the point a little, so as to engage it in the membranous opening.

The resistance of the membranous urethra is overcome by gentle pressure, and the point enters the prostatic urethra. There may be a further slight resistance at the entrance of the bladder. In cases where instruments have been passed for many years, the bougie may be arrested in a pouch of the prostatic urethra, just behind the entrance into the bladder. In such a case a curved metal instrument can be passed by pulling gently upon the handle as it is being depressed between the thighs.

4. Urethroscopy.—The urethroscope consists of a tube which is introduced into the urethra and an apparatus for illumination. There are two varieties. In one the light is reflected from a lamp at the proximal end of the tube; in the other the lamp is placed in the lumen of the tube at its distal end. ..

I use Casper's and Wyndham Powell's patterns, in which the light is reflected into the tube by a mirror contained in the lantern. The part of the lantern that fits into the upper end of the urethral tube is provided with a window which is opened by a spring.

Below this is a tap which is connected with a rubber balloon for air-inflation of the urethra. (Fig. 172.) The electric current may be obtained from the main, the current being reduced by a transformer. For travelling, a small battery or accumulator which gives the required voltage for the urethroscope lamp is necessary.

For the anterior urethra the urethroscopic tube is straight, $5\frac{1}{2}$ in. long, and is provided with an accurately fitting metal obturator. A number of tubes of different calibre are necessary; Nos. 23 to 26 Charrière are useful sizes. The edge of the distal end should be smoothly rounded, and the end may be cut transversely or obliquely, the latter giving a slightly larger field. The tubes may, for convenience of noting the position of diseased areas, be marked in

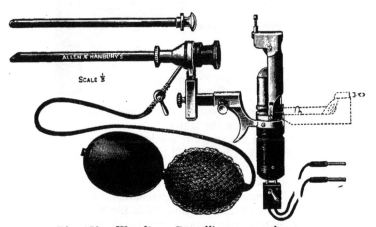

Fig. 172.—Wyndham Powell's aero-urethroscope.

half-inches. It is convenient to have one or two short tubes for examination of the outer portion of the penile urethra. A wire speculum (Smith's), or the slightly more elaborate speculum of Watson, may be used with reflected light for the first inch or so of the urethra.

The urethroscopes of Luys and Valentine are the most perfect of those with an internal lamp. They are open to the objections that the lamp tends to become overheated in a prolonged examination, and may scorch the mucous membrane; that applications of fluids tend to obscure the light; and that the lamps are very small and sensitive, and are quickly destroyed by variations in the electric current.

For operations on the anterior urethra the open urethroscopic tube is used. It is occasionally of benefit to have the urethra distended during the incision of a lacuna or small abscess, and for this purpose Wyndham Powell has introduced a modification of his urethroscope (Fig. 173). Attached to the lantern between the glass window and the nozzle which fits into the urethroscopic tube is a soft indiarubber cylinder which allows the lantern to be manipulated vertically while air-pressure is maintained. The fine

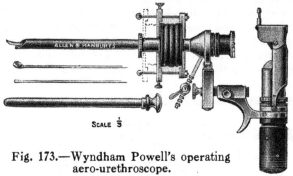

Fig. 173.—Wyndham Powell's operating aero-urethroscope.

urethral knife or probe or electrode is attached inside this, and is controlled by manipulating the lantern.

For examination of the prostatic urethra a longer tube (6¾ in.) with a well-curved beak (1 in.) should be used (Fig. 174). An open window is situated at the convexity of the junction of beak and shaft. The tube is fitted with an obturator during introduction. More elaborate instruments for the examination of the prostatic urethra are the urethroscopes of Goldschmidt and Wossidlo. These consist of a beaked tube with an opening in the shaft near the beak.

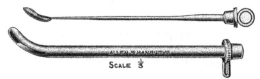

Fig. 174.—Tube for examining prostatic urethra.

Illumination is supplied by a fixed lamp at this opening, which is cooled by a water circulation. A telescope is introduced along the tube after removing the obturator. These tubes have the disadvantage of a large calibre, 23 or 24 Charrière.

Operations upon the posterior urethra are carried out through the open tube of the prostatoscope by means of fine electro-cauteries, curettes, alligator forceps, and other specially constructed instruments. (Figs. 175, 176.)

The Wossidlo urethroscope (Fig. 177) has been modified by H. E. Wossidlo to permit of free manipulation of the probe, fine cautery, or curette in view of the window of the telescope. These instruments pass along the lumen of the tube below the very fine telescope, and there is room for some excursion of the point of the instrument in all directions.

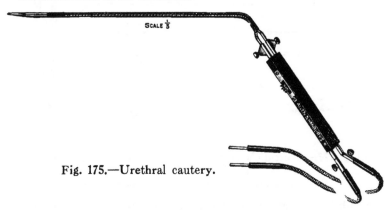

Fig. 175.—Urethral cautery.

A number of long, fine, metal wool-carriers are necessary for swabbing the urethra clear of lubricant, pus, etc. Fine urethral knives, probes, snares, and syringes complete the armamentarium. (Fig. 178.)

Technique of urethroscopy.—For anterior urethroscopy the patient lies flat on a high table, and the surgeon stands on his right side; or the patient may be recumbent, with the buttocks at

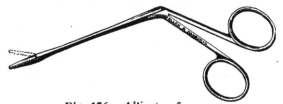

Fig. 176.—Alligator forceps.

the end of the table, the thighs horizontal, the knees bent, and the feet in inverted stirrups, the surgeon standing between the thighs. All parts of the urethroscope are carefully examined, the lamp tested, and the air-bulb blown up with the tap closed. The glans and meatus are cleansed, and the anterior urethroscope tube, with the obturator in position, lubricated with sterilized olive oil and very gently introduced. The instrument sinks as far as the membranous opening, the obturator is removed, a pledget of cotton-wool on a carrier introduced to remove the oil, the lantern applied to the tube, and the light switched on. The urethra is examined as the tube is slowly withdrawn. The tap of the

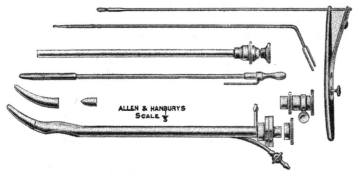

Fig. 177.—Wossidlo's urethroscope for examination of the prostatic urethra.

A snare and a fine cautery are shown, for urethroscopic operations.

air-bulb is now opened, and the urethra is distended like a tunnel. If during the introduction an obstruction is felt, the examination commences here. Air distension is especially useful in examining strictures, particularly multiple strictures and those of large calibre.

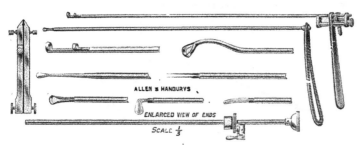

Fig. 178.—Armamentarium for use in operation through Wossidlo's urethroscope.

A punch, cautery, probe, and curette are shown.

In the normal urethra the mucous membrane varies from pink to red, the colour being deeper in the bulbous urethra. It is supple and light-reflecting, and shows longitudinal folds, and the vessels appear as longitudinal red markings. The membranous opening appears as a central depression from which radiate numerous fissures. Under air-distension the wall recedes and the upper lip of the opening forms a sharply cut, rounded arch, while the floor rises sharply and passes behind this. There may be a momentary relaxation of the opening as it swallows a gulp of air, and then it closes again. On withdrawing the tube slowly and keeping up the air pressure, the longitudinal striation of the mucous membrane is seen to be well marked on the floor of the bulbous portion. A central ridge may be found passing along the centre of the floor for about an inch. This is formed by the ducts of Cowper's glands, the openings of which can sometimes be seen about an inch from the membranous opening.

As the tube is withdrawn the air pressure may be relaxed and then re-established, and the mucous membrane is seen to be supple and to fall evenly over the end of the tube. Collapsed, it forms a central point from which radiate several fine fissures, and the longitudinal striation can be clearly seen. If the penis is not held in line with the bulbous urethra, a transverse fold appears on the floor at the peno-scrotal junction, which might be mistaken for a stricture. It disappears on making the urethra tense. On the roof of the bulbous and penile urethra the openings of lacunæ are seen (Plate 40, Fig. 1, facing p. 626), varying in size from a minute point to a pin's head. They are red and open, but are not normally surrounded by inflamed or œdematous mucous membrane, and no discharge issues as the urethroscope tube passes over them. In full air-distension numerous whitish transverse arches appear on the roof. These bands should not be mistaken for strictures of large calibre. The fold of Guérin is seen at the base of the glans, either as two lateral folds or sometimes as a circular narrowing, and the opening of the lacuna magna is found on the roof of the fossa navicularis. The latter is the largest opening on the roof of the urethra, and is bounded below by a transverse fold of mucous membrane.

For examination of the prostatic urethra a local anæsthetic is necessary, and a solution of cocaine sulphate (1 per cent.), or of alypin with suprarenal extract or of eucaine with suprarenal extract, is used. Twenty minims of the solution are introduced into the prostatic urethra by means of a Guyon's syringe. The patient lies on a high couch with the pelvis raised on a cushion, or, better still, is placed on a special chair with the hips and knees flexed. The posterior urethroscope tube, well lubricated, is passed through the anterior urethra and depressed so that the beak passes into the prostatic urethra and enters the grasp of the sphincter vesicæ.

The obturator is withdrawn and a tampon of wool introduced.

2 K

The lantern is applied with the glass window open and the light switched on.

The verumontanum is seen projecting into the window, and the sinus pocularis can be clearly seen, but the openings of the ejaculatory ducts are not visible. On either side are the prostatic sinuses. Below the verumontanum the inframontanal ridge is seen.

Only the posterior and part of the lateral walls can be seen, but in practice this is all that is necessary, as diseases of the prostatic urethra are confined to this area. In the most recent forms of prostatoscope the supramontanal ridge and the junction of the urethra and bladder can be inspected.

Pathological conditions which may be observed include swelling and redness of the lips of the sinus pocularis and the presence of pus at this orifice, distortion of the verumontanum and prostatic urethra from long-standing inflammation, polypi, and granulation tissue due to chronic posterior urethritis or to tuberculons disease spreading from the bladder or prostate.

After examination of the prostatic urethra the patient should rest in bed for at least twenty-four hours, and should take a diuretic mixture containing urotropine.

Female urethra.—The female urethra can be palpated on the anterior wall of the vagina, and should be examined for tenderness, thickening, or the presence of new growths or foreign bodies.

The urethroscope can be used as in the male, but without air-distension.

LITERATURE

Buerger, *Folia Urol.*, 1911, Heft 1.
Dreyer, *Zeits. f. Urol.*, 1909, Nr. 5.
Fenwick, *Obscure Diseases of the Urethra.* 1902.
Goldschmidt, *Folia Urol.*, 1907, Heft 1 ; 1910, Heft 9.
Kollmann und Oberländer, *Die chronische Gonorrhoe der männlichen Harnröhre*, 2 Auf. 1905.
Oberländer, *Lehrbuch der Urethroskopie.* 1893.
Oberländer, Wossidlo, und Frank, III. Kongress Verhandl. d. deuts. Gesell. f. Urol., 1911.
Walbarst, *Med. Rec.*, 1906, p. 627.
Wossidlo, E., *Berl. klin. Woch.*, 1912, Nr. 25 ; *Folia Urol.*, 1912, S. 40.
Wossidlo, H., *Folia Urol.*, 1911, S. 445.

ASEPSIS IN URETHRAL INSTRUMENTATION

The rules of asepsis which guide the surgeon in regard to the sterilization of his hands and the surroundings of the patient in general surgery apply with equal force to instrumental interference in the urethra and bladder. In addition to this, special care must be given to the instruments, the lubricant, and the urinary tract of the patient.

Solid metal instruments should have a smooth plated surface. If this becomes rough from wear, or chipped or cracked, the instrument should be replated. These instruments are boiled for ten minutes in water containing 1 per cent. of soda (sodium carbonate), and then placed upon a dry sterilized towel, or in a shallow tray containing weak carbolic lotion, 1 in 80, or biniodide of mercury, 1 in 5,000, care being taken to remove the lotion with a sterile mop before using the instrument. After use the lubricant is removed and the instrument again boiled, and stored dry.

Metal catheters should have the terminal portion beyond the eye solid, otherwise this forms a pocket for the collection of septic material. They are treated in the same manner as solid metal instruments, care being taken, especially in the smaller sizes, to see that the lumen is free by passing a stream of lotion through it. After use the interior should be washed by injecting lotion by means of a syringe, the lubricant is removed, and the instrument is then boiled, dried, and stored.

Rubber, gum-elastic, and silk-wove instruments require very careful attention. The surface must be absolutely smooth, without cracks, and the covering material flexible. On the first appearance of roughness at the tip or cracking of the body the instrument should be discarded. Such damaged instruments are very dangerous; they harbour germs, and rubber instruments in this condition are very brittle, and portions may be broken off and left in the bladder or urethra. In flexible catheters the terminal portion beyond the eye must be solid, and the interior of the catheter as smooth as the exterior. Information in regard to the state of the interior can be obtained by the sense of touch in passing a stilet with a fine pledget of cotton-wool along the lumen. If any doubt remains, the proximal end of the catheter should be cut off obliquely and the interior examined. These instruments, if well made, withstand boiling. Rubber catheters after repeated boiling tend to become soft.

Flexible bougies and catheters should be placed in boiling saturated solution of ammonium sulphate or in water to which sodium chloride has been added. Care should be taken that the air is expelled from the interior of the catheters, and they should lie upon a wire tray, so that contact with the bottom of the sterilizer is prevented. In removing a catheter from the sterilizer it must not be seized in the middle with forceps or other metal instruments, as the covering is soft and will certainly break. The tray of the sterilizer should be removed, and the catheter tilted into cold sterile water in a tray, or a piece of tape may be tied round the catheter to facilitate removal, or the open trumpet end may be picked up with forceps and the instrument dropped into a tall glass jar filled with cold sterile water. A very useful and easily carried sterilizer for catheters is that introduced by Prof. Zuckerkandl.

After use the catheter should be syringed through with carbolic or biniodide lotion, or it may be attached to a water-tap by an apparatus, and water passed through it in this manner. The lubricant is carefully removed from the surface, and the instrument washed in soap and water and dried. A mop with a drop of sterilized olive oil should then be passed over the surface (except in rubber catheters), so that a trace of oil remains on the catheter and keeps it from cracking. The catheters are stored in a japanned tin tray or in a glass tube, a little lycopodium powder being dusted over them. Special sterilizable metal boxes for carrying catheters, and containing a bottle of lubricant, may be obtained at any good instrument maker's. It is very important that the instruments should be absolutely dry, for even a trace of moisture will make the surfaces of the catheter adhere and become rough. On this account glass tubes should be open at both ends, with rubber stoppers, to allow of thorough drying of the interior. Condensation of moisture on the interior is prevented by leaving the stoppers out occasionally.

Formalin may be used as an antiseptic, and when large numbers of flexible instruments are employed this is a convenient method of sterilization. The formalin sterilizer consists of a metal box containing perforated trays in which the instruments lie. A cup on the floor holds the formalin, and under this is a spirit-lamp. The formalin is vaporized, and the box kept closed for several hours, and then filtered air pumped through it to remove the irritating vapour. A glass tube with a perforated box in the stopper containing a granular preparation of formalin may be used for a small number of catheters, but there is a tendency for moisture to collect and destroy the catheters.

A cystoscope may be sterilized by washing it with methylated spirit or ether soap, and then with carbolic lotion, 1 in 20, or biniodide of mercury, 1 in 2,000. In the irrigation cystoscope care should be taken to clean the interior of the irrigating tube, and especially the valve at the end of this, which should be detached and boiled. In the author's pattern of irrigation cystoscope the irrigating tube can be boiled, and the valve is so constructed that the spring lies outside the lumen, and there is no dead space for the collection of septic material.

The lubricant should be aseptic. Boiled olive oil is the best lubricant, and may be kept in a wide-mouthed, stoppered jar, float-

ing on biniodide solution. Liquid paraffin or vaseline may also
be used, or the following formula : Phenolis, 1 part; olei ricini,
7 parts; olei amygdalæ, 8 parts.

For cystoscopy no greasy lubricant can be used, as it would
obscure the window of the telescope. Glycerine is the best lubricant for this purpose, and 1 drachm of biniodide of mercury
solution (1 in 2,000) should be added to each ounce.

Urinary antiseptics should be used. . If instruments are being
passed once or twice a week, urotropine (5 or 10 grains thrice daily)
should be given continuously ; if the intervals between instrumentation are longer, the medicine should be given for two days before
and two days after each operation. A· diuretic water such as
Contrexéville may be given with advantage during the same period.
Before an instrument is passed the penis should be washed ; and
if there is urethral sepsis the urethra should be irrigated with
permanganate of potash solution, 1 in 5,000, or solution of nitrate of
silver, 1 in 10,000.

URETHRAL SHOCK

A mild degree of urethral shock is not uncommon in nervous
individuals. It occurs especially on the first instrumentation, but
may recur on subsequent occasions. In such patients the urethra
is usually hypersensitive. The patient feels faint and sick, his
pupils dilate, the skin becomes pale and clammy, and the pulse
rapid and feeble, and he may faint.

True urethral shock is rare, and is a much more serious
condition.

After an immunity of eight years, during which instruments
were passed on an average of well over one hundred cases each
week, three cases occurred in a month in middle-aged men in
my out-patient department at St. Peter's Hospital, two of which
were fatal. In all these cases a stricture was present and had
been examined with the urethroscope under air-distension without roughness, and no instrument had been passed through the
stricture ; after withdrawal of the instrument the patient gave
a few short gasps and became unconscious, one or two inspiratory
stridors followed, and breathing stopped. Half a minute later
a single loud expiratory effort, like the commencement of a violent
sneeze, occurred; the pupils became dilated, the pulse imper-
ceptible at the wrist, and after about a minute the heart sounds
ceased. Stimulation, tracheotomy, and artificial respiration were
unavailing. Post mortem the heart muscle was thin and friable,
but there was no valvular lesion. There was a moderate degree
of interstitial nephritis secondary to the stricture.

URETHRAL, URINARY, OR CATHETER FEVER

After the passage of an instrument a rise of temperature may take place, when urinary or catheter fever is said to be present.

Two theories were formerly held to explain the occurrence of urethral fever when the urethra is intact. In one, the rise of temperature was ascribed to a nervous origin; in the other, it was held to be due to sepsis. The two conditions were supposed in some cases to act in combination; in others, apart. Our present knowledge of the absorption of toxins and the access of bacteria, especially from the intestine, into the circulation through minute lesions, or even through apparently intact membranes, renders the nervous theory unnecessary, and it is now generally accepted that urethral fever in all its forms is septic in origin.

The infection either originates in a septic instrument, or the urethra is already infected, or becomes infected by septic urine. Infection is most frequently produced by a septic instrument. The following conditions may be present :—

1. The urethra is healthy and the urine aseptic, and the infection is introduced by the catheter. 2. There is obstructive disease in the urethra (stricture, enlarged prostate), but the urine is aseptic, the infection being introduced by the catheter. 3. The urine and urethra are already infected, with or without the presence of an obstructive lesion (chronic urethritis, chronic prostatitis, cystitis, stricture, enlarged prostate).

The surgical interference in the urethra is usually the passage of a catheter; but the passage of solid instruments, and operations on the urethra, such as internal urethrotomy, are also causes of urethral fever.

Infection is more likely to take place when an obstructive lesion is present than in an unobstructed urethra, in lesions of the bulbous than of the penile urethra, and in lesions of the prostatic than of the anterior urethra.

A rough, inexperienced hand is more likely to produce urinary fever than a gentle, educated touch. Fever tends to follow sudden or gradual increase in urinary pressure when sepsis is already present. Thus it appears on the sudden impaction of a stone in the ureter or urethra, on the blockage of a kidney the seat of pyelonephritis, as by sudden swelling of the mucous membrane due to an excessive dose of vaccine, and also during the first few days after the closure of a suprapubic wound when sepsis is present.

Types of urethral fever. 1. Urethral fever without suppression of urine.—(a) A rise of temperature to 100° or

101° F. may occur with slight malaise, and the temperature fall again to normal.

(*b*) A single severe rise. A few hours after the passage of an instrument the patient has a rigor, and the temperature rapidly mounts to 102° F. or higher. The patient is restless and ill, the tongue dry, the mouth parched, and there is burning thirst. The urine is scanty and high-coloured. In twenty-four or thirty-six hours, after profuse perspiration, the temperature falls to normal.

(*c*) In a third type the fever is prolonged (acute remittent type). After an initial rigor the temperature rises to 102° F. or higher, remaining high for several days, and then falling gradually to normal, sometimes rising again, but eventually falling to normal.

(*d*) A rigor follows internal urethrotomy or the passage of instruments, and the temperature rises to 103° or 104° F., and falls in a few hours or after a varying interval. A second rigor occurs with another rise of temperature, and the rigors are repeated at irregular intervals. The quantity of urine is diminished during the high temperature, but suppression does not take place. Venous thrombosis, pneumonia, or other complications eventually supervene, and the patient dies after several weeks.

2. **Urethral fever with suppression of urine.**—(*a*) There is a rigor within a few hours after internal urethrotomy, and the temperature rises to 104° F. or even higher. A few ounces of bloody urine are passed, and the secretion becomes completely suppressed. The patient is restless and wanders. He becomes rapidly comatose, and dies within eighteen to thirty-six hours of the operation. The condition is one of sudden and very profound toxæmia, of which the suppression is the result. (Chart 17.)

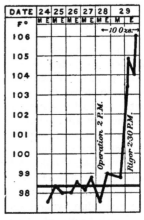

Chart 17.—Temperature chart in suppression of urine following internal urethrotomy.

(*b*) After the passage of a catheter in a case of enlarged prostate there is a rise of temperature, and the tongue is dry and glazed.

The patient is drowsy and heavy, and wanders at night. The temperature remains high; buccal dysphagia, hiccough, and vomiting follow; the quantity of urine, previously large, diminishes, and complete suppression may supervene. Death frequently results from this form of catheter fever, which is a grave danger at the commencement of " catheter life."

Treatment.—Prophylactic measures are very important. The sterilization of all instruments should be carefully carried out. When the passage of instruments is to be undertaken in cases where the urine is septic, previous treatment should, if possible, be carried out, such as washing the urethra with weak nitrate-of-silver solution or other antiseptics, and the administration of urinary antiseptics by the mouth. Diuretics such as Contrexéville water should also be given.

The prophylactic treatment that should be adopted before and after the operations of internal urethrotomy and litholapaxy is described under those operations.

The precautions necessary for the emptying of a distended bladder obstructed by an enlarged prostate are given under that head (p. 703). When infection has occurred, a smart purge should be administered, diuretics, such as large quantities of Contrexéville water, or barley water, freely given, and urinary antiseptics (urotropine, hetralin, helmitol) administered. If the infection is due to the bacillus coli in pure culture, large doses of alkalis (potassium citrate) should be given.

A catheter should be tied in the urethra, and kept in until the temperature has fallen. In severe cases, when this method is unsuccessful, suprapubic drainage with a large rubber tube in the cystotomy wound should be installed.

Vaccine and serum treatment may be tried.

The abdomen should be carefully examined for evidence of pyelonephritis; and should the kidney be found enlarged or tender, and the temperature persist, nephrotomy and drainage of the kidney should be rapidly performed. If there is urethral obstruction, suprapubic cystotomy should be performed at the same time.

CHAPTER XLIV

CONGENITAL MALFORMATIONS OF THE URETHRA

THE development of the urethra has already been described (*see* p. 392).

CONGENITAL ABSENCE OR OBLITERATION OF THE URETHRA

This is rare. The penis is absent or rudimentary, and other malformations are present. A communication frequently exists between the bladder and rectum, which opens just inside the anus. Absence of the urethra has also been observed in female subjects, the urine being discharged at the umbilicus or passing through a fistula into the distended uterus, and thence by another fistula into the rectum. The children are usually stillborn, or die soon after birth. Distension of the bladder may give rise to difficulty in parturition.

No operative treatment is possible, and the treatment consists in the administration of urinary antiseptics and other palliative measures.

PARTIAL OBLITERATION OF THE URETHRA

This may be found at the glans, in the bulbous, membranous, or prostatic urethra.

The prepuce may be adherent and the orifice closed, or there may be atresia of the orifice of the glandular urethra, or absence of a canal in the glans penis, the urethra ending blindly at the base of the glans. In such a case there may be a depression on the end of the glans.

Obliteration of other parts of the urethra is less common. Kauffmann found that the order of frequency was—spongy urethra (11), membranous urethra (7), and prostatic urethra (1).

Multiple obliteration of the male urethra has been observed, and the female urethra may be obliterated. The results of the obliteration depend upon the presence or absence of an outlet for the

569

urine other than the urethra. If no outlet is present and the kidneys are active, the bladder becomes greatly distended and fills the abdomen, causing difficulty in parturition. The ureters and kidneys also become dilated. The kidneys, too, may be the seat of congenital malformation or of interstitial changes, and be inactive, and distension of the urinary passages does not take place. An outlet for the urine may be present in the form of a patent urachus, or a communication with the rectum either direct or through the uterus. In the latter case urine may escape through the Fallopian tubes into the peritoneal cavity, or by a penile or vaginal fistula.

Diagnosis.—In children that survive birth no urine is found in the diapers, and on examination there is atresia of the urethra and distension of the bladder.

The anterior part of the urethra may be normal, but on passing a fine bougie it is arrested.

There is no distension when the urine can escape from the umbilicus or into the bowel. In the latter event urine is passed with a motion from the rectum.

In the majority of cases the child is stillborn, or dies soon after birth. In a few, when the urine can escape, life is prolonged for a few years, but death takes place from ascending infection.

Treatment.—When atresia of the glandular urethra only is present the dilated portion of the canal behind this may be opened and a penile fistula established, a plastic operation being carried out later for the formation of a glandular urethra. In some cases the glans has been tunnelled with a trocar, and the canal kept open by the passage of catheters or bougies. When the obliterated portion lies deeper, the urethra may be opened from the perineum behind the obstruction, and the bladder drained, a communication between the posterior and anterior portions of the urethra being established. Recontraction of the new canal does not, apparently, follow in all cases, as might be expected, but every precaution should be taken to prevent this happening. Suprapubic puncture and cystotomy are emergency operations to relieve distension.

DOUBLE URETHRA AND ACCESSORY TRACKS OF THE PENIS

Double urethra is a very rare condition, and may be combined with double penis, double scrotum, double bladder, atresia ani, or other congenital malformations.

The second urethra may open on the perineum or in the inguinal region. A more frequent condition is where a canal

opens on the glans or below the penis, and runs backwards on
the upper or under surface of the penis. Burckhardt has collected 22 such cases, in 18 of which the abnormal canal ran parallel
with the urethra and opened on the dorsal surface of the penis
in the sulcus coronarius or farther back, and in only 4 did the
canal open on the ventral surface of the organ. Rarely the glans
penis is split. The track varies in length from ½–5½ in., and
usually ends blindly either at the base of the glans penis or at
some part of the penis, but occasionally it passes back to the
triangular ligament, and even pierces this,
and ends behind the pubic bones. In a few
cases the abnormal canal joins the urethra,
and rarely it passes back into the bladder.
The accessory canal is usually single, but
it may be branched. It is lined with
squamous epithelium, and occasionally the
deeper part is lined with columnar epithelium.

A double urethra, either uniting or opening separately into the bladder, has been
described in the female subject.

When the second canal communicates
with the urethra or bladder, urine escapes
from both orifices. Poisson mentions that
the penis may swing from side to side during micturition.

In gonorrhœal infection there is discharge from both orifices. In a case that
came under my care (Fig. 179) a bhud canal,
2½ in. in length and admitting a No. 7 Fr.
bougie, opened on the dorsum of the glans
penis above the meatus. The patient con-

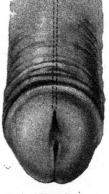

Fig. 179.—Double
urethra.

Dotted lines show position
of false urethra, which opened
above the meatus and ex-
tended backwards for 2½ in.

tracted a gonorrhœal infection of the abnormal canal, but the
urethra escaped infection.

Treatment.—Operation becomes necessary when the abnormal
canal is the seat of chronic inflammation, which is usually intractable. The track may be laid open in its entire length, and the
lining membrane destroyed with the electric cautery. Healing
takes place by granulation, and a thick scar may result, which
interferes with erection. Extirpation of the unopened track by
dissection is more difficult, but the after-result is better and the
convalescence quicker.

If the canal lies immediately above the normal urethra it may
be laid open into it with scissors.

CONGENITAL NARROWING OF THE URETHRA

The points most frequently affected are the external meatus, the junction of the fossa navicularis and the penile urethra, or some part of the membranous or the prostatic urethra. Narrowing of the external meatus is the most common of these.

All grades may be observed, to an opening the size of a pinhole. A probe passed through the opening, and held vertically so that the point is on the floor of the fossa navicularis and hooked forwards, will show the extent of the narrowing.

In rare cases there is a stenosis of the meatus extending into the fossa navicularis. At the junction of the fossa navicularis and penile urethra the fold of Guérin forms a narrowing in the normal urethra. At this spot stenosis may be found, and this may be continued with one or several narrowings of the penile urethra. At the opening of the membranous urethra into the bulb, and at the junction with the prostatic urethra, annular contraction, folds and valves are found, and these may occasionally be found between the verumontanum and the internal meatus. These folds are concave towards the bladder, and give rise to pronounced obstruction to the flow of urine. Valve-like narrowings are also found in the bulbous urethra.

Symptoms.—The symptoms are those either of obstruction to the outflow of urine or of interference with the secretion. Burckhardt points out that the more centrally the obstruction is situated the earlier are symptoms of interference with the secreting apparatus found; the more peripheral the obstruction, the more prominent are the symptoms of mechanical obstruction, while changes in the quality of the urine are delayed.

The symptoms of obstruction are those of a stricture. In severe grades, when the obstruction is in the membranous or prostatic urethra, there is dilatation of the urethra behind the narrow point, dilatation of the bladder, ureters, renal pelvis, and kidney. There is usually dribbling of urine, and, later, infection is superadded.

Diagnosis.—Stenosis of the meatus is readily seen. Deeper valves or folds may be discovered with the sound or in the adult urethra with the urethroscope. Not infrequently a valve which causes obstruction to the outflow of urine does not interfere with the introduction of an instrument. In adults the dilated portion of the urethra behind the stenosis may be seen or felt. In making a diagnosis of congenital stricture in children the possibility of gonorrhœa or traumatism at an early age must be remembered.

Treatment.—Stenosis of the meatus is treated by meatotomy. A general anæsthetic may be given, but local anæsthesia usually suffices. The meatus is split downwards from within the urethra, and two or three catgut sutures are introduced to bring the mucous membrane of the urethra and the skin together. If this is not done the wound will heal rapidly, leaving the stenosis as narrow as before.

In deeply situated stenosis dilatation with graduated bougies should be tried, and, that failing, external urethrotomy with division of the stricture, followed by the regular passage of instruments. When the bladder, ureter, and kidneys are dilated, surgical interference is unavailing.

CONGENITAL DILATATION OF THE URETHRA

This condition is independent of stenosis of the urethra. The dilatation affects the under surface of the penile urethra; very rarely there is dilatation of the bulbous urethra, and the swelling appears in the perineum. Lawson Tait recorded five cases of congenital diverticulum of the female urethra. (*See also* p. 586.)

The communication between the urethra and the diverticulum may be very small, or there may be a large opening.

Symptoms may appear soon after birth, or may be delayed. There is frequent micturition, with a poor stream, pain during the act, and after-dribbling. Incontinence is a later result. A swelling on the under surface of the penis appears during micturition. The stream may dribble after the diverticulum has become distended, and the penis is sometimes twisted to one or other side or becomes erect. The sac is usually only partly emptied at the end of micturition, and after-dribbling follows.

Treatment.—The sac should be excised, the urethra repaired, and the skin stitched separately. A catheter is tied in after the operation. Should a fistula result, a second operation is performed for its closure, and temporary suprapubic drainage of the urine may become necessary to allow the wound to heal firmly.

HYPOSPADIAS

In hypospadias (Fig. 180) the external meatus is situated at some point on the under surface of the penis or on the perineum. Three grades are described, in the following order of frequency:

1. Hypospadia glandis.
2. Hypospadia penis.
3. Hypospadia perinealis.

Hypospadias is the most frequent congenital malformation of the urethra. Mayo found 1 case in 350 men, and Burckhardt 22 cases in 1,849 male patients.

Etiology.—There is no exact knowledge of the origin of the malformation, but two theories are advanced. According to one, the lateral ridges on the under surface of the genital tubercle fail to close over the ventral groove. By the second theory, the hypospadias is due to scarring of the urethra, followed by rupture ; and this explains the scar tissue and pigmentation round the abnormal meatus and the bent form of the penis.

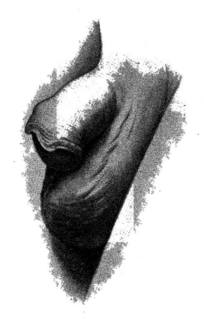

Fig. 180.—Hypospadias, showing downward curvature of penis and apron-like prepuce. (*See also* Fig. 181.)

The different degrees of hypospadias closely correspond to the stages of development of the urethra (*see* p. 392), and it seems certain that the condition results from an arrest of development, due perhaps, as Hunter believed, to some imperfection in the development of the testicles. In the slight degrees of urethral and penile malformation these organs are functional, but in the severe grades (gynæcoid males) the testes are imperfect.

Heredity is an important factor. Lesser found eleven cases of hypospadias in one family. These were confined to the second and fourth generations, while the third and fifth generations were free.

Artificial hypospadias is the result of accident or operation, and will be described under the heading of acquired defects of the urethra (p. 651).

Pathological anatomy.—1. Hypospadia glandis is the most frequent form and the lowest grade of hypospadias. Burckhardt found 16 cases of this degree in 22 cases of hypospadias.

The opening of the urethra is situated on the under surface of the glans, or at its junction with the body of the penis, and is frequently hidden by a fold of skin under the bent glans. Phimosis may exist with this degree of hypospadias. The meatus is a small transverse slit, or it may be contracted to a small round opening. Rarely there is complete atresia of the urethra.

There is not infrequently scarring and pigmentation round the orifice, which is hard and rigid, and this may extend for a short distance along the urethra and give rise to urinary obstruction. The under surface of the glans penis is split, and the fissure varies in depth. With the two sides in apposition, the external meatus appears to be in the normal position. On separating them a deep fissure lined with mucous membrane is opened. This corresponds to the sides and roof of the fossa navicularis. The groove may be shallow and open. Opening at the bottom of the groove are one or several lacunæ, varying in depth. A single lacuna may be half an inch or more in depth, and it may be difficult to distinguish the true urethral opening without sounding. It is always the lowest opening. Usually the lacunæ, when several are present, are arranged in a line at the bottom of the groove, and do not lie beyond the point which would represent the meatus were the urethra normal. Rarely a lacuna in the sinus opens on the dorsum of the glans.

In a second form of hypospadia glandis (Fig. 181) the glandular urethra is normally formed, but there is a defect at the base of the glans, and the urine is discharged from the meatus in this situation. In a third variety there is a depression at the end of the glans, but no groove or canal has formed which would correspond to the glans urethræ. The foreskin is represented by a fold at the base of the glans on the dorsal and lateral surfaces. The glans is usually bent downwards, and the shaft of the penis may also be curved towards the scrotum, and may be adherent to it either by a narrow fold or a broad band. The median raphe on the under surface of the penis is frequently displaced to the right or the left.

Undescended testis, hernia, and other malformations may complicate hypospadias.

2. In hypospadia penis (Fig. 182) the meatus lies on the under surface of the penile urethra, or at the peno-scrotal junction; and there is a long area, traversed by an open channel or groove, or sometimes by a smooth surface level with the rest of the skin. The openings of lacunæ on this may be numerous. The penis may be normal in size, but a diminutive curved organ is frequent with this degree of hypospadias. The glandular urethra, which is

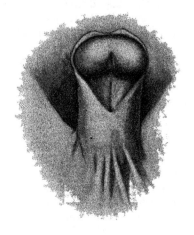

Fig. 181.—Glandular and partial penile hypospadias.

View of under surface of penis. (*See also* Fig. 180.)

developed independently of the penile urethra, may be normal, and open at the normal meatus and at the base of the glans.

3. Hypospadia perinealis is the rarest form. The scrotum is split, and the urethra opens between the halves or in the perineum. When the penis is rudimentary, the two portions of the scrotum poorly developed, and the testicles ectopic, the external genitals may resemble those of the female, and the sex may be mistaken until puberty.

A form of hypospadias has been described in the female subject in which the part of the urethra is split on its vaginal aspect and the meatus opens within the vaginal orifice.

Symptoms.—Narrowing of the abnormal meatus frequently produces a fine or twisted stream, or this severe obstruction causes difficult micturition. In perineal hypospadias urine must be passed in the sitting posture.

Normal coitus is possible in all but cases where the penis is acutely bent and adherent to the scrotum. When the urethral orifice is situated far back on the penis the probability of impreg-

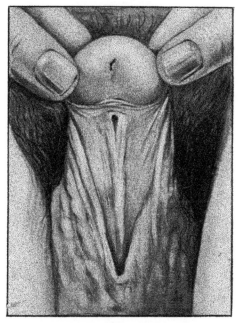

Fig. 182.—Penile hypospadias, with completed glandular
urethra.

The anterior and posterior openings of the glandular urethra are seen. The urinary meatus
is at the peno-scrotal junction.

nation is small. Gonorrhœal infection takes place more readily in glandular hypospadias than in the normal urethra.

Treatment.—Treatment may become necessary on account of narrowing of the orifice of the urethra, for cosmetic reasons, or with the view to ensuring fertility. For the first, dilatation or meatotomy may be sufficient, but usually, if any operative interference is necessary, a more complete restoration to the normal state is desired. In partial or complete glandular hypospadias the probability of a fruitful marriage is slightly, if at all, reduced,

2 L

but at the same time repair of the defect is a simpler and more certain procedure than in the more extensive malformations present in penile and perineal hypospadias, where lack of fecundity is practically certain.

In 22 cases observed by Burckhardt there were 14 married men, of whom 8 had children.

The operation, apart from the relief of obstruction occasion-

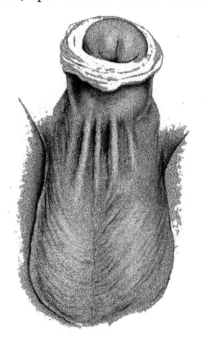

Fig. 183.—Use of foreskin to cover urethral defect in glandular hypospadias.

The glans penis is drawn through a slit in the dorsum of the foreskin.

ally necessary, should not be performed until the child has reached the age of 8 or 10 years. Before that age the penis is small, and the tissues are thin and very delicate, and operation is almost certainly attended by failure from sloughing. Moreover, a second operation is less likely to be successful from the scar tissue produced.

In all plastic operations on the urethra the bladder should

be opened suprapubically and drained for a fortnight after the operation.

1. **Operations for glandular hypospadias.** (*a*) *Beck's operation.*—After introducing a sound into the urethra a circular incision is made round the external meatus, leaving a collar of skin round the actual opening, and the incision is prolonged laterally on each side and extends to one-third of the entire circumference of the organ. A longitudinal median incision is made from this on the ventral surface of the penis for two-thirds of the length of the organ, and the urethra dissected up for a sufficient distance to allow of the necessary elongation. A flap of skin is dissected back on each side. If no groove is present the glans is penetrated longitudinally with a fine scalpel and the isolated urethra drawn through this canal, stitched in position, and the skin flaps united on the ventral surface of the penis. If a groove is present the

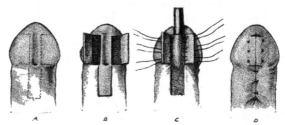

Fig. 184.—Flap operation for glandular hypospadias.

mucous lining is dissected out and the urethra laid along the raw surface. There is a danger of the isolated urethra sloughing.

(*b*) The use of the redundant dorsal prepuce, as shown in Fig. 183. The hooded prepuce is put on the stretch and a transverse buttonhole opening made in it near the corona glandis. Through this the glans penis is delivered so that the prepuce forms an apron below it. A small rubber catheter is laid in the groove on the under surface of the glans, and a longitudinal incision made on each side of this, and two corresponding longitudinal incisions on the anterior surface of the preputial apron. These raw surfaces are then approximated on each side of the catheter so that the floor of the urethra is formed by the anterior surface of the prepuce between the longitudinal incisions, and held in position by stitches. The fistula at the posterior edge of the preputial apron and the abnormal meatus is carefully repaired. The new meatus is carefully finished with additional stitches.

(*c*) The formation of skin flaps (Fig. 184). A longitudinal skin flap, with its base at the abnormal meatus, is raised from the under surface of the penis. A longitudinal shutter-like flap, hinged at its margin parallel to and farthest away from the gutter under the glans, is raised on each side. The first flap is turned forwards and stitched down, and then covered by the lateral flaps.

2. **Operations for penile hypospadias.**—The operation will usually be divided into two stages, and the whole period covered by the necessary operative measures may extend over a year or eighteen months.

The first stage consists in releasing the bands which hold the penis bent downwards. These usually consist of skin and fibrous tissue in the median line, but the corpus spongiosum may also be contracted. After putting the penis on the stretch these bands are divided transversely, and the skin either united transversely or the raw area skin-grafted. In order to prevent recontraction during healing, Burghard recommends that the penis be laid on the anterior abdominal wall and secured there by two stitches, a layer of boric lint being interposed between the skin surfaces. A rubber catheter is placed in the urethra.

For the formation of a penile urethra many operations have been introduced. That of Duplay is well known. Bucknall's and Russell's operations are easier and more successful.

(a) In *Duplay's operation* a catheter is laid along the ventral groove, and a longitudinal incision made on each side and parallel to it. Two longitudinal flaps are raised and united across the catheter, and these again are covered by flaps obtained by under-cutting the skin beyond. There is a great tendency to sloughing and tearing of the sutures, as there is usually a good deal of tension.

(b) *Bucknall's operation* (Fig. 185) consists in forming a floor for the urethra from the scrotal skin. The abnormally placed orifice is the centre, and two parallel incisions are made in front of this on each side of the ventral groove, and carried an equal distance beyond the meatus backwards, on to the skin of the scrotum. The roof and floor of the new urethra are then marked out. Longitudinal lateral flaps are raised for the whole length of these incisions by dissecting outwards. These are turned outwards and the penis laid down over a small rubber catheter, so that the isolated penile groove lies upon it and the isolated strip of scrotal skin beneath it. The raw surfaces of the lateral penile and scrotal flaps are now in contact, and these are stitched together with a double row of sutures, the first row uniting the edges of the new urethra, and the second the redundant skin along the outer edge of the penile and scrotal wounds. After a week, incisions are made in the skin of the scrotum parallel to the penis and wide of it, so that two lateral flaps are raised which adhere to the lateral borders of the penis when the organ is dissected off the scrotum. These flaps are now united on the ventral surface of the raised penis, and the skin of the scrotum brought together. Burghard recommends that these scrotal flaps be made very wide, as there may be difficulty in uniting them round the penis. He records three successful cases.

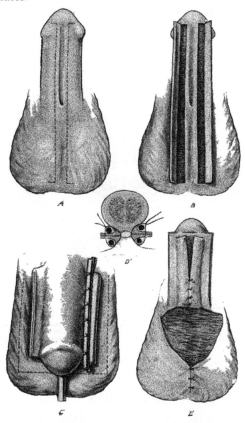

Fig. 185.—Bucknall's operation for penile hypospadias.

A. Lines of incision. B, Lateral flaps turned up. C, Penis laid on scrotum with penile and scrotal flaps approximated by interrupted sutures tied over a rubber tube ; dotted lines show outline of final scrotal flap. D, Details of sutures. E, Penis dissected off scrotum with final scrotal flaps approximated.

(c) *Hamilton Russell's "stole" operation* (Fig. 186). *First operation.*—Step 1 : Incision through the frænum which binds down the penis. This is carried round the dorsum, dividing the prepuce near the corona. The penis is straightened by cutting all tense bands.

Step 2: Glans tunnelled with tenotomy knife. Step 3: Incision as in dotted lines *b, b* (Fig. 186, A, B). A strip of prepuce like a clergyman's stole is thus marked out. This is detached, except at its base, and slipped over the end of the penis. The end is manipulated into a skin-lined tube and pulled through the tunnel in the glans and there fixed. Step 4: Suturing of flaps as in Fig. 186, C. *Second operation.*—Suprapubic cystotomy and closing of perineal urethra.

3. Operation for perineal hypospadias.—Monsarrat raises a large flap from the scrotum below the orifice of the urethra and

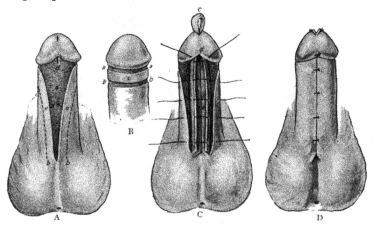

Fig. 186.—Hamilton Russell's "stole" operation for perineal hypospadias.

A, Under surface of penis showing (*a*) raw area made by first incision, (*b, b*) line of second incision, (*d*) opening of tunnel through glans (*c, c*) flaps which will form the tails of the stole and will be approximated (arrows) in the middle line. B, Dorsum of penis showing (*a, a*) first incision, (*b, b*) second incision, (*c*) dorsal portion of the stole. C, (*c*) Dorsal portion of stole, pulled through tunnel in glans; stitching shown. D, First operation completed.

wraps it round a catheter, and sinks this into a groove cut on the ventral surface of the penis over which he sutures the skin.

EPISPADIAS

The opening of the urethra is on the dorsum of the penis. The condition is very rare. Three grades are described:

1. Epispadia glandis.
2. Epispadia penis.
3. Epispadia totalis.

The third form is complicated with ectopia vesicæ, and is referred to under that head.

The following theories are advanced to explain the malformation: Rupture of the urethra resulting from obstruction after the bladder and urethra have closed. This takes place in the fourth to sixth week of fœtal life, before the corpora cavernosa have united, so that these bodies unite underneath instead of above the uro-genital sinus. According to Kaufmann, there are obstruction at the glans and gradual distension of the urethra and rupture, which may take place on the ventral surface (hypospadias) or on the dorsal surface (epispadias) of the urethra.

Pathological anatomy.—Glandular epispadias is the rarest form. There may be slight torsion of the penis. The foreskin and frænum are normal. In penile epispadias the urethral orifice, which is usually dilated, is situated at the symphysis, and is usually concealed beneath a fold of skin. On the dorsum of the penis is a broad groove lined with pale mucous membrane, which may become deeper at the glans. The penis is small, the corpora cavernosa are distorted and frequently separated, and the corpus spongiosum may lie on or between the corpora cavernosa.

The penis may be curved upwards and twisted, usually to the left. The foreskin is split, and hangs like an apron below the glans. Other malformations, such as ectopia testis, absence of the prostate, and hernia, may be present.

Epispadias has been described in the female, the urethra opening above the clitoris.

Symptoms.—In glandular epispadias there is no interference with the urinary function, but in penile epispadias incontinence of urine due to imperfect development of the sphincter muscle is common. The incontinence may be only on standing and walking, but in more severe cases it is constant. Eczema of the skin is common. In slight grades there is no interference with the sexual function, but in severe grades reproduction is impossible.

Treatment.—The penis should first be straightened by section of bands and adhesions.

A necessary preliminary to a plastic operation is perineal drainage of the bladder, which is maintained during the healing of the wounds.

Duplay's operation consists in freshening the edges of the dorsal groove and bringing them together over a catheter.

Thiersch's operation consists in (1) turning a longitudinal flap from one side of the groove over a catheter and covering the outer raw surface of this with a second flap from the other side ; (2) repairing the groove in the glans and removing the apron-like foreskin ; (3) turning down a flap from the pubic region to cover the fistula which remains at the base of the penis. The patient may become continent after the operation, but not infrequently incontinence continues, and an apparatus must be worn.

LITERATURE

Allen, *Boston Med. and Surg. Journ.,* April 3, 1902.
Bazy, *Presse Méd.,* 1903, p. 215.
Beck, *N.Y. Med. Journ.,* Jan. 29, 1908, and Dec. 8, 1900.
Bucknall, *Lancet,* Sept. 28, 1907, vol. ii.
Burckhardt, E., *Handbuch der Urologie* (von Frisch und Zuckerkandl), 1906, vol. iii.
Burghard, F., *System of Operative Surgery,* 1909, vol. iii.
Dubot, *Ann. d. Mal. d. Org. Gén.-Urin.,* 1902, No. 1.
Edington, *Brit. Med. Journ.,* Sept. 21, 1907.
Ehrlich, *Beitr. z. klin. Chir.,* 1908, p. 193.
Englisch, *Wien. med. Woch.,* 1889, p. 1513; *Centralbl. f. d. Krankh. d. Harn- u. Sex.-Org.,* vi. 169.
Escat, *Ann. d. Mal. d. Org. Gén.-Urin.,* 1908, p. 1.
Fleischmann, *Morph. Jahrb.,* 1904, p. 23.
Gutmann, *Zeits. f. Urol.,* 1910, p. 575.
Kaufmann, *Deuts. Chir.,* 1886.
Keith, *Brit. Med. Journ.,* Dec. 19, 1908.
Lichtenberg, *Ueber die Entwicklungsgeschichte accessorischer Gänge am Penis.* 1906.
Mayo, *Journ. of Amer. Med. Assoc.,* April, 1901.
Monsarrat, *Med. Ann.,* 1902, p. 339.
Posner, *Berl. klin. Woch.,* 1907, p. 375.
Russell, Hamilton, *Brit. Med. Journ.,* 1900, ii. 1432.
Wilckens, *Zeits. f. Urol.,* 1910, p. 814.

CHAPTER XLV

PROLAPSE OF THE URETHRA—URETHROCELE

PROLAPSE

THIS is a rare condition, which occurs only in women and female children. About 170 cases are on record. More than half the cases are children (66 per cent.) under 15, and most of the remaining cases occur after the menopause. In total prolapse a ring of mucous membrane protrudes from the meatus, while in partial prolapse the mucous membrane of one part of the circumference, frequently the posterior wall, is extruded.

Etiology.—The condition results from the combination of local conditions such as vulvo-vaginitis, gonorrhœa, the introduction of foreign bodies, dilatation of the urethra, tumours of the urethral mucous membrane, and the loss of tone and elasticity of the urethral wall consequent on advanced age.

Straining may be produced by the urethral condition, or may result from cystitis, constipation, coughing.

Heredity may be a predisposing factor. The condition has been observed in mother and daughter and in two sisters.

Symptoms and diagnosis.—The onset is insidious. There are urethral irritation and discomfort, and the prolapsed mucous membrane becomes tender and painful on sitting. Difficult micturition, strangury, burning on micturition, and incontinence have been observed. In old people symptoms may be entirely absent.

There is at first a protrusion of a portion of mucous membrane, or a complete ring of normal mucous membrane appears. This is easily replaced, or may even retract spontaneously. The prolapse gradually increases, and may reach a hen's egg in size. The mucous membrane becomes congested, blue and inflamed, and excoriated or ulcerated, and a purulent blood-stained discharge soils the linen. On straining, the swelling increases in size. A sound introduced into the central opening passes readily into the bladder. In partial prolapse the opening is eccentric.

The diagnosis is made by the position of the swelling and the opening of the urethra. The urethra should be examined for

585

polypi or other growths, and the urine for evidence of cystitis. In prolapse of the bladder there is no central opening, and the lumen of the urethra, ascertained by introducing a sound, surrounds the tumour.

Treatment.—In slight cases the prolapse may be reduced and the cause, such as cystitis, treated. Longitudinal searing with the electric cautery is sometimes followed by contraction of the mucous membrane and disappearance of the prolapsed portion. Several applications are necessary. In more advanced cases the prolapsed mucous membrane should be removed. A partial prolapse is excised by an elliptical incision, and the cut edges of mucous membrane are carefully united. A total prolapse is removed by a circular incision. Care should be taken not to drag down too much mucous membrane, and as the circular incision made by scissors or knife proceeds, fine catgut stitches are passed through the mucous membrane at the upper edge of the incision to prevent retracting; these are used to unite the upper and lower edges of the incision after the prolapsed portion has been removed. The bladder is drained by a fixed catheter.

LITERATURE

Bente, *Münch. med. Woch.*, Dec. 31, 1901.
Glaevecke, *Münch. med. Woch.*, May 28, 1901, Nr. 22.
Herman, *Brit. Med. Journ.*, 1889, i. 296.
Kleinwächter, *Zeits. f. Geb. u. Gyn.*, 1891, Bd. xxii. ; and 1905, Bd. xlii.
Pinkuss, *Berl. klin. Woch.*, 1901, Nr. 19, 21.
Voillemin, Thèse de Paris, 1900 ; *Brit. Med. Journ.*, Nov. 10, 1900.
Warker, *Amer. Med.*, 1904, viii. 273.

URETHROCELE

A pouch-like dilatation of the urethra occurs alike in male and female subjects, and may be either congenital (*see* p. 573) or acquired. The cavity is lined by mucous membrane from the urethra, which may, however, be inflamed and ulcerated. The muscular wall is present, but may be represented by a few fibres of non-striped muscle, or there may be only cavernous tissue between the mucous surfaces of the sac and the vagina. The sac contains purulent urine, and occasionally a calculus.

These cases should be distinguished from false urethroceles in which urine collects in an abscess or other cavity outside the urethral wall and communicating with the urethral lumen. True urethrocele is rare ; Burckhardt collected altogether 31 cases from the literature. The majority of cases occur between the ages of 25 and 45 (74 per cent.). There is usually a history of injury such as occurs in instrumental labour, passage of stones, introduction of foreign bodies, etc. Duplay and Leguen hold that it is a form of prolapse.

Symptoms.—Dribbling after micturition is the most frequent symptom, and this is increased on standing up and walking. Frequent micturition is observed, and the urine becomes infected and alkaline, and eventually incontinence may be present with irritation and excoriation of the skin.

There is pain in coitus, and also in micturition and defæcation, and severe attacks of radiating pain in the back and vomiting may follow. Neurasthenia may eventually supervene.

On examination, in the female a rounded swelling appears on the anterior wall of the vagina in the position of the urethra. This is covered with normal vaginal mucous membrane, and varies in size from a hazel-nut to a hen's egg. On pressure it is tender and fluctuating, and urine can be expressed from the external meatus. This is alkaline and ammoniacal, and on passing a catheter into the bladder clear or slightly turbid urine is withdrawn. A curved probe or stone sound can usually be manipulated into the pouch and felt from the vagina.

Diagnosis.—The symptoms seldom leave any doubt as to the diagnosis. Vaginal cystocele is situated higher in the vagina, and the urethral tube can be detected below it. Cystocele forms a large swelling, which is emptied by catheter, and the urethroscope and cystoscope render the diagnosis certain. Prolapse of the anterior vaginal wall and cysts of the vagina are not accompanied by any modification of the act of micturition, and the urine is normal.

Treatment.—By washing with solution of nitrate of silver and weak antiseptics, and application of stronger solutions of nitrate of silver through the urethroscope, the inflammatory complications can be cured, but the only radical form of treatment of the sac is by operation. Before operation the sac must be thoroughly washed and the bladder treated, and the vagina also carefully prepared.

A sound is placed in the sac from the urethra, or the sac may be packed with gauze and dissected out and removed with an elliptical area of the anterior vaginal wall. The urethral wall is carefully repaired, and then the vaginal wall accurately united.

LITERATURE

Boursier, *Sem. Méd.*, 1895, p. 379.
Duplay, *Arch. Gén. de Méd.*, 1898, p. 745.
Emmet, *N.Y. Med. Journ.*, Oct. 27, 1888.
Lejars, *Sem. Méd.*, July 28, 1908.
Pouly, *Lyon Méd.*, Feb. 4, 1900.
Routier, *Ann. d. Mal. d. Org. Gén.-Urin.*, 1896, p. 189.

CHAPTER XLVI

INJURIES OF THE URETHRA

WOUNDS

THE urethra may be wounded from within as in the passage of instruments, or from without by cutting weapons, bullets, etc. Injuries made by instruments from within (false passages) are discussed elsewhere (p. 636). Apart from surgical operations the urethra is rarely wounded by cutting instruments. The penile urethra is usually affected; rarely a stab in the perineum wounds the bulbous urethra.

Hæmorrhage is usually severe. A transverse wound of the urethra gapes, while a longitudinal wound does not. Where free exit is afforded to the urine no extravasation takes place, but when the urethral wound does not correspond to the skin wound, or when the wound is in the perineum, widespread extravasation is likely to occur.

Bullet wounds of the urethra are rare, and more often affect the bulbous than the penile. In the American Civil War there were 105 cases. The urethra may be directly wounded, or it may be injured through splintering of the pelvic bones.

Treatment.—Immediate suture of the urethra should be performed in order to avoid extravasation of urine and subsequent stricture. The wound is opened up, a catheter passed along the urethra, and the proximal and distal ends carefully sutured with catgut over this. The corpus spongiosum is then united, and the skin stitched separately. A catheter should be tied in the urethra for four days.

The wound frequently heals by primary union, and no stricture is formed. On the other hand, if the wound is infected and breaks down, and heals by granulation, a thick scar forms, and a stricture of the urethra develops. If suppuration or extravasation has already taken place when the case comes under observation, an attempt to bring the cut ends of the urethra together should still be made. Bullet wounds should be carefully cleaned and the urethra repaired. A catheter is tied in the urethra and the wound drained.

588

In 119 cases of gunshot wounds of the urethra Kaufmann found a mortality of 22 per cent., due to septic complications and extravasation of urine.

RUPTURE OF THE URETHRA

In rupture there are several degrees of injury to the urethra, and any part of the canal may be involved.

Pathological anatomy.—In *interstitial rupture* or bruising of the urethra neither the mucous membrane nor the fibrous sheath of the corpus spongiosum is ruptured. In *partial rupture* there is rupture of the spongy tissue and either the fibrous sheath (partial external) or the mucous membrane (partial internal). In *total rupture* the corpus spongiosum, the mucous membrane, and the fibrous sheath are all ruptured.

The rupture is *incomplete* when a part of the circumference of the urethra is intact, and *complete* when the whole circumference is ruptured. The severed ends contract and retract so that they may be widely separated.

1. Rupture of the *penile urethra* is rare in the flaccid state, but is more frequent when the organ is erect. A direct blow with the fist, or a kick, is the most frequent cause. The injury may be indirect, when " fracture of the urethra " is said to occur. This may result from twists during coitus, forcible bending, or it may occur spontaneously without external violence when erection takes place and the urethra is inflamed, as in chordee during gonorrhœa. The rupture is partial internal, or it may be interstitial. It is never complete. The level of the peno-scrotal junction is the seat of election.

2. Rupture of the *bulbous urethra* is much more frequent. It results from a kick on the perineum, a blow with a lever, a fall astride a beam or trestle, or a blow on the pommel of a saddle. The rupture is usually complete and total, and the severed ends retract some distance. The position of the rupture depends upon the attitude of the body at the time of the injury. Very rarely the urethra has been ruptured in two places. According to Ferrillon the cavernous tissue surrounding the urethra is the least resistant layer, and is always ruptured first, then the mucous membrane, and last the fibrous sheath. The urethra is crushed between the injuring body and the pubic arch and triangular ligament. When the direction of the blow is lateral and the body which produces it small, the urethra is injured against one limb of the pubic arch ; when the blow is median and the injuring body large, the urethra is injured against the pubic symphysis or the triangular ligament, according to the direction of the blow. If the force strikes the

perineum in a direction from before backwards the bulbous urethra is the part injured; but if the blow strikes the perineum from behind forwards the membranous urethra is injured.

3. Rupture of the *membranous urethra* occurs in severe injuries with fracture of the pelvis or dislocation of the pubic bones. The urethra is torn by a fragment of the pubic ramus, or the triangular ligament may be torn. The membranous urethra is also torn by blows upon the buttocks without fracture of the pelvis. Leguen and others suppose that a temporary dislocation of the symphysis pubis takes place, causing tearing of the triangular ligament and rupture of the urethra. Rupture of the membranous urethra is complete, and the two ends are separated and may be much torn by the fragments of the fractured pubic arch.

4. The *prostatic urethra* is very rarely ruptured.

Symptoms.—The symptoms vary according to the position of the injury. In rupture of the *penile urethra* there is hæmorrhage from the meatus, severe at first, but diminishing and disappearing in a few days. There is pain on micturition, but rarely difficulty or retention of urine. Extravasation of urine does not occur, but stricture invariably follows. In interstitial rupture or bruising external hæmorrhage is wanting, and there may be no symptoms until some months or years later a stricture develops.

Rupture of the *bulbous urethra* is the most common form. After a fall astride a beam there is sharp perineal pain, which increases in severity as effusion of blood proceeds. Hæmorrhage from the meatus follows immediately on the injury, and varies greatly in severity. It may cease rapidly, or it may be abundant and continuous. A tumour rapidly forms in the perineum. Some bruising of the skin may be present from the injury, and there is a rounded swelling of variable size over the bulbous urethra. The swelling is tense and tender, and does not extend backwards beyond the transverse perineal muscle, while it is limited laterally by the arch of the pubes. In less severe cases the fibrous sheath is not ruptured, and the large perineal swelling does not appear. There are only hæmorrhage, pain, and tenderness of the urethra. Retention of urine frequently follows the injury, but the patient may pass urine before he comes under observation.

Rupture of the *membranous* or *prostatic urethra* is associated with fracture of the pelvis, and attention may not at first be drawn to the rupture. (Plate 39, Fig. 1.) Hæmorrhage is slight; the blood is effused round the membranous urethra, and finds its way downwards to the perineum, so that some days may elapse before swelling or discoloration of the perineum appears. Retention of urine is absolute, and may last several days; when urine is passed

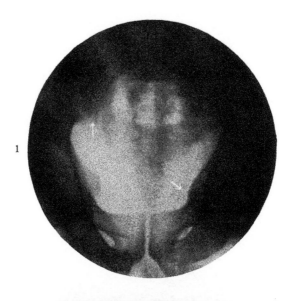

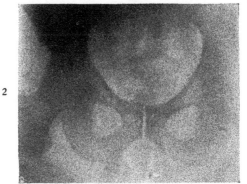

Fig. 1.—Pelvic shadow after fracture of pelvis (arrows)
and rupture of urethra. (P. 590.)

Fig. 2.—Stone in fossa navicularis of urethra (arrow).
(P. 621.)

PLATE 39.

there is pain and straining, and only a few drops escape from the urethra. In the rectum a tender swelling is felt over the membranous or prostatic urethra. The abdominal muscles are frequently rigid. A distended bladder may be felt, or the dullness percussed, above the pubes.

In cases where the rupture lies behind the compressor urethræ and triangular ligament there may be an escape of blood from the meatus. Extravasation of blood and urine takes place into the areolar tissue of the pelvis, and there is rigidity of the abdominal muscles and increasing suprapubic dullness.

Diagnosis.—In rupture of the penile and bulbous urethra hæmorrhage is constant in all but the interstitial variety. This, combined with local tenderness in penile rupture and swelling in perineal rupture, suffices for the diagnosis. When a perineal hæmatoma is present the rupture has affected the fibrous sheath, but it is impossible to say whether the tube is completely torn or a bridge of mucous membrane remains until an operation has been performed. If there is no tumour, Legueu advises that a catheter be passed, and if it glides easily into the bladder it should be tied in place. If the catheter does not pass, operation should be undertaken. In rupture of the posterior urethra the chief difficulty is in distinguishing between this and extraperitoneal rupture of the bladder. On rectal examination there are tenderness and swelling over the membranous or prostatic urethra, and on examination of the abdomen the bladder is usually distended in rupture of the urethra and is collapsed in rupture of the bladder. On passing a catheter there is difficulty at the membranous or prostatic urethra, but in rupture of the bladder the instrument passes easily into the bladder. Operation will be required in either case, but the selection of the suprapubic or perineal route will depend upon the diagnosis.

Course and prognosis.—In rupture of the *penile* urethra the hæmorrhage rapidly ceases and the wound heals, but a stricture forms within a few months. In the *bulbous* urethra, if the patient tries to pass urine he may fail from absolute retention, or he passes a few drops with great difficulty, extravasation of urine into the perineum takes place, and infection follows. The extravasation pursues the same course as in stricture of the urethra, and is accompanied by rigors and high temperature, and the patient may succumb if operation is not promptly performed. In less severe cases the perineal swelling breaks down, and urinary fistulæ form in the perineum. In a case of rupture of the bulbous urethra, in which I passed a catheter and fixed it for three days, no extravasation took place, but some months later a broken ring of phosphatic material, ⅛ in. in thickness, which had formed on the raw area, was extracted from the urethra. Stricture follows unoperated rupture of the urethra within a few weeks or months of the injury, and its extent and density depend upon whether suppuration and sloughing took place, and what distance separated the severed ends. The development of stricture may occasionally be delayed, and Bazy has recorded a case in which the interval between the injury and the onset of symptoms was thirty years.

Treatment.—In rupture of the *penile urethra* the canal should be washed with hot weak solution of silver nitrate, 1 in 10,000. Suprarenal extract, 1 in 1,000, may be introduced if the hæmorrhage continues, and an ice-bag applied. A catheter is passed and fixed in position. The urethra should be washed alongside this daily, and the instrument removed after three or four days. The passage of metal instruments should be commenced after a fortnight and continued regularly.

In rupture of the *bulbous urethra* operation is necessary. A metal catheter is passed gently along the urethra, keeping to the roof of the canal. If it passes the point of rupture and enters the bladder, the urine is drawn off and the instrument kept in position. If it does not pass into the bladder it should be left in the urethra. The patient is placed in the lithotomy position and an incision made into the hæmatoma. If, on attempting to pass the catheter, the rupture be found to lie deeply in the membranous urethra, a curved, transverse, prerectal incision will give the best exposure ; but when the rupture lies in the bulbous urethra a median incision is preferable. The clots are turned out, and a stream of hot lotion from an irrigator is used to stop oozing. If the urethra has not been completely severed there is no difficulty in finding its torn edges, and a catheter is passed along the penile urethra and into the bladder. The edges of the ruptured urethra are trimmed and united as accurately as possible with catgut sutures.

The bladder is now distended with fluid through the catheter, and the patient placed in the horizontal position. The bladder is opened above the pubes, and a large rubber drain introduced. The catheter is now removed, and the lower end of the bed raised to keep the urine from contact with the internal meatus. A suction apparatus (p. 547) may be installed if considered necessary. This method gives much better results than drainage by urethral catheter, where the catheter acts as a foreign body and causes urethritis, and after the first few days the urine commences to trickle alongside the catheter and causes sloughing of the urethral wound and subsequent formation of dense scar tissue.

If the urethra has been completely severed the penile end of the canal is readily found, and a search for the vesical end is commenced. Every depression should be probed under a strong light. The end may be found as a shred of loose tissue; it may resemble the twisted end of a large blood-vessel, or it may be identified by the persistent bleeding of a small vessel in its wall. Should a careful search fail to reveal the stump of the urethra, the gloved forefinger of the left hand should be introduced into the rectum, and when placed at the apex of the prostate will indicate the exact position of the membranous urethra. Lastly, pressure above the pubes will cause some urine to trickle from the over-distended bladder and show the position of the urethral stump.

If the search is successful the ends are approximated over a gum-elastic catheter and united with catgut sutures. In stitching the urethra it is important to put in a continuous extramucous thread of fine catgut and support this by uniting the perineum in layers. Suprapubic drainage is now established.

If the ends cannot be approximated without tension the attempt to suture them must be abandoned.

The cavity is lightly packed with gauze and drained, the perineal muscles and skin are brought together, and the catheter fixed in place. Suprapubic drainage should now be established with a ½-in. rubber drainage tube, and continued for a fortnight. The catheter and perineal drain are removed after a few days.

Should the search for the vesical end of the urethra prove fruitless, suprapubic cystotomy should be performed and a bougie passed along the urethra from the bladder. The vesical end of the urethra is now identified, and the operation completed as before. After healing of the injury, metal instruments should be passed at regular intervals, commencing a fortnight or three weeks after the operation, according to the extent of the injury.

In rupture of the membranous or prostatic urethra a curved prerectal incision with the convexity forwards should be made, and the hæmatoma incised. If the vesical end of the urethra is not found, the bladder should be opened suprapubically and retrograde catheterization of the urethra performed. A catheter is now passed from the bulbous portion into the bladder, and the urethra united over this. In any case the catheter is retained, the wound drained, and suprapubic drainage of the bladder established.

Mortality.—In uncomplicated rupture of the urethra Kaufmann found a mortality of 14·15 per cent. in 205 cases. Urinary infiltration produced a death-rate of 36 per cent. when it occurred.

2 M

Treatment by retained catheter without operation had a mortality of 18·17 per cent. In the latter cases only the least extensive injuries are included, and the mortality is therefore very high. In rupture of the urethra with fracture of the pelvis the mortality in 48 cases was 40 per cent.

In 17 cases, 4 of which were complicated with fractured pelvis, the mortality was 5·7 per cent. All these cases were submitted to perineal section and immediate suture.

After-results.—The formation of a stricture after rupture of the urethra was an almost invariable result in the cases recorded by older writers. Where primary union or rapid healing of the urethra is obtained, the canal either remains uncontracted or the stricture which forms is readily amenable to treatment.

In 7 cases operated on by Rutherfurd the urethra was free from stricture in 5 at periods of sixteen and seventeen months, three, three, and six years respectively. In 5 cases recorded by Cabot no stricture was present from three to five years after the injury.

LITERATURE

Barling, *Birmingham Med. Rev.,* 1891, p. 321.
Birkett, *Lancet,* 1866, ii. 693.
Cabot, *Boston Med. and Surg. Journ.,* 1896, p. 57.
Chambers, *West London Med. Journ.,* 1906, p. 134.
Jacobson, *N. Y. Med. Journ.,* 1900, p. 799.
Legueu, *Ann. d. Mal. d. Org. Gén.-Urin.,* 1907, ii. 1090.
Lennander, *Arch. f. klin. Chir.,* 1897, p. 484.
Martens, *Die Verletzungen und Verengerungen der Harnröhre.* Berlin, 1902.
Oberst, *Volkmanns Samml. klin. Vort.,* Nr. 210.
Poux, *Ann. d. Mal. d. Org. Gén.-Urin.,* 1904, p. 187.
Riche, *Ann. d. Mal. d. Org. Gén.-Urin.,* 1904, p. 1827.
Rutherfurd, *Glasg. Hosp. Repts.,* 1898; *Lancet,* Sept. 10, 1904.
Sczcypiorski, *Ann. d. Mal. d. Org. Gén.- Urin.,* 1907, ii. 1033.
Wasilieu, *Die Trauman der männlichen Harnröhre.* Berlin, 1900.

CHAPTER XLVII

URETHRITIS

THE term urethritis is applied to inflammation of the urethra arising from whatever cause, whether acute or chronic, affecting the whole or only a part of the canal.

Bacteriology.—In the male the portion of the urethra anterior or external to the compressor urethræ is the habitat of bacteria in varying numbers in the normal state, and the varieties have been investigated by Petit and Wassermann, Pfeiffer, and others. Anaerobic bacteria are more abundant than aerobic. The most constant bacteria are Löffler's bacillus, the streptobacillus urethræ, the colon bacillus, and the staphylococcus (albus 42 per cent., aureus 20 per cent., citreus 12 per cent.). The prostatic urethra is aseptic. The female urethra also contains bacteria in the natural state. The bacillus coli has been found by recent observers in from 12 to 66 per cent. of cases, and the staphylococcus albus and aureus in from 14 to 90 per cent.

In the great majority of cases urethritis is primarily due to the gonococcus. Urethritis is described as aseptic when bacteria are completely absent from the discharge. The injection of strong irritating solutions into the urethra, the ingestion of certain urinary irritants such as large quantities of asparagus, and alcoholic excess in some individuals, are occasional causes of urethritis in those who have not previously suffered from venereal disease. Gout and rheumatism are doubtful causes of urethritis. Septic non-gonococcal urethritis is more common, but it also is a rare condition where there has never been gonorrhœal infection. The infection may be carried by instruments such as a catheter or bougie, or the bacteria may be already present and the exciting factor is injury from instruments or an irritating urine as in diabetes mellitus; or an infection with bacteria other than the gonococcus may result from connection with women suffering from leucorrhœa or during menstruation. Septic urethritis following upon gonorrhœal urethritis is very common. After a varying period the virulence of the gonococcus subsides, and it may be replaced by a mixed infection of bacteria already present in the urethra or introduced by means of instruments.

ACUTE GONOCOCCAL URETHRITIS (GONORRHŒA)

The infection in gonorrhœa almost invariably follows connection; rarely it is conveyed indirectly by means of clothes, towels, instruments, etc., which have been smeared with pus containing the gonococcus. Certain individuals appear to be particularly susceptible to the invasion of the gonococcus, and others are unusually resistant. Ill-health, alcoholic excess, hypospadias, and phimosis have a predisposing influence.

Any age and either sex may be attacked. The gonococcus is a diplococcus, each coccus being shaped like a coffee-bean, with the concavity facing the other. It occurs in groups of four or multiples of four, usually numbering twenty, thirty, or forty. They are found free in the discharge or adhering to the surface of desquamated epithelial cells or lying within the leucocytes. In the latter position they lie superficially, and may be so numerous as to obscure the nucleus.

The gonococcus is cultivated with difficulty, and the media most favourable for its growth are " blood agar " and " serum agar." In culture they show a tendency to degeneration, forming single smaller irregularly staining cocci.

Except in artificial conditions such as cultures, the gonococcus does not flourish outside the body, but it may remain alive for several days in thick pus. It stains deeply with methylene blue and other basic aniline dyes, and is negative to Gram's stain (" Gram negative "). The gonococcus produces a toxin which, when introduced into the human urethra, causes an acute purulent catarrh.

After introduction into the meatus the infection travels backwards on the surface of the mucous membrane towards the bladder. The whole length of the anterior urethra becomes involved, and it spreads to the posterior urethra in from 80 to 90 per cent. of cases. The bladder is rarely affected. The lacunæ of the urethra are invaded, and perilacunar leucocytic infiltration is a prominent feature. In the prostatic urethra the glands of the prostate, the sinus pocularis, and sometimes the ejaculatory glands, are invaded. In these recesses the diplococcus may remain for some years after the acute symptoms have passed. In the male the gonococcus finds its habitat in the urethra and frequently invades the prostate, seminal vesicles, and epididymis. In the female it is chiefly found in the urethra, vagina, cervix uteri and Fallopian tubes, and the Bartholinian glands.

The conjunctiva is readily infected with the gonococcus, and the mouth, nose, and rectum may become involved. The gonococcus has been found in pure or mixed culture in inflammation of the bladder, kidneys, peritoneum, endocardium, blood, joints, muscles, subcutaneous tissues, and rarely the lung.

The changes that occur in the urethral mucous membrane have been studied by Finger. The gonococci penetrate between the epithelial cells, which become loosened and are cast off (period of incubation), and eventually reach the subepithelial connective tissue. Here there are signs of acute inflammation; the leucocytes take up the gonococci and pass to the surface, already partly denuded of epithelium, as pus cells, and the purulent stage becomes established. Neither the gonococci nor the leucocytes appear to be adversely affected by this phagocytic action. Penetration of the gonococci to the deeper layers of the mucous membrane, with the consequent changes, is most marked around the lacunæ and glands of the urethra. As the process subsides the cocci are removed from the deeper layers by the leucocytes, but they remain adhering to the epithelial cells, and are especially persistent in the lacunæ.

In chronic urethritis further changes occur which will be described later.

Symptoms and clinical course.—After infection there is a varying period during which the gonococci multiply and penetrate the epithelium of the mucous membrane. During this time there are no symptoms. The period of incubation lasts from three to five days, but there have been exceptional cases where it lasted twelve to fifteen or even thirty days.

There is at first slight irritation or itching at the meatus and adjacent urethra, and some burning on micturition. A little yellowish discharge appears, and the meatal lips are glued in the morning. For two or three days the symptoms increase. The discharge becomes copious and purulent, and may consist of watery pus; but more frequently it has a creamy consistence and a yellow or greenish-yellow colour. The urine now scalds, and micturition may cause severe burning, cutting pain. The urine is milky with pus, which, on standing, quickly settles as a heavy layer with a cloud of mucus on the top. On microscopical examination in the early stage the discharge is found to consist largely of desquamated epithelium with a few leucocytes; but when the discharge has fully developed it consists of pus cells, and few epithelial cells are found. In the late stage epithelial cells again become prominent and are embedded in mucus, while the leucocytes are few in number.

The meatus is red, swollen, and inflamed, with pouting lips, and the glans and foreskin, if there is phimosis, are bathed in watery pus. The urethra is tender and thickened along the penis and in the perineum. The foreskin becomes red and swollen, and this may spread to the skin of the penis, the lymphatics being marked out as red streaks.

The glands of the upper group of lymphatics become painful, tender, and swollen. Erections occur at night and cause intense pain. The thickened, inflamed urethra, from its loss of elasticity, causes downward curvature of the penis (chordee). Following the erections the discharge is frequently blood-stained, and a considerable amount of pure blood may escape. This is due to tearing of the softened, inflamed mucous membrane. The constant discomfort and aching in the urethra, pain and scalding on micturition, and sometimes the frequency of the act and the painful erections, rob the patient of his sleep.

General symptoms are almost invariably present. The patient is pale and feels ill and miserable, the appetite is poor, and there is frequently a rise of one or two points in the temperature. These symptoms develop during the first week or ten days after the discharge has appeared, and increase or remain stationary during the next fortnight, when they begin to subside, and at the end of about six weeks only a slight mucopurulent discharge without symptoms remains, and this quickly disappears.

This is the course followed in a moderately severe case without complications. The duration may be shorter than that described, or it may, owing to complications or to extension of the inflammation to the prostatic urethra, be prolonged; or the inflammation may subside and, as a result of some dietetic indiscretion or other cause, a recrudescence takes place.

The most frequent departure from the course of the disease already described is extension of the inflammation to the prostatic urethra. This occurs in the second or third week, and so frequently that it is sometimes regarded as the natural course in all cases. In about 80 per cent. of cases some degree of posterior urethritis is present, but only in a smaller number of cases are the symptoms at all prominent. Extension to the posterior urethra may occur without apparent cause, or it may follow dietetic indiscretion, exercise, exposure to cold, or any condition which aggravates the inflammation of the anterior portion of the urethra.

The symptoms produced by extension of the inflammation to the posterior prostatic urethra are sudden desire to pass water and constant irritation. There is pain, sometimes of a cramping nature, at the end of micturition, and frequently some bright blood is expressed with the last drops of urine. A heavy aching pain is often present, but when this is marked it is usually due to extension to the prostate gland and the onset of prostatitis.

The occurrence of painful erections is increased, and there are frequent seminal emissions, which may be blood-stained.

Diagnosis.—The onset of symptoms of urethritis a few days after a suspicious connection is, in the majority of cases, due to gonococcal invasion. The only certain test is, however, the discovery of the diplococcus of Neisser. The discharge should be examined in the following manner : A very small drop is placed on a clear glass slide, either by means of a platinum loop, which has previously been sterilized by heating to redness, or by applying the slide directly to the meatus after washing the glans penis. A second slide is drawn edgewise along this so as to leave a very thin film of the discharge. The slide is dried over a spirit-lamp, and a few drops of methylene-blue solution are poured over it. This is gently heated over the flame for a few minutes, and then the slide is washed in running water and again dried. A drop of cedar-wood oil is placed on the stained film, which is examined under an oil immersion lens ($\frac{1}{12}$ in.). The leucocytes are stained a faint blue with deep-blue nuclei, and the epithelial cells and their nuclei are also well stained. The gonococci are deeply stained; they are arranged in groups of ten, twenty, or thirty, and lie inside the protoplasm of the leucocytes or adhere to the surface of the epithelial cells, or they may be found in groups free in the discharge. The diagnosis depends upon the character of the diplococci, the grouping, and the intracellular position. As the cocci are negative to Gram's stain, this should be used if there is any doubt as to the bacteriological diagnosis. When the number of groups of gonococci is large and there are numerous extracellular groups, the infection may be regarded as a severe one.

The diagnosis of extension to the posterior urethra is made by noting the onset of frequent and urgent micturition and other symptoms already described. A valuable method of demonstrating the presence or absence of posterior urethritis is to wash out the anterior urethra with a cold solution of boric acid or with sterile water by means of an irrigator and a glass urethral nozzle. The cold solution promotes contraction of the compressor urethræ and prevents the fluid from passing into the prostatic urethra, and the head of water (2 or 3 ft.) is only sufficient to irrigate the anterior canal without forcing the compressor. After the irrigation the patient passes water. If the urine is turbid the pus must have come from the posterior urethra.

Sir Henry Thompson's two-glass test (p. 610) may be used, but it has little value in acute gonorrhœa.

The filtered urine contains no albumin, or only a trace, in anterior urethritis, while a considerable quantity of albumin is present in posterior urethritis. The origin of this albumin has not been satisfactorily explained.

Staining the discharge with eosin shows the presence of eosino-phile leucocytes, which are said to be especially abundant in posterior urethritis.

Treatment. Prophylaxis.—The prophylaxis of venereal disease has received attention in recent years, and the subject has appealed especially to the medical services of navies and armies, where the results of widespread measures of prophylaxis can be checked in large numbers of cases.

Such measures as the isolation of cases of venereal disease, the inspection of prostitutes, and the education of youths in sexual matters and venereal disease, do not come within the scope of this work.

Certain measures have, however, been successfully adopted to reduce the liability to contagion, and demand mention here. Apart from the use of an impervious condom, certain antiseptics have been used after intercourse. Thorough washing with soap and water and the passage of urine immediately after connection may also prevent infection, and are important adjuncts to the following antiseptic prophylactic treatment.

An instillation of a few drops of protargol solution (5 or 10 per cent.) in glycerine solution (1 in 10), or argyrol (20 per cent.), or albargin (5 per cent.), or mercuric oxycyanide ($\frac{1}{10}$ per cent.), is made into the anterior part of the urethra by means of a glass dropper or a small syringe, as soon after connection as possible.

Abortive treatment.—The gonorrhœal infection commences at the external meatus and spreads backwards, and it is at first confined to the superficial layers of the epithelium. It is possible in the early stage, when the inflammation is still limited to the first inch or so of the canal, to arrest the progress of the disease. When the signs are only a slight tingling or irritation, a little reddening of the meatus, and turbidity and slight increase of the moisture at the meatus, abortive treatment is likely to be successful. When, however, a purulent discharge is fully established, this treatment will certainly fail, and may increase the severity of the inflammation.

The patient passes water. and the urethra is compressed about 2½ in. from the meatus. By means of an irrigator and a glass urethral nozzle (Fig. 187), or of a glass syringe, the anterior part of the urethra is washed with boric solution. A glass pipette with a rubber teat is now taken, and ½ drachm of eucaine solution (2 per cent.) with adrenalin instilled into the urethra and allowed to remain for five minutes. This is followed by an instillation of silver nitrate (2 per cent.) solution made in similar fashion, keeping up pressure with the finger and thumb to prevent the solution from penetrating to a deeper part of the canal. After allowing this to remain for five minutes in the canal it is washed out with boric solution. The application may be repeated in forty-eight hours, and sometimes a third instillation may be made after a similar interval. In the interval between these instillations and following them the irrigation method should be used.

Another method of aborting the disease is that of irrigation of the urethra. This is carried out with a glass irrigator and a glass urethral nozzle. Warm permanganate of potash solution is employed; the strength, commencing with 1 in 5,000 on the first day, rises gradually to 1 in 1,000 at the end of a week. A large quantity of fluid is used—at least 2 quarts at each sitting. The

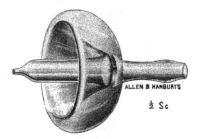

Fig. 187.—Ryall's glass urethral nozzle.

glass reservoir is raised 2 ft. or 3 ft. above the level of the patient. After passing water the patient lies upon a couch, and the surgeon grasps the penis in the left hand and separates the lips of the meatus while he holds the urethral nozzle in the right hand and controls the flow by pressure of the third and fourth fingers on the rubber tube behind it. The stream of fluid is directed to the meatus, which it washes thoroughly. Then the anterior part of the penile urethra, and finally the whole length of the anterior urethra, is irrigated. The utmost gentleness is observed, and the flow of fluid should not be allowed to distend the urethra. This is repeated twice a day, morning and evening, for ten days. After the first two days the discharge, if the treatment is going to succeed, diminishes and disappears, but the washing should not be omitted until the tenth day; after that it is gradually stopped. This method is frequently, but not invariably, successful in cases seen in the very earliest stage. It may be used alone or in com· bination with the instillation method.

Treatment when the inflammation is fully established consists in (1) diet and rest, (2) internal remedies, (3) injections.

The treatment should commence with a smart saline purge, and the patient is placed upon a light diet. Excess of meat, all highly spiced foods, curries, strawberries, tomatoes, asparagus, and rhubarb should be avoided. Wines, beer, spirits—indeed, alcohol in any form—is forbidden. If possible, the patient should be confined to bed for a week or ten days during the most acute stage of the disease, or, if this is impracticable, he should rest as much as possible on a couch. Exercise of any kind should be forbidden; horse-riding and bicycling are especially harmful. A suspensory bandage should be worn, and the penis inserted in a gonorrhœa bag containing wood-wool, which absorbs the discharge and is burnt after use; or a square of aseptic lint, with a central aperture through which the penis is drawn, may be attached with safety-pins to the suspensory bandage and folded around the penis, being secured with a safety-pin or a light elastic band. The foreskin should not be plugged with cotton-wool, as this prevents the escape of the discharge. Sexual excitement and cold must be avoided. The patient should be directed to drink large quantities of fluid: this has the effect of diluting the urine and rendering it less irritating, and is an important part of the treatment. Barley-water, parsley tea, hot water, Salutaris water, and any of the alkaline mineral waters may be taken. Contrexéville water should be prescribed, at least a bottle being consumed each day.

Urotropine and other urinary antiseptics are useless, and may increase the irritation in a sensitive mucous membrane. Certain balsams have long been used as internal remedies—namely, copaiva, cubebs, and sandalwood oil. Of these, sandalwood oil is much the most efficacious and is least likely to cause gastric disturbance, rashes, and renal aching. Pure sandalwood oil should be used, 30 to 40 minims in twenty-four hours, and may be prescribed in the form of capsules or in a mixture containing bicarbonate of potash and spirits of nitrous ether. Indigestion, renal aching, and the appearance of albumin and tube casts in the urine sometimes follow the administration of sandalwood oil and call for the omission of the drug or reduction of the dose. In such cases preparations such as santyl (sandalwood oil with salicylic acid, 10 or 15 minims in capsule thrice daily), gonosan (sandalwood oil with kava resin), santalol or arheol (capsules 5 minims thrice daily), or santalol methyl-salicyl capsules (santalol 4 minims, methyl salicylate 1 minim) may be given with good effect.

Mistura santali composita (Nisbet's Specific), ½-1 drachm in water or milk thrice daily, liquor copaibæ cum buchu et cubeba,

1-2 drachms in a large quantity of water, or liquor santali compositus, in similar doses, are also useful.[1]

Injections should be given from the earliest onset of the discharge. They should be avoided, however, when the urethritis is very severe with marked œdema of the penis and blood in the discharge, and should be omitted when such complications as posterior urethritis or epididymitis supervene.

The method of injection is either by irrigator or by hand-syringe. For lavage of the urethra by means of the irrigator the technique is similar to that already described under abortive treatment. The best solution is weak permanganate of potash (1 in 5,000), and, although the bactericidal action of the drug is very low and the dilution extreme, it frequently exerts a very remarkable effect on the gonococcal infection. The strength may be carefully raised to 1 in 1,000. Nitrate of silver in very weak solution (1 in 10,000 to 1 in 8,000) is sometimes useful. The lavage should be carried out twice daily. Occasionally an intelligent patient may be trusted to carry out the irrigation himself without ballooning the urethra or using too strong solutions, but this is seldom safe and as a rule it can only satisfactorily be done by the medical attendant.

For hand injections a syringe should be chosen with glass barrel, vulcanite mountings, and a rubber piston, and it should have a blunt conical nose and a capacity of 3 or 4 drachms.

The syringe and the penis are washed with carbolic lotion, the injection fluid diluted to the proper strength in a glass and injected slowly into the urethra after the bladder has been emptied. When the anterior urethra is moderately distended with fluid (about 2 or 3 drachms) the syringe is removed and the fluid retained in the urethra for a stated period (three minutes) by grasping the meatus with finger and thumb. This is done several times, and the séance is repeated at regular intervals three or four times during the day. The following solutions are useful, viz. : potassium permanganate, 1 in 1,000 to 1 in 500 ; protargol, $\frac{1}{8}$-1 per cent. ; or argyrol, 3-10 per cent.

In the later stage, when the discharge is subsiding, mineral or vegetable astringents should be used, such as zinc sulphocarbolate, 2-4 gr. to the ounce; zinc sulphate, 1-4 gr. to the ounce; zinc permanganate, $\frac{1}{8}$-$\frac{1}{2}$ gr. to the ounce; alum, 1-2 gr. to the ounce; tannic acid, 1-2 gr. to the ounce ; tincture catechu, 15-20 minims to the ounce ; or extract. hydrastis fl., 30-60 minims to the ounce. The mineral and vegetable astringents may be combined.

When a slight discharge continues for some weeks, in spite of

[1] Martindale, *Extra Pharmacopœia*, 14th ed., p. 501.

injections and other treatment, the anterior urethra should be irrigated, and the urine then passed and examined. If the urine is cloudy and contains shreds, posterior urethritis is present. In this case an instillation of silver nitrate (1 per cent.) by means of a Guyon's syringe usually suffices to clear it up.

When is an acute attack of gonorrhœa cured ?—When the discharge has entirely ceased the injections or irrigations should be continued for a week, and then all treatment omitted. The urine is now examined for gonococci, the first urine passed in the morning being tested. The prostate and seminal vesicles should be massaged and the secretion examined, and this should be free from gonococci. The examination should be repeated in a week after the patient has resumed his ordinary habits and has indulged in alcohol, and if the two examinations are negative the gonorrhœa may be regarded as cured. When marriage is contemplated it is advisable to make a more exhaustive examination. The prostate and seminal vesicles are massaged, and the secretion examined for gonococci. The anterior urethra is dilated with large metal sounds or Kollmann's dilators, and any discharge that can be expressed is examined. Finally, a few drops of silver nitrate solution (2 per cent.) are injected into the posterior and anterior urethra, and the resulting discharge carefully examined. This examination may be repeated after an interval. An injection of gonococcus vaccine is sometimes given, and any resulting discharge examined.

The presence of small numbers of non-bacterial shreds in clear urine does not necessitate treatment. They may persist for many months or even years, and are harmless.

Complications.—The following complications may arise during the course of an attack of gonorrhœa, viz.: balanitis; lacunar abscess; periurethral abscess; inflammation of Cowper's glands; suppurating bubo; spermato-cystitis: prostatitis; cystitis; pyelitis and pyelonephritis; epididymitis; salpingitis; peritonitis; gonorrhœa of the rectum; gonorrhœal rheumatism (gonorrhœal arthritis, gonorrhœal teno-synovitis, gonorrhœal bursitis); endocarditis; gonorrhœal myositis.

Only a few of these need be considered here, most of the conditions being described with the diseases of the organs which they affect.

Balanitis.—This results from accumulation of discharge beneath a long foreskin, but is not directly caused by the gonococcus. The foreskin is red and œdematous, and there may be spreading cellulitis of the skin of the penis. The preputial sac should be thoroughly and frequently irrigated with solution of permanganate of potash, 1 in 5,000, or nitrate of silver, 1 in 5,000.

When the inflammation is intense and is spreading, the foreskin should be slit up and circumcision performed, and the penis enclosed in hot antiseptic fomentations and immersed for half an hour at a time in a bath of hot permanganate solution.

Lacunar abscess.—This usually forms a small, split-pea-sized nodule in the urethral mucous membrane, and occurs more frequently in chronic urethritis than during the course of an acute attack of gonorrhœa. In chronic cases it is readily demonstrated by passing a bougie along the urethra. No special treatment is required in acute cases, but in chronic urethritis the lacunar abscess should be incised from within the urethra by means of a Wagner's urethral knife, or a fine electric cautery passed through a urethroscopic tube.

A larger abscess originating in a lacuna may develop in acute gonorrhœa. This is described under Periurethral Abscess (p. 647).

Bubo and suppurating bubo.—Lymphadenitis of the inguinal glands is usually present, and the .glands are enlarged, tender, and discrete. In some cases they become matted together, and occasionally suppuration occurs. If the lymphadenitis is severe the patient should be confined to bed and fomentations applied. Should suppuration take place a free vertical incision is made, the cavity swabbed with iodine solution, and packed. Healing is sometimes delayed, especially when the patient is unable to rest.

Gonorrhœal rheumatism. 1. *Gonorrhœal arthritis.* — The most frequent form of metastasis of the gonococcus is seen in gonorrhœal arthritis.

Gonococci have been demonstrated in the contents of the joint in these cases. This occurs in women as well as in men, although it is less common in the female. It occurs in 2 per cent. of cases (Besnier and Julien).

The localization to one joint may be influenced by slight injury or strain thrown on the joint.

Gonorrhœal rheumatism appears in the third week of the urethritis. The joint is painful, tender, swollen, and the temperature raised. One joint is usually affected, but exceptionally several joints may be invaded. Finger found the following frequency of the various joints in 376 cases : knee 136, tibio-tarsal joint 59, wrist 43, finger-joints 35, elbow 25, shoulder-joint 24, hip-joint 18, mandibular joint 14, metatarsal joints 7, other joints 15. The changes may take several forms : (1) hydrops, (2) sero-fibrinous inflammation, (3) suppuration, (4) fulminating arthritis. There is a tendency to recurrence in the hydrops form, and the condition may become chronic. In the sero-fibrinous and suppurative types adhesions tend to form and ankylosis may result. In the fulminating form the acute inflammation spreads to all the tissues around the joint. Extreme distortion and ankylosis of the joint follow.

Prognosis is good as regards life, and in the slight degrees complete recovery may be expected. In very chronic and in severe arthritis a stiff joint is frequently the result.

Treatment in the acute stage consists in immobilizing the joint and applying heat and soothing lotions. After the acute stage is over, as soon as possible, gentle manipulation of the joint and massage of the periarticular tissues, tendons, and muscles should be systematically undertaken, and elastic pressure applied by means of crêpe bandages and cotton-wool. Bier's congestion method has given good results. Pressure is applied by an elastic bandage on the proximal side of the joint, and causes venous congestion without obstructing the arterial supply. This should be maintained for several hours daily, depending upon the acuteness of the arthritis and the result of the treatment.

Radiant heat is very efficacious in many cases. The joint is placed in a chamber with incandescent electric lamps, and the heat raised to 200° F. or over for half an hour. This treatment is applied once or twice a week.

Salicylates may be administered, but have no marked effect. Iodide of potash is preferable.

The urethral discharge should be carefully treated. Gonococcal vaccine is of considerable value in these cases, and should always be tried.

2. *Gonorrhœal teno-synovitis.*—This may occur with gonorrhœal arthritis, or it may develop apart from it, especially in the tendon sheaths of the hand and foot, the extensors of the fingers and toes being principally affected. There is slight fever followed by tenderness, swelling, and stiffness of the affected parts, and the skin is red and œdematous.

Gonococci have been found in the turbid exudate.

The condition subsides in a fortnight or three weeks, usually with full restoration of function. Limitation of movement may, however, occur, especially where a neighbouring joint is affected.

The treatment is similar to that used in gonorrhœal arthritis.

NON-GONOCOCCAL SEPTIC URETHRITIS

Septic urethritis has long been recognized, but the condition has been placed on a sound basis by the work of Guiard, Noguès, Vamrod, Hume, and others. All cases where there has been a previous infection with the gonococcus must be excluded from this category, and Hume excludes also cases that have been injected, irrigated, or had instruments passed.

There are two general types of non-specific urethritis :

1. Sexual or infective urethritis. Acute urethritis following coitus after a regular incubation period.

2. Auto-infective or autogenous urethritis. Chronic urethritis which has been chronic from the first.

1. *Acute non-gonococcal urethritis.*—This is a rare condition, which occurred in only 11 out of 493 of Hume's cases.

The incubation period is similar to that of gonorrhœa, lasting from five to nine days, but it is frequently less. The lips of the urethra are puffy and red, and there is a moderately profuse watery yellow discharge. The urine first passed is hazy and contains shreds, while the second glass contains clear urine. Urethroscopical examination shows no infiltration of the mucous membrane in a recent attack.

According to Hume, there are numerous bacteria which are usually in pure culture, or there is a markedly predominating bacterium in a mixed infection. The most frequent organism is the staphylococcus albus. The colon bacillus is occasionally present, but more often an unnamed lanceolate diplobacillus. The streptococcus has also been described.

The prognosis is good, complete recovery following appropriate treatment.

2. *Chronic auto-infective urethritis.*—The urethritis is chronic from the commencement, and is more common than the sexual variety (30 in 493 cases).

The incubation period is ill defined, and the discharge may be discovered some time after connection, or if the patient is observant it may be found when no connection has taken place. It is slight and greyish or white. The first urine is clear, with floating shreds, and the second normal. Examination with the urethroscope shows old-standing infiltration of the urethral mucous membrane. Induration of the prostate and slight chronic seminal vesiculitis may be present.

Hume suggests that the condition may be predisposed to by the presence of a long foreskin, which encourages the growth of bacteria, and that it may commence in early youth and only be discovered when it is aggravated by irritating drinks, acid urine, connection, or other causes which encourage inspection of the urethra. Acute exacerbations frequently occur, and the presence of this condition may adversely influence the course of an intercurrent attack of gonorrhœa.

The prognosis is not so good as in the sexual variety. The

condition may persist for months or even years. Neurasthenia may be present in long-standing cases.

Treatment.—Daily irrigation with permanganate of potash in increasing strength, and an injection of nitrate of silver twice a week, $\frac{1}{2}$–$\frac{1}{8}$ per cent., or injections of protargol, $\frac{1}{2}$ per cent., should be used. Sandalwood oil should be administered internally. An injection of sulphate of zinc, $\frac{1}{4}$–$\frac{1}{2}$ per cent., should be used as the discharge is subsiding.

In chronic auto-infective urethritis circumcision should first be performed, and the urethra treated with irrigations of permanganate of potash or of nitrate of silver, 1 in 10,000 up to 1 in 5,000, and large metal instruments passed or Kollmann's flushing dilators used. Applications of stronger solutions of nitrate of silver, 1 or 2 per cent., may be made through the urethroscope tube. Hume recommends the use of ichthyol or balsam of Peru, in full strength, or with equal parts of lanolin, in sluggish cases.

LITERATURE

Alsberg, *Arch. f. Gyn.*, 1910, xc. 255.
Eitner, *Wien. med. Woch.*, 1909, lix. 2411, 2474.
Finger, *Die Syphilis und die venerischen Krankheiten*, 1896 ; *Wiener Klinik*, 1900.
Hume, *Journ. of Amer. Med. Assoc.*, 1910, liv. 1675.
Leedham-Green, *Treatment of Gonorrhœa.* 1908.
Petit et **Wassermann,** *Ann. d. Mal. d. Org. Gén.-Urin.*, 1891, p. 378.
Pfeiffer, *Arch. f. Derm. u. Syph.*, Bd. lxix., Heft 3, S. 379.
Porosz, *Monats. f. Urol.*, 1904, Bd. ix., Heft 11.
Vamrod, *Ann. d. Mal. d. Org. Gén.-Urin.*, 1905, No. 6.
Wossidlo, *Die Gonorrhoe des Mannes.* 1909.

CHRONIC URETHRITIS—GLEET

Chronic urethritis follows upon acute gonorrhœa, and may be due to the gonococcus, or this may have disappeared and given place to other bacteria. A form of non-gonorrhœal chronic urethritis has already been described.

Etiology.—Want of proper treatment, treatment with too strong applications, the early return to alcohol or sexual intercourse, repeated fresh infection with gonococcus, neglect by the patient to continue treatment until a cure is effected, are recognized causes of chronic urethral infection. Debility, the gouty or tuberculous diathesis, alcoholism, and apparently in some cases idiosyncrasy, act as predisposing factors, while local conditions, such as a narrow meatus, phimosis, stricture, and hypospadias, act mechanically in preventing free egress of the discharge.

Pathology.—In the anterior urethra there are changes in the glands and lacunæ. The lacuna magna, the normally placed lacunæ on the roof of the urethra, or large abnormal lacunæ, con-

tain pus and are surrounded by round-cell infiltration ; occasionally the outlet of a lacuna or of several lacunæ becomes blocked,
and the pus and secretion distend it to form a small cyst or
abscess.   There are patches of infiltration with round cells of varying extent surrounding the urethral glands and with a slightly
raised surface.   Later the patch becomes organized to form scar
tissue.   The surface of epithelium is changed in character, the
transitional epithelium being transformed into a thick layer of
squamous epithelium.   These patches of infiltration are the early
stage in the formation of a fibrous stricture.

Ulceration of the mucous membrane is very rarely, if ever,
seen.   Cowper's ducts are rarely the cause of chronic urethritis,
but they may occasionally be found inflamed with purulent contents.   In the posterior urethra the sinus pocularis is frequently
the seat of chronic inflammation and a continued source of infection of the urethra.   The ducts of the prostatic glands opening
into the prostatic sinuses and the ejaculatory ducts opening on
the verumontanum are channels by which infection is constantly
poured into the urethra in chronic prostatitis and seminal vesiculitis respectively.

Symptoms.—The symptoms of chronic urethritis are discharge, changes in the urine, changes in micturition, and sexual
irritation.

The discharge varies greatly in amount.   There may be a very
slight discharge continuously present, gluing the lips of the meatus
and staining the linen ; or there may be a single drop in the morning and none during the day; or no discharge appears at the
meatus unless the urethra is stripped with the finger.   The discharge is yellow, yellowish white, white, or greyish white.

Changes in the urine consist in cloudiness, due to mucus and
a little pus and the presence of urethral threads.

Urethral threads consist of mucus in which are embedded
epithelial cells and pus cells in varying proportions and bacteria:
The epithelial cells are more prominent in the slight forms of
urethritis, while in the more acute and severe forms the shreds are
purulent.   The threads are formed from the film of discharge which
adheres to an inflamed area.   When micturition takes place the
film is detached, rolled up, and swept away in the urine.   Number-
less long, irregular shreds of varying size are found where the
urethritis is subacute and extensive.   They are usually suspended
in a cloudy urine.   Smaller regular threads of equal size are
found in clear urine in chronic cases.   Very small fine threads,
frequently comma-shaped, are plugs from the gland ducts and
emanate from the prostate.   In some slight cases of catarrhal

2 N

urethritis innumerable flat flakes of epithelium like bees' wings are seen floating in clear urine, and quickly fall to the bottom of the glass. A single long coiled thread is found in some cases where a single localized area of inflammation is present. In slight catarrhal urethritis at the close of a urethral infection the threads become transparent and filmy.

Where the posterior urethra is affected there are urgency and increased frequency of micturition. This may be so slight as to be hardly noticeable, but it may also be severe, and there may be an involuntary escape of urine (active incontinence) from uncontrollable spasm when no opportunity is presented for passing water. The symptoms may amount only to a slight burning during micturition. Seminal emissions may be frequent, and there may be premature ejaculation.

The general health of the patient is frequently depressed from emissions, constant irritation in the urethra, and reflected pain from chronic prostatitis. Sexual neurasthenia is apt to develop.

Diagnosis.—The diagnosis of chronic urethritis consists in ascertaining the position of the lesion, in recognizing its nature, and in forming a conclusion as to when the condition is cured.

1. **History.**—If there has been epididymitis, or the patient gives a history of prostatitis and there are symptoms of sexual irritation and of frequency and urgency of micturition, the seat of inflammation will be found in the prostatic urethra, whereas, if this history and these symptoms are absent, the lesion may be in the anterior urethra, and this is more probable if there is some spot of tenderness in this part of the canal on palpation or on passing urine.

2. **Examination of the urine.**—A large number of clinical tests have been applied to this part of the examination.

i. *Thompson's two-glass test.*—The patient passes urine into two glasses. If the first urine is cloudy and the second clear, the anterior urethra is affected alone and the prostatic urethra and bladder are free. If both urines are cloudy there is said to be inflammation of both anterior and posterior urethra. Certain fallacies reduce the value of this test. Both urines are cloudy not only where there is anterior and posterior urethritis, but also where there is a very copious discharge from the anterior urethra, and where there is severe posterior urethritis without anterior urethritis (an uncommon condition). The turbidity of the second urine is usually due to regurgitation of discharge from the posterior urethra into the bladder, and it has been pointed out that this occurs especially at night, when the urine is long retained in the bladder and the secretion has time to collect. As a result, in mild cases of posterior urethritis the two-glass test will show two turbid urines in the morning and a turbid first and clear second urine during the day.

ii. *Jadassohn's three-glass test.*—The urine is passed into three glasses. The first urine contains the sweeping of the whole urethra, the second any discharge that may have regurgitated into the bladder, and the third the discharge which may be squeezed from the prostate gland by the final contraction of the prostatic and urethral muscles.

iii. The most satisfactory method is to irrigate the anterior urethra with cold boric solution until all pus or threads are washed out. This is best done by an irrigator and glass urethral nozzle, the head of water not exceeding 2 ft. The cold lotion produces contraction of the compressor urethræ, and prevents the wash from penetrating into the prostatic urethra. The patient then passes urine into two glasses. The first glass receives the washing of the anterior urethra, the second the content of the prostatic urethra and bladder washed out by the urine, and the third the discharge expressed from the prostatic gland by the terminal urethral and prostatic contraction and contained in the last portion of urine.

In order to demonstrate more clearly the flakes which come from the anterior or washed portion of the urethra, the fluid may be coloured with methylene blue, or a solution of potassium permanganate may be used, so that the shreds are stained.

iv. *Wolbarst's method* is a further modification of these tests, and is more accurate in differentiating between pus from the prostatic urethra and that from the bladder. It is an easily used and very useful method of localizing the seat of inflammation. (*a*) The anterior urethra is irrigated until the washings are clear. (*b*) A soft sterile catheter, lubricated with glycerine, is passed into the bladder, the contents are drawn off, the bladder is carefully washed, and 8 oz. of fluid are left in it. (*c*) The patient passes 2 oz. of fluid. (*d*) The prostate is massaged, and the patient passes the remainder of the fluid.

Glass 1 represents the anterior urethra, Glass 2 the bladder, Glass 3 the prostatic urethra, and Glass 4 the contents of the prostatic gland.

3. **Palpation and rectal examination.**—Palpation of the penile and bulbous portions of the urethra may show some tender spot, and on passing a bougie along the urethra the patient complains of tenderness at this point. Rectal examination may show induration of the prostate and thickening of the seminal vesicles, and there may be tenderness in the line of the prostatic urethra.

4. Examination of the discharge.—If the discharge is sufficient in quantity a smear is taken on a glass slide after washing the glans and meatus. It may be necessary to strip the urethra by running the forefinger along the perineum and under surface of the penis from behind forwards in order to obtain a bead of discharge. A second glass slide is drawn firmly along the first at an angle of 45° so as to spread the film thinly over the surface. This is then gently heated to dryness and passed three times over the flame of a spirit-lamp to fix the film. Should no discharge be obtainable in this way the urine is centrifugalized, and the deposit containing the threads is sucked into a pipette, placed on a clean slide, and prepared as before.

The prostatic secretion and the contents of the seminal vesicles are obtained by placing the patient in the knee-elbow position on a couch or bending over the back of a chair with his hands on the seat, and systematically massaging these organs towards the middle line, and finally stripping the prostatic, bulbous, and penile urethra from behind forwards. The secretion is prepared in a similar manner to the urethral discharge (p. 599). The usual methods of staining are methylene blue and Gram's stain. The gonococcus is Gram-negative. The shreds are found, on microscopical examination, to consist of mucus in which are embedded pus cells and epithelial cells with bacteria. As the urethritis diminishes, the pus cells become fewer and the epithelial cells proportionally greater in numbers. Gonococci are found adhering to the epithelial cells, within the leucocytes, and free. They have the characters already described. In old-standing cases they may be very scanty in numbers and difficult to find, and many films must be examined lest they be overlooked. In many cases they have completely disappeared and have been replaced by a mixed infection of other bacteria. The gonococcus may persist for as long as three years or even longer after the original infection.

An aseptic non-gonococcal discharge is occasionally observed as a final stage, but is rare.

Should the examination fail to reveal the presence of the gonococcus, an artificial urethritis should be created by injecting a few drops of silver nitrate solution (1 per cent.) into the urethra. When a reaction follows, in a few hours or after a day, the discharge should be examined, and the gonococcus may now be present.

5. Urethroscopic examination.—The urethroscope, the methods of urethroscopy, and the appearances of the normal urethra have already been described (p. 556).

The anterior urethra is first inspected. In the more pronounced

XLVII]   GLEET: DIAGNOSIS   613

and recent forms of chronic urethritis the mucous membrane is swollen and bright or deep red. It has lost some of its refractile power and appears dull and is less easily illuminated, bleeds easily, and the radiating folds are heavier and less supple. The striation, well marked in the normal urethra, is obscured and may have disappeared. Gross forms of ulceration are wanting, but there are areas in which the surface has a granular appearance from denudation of the epithelium. The openings of the lacunæ are slit-like and the lips puffy, and as the urethroscope tube passes over them a little pus wells out. These appearances may extend along the whole anterior urethra, or may be confined to the bulbous urethra or occur in patches at any part of the anterior urethra.

In a less severe form the inflammation is found in patches surrounding inflamed lacunæ. The openings of the lacunæ are large and red, and a small point of pus may exude from them.

In some cases the openings of one or several lacunæ become blocked and the contents accumulate, forming reddish-yellow beads projecting from the roof of the urethra, and best seen under air-distension.

In more chronic conditions there are patches of induration of varying extent. The mucous membrane is dull red and raised, and has lost its suppleness and texture. On withdrawing the urethroscope such a patch distorts the star-shaped folds, so that one segment of the field is occupied by a broad, thick, tough fold, and the central depression of the urethra is displaced towards the opposite side.

As organization of this tissue takes place the surrounding mucous membrane is dragged upon and raised up, and a fine ridge appears, the first stage of an annular stricture.

In the prostatic urethra congestion of the prostatic sinuses is present. The verumontanum is thickened and increased in size, and frequently distorted in old-standing cases. The swollen, inflamed orifice of the sinus pocularis can be distinguished when this is the seat of residual infection.

Treatment.—When the urethritis has followed an acute attack of comparatively recent date the lesions are usually superficial, and are frequently confined to the prostatic urethra. The most useful method of treatment is irrigation of the whole length of the urethra and the bladder with weak solutions of astringent antiseptics, such as nitrate of silver, 1 in 10,000, cautiously increased to 1 in 1,000. This may be carried out by hydrostatic pressure.

Janet's method of urethral irrigation.—The patient lies on a couch on a waterproof sheet with a basin between the thighs, or stands over a basin. An irrigator containing the fluid, which must be warm, is raised to the height of about 3 ft. above the level of the pelvis. A glass urethral nozzle is attached to the rubber tubing and grasped with the right hand, so that the rubber tube is controlled immediately behind it with the third and fourth fingers.

The penis is seized with the left hand. A stream of fluid is first directed against the meatus, and then the terminal portion of the urethra is washed, and eventually the whole anterior urethra, fluid being allowed to distend the canal gently and then escape. The patient is now directed to relax all the urethral muscles and breathe deeply; the flow is controlled by pressure of the fingers, and allowed to pass slowly at first, and gradually with greater volume and force, until the resistance of the compressor urethræ is overcome and the fluid flows through the prostatic urethra into the bladder. When the bladder is distended the patient passes the contents and the irrigation is repeated. Several pints of fluid are used at each sitting. Some practice on the part of the patient may be required before the urethral sphincter can be readily relaxed. The injection of 20 minims of cocaine solution (1 per cent.) by means of a pipette or Guyon's syringe will overcome spasm in difficult cases. Should this prove unsuccessful a soft rubber catheter may be passed through the compressor urethræ, the fluid flowing through this into the bladder. On withdrawal of the catheter the anterior urethra is washed, and the patient then empties the bladder, washing the whole length of the urethra. The irrigations are made daily or every second day.

Instillations.—In chronic urethritis confined to the posterior urethra instillations of stronger astringents and antiseptics are useful. Nitrate of silver solution is employed usually in 1 or 2 per cent. strength, but occasionally stronger solutions, 3 or 4 per cent., may be used. Zinc sulphate solution, 2 to 4 per cent., is efficacious in some cases.

The instillations are made with a Guyon's syringe or an Ultzmann's syringe, and are repeated once a week. The catheter of one of these syringes is passed until the point is felt to hesitate at the membranous urethra. It now passes on into the prostatic portion, and the solution is then injected. This method should be used with great care. There is a danger of prostatitis and of epididymitis following the incautious use of strong solutions in unsuitable cases.

Applications through the urethroscope.—In the anterior urethra patches of chronic inflammation may be treated by pass-

ing the urethroscope tube and applying a solution of nitrate of
silver (2–4 per cent.) to the diseased area by means of a pledget
of cotton-wool on a carrier. This is allowed to remain in contact
with the mucous membrane for one or two minutes, and the excess
of solution mopped up with a dry pledget of wool. Occasionally
a specially resistant spot may be cured by touching it with a fine
head of solid silver nitrate melted on to a fine wire. The same
treatment may be applied to the prostatic urethra and to the
orifice of the sinus pocularis through a prostatic tube.

Inflamed and blocked lacunæ are treated by cauterization with
a fine urethral electro-cautery or slit with a fine urethral knife.

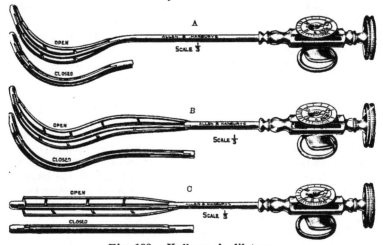

Fig. 188.—Kollmann's dilators.

A, Curved, for prostatic urethra. B, Curved and straight, for prostatic and bulbous urethra.
C, Straight, for anterior urethra.

Dilatation.—1. In chronic induration, apart from the presence
of a stricture, dilatation by large metal sounds (12–14, 14–16) is of
great value. If necessary, the meatus should be slit in order to accommodate the sounds, which should be passed once or twice a week.

2. This dilatation may be followed by *irrigation by Janet's
method* (p. 613).

3. The combination of dilatation with the application of *antiseptic and stimulating ointments* has long been used. The ointment may be smeared on the ordinary smooth conical metal sound,
or a specially constructed sound with longitudinal grooves (four
to six) in which the ointment is used. An ointment suggested
by Mena has the following composition : Bals. peruv. 2, argenti
nitras 1, cera flav. 2, butyr. cacao 100.

4. *Kollmann's dilators.*—A number of forms of graduated dilator have been introduced, the most perfect of which is that of Kollmann (Fig. 188). It consists of smooth metal strips (four in number), which are separated by turning a screw in the handle, the amount of dilatation being indicated by a dial. Straight dilators are used for the anterior, and curved for the posterior urethra. The dilator is smeared with lubricant and introduced. In the earlier dilators a fine rubber covering was used to prevent injury of the mucous membrane by the blades, but no rubber covering is required for the most recent models. The screw is gently turned to 28. or 30 at first, and this is maintained for ten minutes. Later, higher numbers are reached and the length of time is extended. The dilatation is performed once or twice a week.

5. *Irrigating dilators.*—Provision is made in the instrument for irrigation of the urethra with a stream of weak antiseptic (silver nitrate, 1 in 10,000) during the dilatation.

Urethritis and Marriage

This subject assumes a serious importance owing to the grave results of gonococcal infection in the female.

It is necessary to demonstrate the absence of the gonococcus. After an acute gonorrhœal urethritis, when the discharge has entirely disappeared, and the urine is clear and contains no shreds, there is a possibility that gonococci may still lurk in the lacunæ and in the prostate, and that they may reappear on connection. The tests that have already been described must be carefully employed (*see* p. 610).

The examination may be summarized as follows :—

1. Examination of the deposit of centrifugalized morning urine.

2. Urethroscopic examination of the anterior and posterior urethra.

3. Examination of the urine passed or of washing of the urethra after dilatation by sounds or dilators.

4. Examination of the contents of the prostate and seminal vesicles obtained by massage from the rectum.

5. Examination of an artificial discharge produced by instillation of nitrate of silver solution (1 per cent.).

6. Examination for discharge after the injection of gonococcal vaccine.

Should these methods fail to demonstrate the gonococcus, a delay of at least two months should still be insisted upon before marriage is permitted.

In chronic urethritis with the presence of gonococci, similar means should be adopted to ascertain if the gonococcus is present, and a longer period (four to six months) is necessary after the diplococcus has disappeared.

In non-gonococcal infections the same rigid care need not be taken. The urethritis should be treated, and discharge must have disappeared before marriage can be allowed, but the presence of a few flakes in clear urine cannot be looked upon as a bar to marriage provided the gonococcus can be excluded.

CHAPTER XLVIII

URETHRAL CALCULUS—FOREIGN BODIES

CALCULUS

THERE are two varieties of stone in the urethra—(1) primary, when the calculus originates in the urethra ; (2) secondary, when a migrating calculus is· arrested in the canal.

Etiology.—Primary calculi take origin in phosphatic crusts deposited upon a raw surface in the urethra. This is more likely to occur when stricture is present and the urine tends to " hang " in the tube. A small portion of phosphatic deposit detached from such a surface forms the nucleus of a stone on which fresh deposit accumulates. I have seen a case in which a ring-like urethral calculus formed after rupture of the urethra (p. 591).

Calculi which form in pockets connected with the urethra have a similar origin. In the anterior urethra the diverticula may be congenital or result from operation, stricture, or the rupture of cysts or abscesses. Many cases of prostatic calculi are of this nature, and a history can be obtained of a prostatic abscess which ruptured into the urethra at a previous date.

Secondary calculi are passed from the bladder.

In the old operation of lithotrity the fragments of the crushed stone were passed by the patient, and might become arrested and form the nucleus of a urethral calculus.

Pathology.—Primary urethral calculi are always phosphatic. They are composed of calcium and magnesium phosphate, or calcium carbonate, and sometimes ammonio-magnesium phosphate. Secondary calculi contain uric acid, calcium oxalate, or other ingredients found in renal and vesical calculi. This forms the nucleus, usually of small size, around which phosphates are deposited in layers.

Lieblein and Finsterer have described calculi composed of urates, with or without phosphates or oxalates, which they considered from the absence of symptoms of descent to have been formed *in situ ;* and Monsarrat made similar observations in regard to three calculi containing calcium oxalate.

Increase in size is always most extensive at the vesical end of

the calculus. As the calculus grows it becomes moulded to
the shape of the urethra, and the urethra itself is gradually
dilated. Very large calculous masses are occasionally found.
These are usually in the form of two or several calculi, the points
of contact being worn and faceted, the one segment fitting accurately into the other, sometimes in the form of a ball-and-socket
joint. I removed from the urethra of a man aged 50 a calculus which weighed 750 gr., measured 4¼ in. in length, and
consisted of two pieces faceted at the contiguous surfaces. The
entire mass formed a cast of the dilated prostatic urethra, a
narrow neck at the membranous portion, and a long expansion

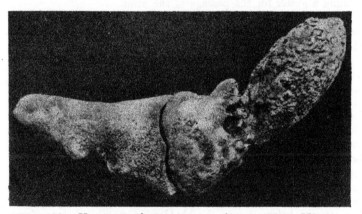

Fig. 189.—Urethral calculus in two pieces, weight 750 gr.,
which formed a cast of urethra.

On the right is seen a cast of the dilated prostatic portion, then a constriction corresponding
to the membranous portion; and to the left a cast of the bulbous urethra as far as the commencement of the penile portion.

filling the bulbous urethra as far as the peno-scrotal junction.
(Fig. 189.)

Multiple stones are due to fracture of a single stone, and a
nucleus only exists in one of them. When a calculus occupies
the prostatic urethra and projects into the bladder, phosphatic
material is rapidly deposited on the intravesical portion, so that
an umbrella- or mushroom-like form is given to the stone.

Calculi may lie in any part of the canal. According to Englisch,
the calculus is lodged in the membranous (and prostatic) portion in
42 per cent.; in the bulbous urethra in 18·6 per cent.; in the
scrotal and penile urethra in 28·2 per cent.; and in the fossa
navicularis in 11·2 per cent. In the majority of cases one or several
strictures of the urethra coexist. The calculus frequently lies

behind a stricture, or between two strictures. Urinary fistulæ
are occasionally present in the perineum.

. I have operated in a case where a large stone·occupied the
prostatic urethra. There was congenital stenosis of the bulbous
urethra and a large congenital urethro-rectal fistula opening behind
the stricture.

A calculus may lie in a pouch communicating with the anterior
urethra either in its bulbous or penile portions, or in a pocket in
the substance of the prostate. A portion of the calculus usually
projects into the urethra, and may be joined to the extra-urethral
portion by a neck. A groove is present on the urethral portion,
forming a gutter for the passage of the urine.

Symptoms.—A migrating calculus most frequently becomes
impacted in the urethra in children, but the accident may occur
at any age.

1. **Impaction of a migrating stone.**—In adults there is frequently a preliminary attack of renal colic when the stone is passing down the ureter, followed, it may be, by a quiescent interval
of several days. In children this is usually absent. The patient
feels something enter the urethra during micturition, and then
there are sudden arrest of the stream, intense pain, and continuous
ineffectual straining, with the passage of a few drops of blood.
Complete retention of urine not infrequently follows. On passing a metal ·catheter to relieve the obstruction, the compressor
urethræ is found spasmodically contracted, and the click of a
stone is felt in the prostatic urethra. The instrument may push
the calculus before it into the bladder, or may pass alongside it.
The calculus may be felt from the rectum. Recurrent attacks
of difficult micturition, or even complete retention, occur when
the stone becomes impacted behind a stricture of the bulbous or
penile urethra. Here the calculus can be felt on palpating the
perineum or the penile urethra. Occasionally the stone becomes
impacted in the fossa navicularis, and can be readily felt.

2. **Stone in the urethra.**—When the calculus has been present in the urethra for a considerable time, it may have reached
a large size without causing great inconvenience. In a case under
my care the stone had been thirty years in the urethra. . There
are pyuria and usually a urethral discharge, difficult micturition
with a small distorted stream, frequent micturition, and discomfort. Urinary fistulæ may be present. Frequently there is a
stricture, to which the symptoms of obstruction may be ascribed.

On palpation of the penile or bulbous urethra, or by rectal
examination, the stone can be felt in either the anterior or the
posterior urethra. On examination with the urethroscope a

greyish-white stone can be seen (Plate 40, Fig. 3), and a metal sound is arrested with a metallic click. If several calculi are present, characteristic grating can be felt.

The X-rays show a shadow in the line of the urethra. (Plate 39, Fig. 2.)

Treatment.—A migrating calculus of the prostatic urethra is usually pushed back into the bladder on passing a catheter. It should then be either evacuated with a lithotrity cannula and bulb, or crushed and removed. If the calculus is not pushed back into the bladder with the catheter, the instrument should be tied in place for a few days, and on removing it the stone will probably be expelled. A calculus at the fossa navicularis can usually be coaxed out of the urethra with a bent probe. If necessary, the meatus should be slit downwards to allow of its removal.

A fixed calculus of the prostatic urethra should be removed by median perineal section, and if it is embedded in a sacculus, care should be taken to destroy the wall of this pocket. The bladder should then be searched for vesical calculi, and these removed with lithotomy forceps. In the bulbous urethra an extensive operation may be necessary for the removal of large calculi, and when fistulæ are present a plastic operation will be required at a later date.

Small calculi in the penile and bulbous urethra can sometimes be removed by urethral forceps when no stricture is present ; but when they lie behind a stricture external urethrotomy is necessary, the stricture being cut at the same time.

LITERATURE

Court, *Lancet,* 1896, i. 1561.
Englisch, *Arch. f. klin. Chir.,* Bd. lxxii., p. 489.
Fenwick, *Trans. Path. Soc.,* 1890, vol. xli.
Kaufmann, *Krankheiten der männlichen Harnröhre und der Penis.* 1886.
Korn, Inaugural Dissertation, Leipzig, 1865.
Lieblein, *Beitr. z. klin. Chir.,* 1896, p. 141.
Monsarrat, *Brit. Med. Journ.,* 1912, i. 3.
Pasteau, *Ann. d. Mal. d. Org. Gén.-Urin.,* 1901, p. 416.
Ziessl, *Ueber die Steine in der Harnröhre des Mannes.* Stuttgart, 1883.

FOREIGN BODIES IN THE URETHRA

A large variety of foreign bodies may be found in the urethra of erotic individuals, and portions of surgical instruments may be accidentally left in the canal during operations. The following is a selection : Large jet button, pipe-stem, glass rod, hat-pin, hair-pin, needle, portion of wood, pencil, rubber tube, feather, blade of straw, roll of paper, coin, portion of a catheter or bougie. Poucet describes the case of an Arab who hid in his urethra two gold chains, a small cross, the handle of a cup, two pieces of bone, two fragments of teeth, a pearl, and a portion of whetstone. Fragments of bone may penetrate and become lodged in the urethra, in fracture of the pelvis, or osteitis of the pelvic bones.

Symptoms.—The foreign body does not usually remain for long in the urethra. Either it is forced out by the urine or removed by the surgeon, or it may pass backwards into the bladder.

When it remains in the urethra there is a purulent discharge, pain, burning, and hæmorrhage, increased by erection. Frequent micturition, difficulty, dribbling, and sometimes complete retention occur. When alkaline cystitis is present the foreign body is quickly encrusted with phosphates. Periurethritis and periurethral abscess may result.

The foreign body is usually lodged in the fossa navicularis or the bulbous urethra, rarely in the prostatic urethra, or partly in the prostatic urethra and partly in the bladder.

Diagnosis.—The patient frequently conceals the fact that he has introduced a foreign body, and the diagnosis is made on palpation of the urethra or on passing a sound or urethroscope tube.

Treatment.—The foreign body may be swept out by the stream of urine if the meatus is compressed during the flow and then suddenly relaxed. A long, firm body may be pressed out from the perineum or penis. Meatotomy is frequently necessary.

A pin with round head lies in the urethra, with the head bladderwards and the point buried in the mucous membrane. The point should be manipulated through the skin and the pin drawn out. The head is then reversed, and pushed towards the meatus until it projects from it.

Small objects or portions of a catheter may be withdrawn by means of long, fine urethral forceps, and a magnet has been used to remove an iron foreign body (Hofmeister).

The urethroscope is used to diagnose and also to remove foreign bodies, urethral forceps being passed along a large urethral tube. If these measures fail, external urethrotomy should be performed and the foreign body removed. When the foreign body lies in the prostatic urethra it will be easier to push it back into the bladder and deal with it as a foreign body of the bladder.

LITERATURE

Brown, *N.Y. Med. Journ.,* July 7, 1900.
Ebermann, *Centralbl. f. d. Krankh. d. Harn- u. Sex.-Org.,* 1895, iv. 8.
Gannau, *Brit. Med. Journ.,* May 2, 1896.
Goldberg, *Centralbl. f. d. Krankh. d. Harn- u. Sex.-Org.,* 1897, p. 113.
Hawley, *Brit. Med. Journ.,* March 17, 1900.
Poucet, *Gaz. Hebdom. de Méd. et de Chir.,* 1893, p. 247.
Tousey, *Med. Rec.,* May 2, 1896.
Wayland, *Brit. Med. Journ.,* 1896, p. 1033.
Wilson, *Brit. Med. Journ.,* Feb. 24, 1900.

CHAPTER XLIX

STRICTURE OF THE URETHRA

STRICTURE of the urethra is congenital, inflammatory, or traumatic. Congenital stricture has already been described (p. 572).

The normal urethra is a collapsed tube with elastic and contractile walls. In stricture the wall loses its elasticity and becomes rigid.

Etiology. — The female urethra is very rarely affected. Acquired stricture has been observed in male infants, but in the great majority of cases the age is between 20 and 40.

The most frequent causes of stricture are traumatism and chronic inflammation, and the latter is the more common.

The chronic urethritis which causes a stricture is gonorrhœal in origin in from 90 to 95 per cent. of cases (Antal). Martens found that 129 out of 186 cases of stricture were of this nature. The urethritis is not necessarily severe in the acute stage, but is prolonged in a chronic form. Any condition which tends to prolong the inflammation in chronic urethritis, such as a narrow meatus, phimosis, hypospadias with contracted meatus, injudicious treatment by means of strong injections, alcohol, and exposure, acts as a predisposing cause. Rarely, chronic urethritis due to tuberculosis of the urethra or diabetes produces stricture. Syphilis has been known to cause stricture in the tertiary stage, or stricture may follow a urethral chancre of the fossa navicularis. Nongonococcal urethritis rarely causes stricture, as the lesions are superficial.

Individual idiosyncrasies exist in regard to the development of thick, dense strictures of the urethra, and the alcoholic habit, exposure to a hard climate, and neglect of regular treatment play an important rôle.

Pathological anatomy.—In traumatic stricture fibrous tissue develops in the space between the severed ends of the ruptured urethra. The extent of this depends upon the distance between the ends of the urethra and upon the subsequent destruction of tissue by necrosis from the injury or sloughing from septic complications. The lesion develops rapidly and is single. Occasionally there is a thin, supple band involving the mucous membrane, but more often there is a thick, tough, sharply defined mass of fibrous tissue involving the mucous and submucous coats and the cavernous tissue, and sometimes also the perineal tissues and skin. The narrowed lumen is eccentric and irregular.

Gonorrhœal stricture is usually multiple. Of 100 cases of stricture examined by urethroscope and bougie, 3 were traumatic and single, and the remaining 97 cases were gonorrhœal. Of these, 23 were single, 42 had two strictures, 27 had three strictures, and 5 had four strictures.

The part most frequently affected (72 per cent.) is the bulbous urethra. Strictures of the penile urethra alone are comparatively uncommon, only 6 per cent. being situated between 1 and 3½ in. from the meatus. Multiple strictures affecting both the penile and the bulbous urethra are, however, more common (22 per cent.). The prostatic urethra is very rarely affected in gonorrhœal stricture.

In explanation of the majority of strictures occurring in the bulbous urethra 5 or 5½ in. from the meatus, it has been held that the bulbous urethra is the most dependent part of the fixed curve of the urethra, and here the discharge of a gonorrhœal urethritis will collect. But in the recumbent position this is not the most dependent part of the curve and there is not necessarily any collection of discharge at this part. I hold the view that the floor of the bulbous urethra just in front of the membranous opening is the point of the fixed curve on which the full force of the stream of urine impinges when the bladder is emptied, and in acute gonorrhœal urethritis damage is produced by this force. Excessive infiltration occurs, and later stricture develops. Analogy may be drawn with the frequent localization of disease to the arch of the aorta.

When multiple strictures are present they may be distributed over almost the whole length of the anterior urethra, but the parts of the canal lying between them are not cicatricial. Extensive fibrosis of the mucous membrane may, however, be found, the strictured part measuring an inch or more, and in rare cases almost the whole length of the anterior urethra appears to be sclerosed. It is rare that the lumen is entirely obliterated, but such cases have been recorded. Short of this, the size of the stricture varies from a lumen admitting a bristle to a fine linear fibrous ring which very slightly diminishes the lumen when the canal is fully distended.

The stricture may be a fine elastic band of fibrous tissues, which either involves the whole of the circumference (annular stricture, Fig. 190) or one part—the floor, roof, or sides of the wall ; or it may form an isolated band stretching across the lumen (bridle stricture). The latter is usually produced from an annular stricture by a false passage (Fig. 191) being made through the stricture tissue by the point of an instrument carelessly handled. The false passage lies below the lumen of the stricture, has a calibre as large as that of the stricture, and is only separated from its lumen by the bridge of tissue which is named a "bridle." In old-standing strictures the fibrous tissue is hard, tough, and avascular (cartilaginous stricture). The lumen is central or eccentric, according to whether the fibrous tissue develops evenly around the whole circumference or is more abundant at one part. In the normal urethra the elastic walls are in close contact ; in a strictured urethra there is a permanent lumen at the stricture. The histological changes consist in proliferation of the epithelium and change from the transitional to a squamous type, and sclerosis of the subepithelial tissue, so that a dense avascular inelastic fibrous layer develops. This invades the submucous tissue and the tissue of the corpus spongiosum.

The earliest stage is an infiltrated patch in the

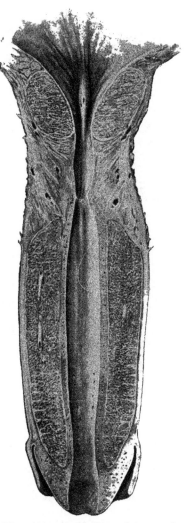

Fig. 190.—Annular stricture of the bulbous urethra.

2 o

mucosa in the course of a chronic urethritis. Sclerosis of this patch is the commencement of the stricture, which increases by circular traction on the mucous membrane. (Plate 40, Fig. 2.)

When the narrowing has progressed so far as to cause obstruction to the flow of urine the force of the stream drags and tears at the stricture during micturition, and, I believe, keeps up and increases the chronic inflammation that is already present. Where the lumen of the stricture is very small and the stricture tissue supple, the stream of urine probably drives the stricture forwards and balloons it inside the urethra at each micturition. In support of this view it will be found that in multiple stricture the narrowest stricture is nearest the bladder, and this is the one which is exposed to the full force of the stream.

The urethra behind the stricture shows chronic inflammation and dilatation. Vegetations and ulceration are frequently present.

The bladder muscle is hypertrophied, and cystitis is common. There may be acute retention of urine, or the bladder may be chronically distended. It is, however, the exception, apart from complete retention, to find residual urine.

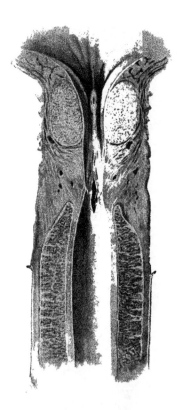

Fig. 191.—Stricture of the bulbous urethra, with recent false passage.

The ureters, and eventually the kidneys, become dilated, and ascending septic pyelonephritis is usually present in old-standing cases.

Symptoms.—In stricture of large calibre the only symptom may be a persistent purulent discharge (gleet).

In stricture with small lumen other symptoms develop. The stream is small, thin, twisted, forked, or sprayed, or it may appear in short jets or only in drops. None of these is characteristic of

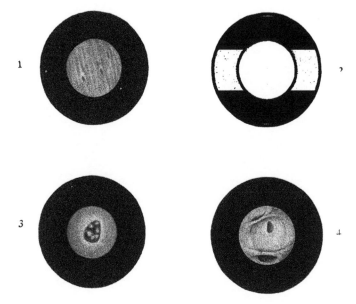

Fig. 1.—Lacunæ and striation of roof of normal urethra. (Pp. 554, 560.)

Fig. 2.—Scar tissue in urethra in old-standing stricture. (P. 626.)

Fig. 3.—Urethroscopic view of stone behind stricture of urethra. (Pp. 621, 628.)

Fig. 4.—Urethroscopic view of stricture with large false passage on floor and another on roof of urethra. (P. 628.)

PLATE 40.

stricture, although they are frequently present. The projection is feeble; instead of the stream performing a full curve it drops vertically. There may be a pause before micturition commences, the latent period lasting for a few seconds to two or three minutes. The patient strains to pass urine, and the stream, poor throughout, tails off at the finish into a feeble dribble.

Frequent micturition is usually due to chronic urethritis of the prostatic urethra or to cystitis; occasionally, however, it develops without inflammation being present.

Pain may be felt at the seat of the stricture during micturition. Usually, however, the patient is unconscious of any urethral sensation. Pain at the external abdominal rings may be due to hernia from straining. In the absence of this cause it is caused by dilatation of the lower end of the ureter. Pain in the posterior renal area is the result of back pressure on the kidney. The patient may feel pain over one kidney each time he passes water, due to loss of sphincter action of the lower ureter.

Pain on ejaculation and reflux of semen into the bladder occur, and are a cause of sterility.

Transient retention may occur, the patient being unable to pass urine for a few minutes to half an hour, or even longer, and then the flow gradually recommences.

Acute total retention of urine is caused by a chill, an excess of alcohol, dietetic indiscretion, or sexual excess. The stricture is usually narrow, but not infrequently the calibre is comparatively large (8 or 10 Fr.). The patient complains of severe suprapubic cramping pain which occurs in paroxysms with intervals of aching. He is pale, the skin often pale and perspiring. The bladder is felt as an oval suprapubic swelling. No urine escapes, or only a few drops are passed from time to time. In some cases there is a remarkable absence of pain, the patient complains of inability to pass water, and the bladder is found distended.

Retention of urine in stricture is due to spasm of the compressor urethræ muscle, or to congestion of the mucous membrane at the stricture, or to both these factors combined. In a few cases it may result from temporary paralysis of the bladder, due to cystitis or over-distension.

Incontinence of urine is observed in narrow strictures and takes several forms. A small quantity of urine may be retained in the urethra behind the stricture and dribble away after micturition is finished. Some escape of urine occasionally takes place on walking or exertion, from distension of the urethra behind the stricture and weakening of the sphincter. Involuntary dribbling of urine is observed when the bladder is chronically over-distended.

In the later stages of stricture chronic cystitis is almost invariably present and the bladder becomes contracted, so that there is frequent and painful micturition day and night. In long-standing stricture dilatation and septic infection of the ureters and kidneys lead to symptoms of urinary septicæmia and of renal failure (p. 133).

Examination of the urethra.—A circumscribed cartilaginous stricture of the penile urethra, and occasionally one situated in the bulbous urethra, can be felt on palpation, and is more distinct when felt upon a bougie. Normally a 25 or 26 Fr. should pass freely along the urethra into the bladder. A large gum-elastic bougie (20 or 21 Fr.) should be introduced gently along the canal, and if it is arrested at any point it should be withdrawn, the distance from the meatus being noted on the bougie. Spasm of the compressor rarely causes obstruction which resists gentle pressure with a bougie of this size. The position of the obstruction may be well in front of the membranous urethra, so that no confusion need arise.

The hard, inelastic sensation given by a cartilaginous stricture is quite distinctive.

A more resilient sensation is imparted by an elastic fibrous stricture. With practice it is possible to distinguish between this and obstruction by a fold of mucous membrane. Smaller instruments are passed until one which will enter the lumen of the stricture is found.

When the stricture is of fairly large calibre a bougie à boule may be used. This has an acorn tip. When this is passed through the stricture and withdrawn the shoulder of the acorn hitches at the stricture and the length of the strictured portion can be measured.

The urethroscope is of great use in the diagnosis of stricture. After introducing the tube and applying the lantern, the air pressure is turned on and the urethra becomes inflated. The stricture is readily diagnosed and examined by this means (Plate 40, Figs. 3, 4); strictures of large calibre are recognized, and through the lumen of the first stricture others may be seen. The opening of the membranous urethra, which is seen as an arch on full distension, should be distinguished from a stricture.

Diagnosis.—1. *Spasm of the compressor urethræ* (spasmodic stricture) is caused by acute or chronic inflammation of the prostatic urethra. The symptoms produced are difficult micturition and increased frequency, with a varying amount of urethral discharge or only urethral threads in the urine. The difficulty in these cases is intermittent in character. At one time the flow of urine is free and the stream good ; at another time there is difficulty and even retention. In organic stricture there is a history of gradually increasing difficulty in micturition.

On passing a large bougie obstruction is encountered at 6 in. from the meatus, but gentle continuous pressure succeeds in overcoming this resistance, and the bougie passes readily into the bladder. Occasionally the spasm is so tense that it is impossible to overcome it by pressure. The urethroscope and air distension will then be necessary to distinguish between spasmodic and organic stricture.

2. *Malignant disease of the prostate* gives rise to symptoms of gradually increasing obstruction. The onset of symptoms in stricture dates from a much earlier age than that of malignant disease of the prostate. The obstruction to the passage of instruments is at the apex of the prostate, and rectal examination shows a hard, nodular prostate.

Complications.—The following are complications that may be observed :—

1. Retention of urine.
2. Septic complications :
   Acute or chronic urethritis.
   Periurethral abscess.
   Acute or chronic prostatitis.
   Epididymitis.
   Cystitis.
   Pyelonephritis and pyonephrosis.
3. Extravasation of urine.
4. Fistula..
5. Stone in the urethra and bladder.
6. Malignant growth of the urethra.

Retention of urine has already been described.

In old-standing and neglected strictures infection of the urine is almost invariably present. This is usually caused by the use of septic instruments, rarely it is hæmatogenous in origin. For many years the infection may be confined to the urethra behind the stricture and to the bladder, with the addition of chronic prostatitis. There are frequent micturition, scalding and pain, and the urine contains pus, mucus, and bacteria. The temperature is normal, with an occasional rise to 100.2° F., or there may be a slight evening rise for some months at a time. At any time acute septic complications may supervene, such as periurethral abscess, extravasation of urine, acute prostatitis, or epididymitis, or an ascending infection causing cystitis and ascending pyelonephritis, and, if obstruction takes place at the upper end of the ureter, pyonephrosis develops. Fistula is a complication of old-standing stricture, and usually follows periurethral abscess. Stone in the urethra is a not uncommon complication, malignant growth is rare. These conditions will be described later.

Prognosis.—An aseptic inflammatory stricture is amenable to treatment by dilatation and operation, and there is a good prospect of cure without permanent damage to the urinary organs.

Traumatic stricture is less favourable to complete cure.

When sepsis has been introduced the prognosis is much less favourable, and when it persists for some years, untreated or intermittently treated, renal complications make the prognosis very serious.

Treatment.—The methods of treatment in use are (1) dilatation, (2) operation.

1. **Dilatation.**—Metal instruments or flexible bougies of silk or cotton web coated with certain preparations are used.

Metal instruments may have a conical or, better, a bulbous end. The graduation varies slightly with the individual instrument-maker, and the instruments bear two numbers which show the size at the tip and at the thickest portion of the shaft. Metal instruments have the advantages of withstanding boiling, so that they last for many years ; and of having a smooth, highly polished surface that is easily kept surgically clean. They are specially useful in certain tortuous strictures, in cartilaginous strictures, and in strictures that have been dilated up to a large size and still require the occasional passage of an instrument. The lower-size metal instruments are apt to injure the urethral mucous membrane, and should be handled with the greatest caution. When not in use metal instruments should be smeared with vaseline before being laid aside. They should be replated on the first sign of cracking or scaling of the nickel.

Gum-elastic instruments or bougies should be pliable or resilient. A good bougie tapers gradually to a bulbous or olivary tip, and presents no abrupt shoulder. The shaft should be stiff, but the half of the instrument next the tip should bend readily to the touch.

Whalebone bougies are dangerous instruments and should not be used. Bougies are graduated according to a French scale which indicates the circumference in millimetres, or to an English scale similar to that used for metal instruments.

The French bougies possess the advantage of an exact and constant measure, and they ascend by finer gradations of size (roughly, 3 French to 2 English).

Pliable bougies are less likely to damage the urethral mucous membrane than are metal instruments. They are especially useful in the smaller sizes, and are preferable for the dilatation of most strictures up to 21 or 22 Fr. size. Beyond this size they are stiff and unwieldy, and should be replaced by steel instruments.

There are three essentials to the satisfactory passage of an instrument in a case of stricture of the urethra ; the instrument must be aseptic, well lubricated, and used with a gentle hand.

The sterilization of urethral instruments and the suitable lubricants are described at p. 562.

It is lack of the third essential—a delicate touch—that accounts for most of the accidents which result from the passage of urethral instruments.

The method of passing instruments is as follows : The surgeon stands upon the left side of the recumbent patient and handles the instrument with his right hand while he manipulates the penis with his left. (Figs. 101-4, pp. 358-9.) In the introduction of a steel instrument the penis is grasped behind the glans by the thumb and forefinger, and the tip of the instrument inserted into the meatus, while the shaft of the instrument lies transversely across the left Scarpa's triangle. The handle of the instrument is now carried gently towards the patient's abdomen and onwards to the middle line, and gradually raised meanwhile, so that the point drops downwards and backwards. During this manœuvre the left forefinger and thumb thread the penis upon the instrument. The handle is lightly held between the right forefinger and thumb, and the slightest hitch receives instant attention. If the instrument is stopped at the stricture, a smaller is tried until one is found that will pass. As the point passes down to the bulbous urethra the left hand leaves the penis and the fingers are used to support the perineum. The point of the instrument passes into the membranous urethra as the handle becomes vertical and swings downwards, and the left forefinger and thumb replace the right, while the handle is gently depressed between the thighs and pushed onwards.

In passing elastic bougies the operator has little power of changing the direction of the point of the instrument, and the passage of the bougie into the membranous urethra depends upon its pliability. The penis is grasped behind the glans by the thumb and forefinger of the left hand, and kept on the stretch to render the urethra straight and obliterate the folds in its walls. The bougie is introduced and lightly held by the corresponding digits of the right hand. If the instrument engages in the stricture it is pushed gently onwards. If the point is arrested it is withdrawn a little and again pushed on. If the attempt fails a smaller instrument should be selected, and so on until the size that will pass is reached. If, on the other hand, the bougie first passed lies loose in the stricture, a larger instrument is passed until the size is reached which is lightly gripped by the stricture. This "fitting" a stricture with an instrument must be distinguished from dilatation of the stricture.

In attempting to pass an instrument through a small stricture,

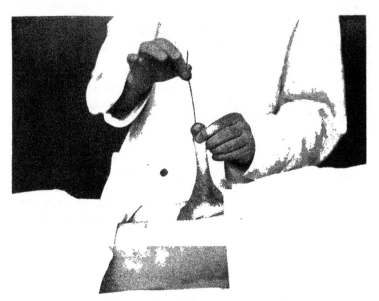

Fig. 192.—Passage of a filiform bougie through narrow stricture of bulbous urethra.

Note the penis put on the stretch with the left hand and the bougie lightly held in the right.

filiform bougies are employed. (Fig. 192.) They should not be used until the operator is satisfied that he is really dealing with a small stricture, for the point of a filiform bougie readily catches in any fold of mucous membrane, and for this reason may fail to pass where a stricture of comparatively wide calibre is present, or where the obstruction is spasmodic in character. If the filiform bougie fails to pass, it is withdrawn and gently advanced again. On further failure the tip of the instrument is bent to an angle and the bougie again introduced. The face of the stricture is now searched by turning the bougie round and testing the different parts of the circumference. If this manœuvre fail it should be repeated with another filiform bougie. A syringeful of oil may be injected into the urethra and the meatus gripped with finger and thumb to retain the oil, while at the same time the searching of the face of the stricture is continued. If this be unsuccessful, a number of filiform bougies should be passed into the urethra, and will engage in any pockets or false passages. By trying each bougie separately, one of them may pass on through the narrow opening.

It is sometimes of assistance to pass a large bougie down to the face of a stricture, and after withdrawing it to pass a filiform one. In this way the opening of the stricture may be centred and obstructing folds of mucous membrane pushed aside. If these attempts fail and no retention be present, the patient should be replaced in bed and a brisk purge administered. A further trial should be made next day, and will usually be successful. An instrument sometimes passes readily when the patient is under an anæsthetic, after all other methods have failed.

When several strictures are present, a bougie smaller than will fit the anterior strictures will be required to negotiate the second narrowing, for if the instrument accurately fits the first stricture it can only be pushed straight onwards without in the least altering the direction of the point. A stricture which lies immediately in front of the membranous opening of the urethra will give rise to difficulty in the passage of instruments, for the membranous opening is on the roof of the bulbous urethra, and the bougie impinges upon the floor of the canal, which rises up towards this opening. In these cases it is often necessary to resort to a rigid metal instrument, the point of which is more easily guided into the membranous opening.

Routine treatment of stricture.—The majority of strictures of the urethra are amenable to dilatation by instruments. Dilatation is carried out in three ways: i. As intermittent dilatation. ii. As continuous dilatation. iii. As rapid dilatation.

i. *Intermittent dilatation* is the best method of treatment of the majority of strictures, and is carried out in the following manner: The diagnosis of stricture having been made by the passage of a bougie of large size (say No. 20 Fr.) down to the stricture, the next step is to " fit " the stricture with its proper size of bougie. A much smaller instrument is at once tried (say No. 10 Fr.), and, if this fail to pass, successively smaller numbers are used, resorting at length, perhaps, to a filiform.

When a bougie is found that passes, it may lie loosely in the stricture; and if so, a larger size is passed until the proper size is reached which passes but can be felt to " fit." This size is noted, no attempt being made to dilate the stricture by passing larger instruments. An interval of four to six days is now allowed, and the size which fitted the stricture is again passed, and is followed by the next larger size in the scale, and this is repeated after a similar interval. The scale is thus gradually ascended until the size of the stricture has reached 21 or 22 Fr. Above this size the gum-elastic bougies become too rigid and too difficult to guide, and steel instruments should be employed.

During the ascent of the scale the interval between the instrumentations should gradually be extended. At 14 Fr. a week may intervene, at 18 Fr. a fortnight, at 20 Fr. three weeks, and with the larger steel bougies (12-14, 13-15, 14-16) a month should elapse. If all goes well this will be extended to two months, three months, and finally the patient will call once in six months or once a year to have an instrument passed.

No absolute rule can be laid down as to the largest size to which the urethra should be dilated. The natural size of the canal varies in different individuals. If necessary, the meatus should be incised in order to let large-sized bougies pass. In most individuals the urethra should admit a bougie of 22 Fr. calibre, and it is advisable to dilate a stricture beyond this if possible.

The urethra should be syringed before and after the passage of the bougie with a weak solution of permanganate of zinc (1 in 5,000) or of silver nitrate (1 in 10,000).

During the dilatation, and especially during the earlier part of the treatment, urinary antiseptics should be administered. Urotropine 5 gr. thrice daily, hetralin 7 gr., helmitol 7 gr., and boric acid 10 gr., are among the best of these.

When the intervals between the passage of instruments are prolonged to a month, the patient may take these medicines for two days before and two days after the operation.

A slight gleet often accompanies stricture, and should be treated by the patient using an injection night and morning with a hand-syringe. Permanganate of zinc, ½ gr. to the ounce, or sulphocarbolate of zinc in the strength of 1 per cent., is a suitable injection.

The dilatation of the stricture will remove the principal cause of the discharge. The time taken for the treatment varies according to the behaviour of the stricture. At the end of three months the patient may be in the position that a large steel bougie is passed once in two months. It is seldom that a case can be dismissed before the end of six months or a year. More often the treatment extends over eighteen months or two years. Some patients, especially those belonging to the hospital class, are careless and irregular in their attendance, and after a time the stricture gets into a callous condition which is beyond the hope of complete cure.

Strictures which have not become tough and leathery from long duration, irregular treatment, and prolonged irritation from chronic inflammation, will be cured by this means. A few of these relapse after a year or two, and require an instrument at long intervals.

In cases in which the patient gives a history of dribbling, and the clothes are saturated and the prepuce sodden with the leakage, the surgeon should at once resort to filiform bougies, for the stricture is of very small calibre. Where a filiform bougie is the largest instrument that will pass, we have to deal with either a very narrow stricture, or a moderate-sized stricture to which congestion or spasm is superadded. After a brisk saline purge and confinement to bed for two days, spasm or congestion will have subsided, a bougie of moderate size (10 to 12 Fr.) will pass, and intermittent dilatation may be commenced. On the other hand, the stricture may still grasp a filiform bougie, and a choice of methods is open, viz. continuous dilatation, rapid dilatation, a cutting operation.

ii. *Continuous dilatation.*—Continuous dilatation is useful in cases in which retention of urine has complicated a very narrow stricture. The patient is confined to bed, and a filiform bougie passed and fastened in by tying a silk ligature round it and fixing the ends to the sides of the penis by means of plaster. The urine trickles alongside the bougie in from one-half to two hours. After twelve hours a slightly larger instrument can be substituted, and after twenty-four hours a 6 or 7 Fr. can be passed. The continuous dilatation is now abandoned and intermittent dilatation commenced.

iii. *Rapid dilatation.*—This consists in forcing bougies of increasing size through the stricture in rapid succession until a large size is reached. This may be carried out by means of conical metal instruments, or, if only a filiform bougie can be passed, a tunnelled instrument is threaded over this and pushed through the stricture. This method ruptures the stricture although the epithelial covering may remain intact. At a later time a denser and more extensive stricture forms. It is not, therefore, recommended as a routine method of treatment, although it may be the only method available owing to lack of instruments or the necessity for at once dilating the stricture to the size that will admit a catheter.

It is not always possible to have the patient in bed for the passage of urethral instruments, nor is it necessary after the patient is accustomed to the operation, but it is essential during the earlier operations until the surgeon is familiar with the " temper " of the stricture with which he has to deal.

Complications of dilatation. (*a*) *False passage.* — Blood appears at the meatus, and a peculiar sensation of fine grating is felt. The further passage of instruments on the occurrence of such an accident must be suspended. The urethra should be washed with a warm boric or permanganate-of-zinc solution, to which a little hazeline or the tincture of hamamelis (B.P.) may be added if the oozing is pronounced. Copious bleeding rarely occurs. An ice-bag should be applied to the perineum. A week should elapse before further attempts are made to pass instruments. Especial gentleness should be exercised in the first passage of instruments after this accident, and the urethroscope is invaluable in demonstrating the position of the urethral opening and the false passage. Where a false passage of old standing is known to be present it may be avoided by passing a fine bougie gently into it and then introducing a second into the urethra alongside the first bougie.

(*b*) *Infection.*—This is prevented by the sterilization of instruments, of lubricant, and of the hands, and the washing of the penis and urethra before the passage of instruments. Urinary antiseptics are also valuable in preventing the occurrence of the infection and in its treatment. An injection with a hand-syringe of a solution of permanganate of zinc, $\frac{1}{2}$ gr. to the ounce, or of sulphocarbolate of zinc, $\frac{1}{2}$ per cent., or a copious daily urethral lavage by means of a douche-can and urethral nozzle with permanganate of zinc (1–5,000), will quickly cure the urethritis.

If a rigor occurs, the patient is confined to bed, surrounded by hot bottles, and hot drinks such as tea or hot Contrexéville water, and drugs such as quinine and urotropine, are given. A brisk saline purge should be administered.

(*c*) *Syncope.*—A sense of faintness or actual syncope may occur during the passage of instruments. For this reason the patient should invariably be in the recumbent position during the operation. The usual remedies for syncope are adopted, and the instrumentation is suspended. On succeeding instrumentations a solution of eucaine, 8 per cent., should be injected into the urethra as a precaution against this accident. Cocaine should not be used as a routine measure, for, besides the danger of absorption of the drug, the surgeon loses a very important guide and check to his manipulation when he abolishes the urethral sensation.

Spasmodic stricture.—The spasm affects the constrictor urethræ, and the obstruction is in the membranous urethra. The obstruction is intermittent; in an organic stricture it is continuous and increasing if untreated.

In spasmodic stricture a large instrument, if gently handled, will pass on after a slight delay. The use of cocaine (10 or 15 minims of a 2 per cent. solution) is permissible and advantageous if the diagnosis has been clearly established.

The cause of the urethral spasm must be diligently sought, for upon it depends the treatment. Causes of reflex irritation, such as anal fissure, inflamed piles, etc., should be treated, when present. Most frequently the spasm results from some urethral irritation, such as subacute inflammation in the prostatic urethra, or a small stone caught in this portion of the urethra in its outward passage. The latter accident will be treated by passing a large steel bougie and pushing the calculus back into the bladder, when it will be dealt with as a bladder stone. Posterior urethritis is treated by the passage of a large metal instrument and the instillation of a few drops of nitrate of silver solution (5 gr. to the ounce) into the prostatic urethra by means of a Guyon's syringe. Two or three instillations at intervals of a week will usually suffice. Retention of urine as a complication of this condition should be treated by a hot sitz-bath and an opiate, and, these failing, by the passage of a catheter.

2. **Operative treatment.**—While the majority of cases of stricture are cured or relieved by the passage of instruments, in a certain number of cases a cutting operation becomes necessary. The **indications for operation** are as follows:—

A. *Gradual dilatation may have failed.*

(1) In cases of hard cartilaginous stricture dilatation may be carried up to a certain size, and no further progress be made.

(2) Resilient stricture. The stricture is readily dilated but quickly relapses.

(3) Rigors follow the passage of an instrument under aseptic precautions.

(4) Hæmorrhage. A few strictures bleed at the slightest touch of a bougie, apart from any lack of skill or want of care.

(5) Repeated attacks of epididymitis.

(6) Recurrent attacks of retention of urine following the passage of instruments in strictures of moderately large calibre.

(7) Periurethral abscess and extravasation of urine.

B. *Cases unsuitable for gradual dilatation.*

(1) The stricture is impassable to the finest bougie, or only admits a filiform bougie with difficulty on several occasions.

(2) In cases of urethral stone, periurethral abscess, extravasation of urine, and urethral fistula.

(3) The stricture may be a complication of some disease of the prostate or bladder, such as enlargement of the prostate, stone, tuberculosis, chronic cystitis, new growths.

(4) In some diseases of the kidneys complicating stricture.

C. *The patient is unable or unwilling to carry out gradual dilatation.*

(1) He may be going abroad out of reach of medical aid.

(2) He may be unable to find time for gradual dilatation.

Internal urethrotomy.—The stricture is cut by means of a guarded knife (urethrotome) introduced along the urethra. (Fig. 193.)

The author's modification of Maisonneuve's urethrotome consists of filiform guides which screw on to the end of a fine grooved staff, and a triangular knife which runs in the groove. The modifications consist in (1) making the metal attachment of the guide taper, and placing it inside the end of the guide instead of having an abrupt metal shoulder from which the flexible guide tends to break; (2) the groove ends just beyond the commencement of the curve, so that the knife does not enter the prostatic urethra; (3) two wings are provided to hold the instrument steady; (4) a metal rod is provided which fits into the groove during introduction and prevents buckling when the stricture is narrow and hard. (Fig. 194.) This rod is removed before the knife is introduced. A general anæsthetic should be given, and the urethra thoroughly washed with a weak solution of nitrate of silver, 1 in 10,000. The surgeon stands on the right side of the patient, and the assistant opposite to him. The guide is introduced through the stricture and the staff screwed into it.

The staff is now made to follow the guide, which is pushed into the bladder and coils up there. The staff is held by an assistant at an angle of 45° with the horizontal. He grasps the wings of the urethrotome with a thumb on the upper surface of each, and holds the instrument absolutely steady in the middle line. The triangular knife is run along the groove and passed sharply through the stricture; as it is being withdrawn resistance is again felt, and the posterior cutting surface of the knife cuts the stricture a second time. Large metal instruments (12-14 to 14–16) are now passed to make certain that the stricture is completely cut.

A coudé catheter (22 Fr.) is passed and the bladder washed out

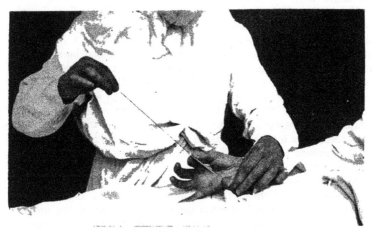

Fig. 193.—Internal urethrotomy.

The metal guide has been passed through the stricture, and its off transverse wing is held by the thumb and forefinger of the assistant's right hand (the assistant's left hand, which should hold the near transverse wing, is not shown). The operator has inserted the triangular knife in the groove of the guide and is holding the penis preparatory to pushing the knife home.

with weak nitrate of silver solution, and the catheter tied in. A roll of gauze is placed around the catheter at the external meatus and fixed with adhesive plaster. The catheter is plugged, and the urine withdrawn every two hours.

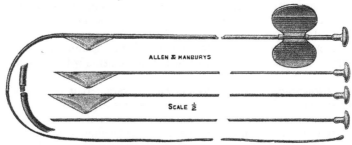

Fig. 194.—Author's urethrotome.

After forty-eight hours the catheter is removed, the urethra washed with nitrate of silver solution, and the patient passes urine himself.

Internal urethrotomy may be performed from behind forwards

by using a Civialé's urethrotome, which is passed through the stricture, the blade projected, and the stricture cut as it is withdrawn. The stricture must previously have been dilated to the size of No. 5 E.

The patient is kept in bed for a week and then allowed up. No instruments are passed for fourteen days after the operation, and then a full-sized metal instrument is introduced. A fortnight later instruments are again passed, and if the surgeon be satisfied that no recontraction is taking place the next visit should be paid a month later, then at intervals of two, three, four, and six months; and eventually the patient returns at the end of a year's interval, when, if no obstruction to the passage of a large metal instrument is detected and no fibrous ring is seen with the aerourethroscope, he may be dismissed as cured. Should recontraction of the stricture take place, instruments must be regularly passed at proper intervals.

Difficulties and dangers.—i. The fine guide of the urethrotome may break across at the metal attachment. This is a rare accident and is due to an imperfect instrument. To prevent it, the metal portion of the guide should be tapered inside the flexible portion. A lithotrite should at once be passed, and the guide caught and withdrawn. Failing this, a Luys' direct cystoscope should be passed and the bougie seized with fine forceps or caught with a hook. Should this fail, perineal cystotomy should be performed and the instrument removed by this route, and a drainage tube placed in the bladder.

ii. After removal of the urethrotome the surgeon may fail to pass a metal sound. The staff of the urethrotome with a small metal bulbous tip attached should be passed, and the stricture again cut. If this fail, a Harrison whip bougie is the instrument most likely to pass. Should the attempt be unsuccessful, the patient should be returned to bed and kept on diuretics and urinary antiseptics for a week, when the instruments will be found to pass.

iii. *Hæmorrhage.*—Serious hæmorrhage is rare. If it occur the lower end of the bed should be elevated, an ice-bag placed on the perineum, and pressure over this applied by means of a large sandbag. If a catheter be in the urethra, it should be allowed to remain *in situ.* A hypodermic injection of ergot and morphia should be given. If these measures fail, the catheter should be removed and the urethra irrigated with a hot solution of silver nitrate, . 1 in 10,000, or a solution containing tincture of hamamelis or adrenalin, and pressure reapplied. If spasm of the urethra appear to be a factor, hot fomentations may be tried. Finally, external urethrotomy should be performed and a large rigid tube introduced into the bladder and packed around with gauze.

iv. *Urethral fever.*—When no catheter has been tied in there is frequently a slight rigor and a rise of temperature some hours after the operation, following the first passage of urine. (Chart 17, p. 567.) This varies in intensity and duration. It may be prevented by tying a catheter in the urethra at the operation, and washing the bladder and urethra with nitrate of silver solution. Rarely a rise of temperature follows the removal of the catheter thirty-six or forty-eight hours after the operation. The urethra should be washed with nitrate of silver solution and the catheter replaced for another twenty-four hours.

v. *Anuria.*—This is a rare but very fatal complication. In from six to twenty-four hours after the operation there is a severe rigor, and the temperature rises to 104° F. or higher. The patient is restless, the face dusky, and the skin clammy. The breathing is rapid and later becomes stertorous; muttering delirium and eventually coma supervene, and the patient dies within eighteen to thirty-six hours of the rigor. A very small quantity of blood-stained urine, or none at all, is secreted after the operation. Prophylactic treatment consists in asepsis and preparatory washing of the urethra with silver nitrate solution and in tying-in a catheter after the operation. When the condition develops, venous and rectal infusion of several pints of saline solution should be given. In one case I performed nephrotomy and decortication of the kidneys, but without restoring the renal function.

Results of internal urethrotomy.—In most cases when death has followed the operation it has resulted from an exacerbation of pre-existing disease, and not from any new factor introduced by the operation itself. During thirteen years (1895–1908) 1,018 patients suffering from stricture were treated by internal urethrotomy at St. Peter's Hospital, and 8 patients died, a mortality of 0·78 per cent. Watson and Cunningham united several series of cases recorded in the literature, and found 53 deaths in 4,686 cases, a mortality of 1·1 per cent.

The causes of death are exacerbation of old-standing pyelonephritis (50 per cent.), anuria and uræmia, septicæmia and hæmorrhage.

After-results.—(1) Complete cure may be obtained without further interference in a small number of cases. In the majority of cases complete cure can be obtained by internal urethrotomy followed by the passage of instruments at long intervals.

(2) Recontraction of the stricture may occur after several

2 P

months or some years, but the occasional passage of a large metal
instrument suffices to prevent this.

(3) The stricture rapidly recontracts, and a cutting operation

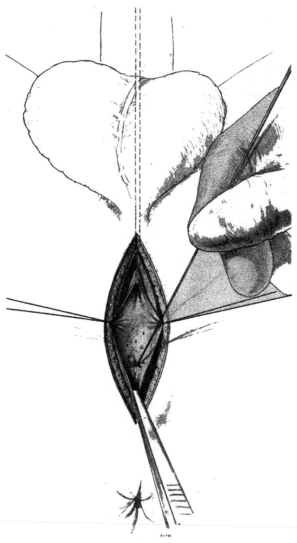

Fig. 195.—Wheelhouse's operation.

The urethra opened in perineum, the lumen of the stricture is being sought for.

must be repeated and dilatation by instruments resumed. Irregular attendance, alcoholic indulgence, exposure, and individual idio-syncrasy account for these relapses.

(4) In cartilaginous stricture operation permits the passage of large instruments, and this must be maintained. In spite of this the stricture may recontract.

External urethrotomy.—A variety of operations may be per-formed, depending upon whether it is possible to pass an instru-ment through the stricture or not.

External urethrotomy with a guide (Syme's operation).—The stricture is dilated to a No. 4 E. gauge by means of bougies, and a Syme's staff introduced. The patient is placed in the lithotomy position and an incision made on the staff just behind the shoulder. The stricture is cut in the middle line and the incision carried back to the membranous urethra, the probe-point of a gorget is introduced into the groove of the staff and pushed into the bladder. The staff is withdrawn and a perineal drainage tube introduced

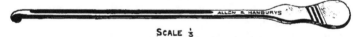

SCALE ⅓

Fig. 196.—Wheelhouse staff.

and tied in position, or a catheter passed along the penile urethra and on into the bladder.

The perineal wound is either left open or brought together with a few stitches.

External urethrotomy without a guide. (a) *Wheelhouse's operation* (Fig. 195).—This and the following operations are undertaken when the surgeon has failed to pass an instrument through the stricture. A Wheelhouse staff (Fig. 196) is passed down to the face of the stricture, and an incision made upon it about an inch from the end. The staff is hooked in the upper angle of the wound and the mucous membrane picked up on each side, and a careful search made for the opening; when this is found a probe is passed through the stricture, which is then slit up, and the operation is finished as in Syme's method.

This operation should not be performed at the end of a pro-longed and unsuccessful attempt to pass instruments through a stricture. In such a case some bleeding is almost invariably going on, and obscures the field in which search is to be made for the opening of the stricture. Unless the case is very urgent the patient should be returned to bed and the Wheelhouse opera-tion performed in a few days.

If Wheelhouse's operation fail, one of the following procedures may be adopted :—

(b) The incision is carried back and exposes the dilated urethra behind the stricture, or a second median incision may be made for this purpose when the first incision has been far forwards, or a curved prerectal incision may be made and the urethra exposed by dissection. A probe is then passed penis-wards through the stricture, and the scar tissue slit up upon this.

(c) Cock's operation, which was originally introduced for cases of acute retention in impassable stricture, may be done. The operation depends upon the presence of distension of the bladder and dilatation of the urethra behind the stricture. The tip of the forefinger of the left hand is placed in the rectum on the apex of the prostate, and a knife entered in the middle line of the perineum ½ in. in front of the anus and pushed straight for this point. The dilated urethra behind the stricture is opened.

(d) Suprapubic cystotomy is performed and retrograde catheterization with a metal sound, and the point of this is cut down upon in the perineum. The operation has little to recommend it over the perineal dissection (b).

Dangers of external urethrotomy.—The dangers are :

(1) Hæmorrhage, which is controlled by packing the wound.
(2) Cystitis and septic pyelonephritis.
(3) Renal failure and uræmia.
(4) Pelvic cellulitis.

Results.—The mortality was 8 per cent. in 100 cases performed at St. Peter's Hospital. Gregory found a mortality of 8·8 per cent. in 992 cases ; Thompson, 6·5 per cent. in 219 cases ; Howitz, 4·3 per cent. in 116 cases.

After-results.—Only a small percentage of cases are cured by the operation. When instruments are passed regularly after the operation the results are much better and correspond to those of internal urethrotomy.

Excision of strictures.—A single stricture of moderate dimensions may be resected. Every effort should be made to get rid of urethral or vesical infection before the operation. With this object the urethra is irrigated daily and, if necessary, cystotomy is performed a week or more before the operation. In all cases a preliminary suprapubic cystotomy is performed, and a rubber tube fixed in position. The patient is placed in the lithotomy position and a gum-elastic bougie passed through the stricture. A median incision 2 in. long is made, with the stricture as its centre. If the stricture is situated in the bulbous urethra the compressor urethræ is divided along the middle line. Goldmann and Hey

Groves have insisted on the necessity of excising the whole thickness of the spongy body with the strictured portion of the urethra. This does not interrupt the circulation of the peripheral end of the spongy body, for the glans and spongy body are supplied by the dorsal artery of the penis as well as by the artery to the bulb. The strictured portion of the urethra, together with the spongy body overlying it, having been removed, the ends of the severed tubes are carefully united with fine catgut on the metal instrument. Over this the fibrous sheath is accurately united and the compressor urethræ and perineal muscles are carefully brought together. The instrument is now removed. The suprapubic wound is drained by means of a suction apparatus for seven or ten days.

The extent of urethra that has been removed by excision has varied. Burckhardt resected 6 cm. (about 2¼ in.), and Goldmann a portion measuring 8 cm. (about 3⅛ in.). The subsequent forward curving of the penis on erection gradually disappears.

Results.—In 18 cases collected by Noguès and Viguard there was no recurrence at the end of periods varying from six months to eight years. Similar results have been described by Heusner, Horteloup, Rutherfurd, and others.

Watson and Cunningham collected 64 cases of resection, but only in 13 was there any information in regard to the urethra more than a year after the operation. In these the result was satisfactory from one year to six and a half years after the operation.

Selection of operation. — The following points must be considered :—

i. *Position of the stricture.*—A penile stricture is unsuitable for external urethrotomy, for a fistula is likely to follow. Internal urethrotomy with subsequent dilatation or resection of the stricture is preferable. Stricture of the bulb is suitable for any operation.

ii. *Character of the stricture.*—Soft annular strictures are especially suitable for internal urethrotomy. A hard cartilaginous inflammatory traumatic stricture may be cut by internal or external urethrotomy, but in either case instruments must be used afterwards. Excision of the stricture will be more likely to give a permanently successful result.

iii. *Thoroughness of the operation.*—Excision is the most radical operation. External urethrotomy cuts through a greater depth, but it only cuts the narrowest stricture, which lies nearest the bladder, and neglects the wider, more peripheral strictures. Internal and external urethrotomy may be combined and overcome this objection.

iv. *Convalescence* lasts a week or ten days after internal and two to three weeks or sometimes longer after external urethrotomy.

v. *Danger.*—The mortality figures are deceptive, since the worst types of stricture are submitted to external urethrotomy. The danger depends rather upon the complications of the stricture than upon the operation.

vi. *After-results.*—Recontraction occurs after both internal and external urethrotomy in almost equal degree.

vii. *Complications.*—External urethrotomy becomes necessary when local complications such as periurethral abscess, fistula, extravasation of urine, or urethral calculus are present.

LITERATURE

Albarran, XIIIe Congrès Internat. de Méd., 1900.
Antal, *Centralbl. f. d. Krankh. d. Harn- u. Sex.-Org.,* ii. 366.
Ballinger, *Med. News,* Nov. 11, 1905.
Berg, *Ann. Surg.,* 1903, No. 4.
Burckhardt, *Handbuch der Urologie* (von Frisch und Zuckerkandl), 1906, Bd. iii.
Goldberg, *Deuts. Zeits. f. Chir.,* 1900, p. 393.
Goldmann, *Beitr. z. klin. Chir.,* 1904, Bd. xlii.
Groves, Hey, *Bristol Med.-Chir. Journ.,* 1910, p. 325.
Hägler, *Deuts. Zeits. f. Chir.,* Bd. xxix.
Heresco, XIIIe Congrès Internat. de Méd., 1900.
Heusner, *Deuts. med. Woch.,* 1883, Nr. 28.
Ingianni, *Deuts. Zeits. f. Chir.,* 1900, Bd. liv.
Le Fur, *Ann. d. Mal. d. Org. Gén.-Urin.,* 1905, i. 1.
Lichtenstern, XVIe Congrès Internat. de Méd., Budapest, 1909, p. 436.
Lydston, *Med. News,* March 4, 1899.
Martel, *Presse Méd.,* 1904, p. 289.
Martens, *Die Verletzungen und Verengerungen der Harnröhre.* Berlin, 1902.
Poussou, *Ann. d. Mal. d. Org. Gén.-Urin.,* 1891, p. 20.
Rutherfurd, *Lancet,* Sept. 10, 1904.
Sawamura, *Folia Urol.,* 1910, Bd. iv., S. 683.
Thomas, *Brit. Med. Journ.,* Nov. 8, 1902.
Walker, Thomson, Burghard's *System of Operative Surgery,* vol. iii. 1909.
Wassermann et **Hallé,** *Ann. d. Mal. d. Org. Gén.-Urin.,* 1894, p. 241.
Watson and **Cunningham,** *Surgery of the Genito-Urinary System,* vol. ii. 1909.

CHAPTER L

PERIURETHRITIS—URETHRAL FISTULA

PERIURETHRITIS AND PERIURETHRAL SUPPURATION

THE source of infection is the urethra, and the inflammation takes various forms, such as abscess, fibrous masses, and gangrenous or phlegmonous inflammation, or extravasation of urine.

Etiology.—In the majority of cases the urethra is the seat of stricture, but injury from the passage of instruments or internal urethrotomy, new growths of the urethra, foreign bodies, calculi, or a retained metal catheter, may be the predisposing cause. There is usually a mixed infection of bacillus coli, streptococcus, and staphylococcus; less frequently the colon bacillus is found as a pure culture, and rarely the streptococcus is present alone. Anaerobic bacteria have been found most frequently mixed with aerobic bacteria, but occasionally alone.

The following varieties were isolated by Cottet, viz. micrococcus fœtidus, bacillus fragilis, bacillus funduliformis, staphylococcus parvulus, bacillus nebulosus, diplococcus reniformis. Anaerobic bacteria, especially the bacillus perpingus, are particularly frequent in the phlegmonous form of periurethritis—extravasation of urine (Jungano).

When a stricture is present, urine collects in the dilated urethra behind it, and the mucous membrane is inflamed. According to Leguen and Noguès, the inflammation spreads to the periurethral tissue by phlebitis and thrombosis in the corpus spongiosum; but Motz and Bartrina support the more widely accepted view that the inflammation spreads along the ducts of the urethral glands —namely, the glands of Littré, Cowper's glands, and also the prostate.

PERIURETHRAL ABSCESS, "URINARY ABSCESS"

The abscess may develop in relation to the penile or the bulbous urethra.

In the *penile urethra* a periurethral abscess occurs most frequently during the acute stage of an attack of gonorrhœa, less frequently in chronic urethritis. It is often situated at the base of the glans penis, but any part of the penile urethra may be affected. A tender swelling appears on the under surface of the penis, the skin becomes red and tense, and the abscess frequently bursts externally at one or both sides of the frænum or nearer the scrotum, according to the position of the abscess. Rupture into the urethra may also take place. A urinary fistula usually follows.

Abscess around the *bulbous urethra* may develop in relation to the perineal or scrotal portion. The abscess may form insidiously, and cause only slight pain on pressure or sitting, and is felt as a firm, tender nodule. The onset and course may be more acute, and there are a rigor, fever, and severe local pain and tenderness, and a hard swelling of considerable size quickly forms in the median line of the perineum over the bulbous urethra. The skin is red, tense, and glazed. As the swelling increases it passes forwards under cover of the scrotum, but is limited posteriorly by the fascia of Colles, which dips behind the transverse perineal muscle at the level of the central point of the perineum, and laterally by the attachment of this fascia to the rami of the ischium and pubes.

Partial or complete retention of urine is often present.

The **diagnosis** of periurethral abscess should be made—from anal abscess and ischio-rectal abscess, by the position; from abscess of Cowper's gland, by the unilateral position and the filling-up of the sulcus at the side of the membranous urethra on rectal examination in the latter; and from a prostatic abscess burrowing into the perineum, by rectal examination. Periurethral abscess rarely forms the starting-point of phlegmonous periurethritis. Rupture into the urethra may occur, and, if untreated, rupture on the surface may also take place, and a urinary fistula is formed.

Treatment.—A *penile* periurethral abscess should be opened through the urethra if it lies in the anterior part of the canal. This may be done with the aid of a wire speculum and reflected light, or a short urethral tube and urethroscope. A fine knife may sometimes be passed carefully along the urethra and plunged into the abscess, which is held between the finger and thumb of the left hand. The urethra should be washed daily with mild antiseptic solutions.

In *perineal* periurethral abscess all intra-urethral treatment should be stopped and hot fomentations applied, and the abscess opened by a free median perineal incision as soon as possible. The cavity is flushed with a large quantity of biniodide solution (1 in 5,000) and all pockets are freely opened, counter-openings being made if necessary. One or more drainage tubes are inserted, and the cavity is lightly packed with iodoform gauze, which is renewed daily. The cavity granulates, and the convalescence will take about five or six weeks.

It is seldom necessary to treat the stricture at the same time. Internal urethrotomy should be performed when the perineal wound is nearly healed. When a narrow stricture and severe cystitis coexist the perineal incision should be used to perform external urethrotomy, and a large rubber drain placed in the bladder.

DIFFUSE PHLEGMONOUS PERIURETHRITIS, "EXTRAVASATION OF URINE"

This is a virulent, rapidly spreading cellulitis, with sloughing of the urethra. It was at one time believed that the condition consisted in infiltration by infected urine which was forced through the urethral wall behind a stricture, but this view is now abandoned. Stricture is usually present, but may not be narrow, and cases occur in which no stricture has existed.

The bacteriology has already been described; anaerobic bacteria are specially common in this disease. The condition may commence in a periurethral abscess, but more commonly the onset is sudden, and the symptoms at once become severe.

After a rigor the temperature rises to 102° F. or higher, and profound toxæmia rapidly develops. The patient is pale and the skin clammy, the tongue and mouth become dry and coated, and delirium appears. The urine is passed with difficulty and in small quantity. A dull-red brawny induration appears in the perineum, and rapidly increases. The spread is limited by the attachments of Colles's fascia to the triangular ligament behind the transverse perineal muscle posteriorly, and laterally to the rami of the ischium and pubes. The scrotum becomes œdematous and red, the penis swollen and distorted, and the infiltration rapidly mounts on to the pubes and abdominal wall. Crepitation from the formation of gas may sometimes be detected. A fatal result from toxæmia is not uncommon, and may occur after operation.

Treatment.—Operation should be performed at the earliest moment. Multiple incisions are made in the skin of the scrotum, perineum, and abdominal wall, wherever the infection has spread. A constant stream of hot biniodide of mercury solution, 1 in 2,000, plays upon the parts, and is made to flow from one opening to another; or peroxide of hydrogen may be used. The skin of the scrotum is grasped and the thin sanious fluid expressed. It is not necessary to insert drainage tubes, as the multiple incisions should lay the sloughing tissues freely open. Hot fomentations

are applied and frequently changed, and the wounds are irrigated
several times in the twenty-four hours with peroxide of hydrogen.
Stimulants should be freely administered, and subcutaneous or
rectal saline infusions given. It is not advisable to place a drainage
tube in the bladder, as this may result in a violent cystitis where
only a mild infection of the bladder was previously present. Sloughing of portions of the bulbous urethra takes place, and urine is
discharged from one or more of the perineal incisions. The convalescence is usually prolonged. As soon as the condition of the
patient will permit he should be placed in a sitz-bath to which
permanganate of potash or solution of iodine is added, and should
sit in it for one-half to one hour at a time several times daily. At
a later date treatment for stricture and fistula may be required.

Chronic Indurative Periurethritis

This condition affects the bulbous urethra, and large masses
of fibrous induration form in the perineum and scrotum. There
is a stricture of the urethra, which is usually of the irregular cartilaginous type. The onset may be gradual, but there is usually a
periurethral abscess which has ruptured on the surface, besides
several urinary fistulæ. Around these, thick masses of fibrous
tissue gradually form. In the indurated mass there is frequently
one, and sometimes there are several small abscesses. Several
fistulæ may open into a common cavity, and this again into
the bulbous urethra.

Calculi may form in the fistulæ or in the urethra behind the
stricture, and a malignant growth has been known to develop.

Symptoms.—There is usually a long history of symptoms
of stricture, and operations may have been performed for its relief.
A perineal abscess has formed and ruptured or been incised, and
then the urethra has been neglected. Urine escapes from one or
several fistulæ during micturition, and the perineum may resemble
the rose of a watering-can: micturition must be performed in the
squatting posture. The fistulæ make tortuous tracks, and frequently intercommunicate. The induration forms a large, irregular
hard mass in the perineum and scrotum. An impassable cartilaginous stricture is frequently present.

Treatment.—If a filiform bougie can be passed, internal
urethrotomy should be performed as a preliminary to operation
on the periurethral induration a week or more later. If the stricture be impassable, external urethrotomy is performed at the time
of the perineal operation.

When a large mass of infiltration exists and internal urethrotomy
has previously been performed, a staff is placed in the urethra, the

patient placed in the lithotomy position, and the indurated mass split down to the corpus spongiosum in the middle line. The mass is seized on one side by forceps and removed, healthy tissue being cut through at the edge of the induration, and then the second half is treated in the same manner, all the fistulæ in the mass being included. If fistulæ or pockets remain, these are freely opened up and scraped, and indurated tissue around them is removed.

The opening into the urethra is found and repaired with catgut sutures. A large raw surface remains after the excision. This is reduced as far as possible by suturing from before backwards, and the remainder left open to granulate. A catheter is tied in the urethra. When the stricture is impermeable external urethrotomy is performed at the end of the operation. There is usually little difficulty in exposing and opening the dilated portion of the urethra behind the stricture.

LITERATURE

Albarran et Cottet, *Presse Méd.*, 1903, p. 85.
Escat, *Ann. d. Mal. d. Org. Gén.- Urin.*, 1904, p. 1761.
Legueu et Noguès, *Ann. d. Mal. d. Org. Gén.- Urin.*, 1903, p. 822.
Motz et Batrina, *Ann. d. Mal. d. Org. Gén.- Urin.*, 1903, p. 1601.
Walker, Thomson, Burghard's *System of Operative Surgery*, vol. iii. 1909.

FISTULA AND OTHER DEFECTS OF THE URETHRA

Urethral fistula may be congenital or acquired, and may open on the skin of the penis, scrotum, perineum, groin, or gluteal region, or into the rectum. There may either be a fistulous track, which may be tortuous and branching, or the opening may be direct.

Etiology.—Congenital fistula may take the form of hypospadias or epispadias (p. 573).

The most common *congenital* form is a fistula of the deep urethra, and is combined with atresia ani. The fistula may open into either the membranous or the prostatic urethra. In a man on whom I operated there had been atresia of the anus at birth, and the rectum had been incised. There was a recto-urethral fistula which admitted the forefinger and opened into the membranous urethra. A large round calculus occupied this portion of the canal, and in front of it were two congenital strictures, between which lay another calculus. The perineal muscles were atrophied, and the recto-urethral septum was as thin as paper.

Acquired fistula is due to trauma, inflammation, or new growth. Traumatic fistula arises from within the urethra from false passages and sloughing due to tying-in a metal catheter, from without by stabs, impalement, bullet wounds, etc., or after surgical operations such as external urethrotomy, perineal prostatectomy, opening (or rupture) of a periurethral abscess, or the incision of gangrenous periurethritis. Tuberculosis and bilharziosis are rare causes of fistula.

Symptoms.—Urine escapes from the fistula during micturition. The symptoms of stricture are also present when the urethra is narrowed. The quantity of urine which escapes varies from a few drops to half or more of the total quantity passed.

Fistula of the *penile* urethra opens directly into the urethra, and is surrounded by a firm ring of fibrous tissue. A fistula opening at the side of the frænum may have an oblique track.

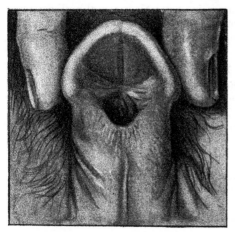

Fig. 197.—Artificial hypospadias due to removal of calculi from the fossa navicularis and penile urethra.

In *perineal* fistula there may be one or several openings. A single fistula is surrounded by a tube of hard, fibrous tissue; where a number of fistulæ are present there is usually a large indurated mass in the scrotum or perineum. A probe shows that the fistula is tortuous, and occasionally a stone can be felt in the fistula or in the urethra. In a small, old-standing fistula the opening may be difficult to discover, being hidden in a depressed and irregular scar. The skin is often inflamed and excoriated by soiling with urine.

In *urethro-rectal* fistula the urine is discharged into the rectum at each micturition, and this produces a watery motion, with or without fæcal masses. Gas may be passed along the urethra, and fæcal matter escapes with the urine. Urethritis and cystitis are usually present from infection. It is important, in view of treatment, to ascertain the presence or absence of stricture, cystitis, urethral calculus, and the number and duration of the fistulous tracks.

Defects of the urethra may follow surgical operations for the removal of calculus from the urethra. (Fig. 197.) The defect may resemble glandular hypospadias or penile hypospadias, or there may be extensive defects of the bulbous urethra. (Fig. 198.) The rite of subincision or *ariltha* (Sturt's rite), which is practised by the aboriginal tribes occupying a large part of South and West Australia, consists in subincision of the penis, by means of a sharp chipped piece of flint, so that the penile urethra is laid open from the meatus right back to the junction with the scrotum. (Fig. 199.) No serious results follow. In regard to the object of this rite, Spencer and Gillen state that " at the present day, and as far back as tradition goes, the natives have no idea of its having been instituted with the idea of preventing or even checking procreation,' which it does not do. Every man, without exception, is subincised, and although the number of children in a family rarely exceeds four or five, the reason for this is not subincision but infanticide.

Treatment.— The treatment of fistula with massive induration has already been described (p. 650). In cases without induration less radical measures may first be adopted. If stricture is present this is dilated, or internal urethrotomy performed, and a

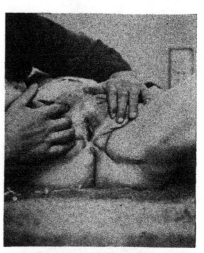

Fig. 198.—Defect of floor of bulbous urethra following removal of calculi of the bulbous and prostatic urethra.

catheter fixed in the urethra for a week or more. The fistula is scraped and cauterized with the electro-cautery or with a fine bead of silver nitrate. If these measures are unsuccessful the fistula should be excised. In perineal and scrotal fistulæ a metal instrument is passed, and the patient is placed in the lithotomy position. The fistulous track is carefully dissected down to the urethra, the opening in the canal carefully sutured with catgut, and the wound closed. A flexible catheter is substituted for the metal instrument, and fixed in place for a week. Should the fistula again open, the bladder should be drained suprapubically during the first ten days after the second operation undertaken to repair the fistula;

and, if the fistulæ are numerous and the operation difficult, it is better to provide suprapubic drainage at the first operation. Fistulæ which open directly into the urethra result from a loss of substance of the floor of the urethra. They are most frequently observed in the penile urethra, but are also found in the perineum, sometimes with extensive defects (2 in. or more) of the floor of the urethra. (Fig. 198.)

The bladder should be drained suprapubically as a preliminary to any of the following plastic operations on the urethra :—

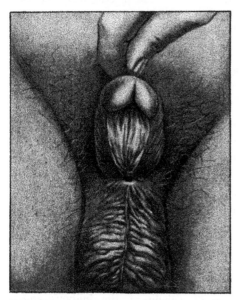

Fig. 199.—Artificial penile hypospadias (subincision) in aboriginal native of Australia.

Fistula at the base of the glans penis. *Dieffenbach's operation.* —The edges of the fistula are excised by a transverse elliptical incision and the raw edges united with fine catgut. A flap is raised from the under surface of the penis with its base at the fistula, and turned forwards over the fistula and stitched to a previously pre-pared raw surface on the under surface of the glans.

Fistula on the under surface of the body of the penis.— The edges of the fistula are excised and the urethra is closed with catgut sutures. This is covered by suturing the skin longitudinally, if necessary, making longitudinal incisions parallel with the wound to relieve tension ; or a quadrilateral flap of skin with its base towards the scrotum may be raised and drawn forwards (Loumeau) ; or a flap with its base towards the fistula turned forwards, and this again covered by lateral flaps (Guyon).

Repair of acquired urethral defects. 1. *Autoplastic methods.*—The cases suitable for these methods are those in which the roof of the urethra remains intact. The defect may be re-paired by undercutting and sliding. A large bougie is introduced along the urethra and lies in the open gutter of the defect. The urethra is dissected free on its under and lateral surfaces at each end of the defect, an incision is carried through the skin on each side parallel to the gutter, and two long flaps are turned over the bougie and united. On each side a longitudinal flap is raised by extensive undercutting, and these are united over the urethra.

2. *Heteroplastic methods.*—These are suitable for cases where portions of the urethra have been completely destroyed or removed.

Portions of tissue from other parts of the patient's body have been used, such as the foreskin, mucous membrane from the lower lip, the long saphenous vein. Mucous membrane has also been transplanted from other human beings, such as the mucous membrane of a prolapsed uterus, and from animals (bullocks, goats) and birds.

Operations similar to those used after excision of strictures may also be employed.

Results.—The results of these plastic operations have not been uniform. Successes have been recorded with all the methods, but on the whole the autoplastic have been more satisfactory than the heteroplastic operations.

Urethro-rectal fistula. — Congenital stricture, calculi, and other complications should be treated before closure of the fistula is attempted. The bladder is drained by suprapubic cystotomy, and the bowels are very thoroughly emptied. A curved pre-rectal incision is made, and the rectum and membranous urethra are dissected apart, the fistula being isolated on all sides and then cut across. The edges of the rectal opening are then united, and also those of the urethral opening.

Ziembieckl and Fuller isolate the extraperitoneal portion of the rectum and twist it round so that the urethral and rectal openings of the fistula are no longer opposite each other.

LITERATURE

Dittel, *Wien. klin. Woch.,* 1895, No. 20.
von Frisch, *Internat. klin. Runds.,* 1891, Nos. 26, 27.
Fuller, *Journ. of Cutan. and Gen.- Urin. Dis.,* April, 1897, p. 166.
Hallopeau, Thèse de Paris, 1906.
Keyes, *Journ. of Cutan. and Gen.- Urin. Dis.,* 1892, p. 401.
Lapiejko, *Ann. d. Mal. d. Org. Gén.- Urin.,* 1894, p. 41.
Le Prévost, *Bull. et Mém. Soc. de Chir.,* Paris, 1890.
Mensel, *Berl. klin. Woch.,* 1888.
Pasteau et Iselin, *Ann. d. Mal. d. Org. Gén.- Urin.,* 1906, ii. 1697.
Pringle, *Ann. Surg.,* Sept., 1904.
Spencer and Gillen, *The Native Tribes of Central Australia.*
Wolfler, *Arch. f. klin. Chir.,* 1888.
Ziembieckl, *Sem. Méd.,* 1889, p. 379.

CHAPTER LI

GROWTHS OF THE URETHRA

GROWTHS of the urethra are comparatively rare; the male urethra is more frequently affected than the female. The benign growths met with are papilloma, fibroma, caruncle, myoma, adenoma, and cysts; the malignant, carcinoma and sarcoma.

Gonorrhœa is said to play an important part in the etiology of benign growths of the urethra.

In the male the most frequent forms of tumour are papilloma and adenoma; and in the female, caruncle.

PAPILLOMA

Papilloma is found in the anterior urethra, especially in the region of the peno-scrotal junction, rarely in the prostatic urethra.

In structure (Fig. 200) the growth resembles those found on the glans penis and foreskin. There is a central blood-vessel surrounded by a very fine layer of areolar tissue, which in parts, and especially in the finer branches, is wanting, so that the epithelium is set directly upon the wall of the capillary vessel. The perivascular cells are regular and vertically arranged, and radiate from the vessel. The epithelium is thick, and towards the surface the cells become large and more flattened, and lie parallel with the surface. On the surface is a layer of flat cells. A few branches pass out laterally, but the complicated system of branching seen in vesical papilloma is wanting. There is a purulent discharge, and sometimes a peculiar sensation during micturition.

The symptoms are not distinctive, and the papillomas are usually found on examining a case of chronic gleet with the urethroscope. (Plate 41, Fig. 1.) The growths bleed very readily, and are easily torn by the passage of instruments.

There may be a few isolated growths, or the urethra may be choked with papillomatous masses. Preputial warts are not present in these cases.

Oberländer states that these warts may disappear if the gleet is cured. This is exceptional, however, and they are known to persist for many years. In a case observed by Oberländer the papillomas spread to the bladder and ultimately became malignant.

Treatment.—The warts should be removed by means of the urethroscope. Ebermann has used a special urethroscopic tube with a lateral eye for the purpose. A wart is manœuvred into the eye, and then shorn off by means of a second, sharp-edged

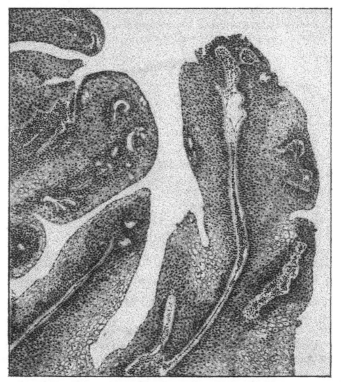

Fig. 200.—Section of papilloma of urethra.

tube passed along the first. Urethral forceps may be used. The base should be touched with a 4 per cent. nitrate of silver solution. Several sittings may be necessary. Recurrence after removal is not uncommon.

POLYPI

Urethral polypi are usually found in the prostatic urethra springing from the verumontanum or close to it, rarely in the anterior urethra. They occur usually in young men or adults.

2 Q

There are two forms—(1) fibroma, consisting of loose fibrous tissue with numerous vessels, and covered with a thin layer of mucous membrane ; (2) adenoma, in which there are numerous gland follicles. (Fig. 201.) Most of the follicles are dilated and may contain intrafollicular projections, and they are lined with columnar cells and set in a stroma of loose fibrous tissue and non-striped muscle. These appearances are identical with those of the " hypertrophied " prostate gland. They occur as small tumours with a short pedicle. In a case of enlarged prostate I have seen a bunch of small adenomas resembling a papilloma, set on the end of a pedicle 2¼ in. long,

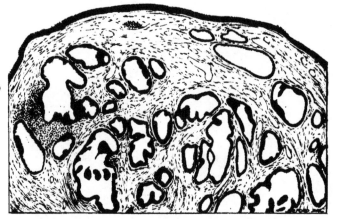

Fig. 201.—Section of glandular polypus of prostatic urethra.

springing from the posterior wall of the prostatic urethra and lying in the bladder.

The fibromas usually arise as a result of trauma, portions of the mucous membrane being torn up by instruments—especially some forms of prostatoscope tube—and these become covered with mucous membrane. At first they may be attached at both ends or are sessile, later they become polypoid. A favourite situation is on the montanal ridge in front of the verumontanum. Both fibroma and adenoma may be present in the same individual. Myoma and fibro-myoma have also been observed.

Labhardt collected 30 cases of benign tumours of the female urethra, which included 22 cases of fibroma, 6 of fibro-myoma, and 2 of myoma.

Symptoms.—A chronic urethral discharge is usually present, but there may be only a few shreds, or the urine may be clear. Tickling and crawling sensations in the urethra are sometimes experienced. Hæmorrhage may follow the passage of an instrument. On examination with the urethroscope the polypus first appears as a round, deep-red or purple swelling closely surrounded by the urethral wall. The pedicle and its attachment are seen when the montanal ridge is exposed to view. (Plate 41, Figs. 2, 3.)

Treatment.—This consists in removal through a suitable urethroscope tube by means of a pair of alligator forceps or a fine electro-cautery. The operation is delicate, but presents no great difficulty.

CYSTS

Small cysts are produced by blocking of the outlet of one of the urethral lacunæ. Cysts of the sinus pocularis are rare, and are usually found after death. The contents are serous. Cysts of Cowper's glands and ducts result from blocking of the ducts. They may be found in children if a few days or months old, or in adults. One or both glands may be affected. Large cysts 2 in. in length may thus be formed. If not opened the cyst ruptures into the bulbous urethra.

The **symptoms** caused are a chronic discharge, obstruction to the flow of urine, and a feeling of weight.

Treatment consists in incising the cyst through the urethroscope tube and applying the electric cautery to the interior of the sac.

CARUNCLE

Urethral caruncles are found in the female urethra on its posterior wall, near or at the meatus. They are vascular tumours covered with squamous epithelium. The chief symptom is pain, which varies very greatly in severity, and is excited by walking and other movements, and causes dyspareunia. There are pain and difficulty in micturition, and occasionally complete retention. Hæmorrhage may occur, usually as terminal hæmaturia.

The caruncle forms a small red tumour which appears at the posterior lip of the urethral orifice, and may extend some distance along the posterior wall of the urethra.

Excision is the only **treatment,** and the operation should be carefully performed by dissecting the whole of the tumour away after dilating the canal. Recurrence is usually due to incomplete removal. I have had to split the urethra into the vagina in order thoroughly to remove a recurrent caruncle. The canal was carefully repaired.

MALIGNANT GROWTHS OF THE MALE URETHRA

Malignant growths of the male urethra are rare. Preiswerk collected 42 undoubted examples, and in a collection made by

Hall there are 6 cases which were not included among these, making a total of 48. Barney records 2 cases, and I have had 3 under my care.

The condition is rare before the age of 40 (Hutchinson, one case at 22; Possi, one at 25), and is most frequently observed between 50 and 60.

Trauma has been noted as a predisposing cause, the new growth developing in a urethra the seat of traumatic stricture. Leucoplakia resulting from chronic urethritis is an important precancerous condition. The columnar epithelium of the urethra becomes transformed into squamous epithelium, forming patches of leucoplakia. Hallé has traced the development of epithelioma from these. Stricture is present in about half the cases.

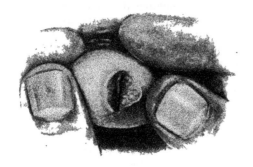

Fig. 202.—Epithelioma of urethra on lateral wall of fossa navicularis.

Pathological anatomy.—The bulbous urethra is the seat of the growth in the majority of cases, the penile urethra (Fig. 202) is less frequently affected, and the prostatic urethra very rarely. The growth may spread from the bulbous urethra to the penile, or from the penile to the bulbous, and a growth removed from the bulbous urethra has recurred four years later in the prostatic.

The growth spreads along the mucous membrane, infiltrating and destroying it, and invades the corpus spongiosum. A stricture is usually present in front of the growth. Posner found that 12 out of 20 cases had pre-existing gonorrhœal stricture. The urethra is dilated behind the stricture with deposits of phosphatic material on the mucous membrane. The periurethral tissues become infiltrated, and fistulæ form on the surface of the perineum. A malig-

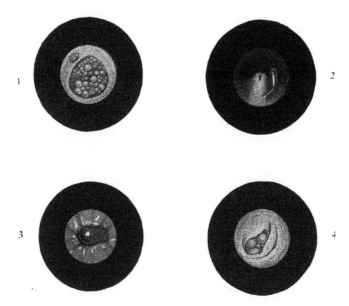

Fig. 1.—Papilloma of anterior urethra.   (P. 656.)

Fig. 2.—Polypus of posterior urethra attached to premontanal ridge.   (P. 659.)

Fig. 3.—Urethroscopic   view   of   polypus   of   urethra.
(P. 659.)

Fig. 4.—Malignant growth of anterior urethra appearing through a stricture.   (P. 661.)

PLATE 41.

nant growth may develop when fistulæ are already present, and is said to originate occasionally in the fistulæ.

The fistulæ may open on the perineum, scrotum, pubis, or buttock, or in the rectum.

The growth takes the form of a squamous epithelioma. Sarcoma has very rarely been observed.

Symptoms.—These vary considerably in different cases.

Increasing difficulty in micturition is usually noted, and is partly due to a fibrous stricture already present. Complete retention may supervene.

Hæmorrhage may occur after the passage of an instrument, or may appear at the meatus as a bloody discharge without instrumentation, or there may be hæmaturia. In one case under my care hæmaturia was severe, and there were several attacks of retention of urine. The growth was situated in the prostatic urethra, and examination by the urethroscope and cystoscope failed owing to hæmorrhage. A purulent discharge, mixed with blood, is very frequently present. In two of my cases this had been mistaken for gonorrhœa before I examined them.

A swelling appears in the perineum in some cases, and the skin becomes red, and either a fistula forms spontaneously, or the swelling is incised for a simple periurethral abscess. The growth then fungates, or progressive destruction by ulceration of the perineal tissues takes place.

In the penile urethra hard induration of the wall of the canal is felt, and this slowly increases and eventually involves the periurethral tissues, spreading towards the dorsum, and the corpora cavernosa become invaded. The penis may be ventrally curved during erection. It becomes swollen and rounded, and, when the growth is at the anterior part of the urethra, may assume a club-like form.

Examination of the urethra with an instrument shows a fibrous stricture in most cases. The instrument may pass this obstruction, but is arrested in an irregular cavity with friable, readily bleeding walls. Nothing abnormal can be detected on rectal examination.

Urethroscopy may give a view of the growth. It is frequently impossible on account of hæmorrhage, as in two cases of my own. In my third case a tough, fibrous stricture was present in the penile urethra, and through this were seen deep-red irregular nodules which were recognized as part of a malignant growth. (Plate 41, Fig. 4.)

Lymph-glands, inguinal and iliac, are enlarged in only one-third of cases, and are affected late.

Course.—The growth may spread very rapidly and death take place some months after the first appearance of symptoms. In other cases the progress is slower and extends over some years. Metastases occur in bones (ribs, vertebræ), liver, and lungs. In one of my cases there was slow growth for two years, and then rapid generalization.

Diagnosis.—From stricture of the penile urethra the diagnosis is usually difficult. Spontaneous hæmorrhage from the urethra, repeated severe hæmorrhage after instrumentation, and persistent hæmaturia are important symptoms.

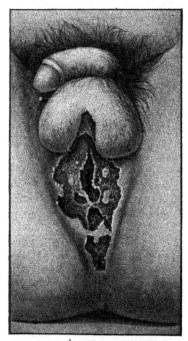

Fig. 203.—Malignant growth of urethra ulcerating on perineum and scrotum, and round anus.

Extensive infiltration of the penile urethra may be observed in subacute and chronic urethritis; when it is progressive, and the discharge is blood-stained, and the patient over 40, the diagnosis of growth is probable.

In cases in which there is a urethral discharge with a swelling in the perineum the diagnosis of periurethral abscess is usually made, and the nature of the disease is only diagnosed after the swelling has been incised, and sometimes not until some weeks later, when healing is delayed and ulceration around the perineal wound has commenced. (Fig. 203.)

Treatment.—Resection of the urethra has been performed in the early stage. In a case recorded by Oberländer, Kuffrecht. excised a growth of the bulbous urethra, with 1½ cm. on each side of it, and united the cut ends of the urethra. Four and a half years later the tumour recurred in the prostatic urethra.

Similar operations have been performed by König, Trzebicki, and others. When the penile urethra is involved by a small growth, amputation of the penis has given good results; but when the growth is extensive, or when it involves the bulbous urethra, complete removal of the penis (Thiersch-Gould operation) is necessary. In the majority of cases the tissues around the corpus spongiosum are infiltrated and the growth is inoperable when they come under observation.

NEW GROWTHS OF COWPER'S GLANDS

These are very rare, only three cases being recorded, two of which were said to be "cylindroma." The symptoms are pain and difficult micturition and complete retention. A tumour appears in the perineum, which can be felt from the rectum, and is at first unilateral. The growths were excised in all cases, but the after-history is unrecorded.

MALIGNANT GROWTHS OF THE FEMALE URETHRA

The condition is rare. Karaki collected 53 cases, 34 being periurethral or vulvo-urethral and 19 primarily urethral. I have met with 2 cases belonging to the latter group. Whitehouse, after careful examination of published cases, found only 43 undoubted cases where a microscopical report was given.

The periurethral growths occur after the age of 50, and the primary urethral growths frequently under that age.

There has been a pre-existing urethral caruncle in several cases, and the malignant growth probably took origin in this. Hallé found that chronic urethritis with leukoplakia preceded the growth in some cases.

The urethral variety may be pedunculated or sessile, appearing as a dark-red grape-like polypus or a nodular ulcerated area. The periurethral variety originates at the external meatus, spreads around the urethra, and extends to the vulva. It may take an ulcerating or an infiltrating character. The majority of the growths are squamous-celled carcinoma (27, Whitehouse), a few are columnar-celled carcinoma (2), and others are adeno-carcinoma (14), analogous to prostatic carcinoma in the male and arising in the periurethral glands. Sarcoma is rare (Kamann).

Symptoms.—There is pain on micturition, on coitus, and on sitting and walking, and the pain radiates down the thighs ; there are also frequent micturition, difficulty in the act, and occasionally complete retention. Incontinence is rare. Hæmaturia is usually present. Hæmorrhage may occur apart from micturition, on coughing or sneezing.

On inspection a growth, pedunculated or sessile, is seen at the meatus or spreading on to the walls of the vestibule. Induration can be detected, and œdema of one or both labia may develop. Lymphatic glands are enlarged.

Treatment.—The urethra may be excised by a longitudinal

incision on the anterior wall of the vagina. The vesical end is, if possible, preserved, and is implanted in the vaginal wall. The patient is continent after this operation, but if it is necessary to remove the whole of the urethra, including the vesical orifice, incontinence results, and it is better in such cases to close the base of the bladder completely and establish permanent suprapubic drainage (see p. 549). One patient was well without recurrence five years, and another one year, after removal of the growth.

LITERATURE

Barney, *Boston Med. and Surg. Journ.*, 1907, p. 790.
Bouzani, *Folia Urol.*, 1909, p. 491.
Cabot, *N.Y. Med. and Surg. Journ.*, 1895, p. 278.
Ehrendorfer, *Centralbl. f. Gyn.*, 1892, Nr. 17.
Englisch, *Folia Urol.*, 1907, p. 38.
Fuller, *Journ. Cutan. and Gen.-Urin. Dis.*, April, 1895.
Gussenbauer und **Pietrzikowski**, *Zeits. f. Heilkund.*, 1885, vi. 421.
Hall, *Ann. Surg.*, 1904, p. 375.
Hallé, *Ann. d. Mal. d. Org. Gén.-Urin.*, 1896, p. 481.
Kamann, *Monats. f. Geb. u. Gyn.*, April, 1906.
Kapsammer, *Wien. klin. Woch.*, 1903, Nr. 10.
Karaki, *Zeits. f. Geb. u. Gyn.*, 1908, p. 151.
Kocher und **Kauffmann**, *Krankheiten der männlichen Harnröhre.* 1886.
Kretschmer, *Trans. of Chicago Path. Soc.*, June 1, 1911, vol. viii.
Labhardt, *Zeits. f. Gyn. u. Urol.*, 1910, ii. 1.
McMurty, *Surg., Gyn. and Obst.*, June, 1908, vol. vi.
Oberländer, *Centralbl. f. d. Krankh. d. Harn- u. Sex.-Org.*, Aug., 1893, Bd. iv. ; and 1900, xi. 454.
Pagnet et **Hermann**, *Journ. de l'Anat. et de la Physiol.*, 1884, p. 615.
Pfannenstiel, *Centralbl. f. Gyn.*, 1901, p. 33.
Posner, *Zeits. f. Krebsforsch.*, 1904, i. 4.
Preiswerk, *Zeits. f. Urol.*, 1907, p. 273.
Soubeyran, *Gaz. des Hôp.*, 1903, p. 1181.
Trzebicki, *Wien. med. Woch.*, 1884, p. 606.
Vineberg, *Amer. Journ. Med. Sci.*, July, 1902.
Wassermann, *Thèse de Paris*, 1895.
Whitehouse, *Proc. Roy. Soc. Med.*, Obstet. and Gynæcol. Sect., Jan., 1912, p. 128.

CHAPTER LII

TUBERCULOSIS OF THE URETHRA AND PENIS

TUBERCULOSIS of the urethra is rare. Primary tuberculosis has been observed, but the infection is almost invariably secondary to tuberculosis of the urinary or genital systems. The female urethra is very seldom affected. The usual form is tuberculosis of the posterior urethra in the male; the anterior urethra is seldom involved.

The prostatic urethra is affected by spread from the prostate gland or from the bladder. A deep tuberculous cavity may open from the substance of the prostate on the posterior urethra, or there may be superficial ulceration or tuberculous granulation tissue. The anterior urethra may be the seat of small superficial ulcers; but if the penis is affected the urethral mucous membrane is involved in the tuberculous infiltration.

The periurethral tissues may be implicated and a "cold abscess" form, and eventually fistulæ appear in the perineum. The prevesical space may also be involved. Englisch has described tuberculosis of Cowper's glands.

Stenosis of the urethra is occasionally observed in the bulbous or penile urethra in cases of urinary and genital tuberculosis. There is seldom a localized stricture such as is found as the result of gonorrhœal urethritis. The wall is infiltrated, and an irregular fibrous thickening of the mucous membrane results.

Symptoms.—A urethral discharge is always present, and is usually thin and pale, but occasionally it is so abundant and purulent and the symptoms are so acute as to suggest gonorrhœal urethritis. Gonococci are, however, absent, and tubercle bacilli are found. Hæmaturia, frequent and difficult micturition, and occasionally complete retention, may be present. There is irregular periurethral induration, and a bougie passed along the urethra meets resistance, and grating may be felt. Hæmorrhage frequently follows.

With the urethroscope infiltration and occasionally ulceration are seen. A deep tuberculous cavity or superficial ulceration or tuberculous granulation tissue may. be found in the posterior urethra.

Tuberculosis of the penis may be confined to ulceration of the glans, usually on the under surface, or the corpora cavernosa of the penis may be invaded. In a case under my care the terminal two-thirds of the penis was greatly enlarged, round, and hard, and the glans penis showed several sinuses through which granulation tissue projected. The first 2½ in. of the urethra were involved. No other tuberculous lesion was detected in the genital or urinary system.

Treatment.—Tuberculosis of the urethra is so seldom an isolated lesion that separate treatment is rarely necessary.

Internal urethrotomy should be performed in stenosis of the urethra, and instruments passed at short intervals afterwards, as there is a marked tendency to recontraction. When a "cold abscess" forms it should be opened, and tincture of iodine applied

Fistulæ are treated by scraping and injection of iodoform emulsion, bismuth paste, or iodine.

Conservative treatment should be adopted when the penis is involved, but amputation may become necessary for extensive lesions. Tuberculin (T.R.) should be given in gradually increasing doses in all cases, and should be persisted in for periods of many months or several years.

Where there is extensive destruction of the urethra, with tuberculosis of the bladder, permanent suprapubic drainage of the bladder may become necessary in order to relieve the constant pain and vesical spasm.

LITERATURE

Asch, *Zeits. f. Urol.*, 1909, iii. 174.
Chute, *Boston Med. and Surg. Journ.*, 1903, p. 361.
Halasz, *Ungarische mediz. Presse*, 1901, p. 762.
Hallé et Motz, *Ann. d. Mal. d. Org. Gén.- Urin.*, 1902, p. 1464.
Hogge, *Ann. d. Mal. d. Org. Gén.- Urin.*, 1901, p. 1491.
Sawamura, *Folia Urol.*, 1910, iv. 683.

PART V.—THE PROSTATE

CHAPTER LIII

SURGICAL ANATOMY—EXAMINATION
CONGENITAL MALFORMATIONS

SURGICAL ANATOMY

THE prostate gland is the size and shape of a Spanish chestnut, and lies with its long axis vertical, its base beneath the floor of the bladder, and its apex at the triangular ligament, ½–¾ in. below and behind the subpubic angle. Its average weight is 4½ drachms, and it measures 1¼ in. in length, 1 in. in the antero-posterior diameter, and 1½ in. transversely. The base lies beneath the floor of the bladder, extending backwards behind the urethra to about the mid-point of the trigone and forwards for ¼ in. in front of the internal meatus. The greatest lateral extent, which measures ¼ in. on each side, is a line drawn from the internal meatus outwards and a little backwards. The glandular tissue of the prostate lies behind and on each side of the urethra, and does not project in front of it.

The arrangement of bladder muscle on the base of the prostate is as follows : The outer longitudinal layer of bladder muscle (Fig. 206) loses itself upon the upper surface of the gland, the muscle fibres becoming incorporated with the non-striped muscle of the stroma of the organ. Lying upon this is the trigone muscle, consisting of a layer of transversely disposed muscle fibres, which forms a thick wedge behind the opening of the urethra and is continued into the outer circular muscular layer of the urethra. Over this muscular layer is a longitudinal layer continuous with the inner longitudinal layer of the ureters and passing into the internal longitudinal layer of the urethra. In front of the urethra the outer longitudinal layer of bladder muscle approaches the anterior wall of the urethra, and becomes lost among the bundles of circular muscle which surround it. The inner or circular layer of bladder muscle is continued well up to the urethra, and then ceases.

Along the anterior wall of the urethra is a thick layer of circular muscle which extends from the base to the apex of the prostate. The true sphincter of the bladder consists of the circular trigone muscle behind the urethra, which spreads out fan-wise on each side of the prostatic urethra and forms the vertical band of circular muscle in front of this portion of the urethra. Surrounding the membranous urethra at the apex of the prostate is the compressor urethræ muscle, and the striped fibres of this muscle are continued upwards (Henlé's muscle) on the anterior surface of the

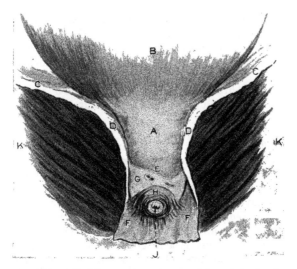

Fig. 204.—Bladder and prostate with pelvic fascia.

A, Part of anterior surface of prostate between reflected lateral layers of sheath. B, Anterior wall of bladder. C, C, Recto-vesical layer of pelvic fascia on upper surface of levator ani muscle. D, D, Vertical line of reflection of fascia on anterior surface of prostate. E, Line of reflection of fascia crossing middle line. F, F, Upper layer of triangular ligament. G, Apex of prostate with termination of dorsal vein of penis. H, Striped muscle round urethra. J, Urethra. K, K, Levator ani muscle.

prostate gland as far as the base. The striped muscle lies between the anterior commissure and the anterior layer of the sheath containing the ascending portion of the prostatic plexus. Laterally some fibres stray among the non-striped fibres of the prostatic stroma, but the layer may be traced on each side on the surface of the capsule as far back as the level of the urethra.

The prostate is surrounded by a layer of fascia, which envelops it except at its basal attachment to the bladder. (Fig. 204.) At the apex the fascia blends with the muscular tissue around the urethra. This sheath is derived from the recto-vesical layer of pelvic fascia, and is formed in the following manner : The recto-vesical layer of pelvic fascia passes inwards from the side wall of the pelvis and meets the lateral aspect of the junction of the bladder and prostate, and from this a strong layer of fascia passes downwards over the lateral aspect of the prostate, forming the lateral portion of the sheath. The lateral layer leaves the gland on each side before it reaches the middle line anteriorly, so that a vertical band on the anterior surface of the prostate is left uncovered. Those layers unite across the middle line at the apex of the prostate to form the upper layer of the triangular ligament. The posterior surface of the prostate is covered by a layer of fascia which splits off from the recto-vesical fascia, and is attached along the base, sending a prolongation upwards to cover the seminal vesicles and the terminal portions of the vasa deferentia and ureters. The fascial sheath can be stripped, without damage to the gland, from the lateral and

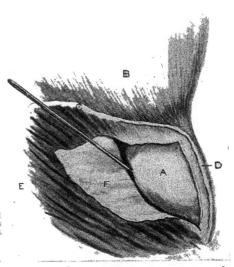

Fig. 205.—Lateral view of prostate and fascia.

A, Right lobe of prostate exposed. B, Bladder. C, Line of attachment of recto-vesical layer of fascia. D, Line of reflection of fascia from prostate. E, Levator ani muscle. F, Lateral layer of fascial sheath thrown back. A probe has been passed behind the prostate within the sheath.

posterior surfaces. (Fig. 205.) It is adherent around the base and at the apex and along the anterior surface.

The prostatic urethra traverses the gland. The first part of the tube from the internal meatus to the verumontanum is straight and vertical. At the verumontanum the urethra begins to curve forwards, and the remaining part of its course is as much forwards as downwards. At the internal meatus the urethra lies on the same vertical plane as the anterior borders of the lateral lobes. From this level it sinks backwards in relation to the gland tissue, so that at the verumontanum it lies midway between the anterior and posterior surfaces of the organ. From this point it passes more and more towards the front of the organ as the gland tubules disappear.

The structure of the prostate gland consists of tubules embedded in a densely woven stroma of non-striped muscle. There is no distinct circular arrangement of the fibres of the stroma around the individual tubules. At the surface of the organ there is an area of stroma in which no gland tubules can be seen, and the fibres are more circular in their arrangement. This is the true

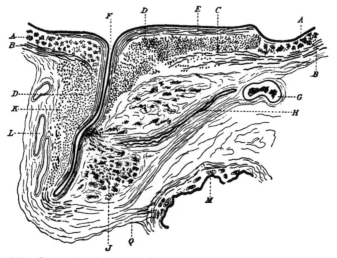

Fig. 206.—Vertical mesial section through bladder base, prostate, and surroundings.

A, A, Circular layer of bladder muscle. B, B, Longitudinal layer of bladder muscle. C, Circular layer of trigone muscle. D, D, Unstriped sphincter of bladder. E, Longitudinal layer of trigone muscle. F, Urethra. G, Seminal vesicle. H, Ejaculatory duct. J, Prostatic gland tissue. K, Striped muscle in front of prostate. L, Veins of prostatic plexus. M, Rectum. Q, Recto-urethral muscle.

capsule of the prostate. The gland tubules are arranged in horse-shoe form around the posterior and lateral aspects of the urethra, and form two lobes. In stained transverse sections of the prostate no division of the gland tissue into two lobes can be seen behind the urethra. (Fig. 207.) In front of the urethra along the whole length of the prostate is a vertical wedge of non-striped muscle and fibrous tissue. This anterior commissure separates the two lateral lobes.

. From the verumontanum a band consisting of the sinus pocularis and the ejaculatory ducts, surrounded by a sheath of non-striped

muscle, passes upwards and backwards through the sheet of gland
tissue which unites the lateral lobes behind the urethra. In a
vertical median section this band appears to isolate a wedge of
gland lying immediately behind the upper part of the urethra.
This is the so-called " median lobe." No separate lobe exists in
the normal prostate. The ducts of the prostatic glands open into
the prostatic sinuses in the immediate neighbourhood of the
verumontanum, and on the posterior wall of the urethra above
this. No gland ducts open into the urethra between the part

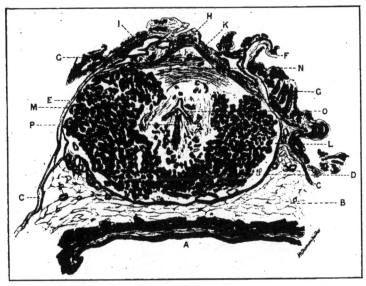

Fig. 207.—Transverse section of prostate and surroundings
at level of verumontanum.

A, Anterior wall of rectum. B, Areolar tissue. C, C, Visceral layer of pelvic fascia. D, Sheath
of prostate formed by pelvic fascia. E, Sheath of prostate. F, Pelvic fascia (sheath) reflected
from anterior surface of prostate. G, G, Levator ani muscle. H, Fibrous tissue on anterior
surface of prostate. I, Large veins of prostatic plexus. K, Striped muscle layer on anterior
surface of prostate. L, M, Capsule of prostate. N, Anterior commissure. O, Verumontanum.
P, Ejaculatory ducts.

immediately adjacent to the verumontanum and the membranous
urethra.

Although the lateral lobes are not separated histologically,
they are physiologically distinct. Acute inflammation and malignant disease may be accurately limited to one lobe, the other lobe
being healthy.

The arteries supplying the prostate are derived from the
vesical, hæmorrhoidal, and pudic arteries.

The veins form the prostatic venous plexus (Figs. 208, 209). This commences in the dorsal vein of the penis, and, passing up the

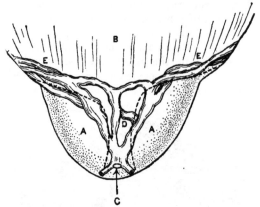

Fig. 208.—Prostatic plexus of veins, anterior view.

A, A, Anterior surface of prostate. B Bladder. C, Termination of dorsal vein of penis. D, Prostatic plexus. E, E, Vesico-prostatic plexuses. The dotted line shows the line of attachment of fascia.

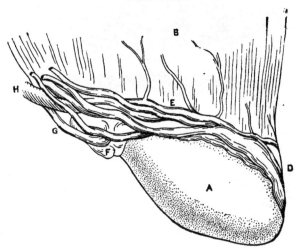

Fig. 209.—Prostatic plexus of veins, side view.

A, Right lobe of prostate. B, Bladder. D, Prostatic plexus on anterior surface of prostate. E, Vesico-prostatic plexus. F, End of right seminal vesicle. G, Vas deferens. H, Right ureter.

anterior surface of the prostate from the apex to the base, here splits into two groups, which pass along each side at the angle formed by the junction of the bladder and prostate. The plexus is thus shaped like the letter **Y**. On the front of the prostate the stem of the **Y** is formed by large intercommunicating venous channels embedded in the anterior layer of the fibrous sheath and separated from the anterior commissure of the prostate by the layer of striped muscle described above. The arms of the plexus receive the vesical veins and those from the seminal vesicles, and pass to the internal iliac vein.

The lymphatics pass in trunks with the veins to glands situated along the internal iliac vessels and at the bifurcation of the iliac artery. A few pass to glands in front of the bladder, and some lymphatic vessels pass round the rectum to a gland in the hollow of the sacrum and upwards to the aortic chain.

The nerves are derived through the hypogastric plexus from the 3rd and 4th sacral nerves.

LITERATURE

Albarran, *Médecine Opératoire des Voies Urinaires.* 1909.
Kalischer, *Die Urogenitalmuskulatur des Dammes.* 1900.
Proust, *La Prostatectomie.* 1904.
Walker, Thomson, *Med.-Chir. Trans.,* 1904, vol. lxxxvii.; *Brit. Med. Journ.,* July 9, 1904; *Journ. of Anat. and Phys.,* 1906, xl. 189.
Ziegler, Thèse de Bordeaux, 1893.
Zuckerkandl, E., *Handbuch der Urologie* (von Frisch und Zuckerkandl), 1904, Bd. i.

EXAMINATION OF THE PROSTATE

Rectal examination (Fig. 210) may be performed with the patient in the knee-elbow position on a couch, or lying on his back with the pelvis raised in the lithotomy position. The former is preferable for routine examination, while the latter is used in examination under general anæsthesia and for bimanual examination.

On introduction of the forefinger, covered with a thin rubber glove and well oiled, a pocket is felt on the anterior wall of the rectum immediately internally to the anal canal. A vertical ridge in the middle line of this pouch is the membranous urethra; on each side of this is a depression in the position of Cowper's glands, which can be felt, when enlarged, by pressing the thumb on the perineum and grasping the tissues between this and the finger in the rectum. The prostate is felt above this anterior pouch, and in the great majority of cases the finger easily reaches above the upper limit of the gland. Difficulty may be experienced when the buttocks are heavy and the perineum deep, and when the patient is nervous and rigidly contracts his muscles. In the middle line of the prostate is a vertical groove, and on each side of this a prostatic lobe is felt.

The consistence of the normal prostate is uniform and elastic,

2 R

and pressure causes a slight desire to micturate. The gland has a moderate degree of mobility, which is best appreciated by comparing it with a prostate the seat of malignant growth. On each side of the gland is a sulcus, the depth of which indicates the antero-posterior size of the prostate. The finger should search for toughness or hardness of the gland, for nodules projecting or buried, for enlargement, lateral spread, vertical spread, for diminution of mobility, for tenderness, for obliteration of the paramembranous depressions.

The track along which lymphatics of the prostate pass is felt as a sling which leaves the upper part of the lateral lobe on each side and passes upwards and outwards. In carcinoma of the prostate thickening may be felt in this situation, and a nodule or

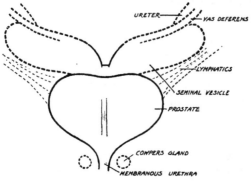

Fig. 210.—Structures in relation to anterior wall of male rectum.
The parts normally felt on rectal examination are shown in continuous black lines ; those felt in disease are shown in dotted lines.

a chain of nodules, representing small lymphatic glands containing deposits. In a very lax bladder the upper surface of the gland can sometimes be palpated.

The seminal vesicles lie immediately above the base of the prostate. They pass transversely outwards and upwards, and are readily palpated by a finger of ordinary length. They may be empty and cannot be felt, or distended and form soft, sausage-like cushions. Nodules and thickening of the wall should be searched for. When malignant growth or chronic cellulitis has obliterated the lateral sulci, a level surface is felt on the anterior wall of the rectum, in which the outline of the organs is wanting.

In bimanual examination the patient is in the lithotomy position, and the left hand presses downwards above the pubic symphysis. An enlarged prostate can frequently be felt in this way.

Rectal examination in the recumbent position may be assisted by the passage of a metal sound, which can be felt in the median furrow.

The length of the prostatic urethra may be measured by passing a coudé catheter. The sensation given to the surgeon's fingers on passing the catheter will show when the point encounters the resistance of the compressor urethræ muscle at the membranous urethra, and passes through this into the prostatic urethra. There is again slight resistance when the point passes through the internal meatus, and the urine now begins to flow, showing that the eye of the catheter is in the bladder. In some forms of enlargement of the prostate the upper part of the prostatic urethra is open and trumpet-shaped, and this test is fallacious. A metal stone sound may be used for this purpose. The beak is turned downwards after entering the bladder, and withdrawn until it hitches on the prostate. A calculus projecting from a pouch in the prostate or lying in the prostatic urethra will be felt with the sound.

The **cystoscope** gives information in regard to the urethral orifice and the upper surface of the prostate. In the normal state the margin of the urethra is slightly concave upwards. In enlargement of the prostate it is convex. A central lobe or lateral intravesical projection may be seen, and the size and extent estimated by the projection hiding part or the whole of the trigone from view and obscuring the view of the ureteric orifices.

An irregular projection is seen in malignant disease of the prostate, and a malignant growth may be seen ulcerating through the bladder base from the prostate.

CONGENITAL MALFORMATIONS

Complete absence of the prostate is rare, and only occurs in combination with other malformations of the genital organs, such as ectopia vesicæ, pseudo-hermaphroditism, hypospadias, absence of the testicle.

CONGENITAL AND ACQUIRED CYSTS

Cysts of the prostate are found in children a few days after birth, due to closure of the opening of the sinus pocularis and retention of the secretion. The verumontanum is enlarged, and the cyst projects into the prostatic urethra. It may attain a considerable size, and can be felt on the rectal surface of the prostate as a rounded swelling. There is a lining of columnar epithelium, and the contents are fluid, with epithelial and round cells. The cyst wall is thin and easily ruptured into the urethra, or it may be thick and resistant. Such cysts cause urethral obstruction and retention of urine. Cysts developing between the prostate and rectum are ascribed by Englisch to vestigial remains of the duct of Müller when their position is median, and of the Wolffian body when laterally placed. They are found in adults, and cause no symptoms when small, but large cysts may give rise to symptoms of pressure on the bladder or rectum, to retention of urine, or to radiating pain in the testicles and thighs. A large cyst may be mistaken for a distended bladder or for a vesical diverticulum. The diagnosis is made by cystoscopy, and by rectal examination with a sound in the urethra, the bladder having been emptied.

Treatment consists in exposure of the cyst from the perineum and drainage.

CHAPTER LIV

PROSTATITIS

ACUTE prostatitis occurs most frequently as a complication of gonorrhœa. Other predisposing causes are stricture of the urethra, cystitis and vesical calculus, sexual excess, various conditions of the intestines, such as constipation, hæmorrhoids, fistula, and dysentery. Bicycling is also said to be a predisposing cause. The exciting cause is frequently the passage of instruments, as in dilatation of a stricture, the use of a lithotrite in vesical calculus, or the injection of strong solutions in the treatment of urethritis, or even irrigation of the urethra with weak solutions.

The infection usually reaches the prostate directly by way of the urethra. Bacteria are already present or are introduced by instruments. A hæmatogenous infection may rarely take place as a complication of parotitis, smallpox, and cellulitis of the neck. Acute prostatitis may occur apart from any known local cause, and is then usually part of a hæmatogenous infection of the urinary tract by the bacillus coli communis in cases of constipation or colitis. The bacteria most frequently found are the staphylococcus, the bacillus coli communis, and the streptococcus ; the pneumococcus is rare. Certain anaerobic bacteria have been described by Albarran, Cottel, and others in phlegmonous inflammation around the prostate. The gonococcus is very rarely found alone ; Casper did not find it in a single instance in 25 cases of prostatic abscess complicating gonorrhœa. Oraison found it in 35 per cent. of cases. In the majority of cases of prostatic abscess complicating gonorrhœa the infection is secondary.

The varieties of prostatitis are acute prostatitis, prostatic abscess, and chronic prostatitis.

ACUTE PROSTATITIS

Symptoms.—A slight degree of acute prostatitis frequently occurs, and is difficult to distinguish from posterior urethritis, with which it is invariably combined.

There is frequent and urgent micturition ; and on passing the urine into two glasses both portions are cloudy. The urine contains comma-threads which are characteristic of prostatic affections. The threads consist of pus cells and columnar epithelium, and are formed in the ducts of the prostatic glands. On rectal examination no enlargement of the prostate gland is found, and there is little or no tenderness on pressure of the gland.

The more severe form of acute prostatitis begins suddenly during an attack of gonorrhœa, or after surgical interference in the urethra. The patient feels ill and may have one or several slight attacks of shivering or a fully developed rigor. The temperature rises to 102° F. or higher, and there are thirst, dry tongue, anorexia, and constipation.

The onset is frequently marked by retention of urine. Occasionally the symptoms commence insidiously.

There is deep, heavy pain in the rectum and perineum and at the end of the penis, which is worse on standing, sitting, or walking, and also on micturition and defæcation. There are frequent and very painful attempts to pass water with straining. If retention is absent small quantities of urine are passed very frequently, sometimes with a few drops of blood.

Rectal examination shows enlargement of one or both lobes of the prostate, the line of enlargement being sharply defined when the prostatitis is unilateral. The consistence is firm and the organ intensely tender.

Course and prognosis.—Resolution may take place. The symptoms subside, and in a week or a fortnight have disappeared, but the prostate remains hard and enlarged, and the infiltration only disappears after some months, or it becomes chronic.

Suppuration may take place. The pain becomes throbbing, the fever continues; the swelling increases, and a sensation of deep-seated fluid may be felt on pressure, and later more distinct softening is detected.

Treatment.—All local treatment, such as irrigation, instillations, passage of instruments, must cease. The patient is confined to bed and hot fomentations are applied suprapubically and to the perineum. A purge such as calomel (4 gr.) should be given, followed by a saline. Hot rectal irrigations should be administered night and morning (110°–115° F.), supplemented by injection into the rectum of a small enema (8 or 10 oz.) of hot water containing antipyrin (20 or 30 gr.) and tincture of opium (10 or 15 minims). Contrexéville water is administered by the mouth, sandal-wood oil in capsules (10 minims), and citrate of potash (20 gr.); belladonna and hyoscyamus may also be given to relieve the irritation and spasm.

PROSTATIC ABSCESS

Latent abscess of the prostate, occurring both in enlarged prostate and in cases in which hypertrophy is absent, has been described. It is rare, and is only discovered on removal of the prostate, or by accident when palpating the gland in routine examination in other conditions such as chronic urethritis.

In the majority of cases the abscess develops in the course of acute prostatitis. The temperature, already raised, increases suddenly after a chill or rigor. There are increased frequency and difficulty of micturition. The pain becomes more severe ; it is constant, heavy, and throbbing, and radiates to the thighs.

On rectal examination the prostate, which was already enlarged, is found to have increased in size, and deep-seated softening may be detected. Later a soft area in the hard mass of enlarged prostate may be easily detected as the pus approaches the rectal surface.

An abscess may form in the neighbourhood of the urethra, or there may be numerous small points of suppuration scattered throughout the prostate, and no sensation of softening is detected with the finger.

Course and prognosis.—1. In a large proportion of cases the abscess, if left alone, ruptures into the urethra, either spontaneously, or after the passage of a catheter for retention of urine, or after rectal examination. A quantity of pus appears in the urine, the temperature falls, the symptoms subside; the prostate diminishes in size and is much softer. The inflammation may now gradually subside. Recurrence of the symptoms may, however, ensue from incomplete drainage and refilling of the abscess cavity.

The persistence of such a cavity may later lead to the formation of an intraprostatic calculus, lime salts being deposited in this paraurethral pouch.

2. The abscess may travel downwards to the perineum, where it appears as a tender swelling immediately behind the bulb, and then passes forwards in the perineum to the scrotum. Rectal examination shows the pouch below the prostate filled up with an inflammatory mass continuous with the gland.

3. The abscess ruptures into the rectum. Pus and blood appear in the stools, but may be overlooked. The track is felt as a firm button in the rectal wall. Healing usually follows, but a fistula may form between the rectum and the urethra.

Treatment.—The abscess should be opened and drained by the perineal route. The curved prerectal transverse incision of

Zuckerkandl is employed, the posterior surface of the prostate exposed, and the rectum displaced backwards. There is danger of wounding the rectum unless the dissection is carefully carried out. The abscess is opened by a vertical incision through the sheath of the prostate, and a large rubber drain introduced and retained for a week, after which it is removed and a gauze drain substituted.

CHRONIC PROSTATITIS

Chronic prostatitis occurs most frequently between the ages of 20 and 40, and may persist after an attack of acute prostatitis, but more often it commences insidiously and gives rise to slight symptoms in its early stage.

Etiology.—Stricture is frequently present; chronic urethritis, cystitis, and pyelonephritis are concomitant if not causative inflammations. Masturbation and sexual excess are also believed to cause prostatitis, and some authorities hold that it may follow bicycling.

Pathology.—In the slightest form the glands and ducts show proliferation and desquamation of epithelium, and the lumen is filled with epithelium and leucocytes. At a later stage there is periglandular infiltration with round cells. Sclerosis of the stroma may take place, and the gland is firmer; and later there is contraction, either destroying the gland tubules by pressure or causing dilatation from obstruction. Rarely small points of suppuration are scattered throughout the prostate.

In most cases the inflammation is postgonorrhœal, but there may be an interval of several years between the acute attack of gonorrhœa and the development of symptoms of chronic prostatitis. It occurs in 35 per cent. of cases of gonorrhœa. Notthaft holds that the gonococcus does not survive longer than three years, and it frequently disappears long before. It is followed by secondary bacteria. Young found that bacteria were present in only 6 out of 19 cases of chronic prostatitis. This author believes that multiple infection is not uncommon.

Symptoms.—These may be so slight as to be overlooked, or they may be combined with those of posterior urethritis and be indistinguishable from them. It must be remembered also that widespread urinary infection may be present, with symptoms of pyelonephritis, pyelitis, ureteritis, cystitis.

The symptoms present great variety, and are conveniently grouped as urinary, nervous, and sexual.

1. **Urinary symptoms.**—Increased frequency of micturition and scalding or smarting during the act are the most common

urinary symptoms. The increased frequency occurs during the day, and in severe cases at night also. It is capricious, varying from day to day and at different hours of the day. The desire to micturate continues after the bladder is empty, and there may be strangury. Urgent micturition may also be noted. Difficult micturition is frequently present, and occasionally an attack of complete retention. Residual urine is said to be present in some cases.

2. **Nervous symptoms.**—Aching pain is characteristic. It may be constantly present, or irregular in its incidence, being present for some part of a day or for some days, and absent for varying periods. It may be increased on movement and exercise, · or on sitting, and sometimes on rising from the recumbent position. The pain is felt in the perineum, along the urethra to the end of the penis, in one or both testicles, in the groins or hips, or at the base of the sacrum. In old-standing cases it may be felt in regions distant from the prostate—namely, in the arms, shoulders, neck, and thighs. Pain on defæcation and during coitus is frequently present. Neurasthenia develops in a considerable proportion of these cases.

3. **Sexual symptoms.**—Nocturnal emissions may be frequent, and there is loss of sexual appetite. Prostatorrhœa is present in a small percentage of cases ; this consists in the escape of prostatic fluid during defæcation or at the end of micturition, or even on exertion. The normal prostatic secretion is a milky fluid, alkaline in reaction or amphoteric (Young), and contains lecithin granules, amyloid bodies, and isolated epithelial cells. In chronic prostatitis the secretion is thick, yellow, alkaline, and contains granules and flakes. The microscope shows columnar cells, single or clumped together, with numerous leucocytes, and a few red blood-corpuscles and amyloid bodies, lecithin granules, and granular phosphates. On the addition of a drop of ammonium phosphate (1 per cent.) large numbers of Böttcher crystals appear. The excess of epithelial cells and the presence of leucocytes are characteristic of chronic prostatitis. According to Goldberg there is a diminution in the lecithin in prostatitis. The urine frequently shows bacilluria, which may be intermittent or constant. When cystitis or pyelonephritis is present the urine has the characteristics observed in these diseases.

In slight chronic prostatitis the terminal portion of the urine is cloudy, with a little mucus and a trace of pus, and contains comma-shreds, small curved flakes formed in the ducts of the prostate.

A slight albuminuria is present in many cases, due to the presence of prostatic secretion in the urine. Terminal phosphaturia is also observed, the last portion of the urine containing a cloud of phosphates.

On rectal examination no change in size, consistence, or sensibility is detected in slight cases. When more extensive changes are present the prostate is slightly tender and the consistence firm. This change may extend throughout the gland, or one lobe may be firmer than the other, or again the gland may be firm at one part and elastic at another. The firm area may be at the periphery. The gland may be fixed, and in the later stages is frequently diminished in size, and may be completely atrophic. The secretion of the prostate should be expressed by massage and examined. It has the characters already described.

The bacteriology is similar to that of acute prostatitis. In some cases no bacteria are found, but it has been shown (Jungano) that anaerobic bacteria are present in all these cases.

Diagnosis.—Prostatic fluid must be distinguished from that derived from Cowper's glands, which may be in excess (urethrorrhœa). The latter is clear, viscid, and glycerine-like.

Schlagintweit introduced the following macroscopic method of distinguishing between prostatic fluid, seminal-vesicle fluid, and pus. The fluid is allowed to drop into a specimen-glass of water. Normal prostatic fluid disseminates and gives an opalescent appearance to the water, pus sinks to the bottom, and the seminal-vesicle fluid floats or hangs in the water and becomes opaque.

The microscope will distinguish between spermatic and prostatic fluid. In order to obtain the prostatic fluid for examination the urethra and bladder should first be washed with saline solution and then several ounces of the fluid left in the bladder. The patient is now placed in the knee-elbow position and the prostate gland is massaged from the rectum and the patient directed to pass the fluid from his bladder. This is centrifugalized and examined.

On rectal examination tuberculous disease and chronic prostatitis must be differentiated. In tuberculous disease the nodule is usually solitary, and it is harder and more sharply defined. There are frequently tuberculous lesions of the seminal vesicles and epididymes, in the urinary tract, or elsewhere in the body. An examination of the expressed prostatic fluid for the tubercle bacillus should be made in doubtful cases.

Malignant disease of the prostate in its early stage may resemble chronic prostatitis. The nodule of malignant growth is harder and more sharply defined, and the symptoms at this stage are usually confined to slight difficulty in micturition without changes in the urine and without the neurasthenic symptoms which characterize chronic prostatitis.

In the more advanced stage of carcinoma there is no difficulty in recognizing the stony, hard, nodular, fixed, insensitive prostate as malignant.

Prognosis.—The removal of an exciting cause such as stricture may be followed by resolution of the prostatitis. Usually, however, chronic prostatitis persists for many years, either in a latent form with recurrent exacerbations, or with little or no improvement. Cases associated with bacilluria are especially resistant to treatment.

Epididymitis is a frequent complication, and may follow too energetic treatment, or sexual excess, or exposure to cold. Atrophy of the prostate may eventually ensue, and it is said that hypertrophy may also result from this cause.

Treatment.—General tonic treatment is indicated, with open-air exercise. Horse-riding and bicycling should be avoided. Ergot and iodide of potash should be given. The bowels should be carefully regulated. If a stricture is present it should be treated.

The regular passage of large metal instruments, even when there is no narrowing of the canal, assists to expel the prostatic discharge by stretching the wall of the urethra. Large instruments should be used (Nos. 14–16 to Nos. 16–18), meatotomy being performed, if necessary, to enable the surgeon to pass the instruments. Kollmann's prostatic urethral dilator is useful for this purpose; the dilatation is carried out once a week, commencing with No. 36 and gradually rising to No. 60, or even No. 70. Simultaneous irrigation of the urethra with weak silver nitrate solutions (1 in 10,000) should be carried out; in the more recently constructed instruments provision is made for this purpose.

Irrigation may be combined with prostatic massage without dilatation. The prostate is first massaged from the rectum with the patient in the knee-elbow position, and then the patient is placed in the recumbent posture and the urethra washed by Janet's method. Large quantities of weak solution are used, such as silver nitrate 1 in 10,000, oxycyanide of mercury 1 in 5,000, permanganate of potash 1 in 5,000.

Instillations into the prostatic urethra by means of a Guyon's syringe of stronger solutions, such as silver nitrate 1, 2, or 3 per cent., are sometimes beneficial.

Young recommends the use of an ointment of 2 per cent. carbolic acid in lanoline in mild cases, or 1 per cent. salicylic acid in cases with epithelial exfoliation. The ointments are introduced by means of an applicator.

Prostatic massage is the most important method of treatment in chronic prostatitis. The patient is placed in the knee-elbow position on a couch, and a rubber glove, well lubricated, covers the surgeon's hand. The forefinger is introduced into the rectum, and first one lobe and then the other is massaged from without inwards to the mid-line, and finally the finger is swept down the interlobar sulcus. The massage lasts five minutes, and is succeeded by lavage of the urethra and bladder, and the treatment is repeated once a week.

Suppositories may be used containing ichthyol 3 gr., extract of belladonna ¼ gr., or iodide of potash 5 gr.

In old-standing cases with severe pain perineal prostatectomy may be performed; it succeeds in relieving the neuralgic pain, but there is a tendency to recurrence after some years. The use of the galvano-cautery (Bottini's method) in some cases has been advocated.

LITERATURE

Bierhoff, *Med. News*, Oct., 1904.
von Frisch, *Krankheiten der Prostata.* 1899.
Gardner, *Arch. Gén. de Chir.*, 1910, p. 482.
Goldberg, *Zeits. f. Urol.*, 1908, p. 814.
Lellei, *Zeits. f. Urol.*, 1907, p. 201.
Notthaft, *Arch. f. Derm. u. Syph.*, 1904.
Schlagintweit, *Centralbl. f. d. Krankh. d. Harn- u. Sex.-Org.*, 1901.
Stern, *Amer. Journ. of Med. Sci.*, Aug., 1903.
Wickert, *St. Petersburg. med. Woch.*, 1909, 6.
Wossidlo, *Zeits. f. Urol.*, 1908, p. 243.
Young, Geraghty, and Stevens, *Johns Hopkins Hosp. Repts.*, 1906, xiii. 271.

PERIPROSTATITIS

Acute periprostatitis is secondary to acute prostatitis and prostatic abscess. In prostatic abscess which ruptures into the rectum there is periprostatitis with adhesions of the prostate and rectal wall. The pelvic cellulitis may spread beyond the neighbourhood of the prostate to the lateral wall of the pelvis and surround the rectum. The symptoms are masked by those of the acute prostatitis. The patient is more seriously ill, the temperature high and swinging, and rigors are frequent and severe. On rectal examination the outline of the prostate is found to be obscured, and the rectal wall fixed in an inflammatory mass anteriorly and laterally. Death from septicæmia or pyæmia may occur.

Treatment consists in free and early drainage of the primary prostatic abscess and of the pelvic cellular tissue by the perineal route.

Chronic periprostatitis follows the acute form, or complicates primary chronic prostatitis. The prostate and seminal vesicles are replaced by a smooth, tough, fibrous surface passing laterally to the pelvic wall. The treatment is that of chronic prostatitis.

CHAPTER LV

TUBERCULOSIS OF THE PROSTATE

Before proceeding to describe tuberculosis of the prostate gland it is convenient to make some remarks in regard to tuberculosis of the genital system—namely, the epididymes and testicles, the seminal vesicles and vasa deferentia, and the prostate.

Genital tuberculosis is very rare in children, although it is occasionally observed as tuberculosis of the testicle at an early age. It is also of rare occurrence in old men, and at this age is usually a recrudescence of some old-standing tuberculous lesion. The great majority of cases occur between the ages of 20 and 50.

A part of the genital system, such as the epididymis, may alone be affected (partial genital tuberculosis); eventually, however, the whole genital system becomes involved (complete genital tuberculosis).

In 100 cases I found the following distribution:—

```
Genital system alone:
    Epididymis alone      ..      ..      ..      ..      16
    Prostate alone ..      ..      ..      ..      ..       7
    Seminal vesicle alone ..      ..      ..      ..       1
    Several genital organs affected      ..      ..      26
                                                         ——      50
Genital and urinary systems      ..      ..      ..      ..      37
Genital system and urethra, periurethral abscess, groin
    glands, or lungs ..      ..      ..      ..      ..       8
Genital and urinary systems with joints, vertebræ, or
    lungs ..      ..      ..      ..      ..      ..      ..       5
                                                                 ——
                                                                 100
```

The average age in these cases was 25·6 years.

Kocher found that in 80 per cent. of 451 autopsies on cases of genito-urinary tuberculosis there were pulmonary tuberculous lesions.

Tuberculosis of the genital system is, compared with urinary tuberculosis, a mild form of infection. The onset is usually insidious and the progress slow. Spread to all the genital organs is common, but not infrequently the tuberculous process is quiescent

685

at one part when the next is affected. Obsolete tuberculous disease of the genital system may again become active after many years, or tuberculosis of the urinary system may develop after a similar interval. The chief danger of genital tuberculosis is that it may become urinary by infection of the bladder or kidney. In the majority of cases the epididymis is the genital organ first affected, and it is therefore more frequently found affected alone than the other genital organs. The infection reaches the epididymis by the blood stream, and also by the vas deferens. The prostate and seminal vesicles may be infected from the epididymis by way of the vas deferens, or they may be infected from the blood stream or from the urethra. In support of his view that the epididymis is always affected first and the prostate later, Salleron states that in 51 cases of tuberculous epididymitis the prostate was only once affected. On the other hand, Keyes and Macfarlane Walker hold that there is always, or nearly always, some abnormal condition of the prostate or vesicles. They admit, however, that these lesions are not necessarily tuberculous. In my statistics quoted above only tuberculous lesions were included. These show that the epididymis was much more frequently affected alone (16 per cent.) than any of the other organs.

Etiology.—In tuberculosis of the prostate there is often a family history of tuberculosis. Gonorrhœal inflammation is said to be a frequent precursor of tuberculous prostatitis, but genital tuberculosis (including prostatic tubercle) is very often found in patients who have not had gonorrhœa. I have only seen 2 cases where tuberculosis of the prostate appeared to follow directly upon an attack of acute gonorrhœal urethritis and prostatitis, and in these cases it was impossible to prove that latent tuberculous nodules had not previously been present. There are cases of tuberculosis of the prostate in which the onset is acute and is accompanied by a fairly copious urethral discharge and symptoms of posterior urethritis. It is possible that such cases have been mistaken for gonorrhœal urethritis, and only in the subsequent chronic stage recognized as tuberculous. Chronic tuberculous nodules are not, in my experience, found in prostates which show clinical evidence of chronic prostatitis. In the early stage the prostate in which the tuberculous nodule is set is elastic and normal to the touch.

The prostate was affected alone in 7 of the 100 cases in the above table. In cases where the genital system alone was tuberculous the prostate was the solitary focus of tubercle in 14 per cent., and in combination with other genital organs in 52 per cent. In 65 per cent. of cases of prostatic tubercle there was urinary tubercle also, and in 18 per cent. of these the prostate was the only genital organ affected. Tuberculous disease was also noted in different cases in the urethra, periurethral tissues, the groin glands, elbow-joints, vertebræ, and lungs. In 100 cases of pulmonary tuberculosis Reclus found only 2 in which the genito-urinary organs were affected.

Pathology. — The tuberculous process commences in the neighbourhood of the acini and gland ducts, the bacilli lying immediately underneath the epithelium. Giant-cell systems form, the periacinous tissue is widely infiltrated, and caseation takes place.

There may be a number of discrete nodules or a single mass. The peripheral portion of the gland is at first affected, but the whole lobe becomes involved. One lobe may be affected and the other remain intact. The caseous masses frequently break down, and a large single cavity or several intercommunicating pockets replace the prostatic tissue. Rupture most frequently takes place into the urethra by one or several openings, or through the bladder base alongside the trigone, a large irregular opening resulting.

Less frequently rupture takes place into the rectum, and occasionally the tuberculous collection infiltrates the periprostatic tissue and passes down along the urethra into the perineum. After rupture into the urethra the tuberculous process usually becomes quiescent, and the lobe of the prostate fibrous and shrunken. Infection of the bladder may take place by the urethra or directly through the base of the organ. After rupture into the rectum the lobe usually shrinks. Fistulæ may form when the abscess invades the perineum.

In late cases the prostate and prostatic urethra are destroyed and a cavity communicating with the bladder is formed. The urethra in front of this is frequently the seat of tuberculous stricture. The infection here is mixed, and secondary phosphatic calculi may form in the cavity or in the bladder.

Symptoms.—There may be complete absence of symptoms, and the tuberculous nodule is discovered on routine examination of the rectum.

Frequent micturition is often present; it is both diurnal and nocturnal, and is little affected by movement.

A urethral discharge may be the initial symptom, and is not infrequently mistaken for a gonorrhœal infection. The discharge is sometimes copious, and may appear suddenly. Hæmaturia may appear at an early stage, or it may indicate the rupture of a tuberculous collection into the urethra. Blood may also appear in the emissions.

These symptoms are, however, often absent. When rupture into the bladder takes place the symptoms of cystitis appear.

The urine is clear in the early stage, and no tubercle bacilli can be detected, but when rupture into the urethra or bladder has occurred the urine contains pus, tuberculous bacilli, and débris, and sometimes blood. A mixed infection of bacillus coli, staphylococcus, and streptococcus introduced by instruments or appearing spontaneously may be found, and the tubercle bacillus may only be discovered after repeated examinations.

In late cases the infection is mixed and the bladder invaded; secondary calculi form, and the urethra anterior to the prostate is narrowed by tuberculous infiltration. The desire to micturate is constant, and there is pain and burning along the urethra, with great straining, and the discharge of a few drops of urine at each attempt. The patient is robbed of his sleep and rapidly loses flesh. The temperature may be raised one or two points.

On rectal examination the prostate is tender, and one or more tuberculous nodules can be felt. The nodule is hard and well defined, and is usually situated at the upper and outer angle, or at the outer and lower part of the gland. It is more sharply defined and harder than a patch of chronic non-tuberculous prostatitis, and is set or buried in a prostate of normal consistence, whereas chronic non-tuberculous prostatitis gives rise to ill-defined firm areas in a prostate of tough consistence.

One or both lobes may be affected. When a tuberculous collection has ruptured into the urethra a hollow is felt in its place, and the remaining lobe is unduly prominent. A small button of induration is felt in the rectal wall where rupture into the rectum has taken place.

The passage of instruments through the prostatic urethra may be difficult, owing to narrowing and distortion of the canal. Cystoscopy frequently shows a prominent congested and sometimes œdematous area on the upper surface of the prostate. After rupture into the bladder an irregular cavity is seen alongside the trigone, and caseous tubercles may be observed around it.

Prognosis.—If septic complications are not superadded and urinary and pulmonary tuberculosis are absent there is a tendency to spontaneous recovery. When rupture into the bladder has occurred, or fistulæ have formed in the perineum and elsewhere, the prognosis is less favourable, but recovery under treatment may still take place. Recrudescence of the tuberculous process may occur many years after it is apparently obsolete.

A fatal result is usually due to urinary tuberculosis and sepsis, or to. tuberculous disease elsewhere. General tuberculosis is rare. Simmonds found that tuberculous meningitis occurred in 30 per cent. of 60 cases, but this complication was rare in my cases.

Treatment.—The passage of instruments through the urethra should, as far as possible, be avoided; and the instillation of medicaments into the prostatic urethra is harmful.

Suppositories of belladonna $\frac{1}{4}$ gr., ichthyol 2 gr., lupulin 4 gr., or other drugs may be given to soothe the irritation and relieve congestion, but they have little effect on the course of the disease. The injection of tuberculin (T.R.) is the most efficacious method of treatment. The dosage should commence at $\frac{1}{8000}$ mg., and the injections are given once a week and gradually raised to $\frac{1}{1000}$ or $\frac{1}{500}$ mg. A reaction, shown by headache, malaise, and increase in the local symptoms, should be avoided. The treatment should be continued for many months, or even several years, either continuously or in courses of three or four months. The patient should at the same time be placed under the best possible hygienic conditions, and should have a free, nourishing diet and take cod-liver oil and malt. In my hands this treatment has given very successful results, and has entirely superseded operative measures.

Operative treatment consists in the exposure of the prostate by Zuckerkandl's transverse prerectal incision, the tuberculous focus being then exposed by incision of the prostatic sheath, thoroughly scraped, and packed with iodoform gauze or gauze soaked in iodine solution.

. Prostatectomy may be performed instead of scraping. In this case the prostatic urethra should not be opened.

After these operations a fistula lined with tuberculous granulation tissue frequently persists. For this the treatment should consist in scraping, applications of iodine or of bismuth paste (vaseline 20, paraffin 10, lanoline 10, bismuth subnitrate 10), and the administration of tuberculin.

Where a mixed infection is present, vaccines should be combined with tuberculin treatment.

In late cases where the prostate is entirely destroyed and the bladder infected, permanent suprapubic drainage gives great relief.

LITERATURE

von Frisch, *Krankheiten der Prostata.* 1899.
Guisy, *Ann. d. Mal. d. Org. Gén.-Urin.,* 1906, p. 1409.
Hallé et Motz, *Ann. d. Mal. d. Org. Gén.-Urin.,* 1903, p. 481.
Hildebrand, *Zeits. f. Urol.,* 1907, p. 827.
Simmonds, *Münch. med. Woch.,* 1901, p. 743.
Walker, Macfarlane, *Lancet,* 1913, i. 435.
Walker, Thomson, *Pract.,* May, 1908.

CHAPTER LVI

SIMPLE ENLARGEMENT OF THE PROSTATE

ENLARGEMENT of the prostate is a disease of advanced life, the frequency of which has been stated at 35 per cent. of men over 60 years.

Cause and nature of the enlargement.—At the present time opinion is unsettled as to the cause and nature of the change in the prostate. A number of theories have been advanced, the more important of .which will be stated.

1. **Adenoma.**—The changes in the gland conform very closely to those found in adenoma of other organs, such as the breast, and carcinoma occasionally develops in the enlarged prostate. Recently this view as to the nature of the enlargement has been pushed into the background by theories advanced to explain the origin of the change. Whatever the origin may be, simple enlargement of the prostate resembles in its gross and histological characters an adenoma with a varying amount of cystic formation.

2. **Hypertrophy.**—Occasionally there is a uniform increase in the gland tubules, resembling those of the normal gland. This might be looked upon as a true hypertrophy, but in the great majority of cases there are changes such as dilatation of the gland tubules, subdivision into nodules, etc., which show that the process is more than a simple hypertrophy.

The so-called hypertrophy has been said by White, Macewen, and others to be secondary to changes which occur in the testicle in old age.

3. **Arterio-sclerosis.**—Based upon researches by Launois, Guyon and others have held the view that enlargement of the prostate is a part of arterio-sclerotic changes which take place in the entire urinary apparatus (kidneys, ureters, bladder). There is interstitial nephritis, sclerosis of the bladder wall, with destruction of the muscular tissue and endoperiarteritis in these organs. According to Guyon, this constitutes the condition of " prostatismus," which is usually, but not always, combined with enlargement of the prostate. Casper has shown that although arteriosclerosis and hypertrophy of the prostate may be present in the

690

same individual, hypertrophy frequently occurs without any change in the blood-vessels of the prostate or bladder ; while Motz found that of 31 cases of hypertrophy of the prostate the blood-vessels were normal in 16, simple congestion without changes in the vessel walls was present in 6, and arterio-sclerosis occurred in 9. The complete restoration of the function of the bladder after removal of the prostate in cases where the patient had been dependent upon the catheter for many years has demonstrated that no such destructive changes take place in the bladder. This view must therefore be abandoned.

4. **Inflammatory changes.**—Recently Ciechanowski has revived and developed the theory that the enlargement is due to inflammatory changes. According to this observer, the inflammatory process exists for years with slight or no appreciable symptoms. There is a chronic inflammation affecting the stroma of the gland. If this involves the portion of the gland immediately adjacent to the urethra and surrounds the principal gland ducts of the prostate, the lumen of these is narrowed and the secretion collects in the acini of the gland and dilates them. At the same time there is proliferation and desquamation of the epithelium. The enlargement of the gland is almost entirely due to dilatation of the gland tubules. To this Ciechanowski adds that if the inflammation principally affects the peripheral portion of the gland the acini are compressed instead of being obstructed, and atrophy of the prostate takes place.

The great frequency of *gonorrhœa* as a cause of chronic prostatitis suggests that this may be the origin of the inflammatory changes ; but Ciechanowski regards this hypothesis as still unproved. Rovsing found that 60 per cent. of his cases of enlargement of the prostate had never had gonorrhœa, and showed no trace of urethritis.

5. Motz and Perearnau have recently advanced the view that the so-called hypertrophy of the prostate is due to **changes in the urethral glands** of the prostatic urethra, and that the true prostatic tubules do not take part in the formation of the tumour, but are crushed aside and atrophy. The arguments in favour of this theory are ably marshalled by Marion, but are unconvincing.

Age-incidence.—The symptoms of enlargement of the prostate commence after the age of 50, usually between the ages of 55 and 60. The change undoubtedly begins earlier, but the statement of Burckhardt that 13 per cent. of cases commence between 36 and 40, and 25 per cent. between 40 and 50, is entirely contrary to my experience. Von Frisch has never seen true hypertrophy of the prostate before 50, and holds that the cases recorded at earlier

ages than this are cases of chronic prostatitis. It is certainly
exceptional to find true enlargement of the prostate before the
age of 50, but cases are occasionally observed. I have removed
a prostate weighing 1½ oz., with a well-developed intravesical projection and the typical structure of the enlarged prostate, from a
man aged 42. The average age of 112 patients on whom I performed suprapubic prostatectomy was 66 years.

In India, according to Freyer, the symptoms of enlargement
of the prostate appear as early as 45 years. In tropical climates
puberty occurs early, and senile changes set in some years before
they commence in a temperate climate.

Pathological anatomy.—The average weight of the prostate
is about 4½ drachms, but the organ varies very greatly in weight
and size in normal individuals, so that the commencement of
enlargement cannot be estimated by relation to this standard.
Enucleated enlarged prostates vary in weight from a few drachms
to 14 oz.; the most frequent size is from 1½ to 3 oz. A prostate of 6 or 8 oz. forms a large mass. In slight enlargement the
earliest changes are the protrusion of a portion of the gland into
the bladder and the macroscopical and microscopical changes seen
on section.

Both lobes are usually enlarged to an equal degree, but one
may be larger than the other, and rarely the enlargement appears
to be confined to one lobe. In all such cases that I have examined,
however, the apparently normal lobe shows changes on section
and microscopical examination which correspond exactly to those
in the large lobe.

The enlarging prostate expands its sheath, and, as it passes
backwards beneath the base of the bladder, strips the seminal .
vesicles from the bladder until they come to lie behind the upper
part of the enlarged prostate instead of above the gland.

I pointed out in 1904 that the enlargement of the gland was
in the majority of cases confined to the portion lying above the
level of the ejaculatory ducts and the verumontanum, and that
the increased space required for the enlarged prostate is obtained
almost entirely at the expense of the structures abutting upon
the upper portion of the gland, little or no change occurring at
the lower part. The verumontanum and ejaculatory ducts
remain fixed. It is not only the upper median portion of the
gland (so-called middle lobe) that enlarges, but the entire upper
portion. Some years later (1911) this point was again raised by
Tandler and Zuckerkandl, who hold that the lower part of the
gland is crushed and flattened and takes no part in the tumour
which is removed by operation. In a few prostates I found that

the glandular substance below the ejaculatory ducts and behind the urethra was the seat of marked enlargement, and in such cases the ejaculatory ducts and seminal vesicles retain their normal relations to the bladder wall and to the prostate as a whole.

A second direction in which the enlarged prostate expands is into the bladder. (Fig. 211.) The upward-growing prostate insinuates itself within the circle of the sphincter vesicæ, which becomes more and more dilated as the projection becomes larger. This upward-projecting portion of the prostate is still covered by the sheet

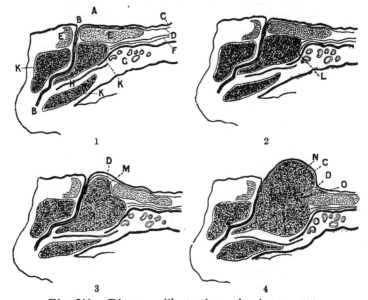

Fig. 211.—Diagrams illustrating enlarging prostate.

1, Antero-posterior section of normal prostate and bladder base. 2, Enlargement of prostate backwards beneath base of bladder. 3, Enlargement of prostate through sphincter. 4, Intravesical enlargement of prostate.—A, Bladder. B, B, Prostatic urethra, C, Vesical mucous membrane. D, Internal longitudinal layer of bladder muscle. E, E, Trigone muscle and sphincter. F, Outer longitudinal layer of bladder muscle. G, Seminal Vesicle. H, Ejaculatory duct. K, K, K, Prostate. L, Prostate pushing seminal vesicle backwards. M, N, Prostate projecting into bladder. O, Groove in enlarged prostate from pressure of sphincter.

of longitudinal muscle fibres which forms the superficial layer of the trigone and passes into the internal longitudinal layer of the urethra. At one point or at several the fibres of this layer separate and allow a nodule of prostatic tissue to appear immediately under the bladder mucous membrane. In grooves on each side of this nodule, or between each of several intravesical nodules, are found these longitudinal muscular bundles crowded together in strong bands.

The upper surface of the prostate is in the form of a horse-shoe around the back and sides of the urethra, and often protrudes into the bladder in this form, the " collar-like " intra-vesical projection. Another form of intravesical projection is the so-called median lobe. I have explained the formation of this lobe as follows : The longitudinal muscle of the ureters passes into the trigone, forming two strong bands which converge and pass over the posterior lip of the urethral orifice to join the internal longitudinal layer of urethral muscle. The enlarged prostate, pressing upwards, pushes in between these two bands and forms a nodule in the middle line posteriorly, which may become pedunculated from the pressure at its base. These bands of longitudinal muscle are readily recognized in the grooves on each side of the median lobe of the prostate after removal.

In 54 enucleated prostates the following was the character of the intravesical projection : Median lobe alone, 9 ; median and lateral lobes as a collar or distinct, 18 ; both lateral lobes, 15 ; one lateral lobe, 12.

The intravesical median lobe in the majority of cases is an offshoot from one of the lateral lobes, but in a few it is found to be distinctly separated from these and to arise from the median portion of the prostate, which lies above the ejaculatory ducts.

Changes in the urethra.—The prostatic urethra is elongated, and may be as much as twice the normal length. A catheter passes in 12 or 15 in. before the eye reaches the bladder. The elongation affects that portion of the urethra which lies between the bladder and the verumontanum, and hardly at all the part in front of this. The canal is compressed laterally and elongated from before backwards, so that it becomes a median antero-posterior slit. The anterior wall remains vertical, but the posterior wall sinks backwards at the level of the verumontanum, so that the part above this point forms an acute angle with that below it. This is probably due to dragging on the verumontanum by the ejaculatory ducts and the surrounding bands of tissue, due to the seminal vesicles being displaced backwards.

Lateral distortion of the urethra is caused by enlargement of one or other lobe, and a median lobe produces a Y-shaped canal or directs the lumen forwards.

At the internal meatus the intravesical projection of the prostate drags the sensitive prostatic mucous membrane up into the bladder. The orifice may be crescentic, Y-shaped, irregular, or trumpet-shaped, according to the shape of the intravesical projection.

On section of the enlarged prostate a milky juice exudes from

the surface. On each side of the long antero-posterior slit which
represents the urethra is a large yellowish-white mass in which
are embedded smaller rounded masses, each surrounded by a
capsule. These contain numerous small cysts. (Fig. 212.)

Microscopically, the enlarged prostate shows closely-set gland
tubules, some of them small and normal in appearance, but the
majority dilated and branched. (Fig. 213.) The dilatation may
be extreme, and numerous small cysts are produced. ˙The epithelium in many of the dilated tubules is heaped up into masses. The

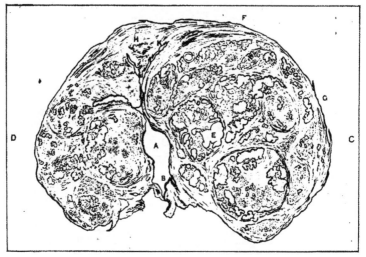

Fig. 212.—Transverse section of prostate removed by
suprapubic prostatectomy.

A, Prostatic urethra. B, Verumontanum. C, D, Right and left lobes. E, Small cyst in
adenomatous nodule. F, G, Capsule. H, Anterior commissure. K, Splitting due to
manipulation.

dilated gland spaces contain desquamated epithelium, granular
material, and amyloid bodies. In some enlarged prostates the
glandular elements are less abundant, the stroma more prominent,
and the consistence firmer. Inflammatory changes in the stroma
are usually absent, but perivascular round-cell infiltration may
be observed. A nodule of circularly disposed non-striped muscle
fibres (myoma) may be found in the substance of a glandular
enlargement.

Secondary changes in the urinary organs take place,
and are due to obstruction and infection. The projection of
the prostate into the bladder raises up the base of the bladder

around the urethral orifice, and behind this there is a hollow, the postprostatic pouch, in which calculi may be lodged. The bladder shows hypertrophy and later sacculation between the thick trabeculæ, or there may be a single or several larger diverticula.

The ureteric orifices usually remain intact and are not dilated. There is slight dilatation of the renal pelvis and kidney, and chronic interstitial nephritis develops. When sepsis is superadded, by the passage of a catheter or other means, cystitis and secondary

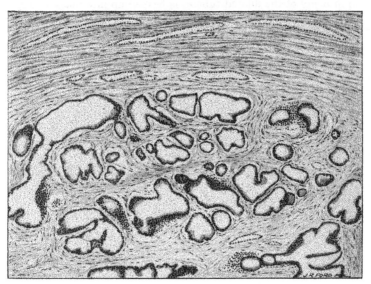

Fig. 213.—Section of enlarged prostate removed by
suprapubic operation.

At upper part is capsule containing blood-vessels; at lower part are dilated gland tubules
with proliferation of epithelium.

stone formation follow. Ascending pyelonephritis develops, and may be acute or chronic.

Symptoms.—Enlargement of the prostate may be latent for several years until it has reached a large size, and then complete retention may occur. Usually, however, symptoms commence gradually, the first being those of vesical irritation. Later, symptoms of increasing obstruction appear, and in advanced cases symptoms of renal failure develop. Septic complications may supervene.

Frequent micturition is usually the earliest symptom. It begins insidiously and increases progressively, and is both nocturnal and diurnal. The nocturnal frequency is characteristic.

The patient rests for four or five hours during the first part of the night, is disturbed at 2 or 3 a.m., and may pass water several times after this. If cystitis is present the frequency loses this character. There is urgency to pass water, and a little may escape involuntarily, but usually, when the attempt is made, there is delay in commencing micturition.

The stream lacks force; it commences feebly, gradually increases in power, and falls away again to a dribble at the end of the act. Intermittent micturition is frequently observed, the pause lasting a few seconds, or as long as a quarter of an hour. Micturition may be best performed when at stool, or special attitudes may be adopted by different patients, such as the knee-elbow position, in order to facilitate the flow of urine. The difficulty is increased on holding the water for some time, also in cold weather, and after taking alcohol.

Retention of urine occurs in many cases. There may be partial retention, the residual urine amounting to 4–10 oz., but the patient is able to micturate and the bladder is not distended. Occasionally there is chronic distension of the bladder, which may reach the level of the umbilicus. The patient is usually unaware of the distension, although he may have noticed an increase in the girth of his abdomen. Urine is passed frequently and in small quantities day and night, and there is often some involuntary dribbling of urine during sleep. Sudden complete retention may occur when a few ounces of residual urine had previously been present or none had been known to exist. The distension of the bladder is painful, and the patient is usually in great distress. After a time the urine begins to dribble away involuntarily, micturition becomes gradually restored, and the patient returns to his original condition. The attack of retention may last an hour or several hours, or it may be relieved only by the passage of a catheter. Occasionally such an attack is followed by permanent inability, which is only cured by removal of the prostate. Such an attack usually follows exposure to cold or wet or dietary indiscretions. Acute retention may suddenly supervene when no symptoms of enlargement of the prostate have previously been noticed.

Hæmaturia is not usually present apart from instrumental interference, but in some cases it is the principal and most urgent symptom, and operation may become necessary on this account alone.

Pain is usually due to secondary conditions. There are discomfort and burning on micturition, not amounting to pain. Suprapubic pain and renal pain are due to obstruction. There may be pain in one or both kidneys on micturition, caused by dilatation of the ureters. There is a sensation of heaviness and weight in the perineum and rectum. Sexual irritation is not infrequent, and may be a very distressing symptom. Constipation is almost invariably present.

Symptoms due to secondary conditions may appear. In retention of urine there are suprapubic pain, dullness on percussion, and a globular swelling.

When interstitial changes are occurring in the kidneys the symptoms of renal inefficiency develop. These are headache, burning thirst, especially at night, dry tongue, loss of appetite, nausea, a harsh dry skin, polyuria, and general malaise (p. 10).

Hæmorrhoids, prolapse of the rectum, and inguinal hernia result from constant straining to pass water.

Examination.—After obtaining an account of the history and symptoms the surgeon will proceed to examine the patient.

The general condition in regard to emaciation, sallowness of the skin, absence of sweat, etc., is noted. The abdomen is examined for distension of the bladder, and the loins are palpated to ascertain if there is enlargement or tenderness of the kidneys.

Rectal examination is then carried out The patient is examined first in the knee-elbow position, and the posterior or rectal surface of the prostate is palpated. The size of the gland is found to be increased. The gland may reach a very large size and form a large prominence in the rectum, obstructing its lumen. The consistence is uniform and usually elastic, occasionally it is firm. The gland is movable, the surface smooth, and the outline well defined. The median vertical sulcus may be obliterated. In some cases the gland is found to be little enlarged on rectal palpation, the symptoms being caused by an intravesical projection.

Bimanual palpation is performed with the patient lying on his back and his knees fully flexed, the feet being firmly planted on the couch. The bladder must be empty. The right forefinger is introduced into the rectum and the fingers of the left hand press deeply immediately above the pubic symphysis. Assistance may be obtained by placing the patient in the Trendelenburg position. A large prostate can be felt between the two hands and its mobility estimated.

Examination for residual urine.—The passage of a catheter or other instrument in a case of enlargement of the prostate should be carried out with the greatest care in regard to asepsis and the avoidance of injury to the urethra. The examination should be made with the patient in bed, and, if possible, he should be prepared by the administration of urotropine and some diuretic such as Contrexéville water or tea.

To ascertain if there is residual urine the patient is directed to pass water standing up and then to lie on his bed. A soft rubber catheter or a coudé catheter is gently passed, and the urine which remains in the bladder is drawn off and measured.

Sounding.—Information may be obtained by the passage of a metal instrument such as a calculus sound. Obstruction is felt by the experienced touch in the prostatic urethra. The instrument must be depressed deeply between the thighs before the beak will enter the bladder. The length of the urethra is increased, and the instrument may sink in to the handle before the beak rides over the prostate at the internal meatus. When the beak is in the bladder the handle can be freely turned from side to side. On turning the beak downwards and withdrawing the instrument it will hitch when the beak comes in contact with the bladder surface of the prostate, and the length of the urethra can thus be estimated.

Cystoscopy.—The cystoscope shows the condition of the upper or bladder surface. The outline of the normal margin of the urethral orifice as seen by the cystoscope is slightly concave. A convex surface surrounds the orifice when a collar-like intravesical enlargement is present. One lobe may be seen to project into the bladder as a round swelling like the end of an egg, or there may be a median globular swelling when a median lobe is present. When both lobes project into the bladder the opening between them into the bladder is **V**-shaped when viewed with the cystoscope partly withdrawn into the urethra. The size of the projection may be estimated by noting whether it obscures the ureteric orifices. On the surface of the intravesical portion may be seen large raised veins; occasionally there are tags of mucous membrane, each containing a vessel, or there may be sago-grain-like swellings due to blocked glands.

Trabeculation and sacculation of the bladder are noted.

Cystitis, dilatation of the ureteric orifices, and calculi may be observed.

Examination for evidence of renal failure should be made (*see* p. 10).

Complications.—During the course of the disease certain complications may arise, viz. retention of urine, septic infection, hæmorrhage, renal failure, epididymitis, stone, stricture.

Several of these complications have already been described in discussing the symptoms, and need no further notice.

Septic infection.—The obstructed bladder is congested, and its powers of resistance are diminished. It therefore forms a ready field for the culture of bacteria if they are introduced. Infection usually follows the use of the catheter. The onset of symptoms may be sudden and severe, or insidious.

In the former case, a few hours after the passage of a catheter there is a rigor, and the temperature rises to 102° F. or higher, and continues high. The urine rapidly becomes cloudy and alkaline, and may be ammoniacal. There is increased frequency of micturition, with scalding and straining, and sometimes retention of urine occurs, with great pain. There is renal aching or actual renal pain, usually confined to one side. Tenderness is present over the kidney on one or both sides. The tongue becomes dry, the mouth parched, and the patient complains of burning thirst. There are nausea and anorexia and constipation, and all but fluid food is refused. The patient becomes drowsy, sometimes with intervals of restless delirium ; these occur especially at night, when he shows great anxiety to get out of bed and to remove dressings or the catheter if one be tied in the urethra. The urine becomes scanty ; vomiting and hiccough supervene, and eventually death, with partial or complete suppression of urine.

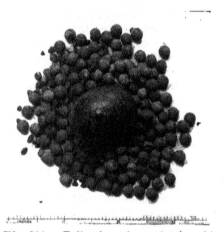

Fig. 214.—Collection of round uric-acid calculi from postprostatic pouch.

But the onset may be insidious and the course less rapid. A slight degree of pyelonephritis is present, and the most prominent feature is cystitis.

Renal failure may be acute or chronic. After rapid and complete removal of the urine from an over-distended bladder, whether the distension is acute or chronic, suppression not infrequently occurs. The urine may be only partly or completely suppressed, the patient becomes drowsy, and gradually sinks and dies a few days after the passage of the catheter (*see* Anuria, p. 15). Chronic renal failure is a common complication of untreated enlarged prostate. There are thirst, headache, nausea, anorexia, constipation, loss of weight, a dry tongue, and sallow complexion. Renal aching is often observed, and polyuria constantly present.

Epididymitis is a frequent complication when sepsis has been introduced. It occurs usually in cases in which a catheter is in constant use.

· **Calculi** are present in the bladder in 7 per cent. of cases. They are composed of oxalate of lime, or uric acid, or phosphates. The phosphatic calculi are found with alkaline or decomposing urine. There may be one or many calculi (thirty or forty). Uric-acid and oxalate calculi assume their characteristic shapes (Fig. 214), phosphatic calculi are faceted (Fig. 215). The stones usually lie in the postprostatic pouch, where they may be fixed and give rise to no symptoms. Larger calculi may, however, move freely and give rise to the characteristic symptoms of stone.

Stricture is an infrequent complication of enlarged prostate.

Course and prognosis.—Enlarged prostate is a progressive condition which, if untreated, leads to a fatal termination. It is serious because of the urinary obstruction which it produces, and the septic complications which are

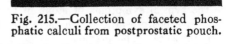

Fig. 215.—Collection of faceted phosphatic calculi from postprostatic pouch.

so frequently superadded. Rarely the simple enlargement takes on malignant characters.

The earliest stage is that of irritation, and this is followed by increasing obstruction, against which the bladder contends for a variable time, lasting usually some years. Eventually the bladder muscle is unable to overcome the obstruction, and complete retention ensues. During the period of increasing obstruction a moderate degree of dilatation of the kidneys, and with it interstitial nephritis, develops. Sepsis introduced by means of the catheter causes cystitis and ascending pyelonephritis, which leads immediately or after some time to a fatal result. Occasionally there is complete retention from the first onset of symptoms.

Diagnosis.—The characteristic features of enlarged prostate are that the symptoms commence at or after the age of 50, that the first symptoms are those of bladder irritation, that there is rarely sudden complete retention, that the frequent micturition is of the " prostatic " type, and that the rectal examination shows an elastic uniform enlargement of the organ, while cystoscopic. examination demonstrates an intravesical projection.

In urethral stricture the symptoms commence before the age of 50, usually before the age of 30, there is gradually increasing difficulty in micturition without increased frequency, the prostate is not enlarged per rectum, and there is obstruction in the penile or bulbous urethra to the passage of instruments.

Malignant disease of the prostate may begin at an earlier age than simple enlargement, but the average age is the same. There is gradually increasing obstruction, usually without irritation in the early stage; when frequent micturition appears it occurs at regular intervals and is not of the " prostatic " type; hæmorrhage is less frequent than in simple enlargement; loss of weight may be present; the lymphatic glands in the groins are frequently enlarged; the prostate is hard, irregular, fixed, and there may be enlarged glands on each side of it; no intravesical projection is present, or there is irregular elevation of the urethral margin.

Chronic prostatitis usually commences before the age of 50; there are bacteria in the urine; the prostate is not enlarged per rectum, but is tender, firm, and sometimes irregular; there is no intravesical projection of the gland.

When the diagnosis of enlarged prostate is made it is necessary to ascertain—

1. **Are calculi present ?**—In a movable calculus there may be the typical symptoms of stone in the bladder, but in calculi lying in a postprostatic pouch there are no symptoms pointing to their presence. The previous passage of calculi may raise a suspicion; hæmorrhage is usually present; the sound will ring upon the stone if the prostate is not very large, but when the intravesical projection is considerable and the postprostatic pouch deep the sound does not strike the calculi. By raising the pelvis before sounding in such a case the stones may be so displaced as to come within the range of the beak of the sound. The cystoscope will detect calculi lying deeply behind the prostate, but occasionally they are not found until prostatectomy is commenced.

2. **Is the bladder permanently atonic ?**—The view of Guyon that the bladder is permanently disabled by sclerosis is now abandoned, but in rare cases the bladder remains atonic after the prostate has been removed. In these cases there is an entire absence of the irritative symptoms of enlarged prostate, while the inability to pass urine is early manifested. Diverticula of the bladder wall are not infrequently found in such cases. Usually it is impossible before removing the prostate to diagnose this condition.

3. **What is the condition of the kidneys?**—The symptoms of renal failure should be searched for, the specific gravity of the urine ascertained, and the urea estimated quantitatively. The tests for the renal function should be employed (p. 20). It may be accepted that in all cases of chronic retention with distension the kidneys are damaged.

Treatment. 1. Treatment of complications. (a) *Retention of urine.*—This may take the form of complete retention of urine or chronic distension of the bladder with power to pass small quantities of urine voluntarily. It is a serious complication, and if treated injudiciously may lead to a fatal result. The two dangers to be avoided are rapid emptying of the bladder, which is frequently followed by hæmorrhage and suppression of urine, and the introduction of sepsis. The most rigid precautions should be adopted in order to prevent infection, and in chronic distension the patient should be placed upon some urinary antiseptic (urotropine, 10 gr. thrice daily) for several days before the distension is relieved. He should be in bed and in a warm atmosphere, and after the catheter has·been passed is surrounded with hot bottles and should drink a tumbler of hot milk or tea. The catheters, whether gum-elastic or metal, must be boiled, the hands carefully cleansed, the penis washed with antiseptic, and the urethra irrigated with antiseptic solution.

The most useful instruments are the coudé and bicoudé silk-wove catheters ; the latter may be obtained specially long (16 in.) for use in very large prostates. These should be boiled (*see* pp. 354, 562) and placed in cold sterile water. A " prostatic " metal catheter is one with a very large curve, and is often useful. A gum-elastic catheter provided with a stilet may be used ; it can be moulded in hot water into a suitable shape, and fixed in cold water.

The lubricant must, of course, be sterile. A good lubricant is boiled olive oil (*see* p. 356).

The coudé and bicoudé instruments should be tried first, and may pass easily. When a difficulty is encountered the catheter should be pushed on with the utmost gentleness, the beak being inclined to one or other side if necessary.

In passing instruments it should be remembered that the anterior wall of the prostatic urethra remains straight and almost vertical ; that the urethra is pushed to one side when one lobe is more enlarged, and this can be ascertained by rectal examination ; that the verumontanum sinks backwards so that the posterior wall forms a deep pocket or angle at this level ; that the posterior lip of the vesical orifice is raised and projected forwards, and that a middle lobe forms a Y-shaped vesical opening along one limb of which the beak of the instrument travels.

If the coudé and bicoudé instruments fail a metal instrument may be tried, or an English gum-elastic catheter, softened in hot water, so bent that it has a large, sweeping, very full curve, and then fixed in cold water. A method sometimes recommended is to introduce a gum-elastic instrument with the stilet in place, and when the beak is in the prostatic urethra, withdraw the stilet a little, thus pulling the beak forwards.

It is important not to empty the bladder rapidly. Only 10 or 15 oz. should be drawn off; after an interval of half an hour a similar amount is withdrawn, and so on until the bladder is empty, the catheter being retained in the urethra meanwhile and plugged. Another method is to tie-in a catheter of very small calibre (5 or 6 Fr.) and allow the urine to trickle away continuously, the bladder being emptied in about one and a half to two hours. When the bladder is empty a few syringefuls of nitrate-of-silver solution, 1 in 15,000, should be injected and allowed to flow away. Stimulants are usually necessary in these cases. The catheter should be tied in, and the patient kept in bed for several days. At the end of that time a decision will have to be made as to whether "catheter life" is to be commenced or an operation performed.

(b) *Hæmorrhage.*—Hæmorrhage may follow the passage of a catheter. The patient should be confined to bed, and ergot or calcium lactate (10 gr. thrice daily for two days) given, and, if the renal function is not seriously impaired, a little morphia. The bladder should be washed with a large quantity of weak silver nitrate solution, 1 in 10,000. If the hæmorrhage is severe and persistent, suprapubic cystotomy and prostatectomy may be necessary.

(c) *Frequent micturition.*—This symptom is frequently due to the presence of residual urine, stone, and sepsis. Residual urine is treated by catheterism or prostatectomy; stone is removed at the operation of prostatectomy; sepsis is referred to below.

Belladonna must be avoided, as its use will be followed by an increase in the residual urine, and sometimes by complete retention.

(d) *Sepsis.*—The treatment of cystitis is usually ineffectual unless bladder drainage is obtained. Prostatectomy is the best method of obtaining this, but before the operation the cystitis should be reduced as far as possible by washing the bladder or by tying a catheter in the urethra. In severe cystitis which has resisted these measures the operation of prostatectomy should be performed in two stages. The first stage consists in suprapubic cystotomy and drainage by a large rubber tube. This is followed by daily washing of the bladder or continuous irrigation. The second stage consists in removal of the prostate, and is carried out ten or fourteen days later. Where prostatectomy is contra-indicated and pyelonephritis is present, the bladder should be drained by catheter, or, better, by suprapubic cystotomy. Treatment for cystitis and pyelonephritis should then be carried out (pp. 134, 430).

2. Non-operative treatment: catheter life.—Catheter life consists in the regular passage of a catheter to withdraw residual urine. It is, of course, only the treatment of a symptom, and does not cause diminution of the size of the prostate or cure the disease. The catheterization may be carried out by the patient or by a trained attendant.

For practising catheterization the following materials are necessary :—

1. An easily prepared antiseptic solution. Soloids of mercuric potassium iodide, each 1·75 gr., in a bottle of fifty, is a convenient form. One soloid is added to 1 pint of water and forms a solution of 1 in 5,000.

2. Surgical absorbent wool, or prepared surgical swabs.

3. Two or more rubber catheters (No. 7 or No. 8 E.), or a silk-wove coudé or bicoudé catheter.

4. A sterilizer. A spirit-lamp and metal pan will serve, but a more convenient form is Zuckerkandl's catheter sterilizer (p. 355).

5. An antiseptic non-irritating lubricant (p. 356) in a collapsible tube.

6. A glass syringe of 2 oz. capacity for washing the catheter.

7. Two bowls of japanned metal or of ware, which are sterilized by burning in them two teaspoonfuls of methylated spirit.

8. A glass irrigator with a capacity of 2 pints or over, rubber tubing, an easily manipulated clip, and a glass nozzle which will fit the end of the catheter. These are only required if the bladder is to be irrigated.

The patient is taught that bacteria are his chief danger, and that they exist everywhere and on everything that has not been boiled or washed with an antiseptic.

A clean towel is spread over a small table and all the materials are placed upon it. The antiseptic solution is prepared in one bowl, the second being used as a receptacle for the urine. The patient washes his hands and soaks them in antiseptic. The catheter is sterilized and placed in the bowl of lotion. The screw cap of the lubricant tube is removed and the top plunged in boiling water.

2 T

The hands and penis are washed with soap and water and then with antiseptic, and the patient stands over the second bowl placed on the table or on a chair. A little lubricant is squeezed on the end of the catheter, which is held in the right hand 2 or 3 in. from its point. The penis is held between the thumb and forefinger of the left hand and the catheter slowly passed. Resistance is felt at the membranous urethra and in the prostatic portion, and is overcome by gentle steady pressure or by a spiral movement by twisting the outer end. When the urine begins to flow the end is turned down into the bowl, and when it has ceased the lumen of the catheter is occluded by pressure with the finger and thumb and the instrument steadily withdrawn.

The catheter is at once washed in soap and water and antiseptic fluid and syringed through. It is thoroughly dried and placed in a japanned catheter box or a glass tube closed at each end with a rubber plug, or it may be kept in a clean handkerchief.

The patient may pass his catheter lying in bed.

If cystitis is already present it will be necessary to irrigate the bladder once or several times a day. This is done when the urine has been withdrawn. The antiseptic fluid (boric acid solution, 1 teaspoonful of the crystals to a pint of water; potassium permanganate solution, 1 drachm of a saturated solution to 2 pints of water; oxycyanide of mercury, 1 in 5,000) has previously been prepared, and the irrigator is placed on the mantelshelf or on a hook 2 or 3 ft. above the level of the bladder. The nozzle of the irrigator is applied to the catheter, and 4 or 5 oz. run in and then discharged, and this is repeated until the irrigator is empty.

If catheterization is performed by the patient away from home the catheter is sterilized before leaving home and placed in an aseptic metal box (p. 356).

If the residual urine does not exceed 3 or 4 oz. the catheter is passed once or twice a week; if it is in greater quantity the catheter is passed every night, or night and morning. When retention is complete, or there is distension of the bladder with voluntary micturition, the catheter should be passed three or five times in the twenty-four hours. The patient should take urinary antiseptics regularly (urotropine, hetralin, etc.).

The dangers of this method are infection and hæmorrhage. In the majority of cases the method breaks down sooner or later by the introduction of sepsis, or from the difficulty of passing the instrument, or from hæmorrhage. The mortality of 'catheter life has been stated to be 7·7 per cent. in the hands of a competent surgeon. It is many times this figure when the patient uses his own catheter or the medical attendant is unskilled in urethral surgery. It is certainly very high, and to it must be added the cases in which death follows on operation performed in desperate circumstances when catheter life has failed.

In order to carry out catheter life with comparative safety the patient must be wealthy, leisured, methodical, patient, and his health must be sufficiently good to allow him to perform the delicate operation with constant care and every precaution. And for the same reason his hand must not be tremulous nor his eyesight failing; nor must he be so stout that his penis is concealed from his view.

As the age of the patient increases he becomes less able to carry out the necessary routine, while the increasing size of the prostate makes the operation more difficult.

There is no justification for recommending catheter life with a view to operation later, should it fail. If operation is to be performed, it should be done under the best conditions possible—that is, when the urinary tract is aseptic and the general health of the patient good. Catheter life is, in fact, only indicated when operative treatment cannot be carried out.

3. **Operative treatment.** — Only one method of treatment need be discussed, namely, prostatectomy. Prostatotomy, Bottini's galvano-caustic incision, castration, vasectomy, and other methods are of merely historical interest.

Prostatectomy. *Selection of cases for operation.*—The majority of the patients who suffer from enlarged prostate are old men ; the average in 112 of my cases of prostatectomy was 66 years. They are frequently in broken health from loss of sleep, and their strength is sapped by urinary sepsis and deficient elimination. If an optional major operation for some extra-urinary condition were discussed it is certain that it would be refused on account of the general condition of the patient in a very large number of these patients. Prostatectomy ranks as a serious major operation with three immediate dangers — shock, hæmorrhage, and uræmia. It is, however, an operation of necessity in most cases, and the results of skilfully conducted prostatectomy are little short of miraculous in even the most unpromising cases.

Old age does not of itself contra-indicate prostatectomy. The mortality does not increase *pari passu* with the age. In 83 cases the death-rate was greater between the ages of 55 and 60 than between 66 and 70 or over 75. Many patients over 80 have now been operated upon successfully. My oldest patient was 86 years, and had suffered from severe hæmorrhage for six weeks before the operation. Freyer records 19 cases of 80 or over with 2 deaths. Elsewhere he states that he has operated upon 47 octogenarians between 80 and 89 years and upon 9 aged 79.

The feeble resistance of these aged patients must, however, be borne in mind. The operative measures should be carried out with the utmost dispatch, and every care taken to maintain the circulation and prevent bronchitis. Skilled nursing after the operation contributes largely to success in these old patients.

The condition of the lungs is an important factor. Chronic bronchitis is a grave complication, and may contra-indicate prostatectomy. When bronchitis is present spinal anæsthesia should be employed, and the patient placed in the sitting posture and in a warm atmosphere after the operation.

Valvular cardiac disease is not a contra-indication if compensation is perfect. I have operated in cases both of mitral and of aortic disease. Disease of the cardiac muscle is, however, a grave complication, and may lead to cardiac failure some hours or even days after the operation.

Disease of the kidneys is, equally with bronchitis, the greatest danger. Many patients who have been on catheter life suffer from "urinary septicæmia," a combination of septic absorption and uræmia due to urinary obstruction and renal infection. In other cases there is an inefficient renal function from urinary obstruction without infection. In all these cases the operation should be performed in two stages, a preliminary suprapubic cystotomy being first performed, and the prostate removed two or three weeks later. By this method patients suffering from advanced uræmia and profound sepsis have successfully undergone prostatectomy.

Disease of the nervous system does not necessarily contra-indicate prostatectomy. I have operated successfully in a case of multiple sclerosis, and operations have been performed on patients suffering from old-standing hemiplegia.

Cystitis, if severe and chronic, should be treated by bladder washing, and occasionally preliminary cystotomy and drainage for ten or fourteen days are necessary. Vesical calculus does not increase the danger of the operation. Large diverticula are occasionally present. The presence of a diverticulum does not contra-indicate prostatectomy, but in these cases there is usually residual urine after the prostate has been removed.

Prostatectomy should be performed whenever the prostate is recognized as enlarged, while the urine is still aseptic, and before the kidneys are damaged by back pressure. It is unnecessary to wait until residual urine appears, or until the patient is becoming worn out by loss of sleep.

Preparations for the operation.—It is necessary to treat bronchitis, constipation, and other concurrent conditions before the operation.

Urinary antiseptics and diuretics should be freely given when sepsis and renal complications are present.

In cases of chronic cystitis some days or even weeks may be usefully employed in washing the bladder with antiseptic solution.

Preliminary suprapubic cystotomy with drainage should be performed in cases of chronic distension of the bladder after first very slowly emptying the bladder (*see* p. 703), in cases of intractable chronic cystitis, and in cases of uræmia or of urinary septicæmia.

There are two routes by which prostatectomy is performed, the suprapubic and the perineal.

Suprapubic prostatectomy.—The operation of complete suprapubic prostatectomy here described was introduced by Freyer in 1901, and is now universally accepted in Europe as the best and most successful method of operating. In America a constantly increasing number of surgeons, as shown by the literature, are adopting the method, although there still remain a few strong advocates of the perineal route.

A catheter is passed and the bladder emptied and washed with boric solution. From 10 to 12 oz. of fluid are introduced and the catheter left in the urethra and plugged. The surgeon stands on the left of the patient, and the bladder is exposed by a vertical medium suprapubic incision 3 in. in length and opened. A narrow retractor or hook is placed in the upper angle of the bladder wound. If calculi are present they are removed by lithotomy forceps or scoop. The left hand is covered with a rubber glove and the forefinger introduced into the rectum. Freyer stands on the right of the patient and introduces the right forefinger into the rectum.

The forefinger in the bladder feels for the most prominent part of the intravesical projection and commences the enucleation by stripping the mucous membrane from the back or vesical surface of this. This readily peels off without the use of any cutting instrument and without using a sharpened nail. When there is no prominent intravesical portion the forefinger is pushed into the prostatic urethra and ruptures the posterior wall of the urethra and commences the enucleation in this way.

At the base of the intravesical portion the finger, guided by the prostate, passes within the circle of the vesical sphincter between the enlarged prostate and its sheath. (Fig. 216.) The prostate will be found to enucleate rapidly and without difficulty. ` First one lobe is freed by sweeping the forefinger around it, and the finger passes across the middle line behind the prostate, and the second lobe is treated in the same way. There may be difficulty in reaching the lower ends of each lobe, and the prostate should be pushed up with the rectal finger. The second finger of the right hand may be used to assist in enucleating if the prostate is large and difficult to reach. The finger sweeps across the middle line anteriorly, and then the urethra is torn across upon the catheter

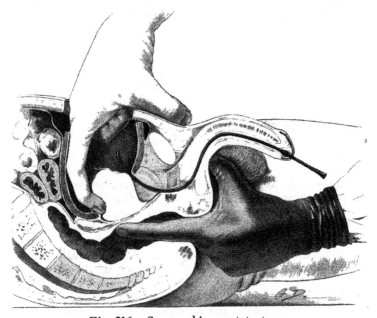

Fig. 216.—Suprapubic prostatectomy.

Left hand, gloved, with forefinger in rectum pressing up prostate. Right hand, ungloved, with forefinger in bladder. The tip of the forefinger has stripped the bladder mucous membrane of the intravesical portion of prostate, and is being insinuated between the prostate and the vesical sphincter.

which still lies in it. (Fig. 217.) The prostate is now projected upwards into the bladder. The left forefinger is removed from the rectum, the glove stripped from the hand by an assistant, and a pair of ovum forceps or lithotrity forceps seized and introduced into the bladder, guided by the right forefinger. The prostate is grasped and removed. A copious stream of hot boric lotion (120° F.) is turned on through the catheter from a reservoir. A large rubber tube, 1 in. in diameter, with one lateral eye, is introduced into the bladder, and the wound in the bladder wall is closed firmly around this by one or two catgut sutures. A small rubber drain is placed in the prevesical space (Freyer uses a gauze wick), and the abdominal wound is closed around these tubes, especial care being taken to bring the edges of the rectus sheath together, either with interrupted catgut sutures or with a continuous catgut thread. The catheter is removed. The lower end of the bed is raised on blocks.

On the following day, and each day until the wound is closed, the bladder is irrigated through the suprapubic wound with boric

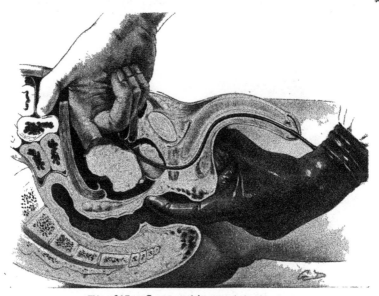

Fig. 217.—Suprapubic prostatectomy.

The prostate has been freed behind, laterally, and in front of the urethra, and the point of the forefinger is in the act of tearing the prostatic urethra on the catheter before dislocating the prostate into the bladder.

solution, or weak biniodide of mercury solution (1 in 8,000), or oxycyanide of mercury solution (1 in 5,000). The tubes are removed on the fourth day. A purge is given after their removal, but care should be taken to prevent the patient from straining. After the operation the urine may be allowed to soak into the dressings, which are changed every four hours. A voluminous dressing, consisting of a few layers of gauze next the wound and much cellulose tissue or large flat pads of wood-wool, is applied, and retained by means of a broad binder or many-tailed bandage extending from the level of the great trochanters to above the umbilicus. The skin is protected by a thick covering of ointment containing boric acid, zinc oxide, lanoline, and castor oil. As an alternative, a Hamilton Irving apparatus (p. 548) may be applied at the end of the operation. It is changed daily and thoroughly cleaned. There is a tendency to eversion of the lips and congestion of the skin with this apparatus, and the wound heals more quickly without it. It is, however, much more economical, and saves the constant soaking and discomfort and frequent dressing.

The wound closes in from three to four weeks. When it is almost closed, healing will be expedited by tying a catheter

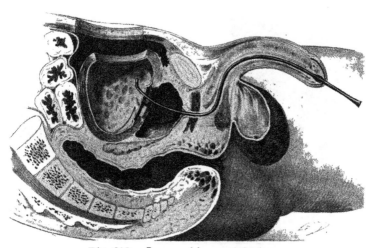

Fig. 218.—Suprapubic prostatectomy.

Condition of parts immediately after removal of the prostate. The cavity from which the prostate has been removed is seen with the catheter passing across it from the membranous urethra to the bladder. The ledge formed by the bladder base, and the portion of the posterior wall of the prostatic urethra left adherent to the wall of the prostatic cavity, are represented.

in the urethra. In one of my cases the patient left the nursing-home, healed, nineteen days after the operation; this is, however, exceptional. Occasionally there is a rise of temperature (100°–101° F.) when the patient first passes urine through the urethra, but this subsides on the following day.

Surgical anatomy of suprapubic prostatectomy.—In 1904 I investigated the surgical anatomy of Freyer's operation, and subsequently (1905) described the anatomical and clinical conditions found after the operation. (Fig. 218.) The structures removed consist of the prostate and prostatic urethra. (Figs. 219–23.) There are two varieties. In one there is an intravesical projection; in the other the prostate is wholly extravesical. The specimen (Figs. 219–21) consists of two lobes enclosed in an envelope of circular fibres, the surface of which is usually smooth. The intravesical portion, when one is present, is marked off from the extravesical portion by a deep groove caused by the sphincter of the bladder. (Figs. 211, 219.) There is a single median lobe behind the opening of the urethra, or two lobes at the sides. When a single median lobe is present a thick band of muscular fibres is seen torn across on each side of it. This is the remains of the longitudinal bands

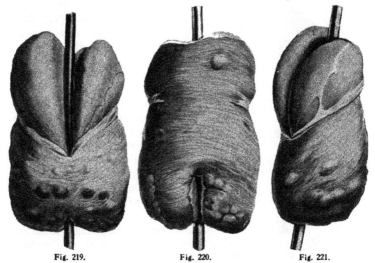

Fig. 219.   Fig. 220.   Fig. 221.

Fig. 219.—Operation specimen of enlarged prostate, anterior view.
Catheter in prostatic urethra.   Bilobed intravesical projection covered by mucous membrane (upper half), and extravesical portion covered by capsule (lower half).

Fig. 220.—Posterior view of same specimen.

Note groove between intra- and extravesical portions, caused by pressure of sphincter.   Edge of vesical mucous membrane is seen at upper margin.   Posterior wall of prostatic urethra from the verumontanum downwards is wanting, having been left adherent to the wall of prostatic cavity.

Fig. 221.—Lateral view of same specimen.

Note bilobed intravesical portion covered with mucous membrane, of which the edge is seen.

of trigone muscle, which pass down from the ureters and enter the longitudinal muscle of the urethra.

The mucous membrane of the bladder is torn across on the vesical surface of the intravesical projection. The anterior commissure between the two prostatic lobes is complete from the vesical orifice of the urethra to the lower end of the specimen, and on the anterior aspect of this may be seen portions of striped muscle fibre, the remains of the vertical portion of the muscle of Henle (Figs. 224, 225), and sometimes portions of the veins of the vertical limb of the prostatic venous plexus. The posterior commissure is complete down to the level of the verumontanum, and from this point downwards the lobes are separate, the posterior wall of the urethra being wanting. The verumontanum can sometimes be seen at the lowest part of the portion of posterior wall removed with the prostate. The anterior commissure may be split during the enucleation, and the lobes part as if hinged posteriorly and display the prostatic urethra (Fig. 223). The prostatic urethra is removed with the prostate, but the portion of the posterior wall extending from the verumontanum downwards is usually left behind. Sometimes a strip of urethral wall measuring $1\frac{1}{2}$ in. is torn out with the prostate and remains attached to the anterior wall of the prostatic urethra.

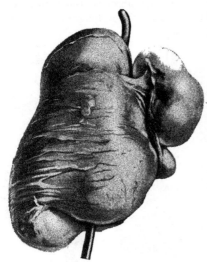

Fig. 222.—Specimen of enlarged prostate after prostatectomy.

Catheter in prostatic urethra. Groove between intra. and extraVesical portions. Torn edge of mucous membrane seen on intraVesical portion, circular fibres of capsule on extraVesical portion.

After removal of the prostate there remains a cavity between the bladder and the membranous urethra. (Figs. 218, 226, 227.) This is partly roofed over by the trigone and sometimes part of the base of the bladder, the opening into the bladder being at the anterior part of the roof. The walls are formed by the fascial sheath of the prostate, on which may be found shreds of the capsule of the prostate, and occasionally a small adenomatous nodule is left adherent. (Fig. 227.) A strip of mucous membrane from the posterior wall of the prostatic urethra from the verumontanum downwards is often adherent to the posterior wall of the cavity, and at the upper end of this the verumontanum may be found.

This cavity contracts gradually to a small size, but even after some years it has not disappeared. (Fig. 228.)

I have shown that after suprapubic prostatectomy the sphincter at the orifice of the bladder becomes active and competent in less

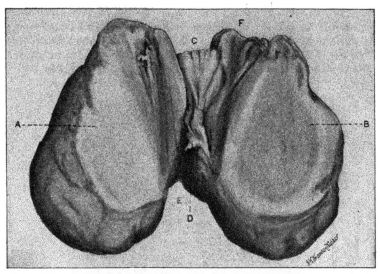

Fig. 223.—Specimen of enucleated enlarged prostate, extravesical variety, open along anterior commissure.

A, B, Mucous membrane of prostatic urethra.   C, F, Torn mucous membrane at internal meatus.   D, Verumontanum.   E Portion of posterior wall of prostatic urethra wanting.

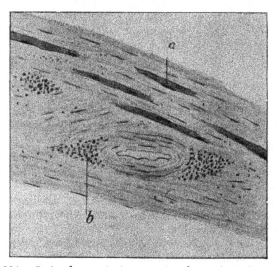

Fig. 224.—Striped muscle in capsule of enucleated prostate.

a, Striped muscle. b, Perivascular infiltration.

than 50 per cent. of cases, and that in the majority of cases the urine is retained by the contraction of the striped compressor urethræ muscle which surrounds the membranous urethra. Further observations tend to show that the number of cases in which the vesical sphincter resumes control is smaller than I had supposed.

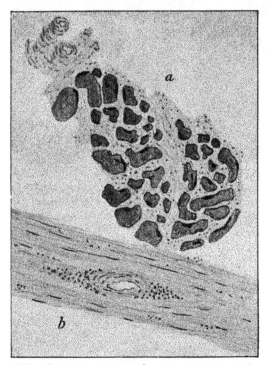

Fig. 225.—Striped muscle lying on anterior surface of enucleated prostate.

a, Striped muscle and areolar tissue. *b*, Capsule of prostate.

Regeneration of the prostate does not occur after Freyer's operation.

Partial prostatectomy, which consists of shelling adenoma from within the prostate, may be followed by recurrence of the growth and the obstruction.

Dangers and complications of suprapubic prostatectomy.—The chief dangers of the operation are :

Shock.

Hæmorrhage.

Uræmia.

Septicæmia.

Bronchitis, pneumonia.

Cerebral hæmorrhage or thrombosis.

Pulmonary embolism.

Prostatectomy ranks high in the list of operations in regard 'to the production of *shock*, but the mortality from this cause is

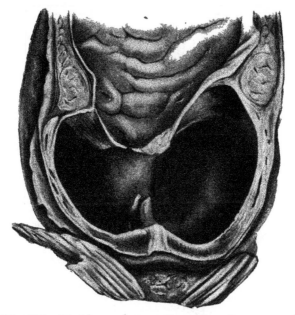

Fig. 226.—Bladder and prostatic cavity after suprapubic prostatectomy.

At upper part is bladder, and on each side the thickened sphincter. Below this is the cavity from which the prostate was removed, roofed over by the bladder base. On the posterior wall of this are a portion of the prostatic urethra and the ejaculatory ducts. In its wall are the prostatic veins, and at the lower part the compressor urethræ and the levator ani.

very small. It is avoided by careful preparation before the operation and by rapid operation, and is treated by saline infusion and strychnine, if necessary, after the operation.

Hæmorrhage is sometimes severe, and may be serious. Flushing with large quantities of very hot water (120° F.) immediately on removal of the prostate is a routine method of treatment. On return to bed the lower end of the bed is raised high on blocks and a hypodermic injection of morphia may be given.

Should severe hæmorrhage continue immediately after remova

of the prostate, or should it occur after the operation, it will be necessary to pack the prostatic cavity with strips of gauze and then introduce the large drainage tube down to the trigone. The packing is removed on the second or third day, a short anæsthesia being sometimes advisable. I do not hesitate to pack the prostatic cavity when there is the slightest anxiety in regard to hæmorrhage. Secondary hæmorrhage may very rarely occur a week or

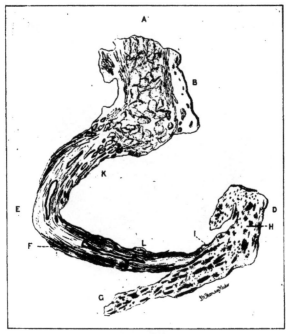

Fig. 227.—Vertical section of bladder wall and wall of cavity remaining after prostatectomy.

A, Bladder muscle. B, Bladder mucous membrane. C, Prostatic cavity. D, H, Membranous urethra. E, Fibrous wall of cavity containing veins (F) of prostatic plexus. G, Compressor urethræ muscle. I, Striped muscle in wall of cavity. K, Bladder muscle in wall of cavity. L, Small portion of prostate adherent to sheath.

ten days after the operation, and is due to sepsis, or to allowing the patient too much liberty in sitting up, raising himself, and moving about. If the urine remains blood-stained after the third day, or if it becomes blood-stained after being clear, the patient should be kept flat, with the lower end of the bed raised, and morphia administered hypodermically.

Severe secondary hæmorrhage is treated by packing the prostatic cavity and reintroducing the bladder drainage tube.

Urœmia results from preoperative disease of the kidneys. When there is evidence of renal disease the operation should be performed in two stages, the preliminary cystotomy preceding the prostatectomy by a week or longer.

Energetic diuretic treatment should be adopted when uræmia is threatened or is present. Large quantities of fluid are administered by the mouth and diuretics given (theocin sodium acetate,

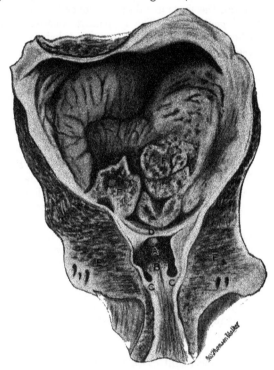

Fig. 228.—Bladder and urethra two years after suprapubic prostatectomy.

A, Cavity from which prostate was removed. B, Portion of posterior wall of prostatic urethra. C, C, Junction of prostatic cavity and membranous urethra. D, Junction of prostatic cavity and bladder. E, E, ,Fibrous and muscular tissue surrounding cavity. F, F, Malignant growth in bladder.

10 gr., every four hours). Rectal and hypodermic infusion of glucose solution (2 per cent.) and intravenous infusion of the same solution should be used. Dry cupping and hot fomentations are applied over the kidneys, and a hot pack is given to promote perspiration.

Septic infection usually results from an exacerbation of preoperative cystitis, and takes the form of ascending pyelonephritis ; it is frequently complicated by suppression of urine. Preventive treatment should be carried out before prostatectomy is performed. This consists in the administration of urinary antiseptics and in bladder-washing, continuous drainage by catheter, or suprapubic cystotomy and free daily irrigation of the bladder. When ascending infection has occurred urinary antiseptics should be administered and the measures detailed under Uræmia adopted.

Bronchitis and pneumonia.—The treatment consists in the use of spinal anæsthesia when bronchitis is present before the operation, in the use of chloroform and not ether where a general anæsthetic is necessary, in rapid operation, and in free administration of stimulants and cardiac tonics such as ergot and strophanthus.

Epididymitis may appear at the end of the second or third week, and last for seven to ten days.

Results of suprapubic prostatectomy.—The operative mortality of 112 consecutive cases in which I performed complete suprapubic prostatectomy was 5 per cent. (1910). This included all my earliest cases, performed soon after the introduction of the operation. In 1,000 cases recorded by Freyer the operative mortality was 5·5 per cent. This observer found that the mortality gradually decreased from 10 per cent. in the first 100 cases to 3 per cent. in the last.

Death is due to shock, hæmorrhage, cardiac failure, uræmia, septicæmia, bronchitis, pneumonia, pulmonary embolism, cerebral hæmorrhage, cerebral thrombosis. In a large proportion of these cases the fatal result is only indirectly connected with the operation, such as those from cerebral hæmorrhage and syncope during convalescence ; in others it is due to an exacerbation of previous disease of the kidneys or other organs which would have proved fatal within a short time had the operation not been performed.

In many of the successful cases the operation was performed when the patient was desperately ill, and in some even supposed to be moribund.

The *late results* are very satisfactory. The patient is able to pass urine naturally, and wholly empties his bladder, even in cases where there has been complete catheter life for many years (six to ten). In a rare class of cases removal of the prostate by the suprapubic or perineal routes is not followed by restoration of the bladder function ; these belong to a group which I have described elsewhere (*see* p. 537). The patient has complete control over the retention of urine after suprapubic prostatectomy ; I have not seen any case in which incontinence was present.

Cystitis present before the operation is usually cured, unless due to septic pyelonephritis, or in sacculated bladders or those in which one or several diverticula are present, when it tends to persist. When stone is present before the operation and the urine is not decomposing, there is no recurrence after the operation. If, however, the urine is decomposing and does not improve after the operation, there may b꞉ a recurrence of stone formation. Calculi of the former type are usually composed of uric acid or oxalate of lime ; those which recur are phosphatic. Suprapubic fistula is rare after prostatectomy. When it persists it can be cured by operation (p. 522). In 112 consecutive cases there were 2 in which a fistula persisted; both were cured by excision of the fistula and repair of the bladder wall. Hernia of the suprapubic scar develops in rare cases, and is due to too prolonged drainage, to neglect to repair the abdominal wall after removing the prostate, or to allowing a heavy patient to get about too soon.

The sexual function was unimpaired in 47·5 per cent. of cases ; in 32·5 per cent. desire and erection were normal, but there was no discharge of semen ; in 7·5 per cent. a failing function before operation showed diminished desire after operation ; and in 12·5 per cent. the sexual function, which was very feeble or abolished before, showed no improvement after the operation. Where the function is normal except for the emission, the semen remains in the prostatic cavity, or finds its way into the bladder and is discharged with the urine at the next micturition.

Stricture has been said to develop after operation at the vesical outlet, but it must be very rare. I have seen one case in which it might have formed but was prevented by tying-in a catheter for a week.

Perineal prostatectomy.—The transverse prerectal incision of Zuckerkandl is that used for perineal prostatectomy. Proust has elaborated the details of this operation, and his technique is widely followed.

The patient is placed in the lithotomy position, the pelvis being raised by putting a hard cushion under the sacrum. Proust described a position (*périnéale inverse*) in which the dorsal and lumbar regions are supported on an inclined plane, the thighs flexed, and the legs held vertically by a framework. In this position the perineum is horizontal. This is not usually considered necessary for the operation. A staff is placed in the urethra and a transverse prerectal or curved incision with the convexity forwards is made from one ischial tuberosity to the other, 1½ in. in front of the anus. The posterior end of the bulb is exposed, the ano-bulbar raphe seized and cut across, and the

2 U

two forefingers are introduced into the wound, separating the
levatores ani muscles and pushing back the rectum. A large
retractor is now placed in the lower part of the wound and pulled
backwards to the coccyx (Fig. 229), displacing the rectum back-

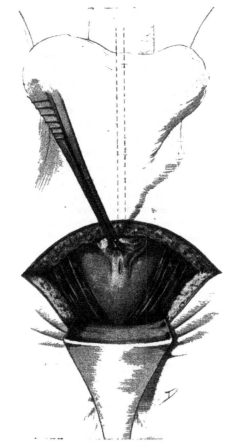

Fig. 229.—Perineal prostatectomy.

The bulb has been exposed and pulled forwards, and the membranous urethra incised, preparatory to introducing the prostatic retractor. The levatores ani muscles and part of the
prostate are seen.

wards and exposing the posterior surface of the sheath of the
prostate. The urethra is opened at the apex of the prostate,
and the walls are picked up in forceps. The staff is withdrawn
and a depressor is introduced through the prostatic urethra into

the bladder. The blades are separated and the handle is raised so that the prostate and bladder base are made to protrude into the wound (Fig. 230).

The prostatic urethra is split backwards to the region of the

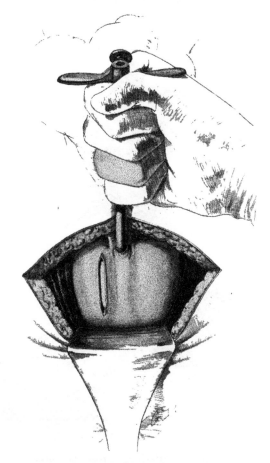

Fig. 230.—Perineal prostatectomy.

The prostatic retractor has been introduced and is being pulled towards the surface and forwards. The leVatores ani muscles haVe been pushed to the sides. A vertical incision through the prostatic sheath has been made, parallel to the prostatic urethra. (*Young's operation.*)

vesical sphincter, the sheath of the prostate is peeled off each lobe, and one lobe seized with forceps. This lobe is dissected off the urethra with scissors, working outwards, and finally hangs by a pedicle formed by the prostatic vessels. The pedicle is tied and cut and the lobe removed. The same dissection is carried out on the other side; an intravesical lobe is hooked down with the finger and removed. The margins of the urethra are approximated by catgut sutures, leaving a space through

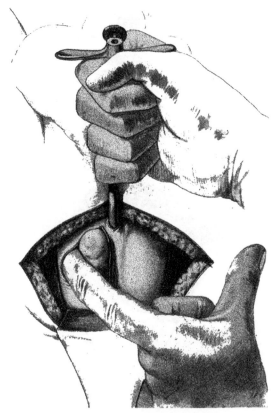

Fig. 231.—Perineal prostatectomy.

The right lobe is being shelled out with the finger. (*Young.*)

which a drainage tube is introduced into the bladder, and some packing into the cavities from which the prostatic lobes were removed. The structures of the perineum are now brought together with catgut sutures. The packing is removed in forty-eight hours, and the perineal tube at the end of a week, when a catheter is tied in the urethra. Healing is complete in five or six weeks.

Albarran performs a similar operation, but removes each prostatic lobe from the apex backwards in two or several portions.

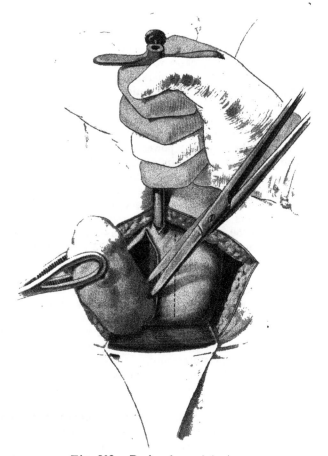

Fig. 232.—Perineal prostatectomy.

Removal of right lobe: cutting along the urethral aspect. The dotted line shows the incision for removal of left lobe. (*Young.*)

Young uses a **V**-shaped incision, and introduces his prostatic retractor through an incision in the membranous urethra. This part of the operation is frequently attended with difficulty. He then makes a longitudinal incision 1·5 cm. deep through the whole length of the prostatic lobe on each side of the urethra, the two incisions being 1·8 cm. apart, and leaves the vertical wedge of tissue between these incisions with the view to preserving the ejaculatory ducts. The lobes are then dissected away. (Figs. 230–2.)

Perineal operations have also been described by Nicoll, Alexander, Freyer, and others, but they require no special notice here.

Results of perineal prostatectomy.—Young shows a mortality of 3·7 per cent. in 450 cases. Other observers are less fortunate. Watson found the mortality 6·2 per cent., Proust 5·8 per cent., and Legueu collected 1,026 cases with a mortality of 8 per cent.

The *late results* show a considerable proportion of cases of urinary fistula; Judd found 6 in a series of 323 cases. Incontinence of urine may follow the operation. Of 323 cases of perineal prostatectomy performed at St. Mary's Hospital, Rochester, U.S.A., Judd found that 7 had "some degree of incontinence," and that in 11 "the retentive power was not strong." Several patients had not good control immediately following the operation, but regained it in a few weeks. Recto-urethral fistula, temporary or permanent, is sometimes observed. In the usual perineal prostatectomy the sexual powers are abolished. Young's operation endeavours to overcome this grave objection. In this observer's statistics 59 per cent. of recent cases are stated to have had a complete return of sexual power, and in 75 per cent. erections returned. Apparently, in the remainder the sexual function was destroyed.

Epididymitis occurs as a complication during convalescence in from 10 to 30 per cent. of cases. Stricture is observed after perineal prostatectomy, and necessitates dilatation over long periods. The operation is always incomplete, and recurrence of the obstruction due to enlargement of the residual portions may necessitate suprapubic prostatectomy.

Choice of method.—Suprapubic prostatectomy can be performed in all forms of simple enlargement of the prostate, while perineal prostatectomy is unsuitable in cases where there are numerous vesical calculi, or the intravesical projection is large or the prostate of considerable dimensions. It follows that when perineal prostatectomy is practised as a routine method the more serious cases are submitted to the suprapubic operation. The mortality of suprapubic prostatectomy at the present time varies from 4 to 6 per cent. for all cases, that of perineal prostatectomy from 3·7 to 5·8 per cent. for the selected cases noted above.

The after-results of perineal prostatectomy are unsatisfactory when compared with those of the suprapubic operation. In the perineal method urinary fistulæ are twice as numerous and the fistula cannot be cured by operation; recto-perineal and recto-urethral fistulæ occur; stricture is frequently observed, and incontinence of urine results in a number of cases. Epididymitis complicates the perineal operation much more often than the suprapubic. The sexual function is abolished in perineal prostatectomy unless a portion of the prostate is left, as in Young's operation; in suprapubic prostatectomy it is completely preserved in a large proportion of cases. Recurrence of the prostatic tumour has been observed after perineal prostatectomy; it cannot occur in complete suprapubic prostatectomy. The convalescence after suprapubic prostatectomy is longer than after the perineal operation.

For simple enlargement of the prostate the complete suprapubic operation is more widely applicable, and the results are infinitely superior to those of perineal prostatectomy. It should therefore be the method adopted in all cases. In the so-called fibrous enlargement the perineal route is preferable, but this condition is a purely inflammatory one, and cannot be considered as a type of enlargement of the prostate.

LITERATURE

Casper,' *Virchows Arch.*, lxxvi. 139.
Ciechanowski, *Anatomical Researches on Prostatic Hypertrophy.* Translated by Greene, 1903.
Daniel, *Brit. Med. Journ.*, 1904, ii. 1140.
Freyer, *Brit. Med. Journ.*, July 20, 1901, and Oct., 1912, p. 868 ; *Lancet*, 1911, i. 923. *Surgical Diseases of the Urinary Organs.* 1908.
Judd, *Journ. of Amer. Med. Assoc.*, 1911, p. 458.
Launois, Thèse de Paris, 1885.
Marion, XVe Sess. Assoc. Franç. d'Urol., 1911.
Motz, *Ann. d. Mal. d. Org. Gén.-Urin.*, 1897, p. 1117.
Motz et Perearnau, *Ann. d. Mal. d. Org. Gén.-Urin.*, 1905, ii. 1521.
Proust, *La Prostatectomie dans l'Hypertrophie de la Prostate.* 1904.
Tandler und Zuckerkandl, *Folia Urol.*, 1911, p. 587.
Walker, Thomson, *Med.-Chir. Trans.*, 1904, lxxxvii. ; *Brit. Med. Journ.*, July 9 and Oct. 29, 1904, Oct. 7, 1905 ; *Arch. of Middx. Hosp.*, 1905, vol. iv. ; *Clin. Journ.*, July, 1912, p. 261.
Ward, *Birmingham Med. Rev.*, March, 1908.
Watson, *Boston Med. and Surg. Journ.*, 1904, p. 453.
Young, *Med. Press and Circ.*, 1911, p. 148.
Discussion at British Medical Association—*Brit. Med. Journ.*, Nov. 8, 1902.
Discussion at II. Congress of the International Association of Urology, London, 1911.

CHAPTER LVII

ATROPHY OF THE PROSTATE

Etiology.—Atrophy of the prostate occurs under a variety of conditions. Congenital atrophy is strictly arrest of development of the gland. It is found in combination with other congenital malformations of the genital organs, especially imperfect development and misplacement of the testicles. When one testicle has failed to develop there may be a corresponding arrest of development in the prostatic lobe of the same side. Not infrequently, however, both lobes of the prostate are fully developed when one testicle is infantile.

Castration before puberty results in arrested development of the prostate gland. Castration after puberty is followed by shrinking and diminution in size of the prostate. After removal of one testicle the prostate may, however, remain for long unchanged in size on rectal palpation.

Castration was at one time supposed to be followed by diminution in size or atrophy of the hypertrophic prostate, and was practised as a method of treatment for this disease. It is admitted that a reduction in congestion of the organ is produced, but the belief that shrinkage from atrophy of the enlarged organ takes place is no longer held.

Atrophy may follow inflammatory diseases of the gland, such as acute and chronic gonorrhœal prostatitis and tuberculous disease, or pressure from calculi or from cysts, and is not infrequently present in old-standing stricture of the urethra as a result of chronic prostatitis.

Senile atrophy develops after the age of 50, and occasionally earlier. The average age in 13 advanced cases under my care was 61¾ years, the youngest patient being 52. The condition in an advanced state is comparatively rare. According to Ciechanowski, atrophy results from pressure caused by fibrosis due to peripherally distributed chronic prostatitis.

Pathological anatomy.—In advanced cases the lobes are reduced so as to be hardly distinguishable. On section a firm, opaque, white or greyish surface is found, and traces of gland

728

tissue can only be found microscopically. Occasionally small cystic spaces are present, which may contain corpora amylacea. The muscle fibres are replaced by fibrous tissue. The prostatic urethra may be tough and leathery, and fibrous infiltration of the tissues around the vesical orifice ("contracture of the neck of the bladder") may be observed.

Symptoms.—Frequent micturition is the most constant symptom. It is present both day and night, and amounts to six or eight times during the day and twice or thrice at night. Occasionally there is great urgency and constant desire to micturate. Nocturnal enuresis is not uncommon, and in a few cases complete incontinence develops. Difficult micturition, or gradual or sudden onset, is often present.

The stream is poor and may be reduced to a dribble. Complete retention is rare.

In the early stage and in moderate degrees there is no residual urine, but later several ounces of urine may remain after micturition, and occasionally the bladder is chronically distended. The urine may be clear, but usually contains evidence of chronic urethral or vesical inflammation.

An instrument may pass easily into the bladder, and the total length of the urethra is found to be reduced. In some cases there is obstruction at the internal meatus, due to fibrous induration of this portion of the canal or to a fold of mucous membrane.

On rectal examination the prostate is greatly reduced in size, and is flat and smooth, with an ill-defined outline, or the finger may fail to detect any remains of the gland. The membranous and prostatic portions of the urethra can be felt, and sometimes the seminal vesicles, but the lobes of the prostate are wanting.

Diagnosis.—The symptoms may closely resemble those of hypertrophy of the prostate, but on rectal examination the atrophy is readily recognized.

In chronic periprostatitis the prostate is obscured on rectal palpation, but here all the structures on the anterior wall of the rectum, such as the seminal vesicles, membranous and prostatic urethra, are also hidden. Examination with a sound in the urethra assists the diagnosis. In atrophy of the prostate it is felt in the prostatic urethra ; in chronic periprostatitis it is felt with difficulty or not at all.

The " atrophic " type of carcinoma of the prostate may give rise to difficulty in diagnosis from simple atrophy of the organ. In the malignant growth the gland, although small and flat, is hard and fixed, and a sound in the prostatic urethra cannot be felt from the rectum. The early appearance of metastatic growths will put an end to any doubt.

Treatment.—When possible, the cause, such as stricture or prostatic calculus, is removed. The use of the catheter is necessary when there is residual urine or complete retention.

Incontinence of urine may necessitate the wearing of a rubber urinal. Barth recommends perineal prostatectomy, and holds that good results follow the removal of scar tissue from around the prostatic urethra. The regular passage of large metal instruments is of benefit, and where there is obstruction at the vesical outlet good results may be obtained by incision and dilatation of the internal meatus through a suprapubic cystotomy wound. Perineal prostatotomy has also proved useful, and Bottini's galvanocaustic operation has been recommended.

LITERATURE

Barth, *Arch. f. klin. Chir.*, 1911, Heft 3.
Englisch, *Zeits. f. Heilk.*, 1901, Heft 12.
Fuller, *Amer. Journ. of Med. Sci.*, 1897, p. 440.
Launois, *Ann. d. Mal. d. Org. Gén.-Urin.*, 1894, p. 721.
Rörig, *Centralbl. f. d. Krankh. d. Harn- u. Sex.-Org.*, 1903, S. 243.
Strauch, *Centralbl. f. d. Krankh. d. Harn- u. Sex.-Org.*, 1894, S. 227.

CHAPTER LVIII

MALIGNANT DISEASE OF THE PROSTATE

THE ratio of cancer of the prostate to other forms of cancer was 2·3 per 1,000 in 6,732 cases of cancer at the Middlesex Hospital. The relative frequency of malignant disease of the prostate in 242 consecutive cases of prostatic enlargement under my care was 16·5 per cent.

Etiology.—There is no certain knowledge as to the cause of prostatic carcinoma. Calculus of the prostate is a rare precancerous condition. Malignant disease rarely develops in a prostate the seat of hypertrophy or simple enlargement. A number of cases are, however, on record where examination of a specimen of enlarged prostate after enucleation showed undoubted malignant characters in some part of it. Albarran and Hallé have stated that 20 per cent. of cases of supposed simple enlargement of the prostate are malignant. The proof of malignancy in these cases, however, rested upon epithelial changes the significance of which is open to doubt.

Pathological anatomy and histology.—Carcinoma is the common form of malignant disease of the prostate, while sarcoma is rare.

Carcinoma occurs most frequently between the ages of 50 and 70 ; the average in 40 cases was 65 years. In one patient the symptoms commenced at the age of 44, and in another at 48. The enlargement may be slight, and von Recklinghausen pointed out that the cancerous prostate might be scarcely enlarged, or even smaller than the normal gland. In the greater number of cases, however, the organ is considerably enlarged, and it may reach very large proportions. It is hard, and may be cartilaginous to the touch. Less frequently it forms a soft, very rapidly growing tumour. On section it presents a thick, fibrous stroma with whitish nodules, or it may be hard and scirrhous throughout. The commonest form retains the outline of the prostate, but there may be a diffuse carcinomatous infiltration of the areolar tissue of the pelvis, matting the pelvic organs together in an inseparable mass ("*carcinose prostato-pelvième diffuse*"—Guyon).

The structure of the majority of carcinomas of the prostate is a small round or polygonal type of spheroidal-celled carcinoma (Fig. 233), and they are peculiar in that the stroma is infiltrated with fine rows of cells or small isolated clumps. The entire tumour may thus in the gross specimen appear peculiarly fibrous, while under the microscope it is strikingly rich in cellular elements. Even in the common spheroidal-celled carcinoma there are certain parts where there is a development of cylindrical-celled adeno-

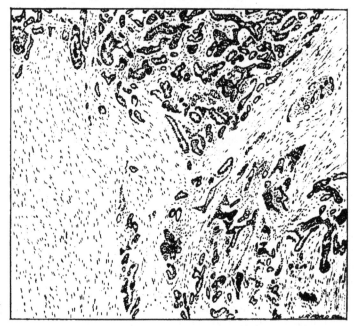

Fig. 233.—Carcinoma of prostate.

carcinoma. In other cases the structure is largely that of a cylindrical-celled adeno-carcinoma. In these some parts may reproduce the structure of a spheroidal-celled carcinoma.

The direction of spread may be towards the bladder cavity, into which the carcinoma fungates. Clinically this form is relatively uncommon, but it frequently occurs in later stages, and is found in a large proportion of cases post mortem (57 in 100 cases—Kauffmann; 80 per cent. in 17 cases—Thomson Walker). Spread along the outer surface of the bladder is common, the growth surrounding the seminal vesicles and lower ends of the ureters and occluding the latter. The growth may also spread laterally in the areolar tissue of the pelvis, obliterating the lateral sulcus on each side of the prostate. In a few cases the growth spreads towards the rectum, and may cause ulceration of the rectal mucous membrane. More frequently it spreads round the outside of the rectum, narrowing the lumen. The pelvic peritoneum may be involved. Deposit in lymph-glands takes place comparatively early, those along the internal iliac vessels being first affected. The lowest lymph nodules of this chain lie in a band which passes out from the base of the prostate on each side and can be felt with the finger in the rectum. The inguinal glands are involved in 16 per cent. of cases. The liver, lungs, kidneys, suprarenal glands, pancreas, and less frequently other organs, may be the seat of metastatic deposit. There is a peculiar tendency for prostatic carcinoma to produce metastases in the bony skeleton, forming osteoplastic nodules or widespread infiltration (70 per cent.—Kauffmann). The vertebræ are most frequently affected, and then the femur, pelvis, ribs, skull, sternum, humerus, fibula, tibia, radius, and ulna.

Sarcoma of the prostate is rare. It may occur at any age, but in most of the recorded cases the age has been under 10 years, and the tumours have grown rapidly and attained a large size. The usual forms are round- and spindle-celled, but 4 cases of rhabdo-myo-sarcoma (Kauffmann 3, Greig 1) are on record.

Symptoms.—Difficult micturition is the most frequent (92 per cent.) and often the first (55 per cent.) symptom. The onset is gradual. The stream is delayed and is small, and the projection feeble, and there is after-dribbling. With this there may be one or several attacks of retention, and eventually the patient may become partly or completely dependent on the catheter. In other cases the onset of difficulty is sudden, and there may be an initial attack of complete retention.

Frequent micturition occurs in 87·5 per cent. of cases, but is rarely the first symptom. The increased frequency occurs during the day, and it is also necessary to pass water at night, usually at equal intervals of two or three hours.

In a few cases there is dribbling of urine from a bladder which is not distended. In these the growth has spread widely and the whole bladder base is rigid, so that the internal meatus is open and rigid and control by the sphincter is lost.

Pain occurs in 72·5 per cent. of cases, and is sometimes the initial symptom. The characteristic pain of prostatic carcinoma is unconnected with micturition or with obstruction to the flow of urine. It is felt in one or several of the following situations—

viz. the penis or urethra, rectum, anus, sacrum, sacro-iliac syn-chondrosis, hip-joints, suprapubic region, perineum, groins, thighs, legs, testicles. The pain is a dull, constant aching, which persists over months or years ; it is unconnected with micturition, defæca-tion, or movement, and is little affected by drugs. It may take the form of sciatica, which may be the prominent symptom, while prostatic symptoms are insignificant.

Hæmaturia is absent in the majority of cases. When it is present (12·5 per cent.) the urine may be bright or dark, and is usually in small quantity.

Emaciation is late and usually slight. There may be emacia-tion from urinary septicæmia which is not directly due to the malignant growth.

Intestinal symptoms are comparatively frequent. There is constipation, and in the later stages intestinal obstruction may supervene. Occasionally where the growth surrounds the rectum the symptoms of intestinal obstruction occur comparatively early and overshadow the urinary symptoms, leading to a diagnosis of malignant disease of the rectum.

On rectal examination the prostate is hard, irregular, and fixed. The malignant infiltration, whether in nodules or diffuse, is stony-hard. Small points or ridges may appear in the rectal surface, as hard and sharp as the edge of a flint.

Occasionally a malignant prostate is small and tough, and rarely it forms a large, soft tumour. The most frequent form is a moderate enlargement made up of numerous hard nodules separated by clefts and fissures, with at some part a hard, sharp ridge or point, which appears to project through the rectal wall. In a few cases (20 per cent.) the gland retains its normal contour and is enlarged, smooth, and stony-hard throughout. A single nodule of malignant growth may be buried in one lobe.

In advanced cases the prostate projects into the rectum as a large mass spreading over and surrounding the seminal vesicles and infiltrating the bladder base beyond the reach of the finger. This upward spread may be more marked on one side. Lateral spread of the growth fills up the sulcus on each side of the pros-tate, so that the gland on rectal palpation appears to be diminished in size. Spread round the rectum may form a thick ring which contracts the rectal lumen and is occasionally mistaken for a new growth of the rectum.

Enlarged lymph-glands are first felt as small shotty nodules in the band which passes outwards on each side at the base of the prostate.

On passage of an instrument there is obstruction in the prostatic urethra, and the tough character of the gland may be felt. Occasionally the prostatic urethra becomes distorted by the growth, so that the obstruction lies at the membranous urethra. On cystoscopy the gland projects into the bladder only to a small extent. The edge of the internal meatus is usually irregular and opaque; rarely the growth may be seen infiltrating the bladder mucous membrane.

Diagnosis.—Malignant growths of the prostate most closely resemble stricture of the urethra in their symptomatology, and stone in the prostate on rectal examination; but simple enlargement and atony from disease of the spinal cord may also give rise to difficulty.

In *s'ricture* of the urethra pain and emaciation are absent, and the symptoms commence at a much earlier age. The usual age at which symptoms of stricture appear is between 20 and 40; the average age in malignant growth of the prostate is 65. The use of the urethroscope, the passage of a large-sized bougie, and rectal examination will differentiate between these diseases. In *stone* in the prostate there is frequently an abundant pyuria and the grate of the stone may be felt on passing a metal instrument, if the cavity containing it communicates with the urethra. On rectal examination stone forms a single mass, even where a number of stones are present, while the malignant prostate has a number of irregularly shaped nodules with sulci between, and ridges and sharp points on the surface. The prostate is usually movable in stone, and crepitation is characteristic of a collection of prostatic calculi. The latter symptom is easily overlooked, and should be carefully searched for in doubtful cases. The X-rays give a dark shadow in the position of the prostate in stone, and no prostatic shadow in carcinoma. In *simple enlargemen!* the symptoms are usually those of irritation rather than obstruction in the early stage; the prostatic type of nocturnal frequency is typical of simple enlargement. Pain is absent, and rectal examination discloses an elastic, sometimes firm, but always movable enlargement of the gland, while the cystoscope reveals a rounded projection of one or both lobes. Hæmaturia is more frequent in simple than in malignant disease of the prostate. *Bladder atony* is diagnosed by examination of the spinal reflexes and exclusion of obstruction of the urethra. The cystoscope shows a trabeculated bladder of the atrophic type in atony from spinal disease (p. 533).

Treatment. 1. Palliative.—The majority of cases have progressed too far when the diagnosis is made for any radical operation to be considered. Treatment then consists in relieving symptoms. The administration of ergot (liquid extract, 15 minims)

and strychnine (liquor, 5 minims) increases the contractile power
of the bladder and assists in the expulsion of urine. The passage
of large metal instruments into the bladder at intervals of a week
or a fortnight gives much relief. In the majority of cases this
is unattended by any danger of bleeding; but when hæmaturia
is already a feature of the case, dilating instruments should be
avoided. With increasing obstruction and retention of urine
the catheter may become necessary. The passage of a catheter
is usually difficult, and the urethra may become so distorted that
self-catheterization is impossible. In such cases permanent suprapubic cystotomy becomes necessary. The bladder is exposed by
a vertical median suprapubic incision, which cuts through the
rectus sheath, and separation of the recti muscles. The bladder
is drawn up to the level of the skin, opened, and stitched to the
skin with catgut, and the recti muscles and sheath are closed
above it. In doing this the bladder should be drawn through the
rectus muscle on one side so as to obtain some amount of valve
action (p. 549). A tube is placed in the bladder through the cystotomy wound and retained there until the opening has contracted
down to the size of a No. 12 E. catheter, when an apparatus is fixed
consisting of a metal plate retained in position by elastic straps
and carrying in a tube a No. 12 E. rubber catheter, which lies in
the suprapubic wound and ends in a rubber urinal strapped to
the thigh. For the pain, phenacetin (10 gr.), antipyrin (10 gr.),
caffeine (3 gr.), or aspirin (10 gr.) should be given in cachet. Should
these fail, opium or morphia in some form should be allowed.
The injection of 20 minims of tincture of opium into the rectum
sometimes gives greater relief than hypodermic administration of
morphia. Radium-therapy has been used in several cases and has
given encouraging results, but at the present it is still under trial.

　　2. **Operative treatment.**—Only those cases in which the
growth is confined to the prostate should be submitted to radical
operation, and the patient must be sufficiently strong to withstand
a severe operation. Many operative procedures have been recorded,
but it is unnecessary to describe them here.

　　Suprapubic operations.—These consist in enucleation of the
malignant prostate with the finger after Freyer's method (p. 709).
In certain cases it is possible to enucleate a malignant prostate by
this method. These are cases of adenomatous enlargement which
have become malignant. In one type of case the enlargement
appears to be benign and is easily removed, and the presence of
malignant degeneration is only discovered on histological examination. In another type some part of an adenomatous prostate
can be felt to be tough and firmer than the rest of the gland. On

enucleation the prostate is found to be densely adherent to its sheath at one part, and after enucleation a dense leathery plaque remains adherent to the wall of the cavity.

The great majority of cases of malignant prostate are, however, quite unsuited for suprapubic enucleation. On opening the bladder the finger feels the base tough and adherent to the underlying prostate. There is much difficulty in commencing the enucleation in the region of the internal meatus, and when it is begun there is no line of cleavage into which the finger can sink. Eventually one or two portions of tissue of tough, indiarubber-like consistence are removed, together with the wall of the prostatic urethra. A conical cavity is left, with tough, irregular walls. There is little bleeding. The result of such operation is rapid recurrence, very frequently with sepsis superadded, and the period of existence is probably shorter, and certainly less comfortable, than it would have been without operation.

In yet another type one lobe is malignant and adherent while the other is adenomatous. The adenomatous lobe shells out. leaving the tough, malignant lobe adhering to the wall of the cavity. Some cases of so-called fibrous prostate are malignant in nature. Only shreds of indiarubber-like consistence can be removed by this method, and the operation is entirely unsuitable for such cases.

Perineal operations.—i. Prostatectomy may be performed in the same manner as for the perineal removal of benign enlargement of the prostate. It is wise in these cases to remove the sheath with the prostate, and to dissect the prostatic tissue from the urethra as thoroughly as possible.

ii. Young's operation consists in the removal of the prostate and its sheath, the prostatic urethra, the portion of bladder wall overlying the prostate, the seminal vesicles, and the lower end of the vasa deferentia. This is carried out by an inverted V perineal incision and exposure of the membranous urethra, which is opened on a grooved staff. A Young's prostatic depressor is now introduced and the posterior surface of the gland freely exposed. The membranous urethra is cut across, and the apex of the prostate depressed and pulled downwards and separated from the posterior surface of the pubic symphysis. A transverse incision is now made through the anterior bladder wall at the base of the prostate, and by further depressing the prostate this can be extended laterally so as to expose the upper surface of the gland, covered by bladder base. A transverse incision is made immediately in front of the ureteric orifices, and the bladder wall carrying these is pushed back, exposing the seminal vesicles and vasa deferentia.

2 v

The latter are cut across, and the prostate is now free. The opening in the bladder wall is closed with catgut sutures from behind forwards, leaving a small opening at the anterior angle, and this is brought down and united to the stump of the membranous urethra. The perineal structures are united, a rubber drain is placed in the wound, and a catheter tied in the urethra. At first there is complete incontinence, and a rubber urinal is worn ; but if care is exercised almost perfect control is regained by the action of the compressor urethræ, and every care should be taken to preserve this muscle as far as possible during the operation.

Results.—After suprapubic enucleation recurrence is usually rapid, few of the patients living longer than eighteen months to two years. Perineal prostatectomy gives temporary relief from symptoms, but the growth recurs in from one to two years.

Of 3 of my patients operated on by Young's method, 2 died of recurrence two years and the third three and a half years after the operation. Young has performed the operation 6 times, and 2 of his patients are alive and apparently well, one six years after the operation and the other two years.

LITERATURE

Adenot, *Ann. d. Mal. d. Org. Gén.- Urin.*, 1901, p. 596.
von Frisch, *Krankheiten der Prostata.* 1899.
Fuller, *Journ. Cutan. and Gen.- Urin. Dis.*, 1898, p. 581.
Greene, *N.Y. Med. Journ.*, 1903, p. 285.
Greig, *Brit. Journ. Child. Dis.*, May, 1908.
Harris, *Ann. Surg.*, 1902, p. 509.
Motz et Majewski, *Ann. d. Mal. d. Org. Gén.- Urin.*, 1907, i. 161.
Oraison, *Ann. d. Mal. d. Org. Gén.- Urin.*, 1903, p. 641.
Petit, Thèse de Paris, 1902.
Pousson, *Ann. d. Mal. d. Org. Gén.- Urin.*, 1904, p. 881.
Proust, *Prostatectomie Périnéale totale.* 1900.
Socin und Burckhardt, *Krankheiten der Prostata.* 1902.
Walker, Thomson, *Arch. of Middx. Hosp.*, 1905, vol. v. ; *Lancet*, April 11, 1908 ; *Pract.*, Feb., 1908.
Young, *Johns Hopkins Hosp. Repts.*, 1906, vol. xiv. ; IIe Congrès de l'Assoc. Internat. d'Urol., London, 1911.
Zuckerkandl, *Wien. med. Presse*, 1889, Nr. 7, p. 19.

CHAPTER LIX

CALCULUS OF THE PROSTATE

PROSTATIC calculi occur in middle life and old age. The average in 29 cases under my care was 50·6 years. The oldest patient was 72, the youngest 21 years.

Etiology.—There are three chief classes of prostatic calculi :

1. Calculi originating in the substance of the prostatic gland.
2. Calculi in the prostatic urethra.
3. Calculi in pouches communicating with the prostatic urethra.

1. Small bodies varying in size from a grain of sand to a millet-

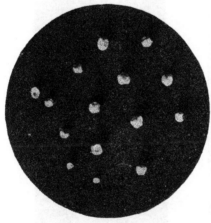

Fig. 235.—True prostatic calculi removed from prostate.

Fig. 234.—Collection of true prostatic calculi removed from prostate.

seed are found *in the prostate* at any age after puberty ; they are larger and more numerous in old age. They are round, oval, or polygonal (Figs. 234, 235) ; at first they are colourless, then yellow, brown, and finally black. The nucleus is homogeneous or granular, and shows remains of cell nuclei, and the periphery is laminated. These bodies are named *corpora amylacea,* from their starch-like consecutive laminations, and from taking a violet colour on the addition of potassium iodide.

In their composition two substances are present, an albuminoid and lecithin, the latter being a constituent of the prostatic secretion. The bodies may increase in volume and form split-pea-sized calculi scattered throughout the substance of one or both lobes, or a number may become cemented together to form irregular or nodular concretions the size of a split pea or even larger; or a number of small, polished, round, or faceted black prostatic

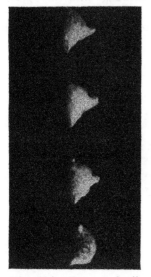 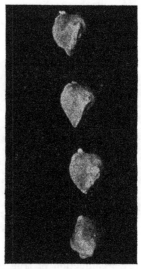

Fig. 236.—Four calculi, identical in size and shape, removed from prostate at intervals of 12 or 18 months.

Fig. 237.— Lateral view of the same calculi as in Fig. 236.

concretions, resembling small gall-stones, collect in a cavity in the substance of the prostate.

A small prostatic calculus of this nature may receive phosphatic deposits and form the nucleus of a large phosphatic calculus. These calculi are composed of phosphates, and they contain a considerable proportion of organic matter and calcium carbonate.

2. Calculi *in the prostatic urethra* are secondary, and are derived from the bladder or kidneys, having the composition of vesical and renal calculi. By phosphatic deposit the calculus increases in size and eventually projects through the vesical sphincter into

the bladder. The portion exposed to the urine in the bladder increases rapidly, and a mushroom form is produced.

3. Calculi *in pouches communicating with the prostatic urethra* are formed by the deposit of phosphatic salts from the urine. The origin of these pockets is sometimes obscure, but occasionally a history of the rupture of a prostatic abscess into the urethra can be obtained.

Such a cavity acts as a mould, and if, after removal of the calculus, the pocket is not destroyed a calculus again forms, and the successive calculi resemble each other to the smallest detail (Figs. 236, 237). The shape of these calculi conforms to that of the cavity. They usually project from it into the urethra, and a gutter is found on the urethral portion (Fig. 238), which is united with the prostatic portion by a neck. These calculi occur most frequently in young men.

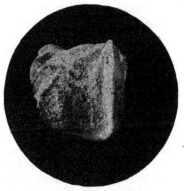

When calculi are present in the prostate the prostatic tissue becomes fibrous, and is reduced, in large calculi, to a mere shell which is adherent to its sheath.

Symptoms.—These are frequently obscure. Pain is usually present; it may be felt only during and after micturition, and is sharp and pricking; or it is a constant aching, un-

Fig. 238.—Prostato-urethral calculus, showing vertical groove along which urine passed.

connected with micturition and sometimes relieved by it, referred to the rectum, testicle, perineum, groin, or thigh. The pain is usually aggravated by defæcation. Hæmaturia is often present, as an occasional attack or as slight terminal hæmaturia.

In many cases there is purulent urethral discharge, which may be copious. Frequent micturition is a constant symptom, and is present day and night. Small stones may be passed when a collection occupies a pocket communicating with the urethra. As many as twenty calculi may be passed in this way. Difficult micturition and occasionally retention of urine are observed.

When the calculi are buried in the substance of the prostate their discovery may be accidental. The symptoms are usually those of posterior urethritis or chronic prostatitis. When the stone lies in the prostatic urethra or in a cavity communicating with it there are pyuria, frequent and difficult micturition, and sometimes retention.

On rectal examination a small collection of prostatic calculi is felt as a nodule in one lobe of the prostate.

A large stone, or a collection of stones, forms a mass in one or both lobes. The prostate is tender on palpation. Crepitation is usually present, and is elicited by pressure with the finger-pulp on the hard mass. It closely resembles the sensation given to the finger by emphysema of the skin or by teno-synovitis.

Diagnosis.—The passage of a sound gives no information if the calculus is buried in the substance of the gland; but if the stone lies in the prostatic urethra or in a pocket communicating with it, the metal instrument grates on its surface. When the stone is small and free in the urethra the sound may push it back into the bladder, and a second attempt may fail to find it until the bladder cavity is sounded.

On rectal examination a small collection of calculi may resemble inflammatory thickening in chronic prostatitis, or a tuberculous nodule. Crepitation may be obtained even in a small collection of calculi. The X-rays give a definite shadow in prostatic calculi (Plate 42), and none in chronic prostatitis or tuberculous nodules. In tuberculous disease there are frequently nodules in the epididymis. The nodules of chronic prostatitis are rarely so definite as to lead to a mistake in diagnosis.

Larger calculi may be confused with a malignant growth of the prostate. In malignant growth there are frequently multiple hard nodules, with deep sulci between; a hard, sharp ridge or point projecting on the rectal surface of the prostate is part of a malignant growth and not a calculus.

The gland is almost invariably fixed in carcinoma, but movable in calculus. Exceptions to this, however, occur. Crepitation is characteristic of calculus. The X-rays throw a heavy shadow in calculus, but no shadow in the prostatic area in malignant disease.

Treatment.—The method of removal of the calculus varies in different cases.

If the calculus is in the prostatic urethra and does not project into the bladder, the membranous urethra should be opened by a median perineal incision, and the stone removed by the finger aided by a suitable stone scoop. In mushroom-shaped calculi the suprapubic route should be chosen. A collection of small calculi in one lobe of the prostate should be removed by the perineal route. The posterior surface of the prostate is exposed by a transverse perineal incision, the sheath incised over the collection,

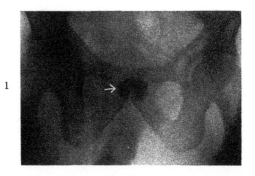

1

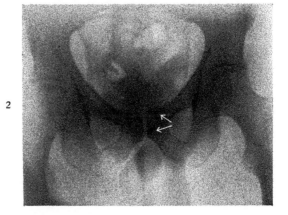

2

Fig. 1.—Shadow of large single prostatic calculus.

Fig. 2.—Shadows of small irregular scattered prostatic
calculi.

PLATE 42. (P. 742.)

and the calculi removed by means of a scoop and forceps without opening the urethra. When the prostate is slightly enlarged and calculi are present in both lobes, prostatectomy should be performed by the perineal route. If the enlargement of the gland is pronounced, suprapubic prostatectomy should be performed. When the calculus occupies a pouch communicating with the urethra the perineal route should be chosen and an endeavour made, by scraping with a sharp spoon and cutting with scissors, to destroy the pouch and prevent recurrence.

LITERATURE

Bonneau, *Ann. d. Mal. d. Org. Gén.- Urin.*, 1908, i. 1046.
Burckhardt, *Krankheiten der Prostata.* 1902.
Englisch, *Centralbl. f. d. Krankh. d. Harn- u. Sex.-Org.*, 1904, p. 19.
Falcone, *La Clinica Chirurgica*, 1909, p. 37.
Fürbringer, *Zeits. f. Urol.*, 1911, v. 169.
Pasteau, *Ann. d. Mal. d. Org. Gén.- Urin.*, 1901, p. 416.

PART VI.—THE SEMINAL VESICLES AND COWPER'S GLANDS

CHAPTER LX

ANOMALIES AND AFFECTIONS OF THE SEMINAL VESICLES—COWPER'S GLANDS

Anatomy.—The seminal vesicles are two hollow organs lying above the base of the prostate on the bladder wall between the bladder and the rectum. They are 2 in. long and ½ in. broad, lie transversely along the upper border of the prostate, and incline upwards, especially at the outer end. They are bound to the bladder wall by a layer of recto-vesical fascia continued upwards from the back of the prostate. Above and internally to the vesicles, and closely united to them, are the ampullary dilatations of the vasa deferentia. The ureter enters the wall of the bladder under cover of the seminal vesicle on each side. The recto-vesical pouch of peritoneum descends so as to cover about one-half of the breadth of each vesicle. The relation to the bladder cavity is shown by a line drawn from the mid-point of the trigone outwards and backwards so as to round the ureteric orifice and pass inwards parallel with and immediately behind the base of the trigone to the middle line.

Each seminal vesicle consists of a coiled and folded tube about 6 in. long, which has numerous diverticula. At the inner and lower end it unites by a narrow duct with the corresponding vas deferens at an acute angle to form the common ejaculatory duct, which opens on the verumontanum. The function of the seminal vesicle is to store spermatic fluid, to which it adds a secretion supposed to stimulate the activity of the spermatozoa.

CONGENITAL ANOMALIES AND ATROPHY

Congenital absence is rare, usually affects one side only, and is combined with other anomalies of the genital system such as malformation of the urethra and prostate and absence of the testicles. The condition of the vesicles is not so closely connected with that of the testicle as is the condition of the prostatic gland. The testicle and epididymis may be absent or rudimentary while the seminal vesicles are present and well developed, or the testicles may be well formed and the seminal vesicles absent. Multiple seminal vesicles have been described, the vesicle being double on one side. Atrophy has been noted in old age and after inflammation; it is independent of the condition of the testicles. The ejaculatory ducts may be absent or fused, or may open in some abnormal position.

SPERMATOCYSTITIS, VESICULITIS

Inflammation of the seminal vesicles may be either acute or chronic, and is invariably secondary to inflammatory disease of the urethra.

Etiology.—Sexual excesses and irregularities, the presence of stricture of the urethra, or chronic urethritis, prostatitis, or cystitis, are predisposing causes. The exciting cause is most frequently the gonococcus, and the vesiculitis usually complicates the course of an acute attack of gonorrhœa; but the infection may be due to other bacteria, such as the bacillus coli, staphylococcus, or streptococcus.

Pathology.—The wall of the vesicle is greatly thickened, and the mucous membrane swollen and bright red. The secretion is retained and mixed with epithelial débris, spermatozoa, and pus. The amount of pus produced is moderate, and empyema of the seminal vesicle is uncommon.

In chronic vesiculitis fibrous thickening of the wall takes place and perivesiculitis is commonly present. Atrophy of the mucous membrane occurs in some cases, and may affect the whole vesicle. If the outlet is obstructed the muco-purulent secretion is retained and the vesicle becomes distended. This may be combined with great thickening of the walls of the vesicles.

ACUTE SPERMATOCYSTITIS

Symptoms.—The symptoms of acute spermatocystitis are usually obscured by those of acute inflammation of the prostatic urethra. During an attack of gonorrhœa there are frequent and urgent micturition, discomfort at the neck of the bladder, scalding during the act, and there may be terminal hæmaturia.

Fever is sometimes present, but the temperature is rarely raised more than one or two degrees.

The symptoms which are specially produced by the spermatocystitis are painful erections and frequent emissions. The seminal fluid is stained dark brown with changed blood, or may contain bright blood in considerable quantity (hæmospermia).

There are deep-seated heavy pain in the perineum, pain and fullness in the rectum, and intense pain on defæcation. Heavy aching pain is felt at the base of the sacrum and in the region of the sacro-iliac synchondrosis, and testicular aching is common. A sensation of fullness in the bladder and rectum is usually present, and is unrelieved by emptying the bladder or rectum.

The patient is examined in the knee-elbow position on a couch. At the base of the prostate, passing upwards and outwards on one or both sides, a sausage-shaped swelling is felt. It is doughy and very tender.

Course and complications.—The inflammation is more often subacute than acute, and the symptoms detailed above are present in a slight degree. The spermatocystitis subsides as the inflammation of the posterior urethra becomes less acute. Pelvic cellulitis by spread to the surrounding cellular tissue is an occasional complication, and more severe general symptoms then develop. Prostatitis and epididymitis are frequent complications. Peritonitis and even pyæmia have occurred in rare cases. Rarely the vesicle becomes distended with pus, or an abscess may develop in the perivesicular tissue. The vesiculitis and perivesiculitis often become chronic.

Treatment.—In the acute stage active local treatment of the urethral inflammation should be suspended and the treatment confined to diuretics such as Contrexéville water and sandalwood oil. If the inflammation is severe, and if there is a rise of temperature, the patient should be confined to bed. The rectum should be emptied by a large soap-and-water enema. Severe pain and irritation are allayed by hot rectal douches or by the injection of a small quantity (10 oz.) of hot water containing antipyrin (20 gr.). Suppositories containing morphia (¼ gr.) and extract of belladonna (¼ gr.) should be introduced night and morning in an acute case. The acute stage lasts from a week to a fortnight, unless periprostatitis is present as a complication, when the duration will be more prolonged.

Chronic Spermatocystitis

Symptoms.—Chronic spermatocystitis is usually combined with chronic inflammation of the prostatic urethra.

There is a slight increase in the frequency and urgency of micturition, and the urine contains mucus and flakes. If posterior urethritis is absent the urine is clear. There may be slight urgency of micturition and scalding during the act.

The symptoms are chiefly sexual and nervous. There are frequent erections and emissions; the seminal fluid is mixed with pus, and may contain brown pigment from degenerated blood. The nervous symptoms are pain, depression, lassitude.

There are discomfort in the urethra and aching pain in the perineum, rectum, groins, thighs, sacral base, sacro-iliac synchondrosis, and frequently pains are felt in more distant parts such as the shoulders and neck.

In old-standing cases the patients become neurasthenic, dyspeptic, and sometimes almost melancholic.

Spermatorrhœa may be present, but this condition may occur without vesiculitis. It consists in the discharge of seminal fluid containing spermatozoa and other elements without erection or desire. The fluid is mixed with pus cells, and sometimes with red blood-corpuscles.

On rectal examination the vesicles are found to be thickened and tough, and their outline can be defined.

An atrophic type is also described.

Diagnosis.—The local symptoms may be slight and neurasthenia well developed, so that the vesiculitis is overlooked. The rectum should therefore be examined in all doubtful cases.

A dilated normal seminal vesicle can frequently be detected as a soft, sausage-shaped cushion. In chronic vesiculitis the wall is uniformly thickened and tough, and tenderness is in many cases present.

In tuberculous disease the vesicle is hard and nodular, and only a part of the vesicle may be affected. The vesicle frequently feels like a string of small beads, or there may be one or two separate nodules.

Chronic urethritis is often present and obscures the symptoms of chronic vesiculitis. The diagnosis is made by rectal examination, and by microscopical examination of the fluid obtained from the vesicles by massage.

If chronic urethritis is present the urethra is first washed by Janet's method. The patient is then placed in the knee-elbow position with a receptacle under the penis and the vesicles are massaged. The fluid may drop from the urethra into the receptacle, or may be expressed from the urethra by stripping it forwards. The presence of pus and blood in the expressed fluid indicates vesiculitis.

Treatment.—It is important to empty the vesicles of inflammatory products which accumulate in the branches and pockets of these hollow organs. This is done by massage. The patient is placed in the knee-elbow position, the forefinger of the gloved right hand is introduced into the rectum and feels for the vesicle above the corresponding lobe of the prostate. Unless the surgeon's finger is unusually short or the perineum of the patient deep, the forefinger reaches to the tip of the vesicle without difficulty (*see* p. 674). The finger strips the vesicle from without inwards and downwards with a firm, even pressure. This is done several times, and the second vesicle then treated similarly. The contents of the vesicle appear at the external meatus, or they may be expressed from the urethra, and are examined microscopically. Thomas recommends that the massage should be carried out with the patient standing with the legs widely. apart. When chronic urethritis is present the massage is followed by irrigation of the urethra by Janet's method. A metal shield or thimble to assist and extend the reach of the forefinger has been suggested, but is unnecessary. The treatment is repeated once or twice a week, and extends over several weeks. Great care should be taken to select the proper cases. Acute and subacute cases are unsuitable, and an exacerbation of subacute or acute symptoms should be. the signal for abandoning the treatment. Tuberculous disease of the prostate and seminal vesicles must be excluded with absolute certainty before undertaking vesicular massage ; much harm is done by applying it to tuberculous cases.

Suppositories containing ichthyol, 3 gr., or potassium iodide, 5 gr., should be introduced night and morning. Rectal irrigations of hot water are occasionally of benefit where pelvic cellulitis is present or where pain is a marked feature ; they are given each night. Occasionally cold douches are found more effective. Iodide of potash, 10 gr., is the best drug for internal administration. The treatment of chronic urethritis (p. 613) should run concurrently with that of vesiculitis.

Vaccine treatment should be resorted to in chronic cases. A vaccine is prepared from cultures obtained from the fluid expressed from the vesicles.

Operative treatment.—This may be called for in chronic vesiculitis which persists in spite of other treatment, but the cases in which it becomes necessary are rare. Fuller has strongly advocated vesiculotomy in intractable cases.

The vesicles are exposed by the curved prerectal incision of Zuckerkandl used for perineal prostatectomy. The patient is placed in the lithotomy position with a cushion under the sacrum, and the posterior surface of the prostate exposed. Further separation of the rectum from the base of the prostate with the forefingers exposes the vesicles. The rectum is displaced backwards with a suitable retractor and the cavity illuminated with a powerful head-light. The fascia over the seminal vesicle is incised and the organ separated by blunt dissection, care being necessary at the outer extremity, which is in close relation to the trunks of the prostato-vesical venous plexus. The vesicle is either laid open and drained or it is dissected up from without inwards and removed.

In Fuller's operation the patient is placed in a kneeling position with the chest on the table, and supported by assistants. An incision is made alongside the anus from the border of the coccyx downwards and inwards just within the inner border of the ischium to ¾ in. in front of the anus. A similar incision is made on the other side, and the anterior extremities of the two incisions are joined across the perineum. The rectum is separated from the urethra and prostate. The tip of the right forefinger searches for the apex of the seminal vesicle, and along it a grooved director is slipped. A knife is passed along this, and the point enters the apex of the vesicle, the vesicle being then laid open; and this is repeated on the second side. The cavity is curetted and packed. Fuller has performed this operation 126 times without a death.

The seminal vesicle may also be exposed by an incision above and parallel with Poupart's ligament; the steps are the same as in exposing the pelvic portion of the ureter. The exposure is not good, and the operation may be difficult in a stout subject. The seminal vesicles can be exposed at the bottom of the recto-vesical pouch after opening the peritoneal cavity by a vertical median suprapubic incision. The patient is placed in the Trendelenburg position and the intestines are packed off. A transverse incision through the peritoneum at the lower part of the recto-vesical pouch exposes the vesicles.

LITERATURE

Barnett, *N.Y. Med. Journ.*, May 21, 1910.
Eastman, *N.Y. Med. Journ.*, Oct. 27, 1900.
Fuller, *Med. Rec.*, 1909, p. 717: *N.Y. Med. Journ.*, May 30, 1908.
Gruber, *Münch. med. Woch.*, 1911, Nr. 19.
Lloyd, Jordan, *Lancet*, 1891, ii. 975.
Swinburne, *Journ. of Cutan. and Gen.-Urin. Dis.*, March, 1898.
Thomas, *Internat. Med. Mag.*, Jan., 1901.

TUBERCULOSIS OF THE SEMINAL VESICLE

The seminal vesicle is seldom affected alone. Most frequently either the epididymis or the prostate, or both, are also tuberculous. Of 94 cases of genital tuberculosis under my care the seminal vesicle was affected in 37 (39·3 per cent.), the infection being unilateral in 26 and bilateral in 11.

In only 3 cases was the seminal vesicle the only genital organ affected, and in but 1 was it the solitary focus of tubercle, the bladder being affected in the other 2.

The organ most frequently affected alone with the seminal vesicle was the epididymis (14 cases); the prostate was affected alone with the seminal vesicle in 5 cases, and both the prostate and epididymis with it in 16 cases.

The average age was 30 years, the youngest being 18 years.

The tuberculous process is very rarely in the form of miliary tubercle. In most instances caseous nodules are formed. The inner end of the vesicle is first affected, and later the whole organ becomes a nodular mass. The disease is chronic, and the wall may undergo fibrous induration, the vesicle shrinking to form a hard, rigid mass. Rupture of the tuberculous collection may take place after adhesions into the rectum or through the bladder wall into this viscus. Less frequently the abscess tracks downwards into the perineum, or unites with a prostatic collection and ruptures into the urethra.

Symptoms.—Usually the symptoms are slight, and they may be entirely wanting. The affection of the vesicle is generally discovered on examining a case in which tuberculous epididymitis or prostatitis is present, or vesical tuberculosis.

In rare cases the onset and course are acute, and acute gonorrhœal spermatocystitis is simulated.

The symptoms which point to tuberculous cystitis are sexual irritation, frequent erections, and painful and bloody emissions. There may be pain at the root of the penis or in the groin.

Frequent micturition is often present, and is due to involvement of the prostate and bladder base. Spread to the bladder may be slow, or a tuberculous collection may rupture into the bladder. In the latter case there is a history of hæmaturia, which may be severe, and of frequent micturition.

Rectal examination in the knee-elbow position shows a nodular vesicle. There is a single nodule at the inner extremity of the vesicle, or a series of nodules closely set, and when the whole organ is affected a hard, craggy, elongated body is felt lying just above the prostate and extending outwards and upwards. The vesicle is tender on palpation. The prostate may contain nodules.

On cystoscopy the bladder is normal, or if it has been infected from the vesicle it shows tuberculous lesions immediately behind the base of the trigone.

Course and prognosis.—In the majority of cases the course is very chronic. The vesicle may shrink and remain as a small, hard band for years without any change. After some years' quiescence renewed activity may lead to spread of the tuberculous process. The chief danger is that it may spread to the bladder, and the genital become urinary tuberculosis. This had occurred in 14 out of 37 cases under my care. Less frequently the kidney is affected alone with the seminal vesicle and other genital organs (2 cases).

Treatment.—The general condition of the patient should be improved by a nourishing diet with plenty of milk and cream, and cod-liver oil and malt, and he should live an outdoor life in a warm, dry climate.

Tuberculin treatment should be commenced as early as possible and continued for two or more years (see p. 689). The results of this treatment are good ; the tuberculous vesicle shrinks and becomes quiescent.

Operation.—Excision of the seminal vesicles has a small mortality (2 per cent.). The cases in which the seminal vesicles alone are affected being rare, it will usually be necessary to remove the prostate and epididymis at the same time.

The perineal route should be chosen (see p. 748). A sinus remains in a considerable number of cases, due to tuberculous infection of the wound. Urinary fistulæ have also been recorded.

The cases suitable for this operation are not very numerous. It should be followed by a prolonged course of tuberculin.

Where the epididymis is tuberculous on one or both sides, epididymectomy or castration may be performed in addition to this operation. It has usually been found that removal of the tuberculous epididymis or testicle has a beneficial effect on the seminal vesicle, and operation upon the vesicle may not be required. Heroic operations for the removal of the testicles, vasa deferentia, seminal vesicles, and prostate have not given satisfactory results and have been abandoned by most surgeons.

LITERATURE

Cholzoff, *Folia Urol.*, 1908, p. 555.
Guelliot, *Presse Méd.*, 1898, p. 193.
Legueu, *Bull. et Mém. de la Soc. de Chir., Paris*, 1905, p. 136.
Walker, Thomson, *Pract.*, May, 1908.

VESICULAR NEW GROWTHS AND CONCRETIONS

The seminal vesicle is occasionally invaded by carcinoma of the prostate. More frequently the ejaculatory ducts are obliterated, and the vesicles become distended and the walls thickened. Only two or three cases of primary carcinoma of the seminal vesicles are on record. I have diagnosed the condition clinically in two cases in which a growth that pursued a malignant course commenced in the region of the seminal vesicle.

Two cases of sarcoma have been described.

Single or multiple concretions are sometimes found in the seminal vesicles in middle or old age. They are fawn-coloured, yellow, brown, or black. At first they are soft, and consist of spermatozoa, mucus, and epithelium; on this phosphates and carbonate of lime are deposited, and a hard concretion is formed which may reach the size of a cherry. The ejaculatory ducts are frequently obstructed. There are sexual irritation, painful ejaculation, pain in defæcation, and occasionally aspermia. The concretion is felt as a round nodule in the seminal vesicle.

Soft concretions may be crushed with the finger and small calculi expelled by massage. It has not been found necessary to remove the concretions by operation.

COWPER'S GLANDS

Cowper's glands are two small tubular glands lying on each side of the membranous urethra between the bundles of the compressor urethræ. The ducts pass for an inch to open on the floor of the bulbous urethra; occasionally they unite to form a single duct which opens in the middle line. With the urethroscope and air distension of the urethra the ridge formed by the ducts can usually be seen on the floor of the bulbous urethra. Cystic dilatation of the duct has already been described (p. 659). With the forefinger in the rectum at the side of the membranous urethra and the thumb pressing up from the perineum, the gland of one side is between the finger and thumb, but it cannot be felt in the normal state. (*See* p. 555.)

Acute inflammation (badly named Cowperitis) occurs as a complication of acute urethritis, and is usually due to the gonococcus. An abscess may form, and points alongside the bulb in the perineum, or it may open into the bulbous urethra or rectum.

Chronic inflammation causes discomfort and pain on sitting. The gland can be felt as a hard, tender, pea-sized body.

If troublesome the gland should be removed, either by a transverse prerectal incision, or by an oblique antero-posterior incision alongside the bulb.

Carcinoma of Cowper's gland has been described, but is very rare.

PART VII.—THE TESTICLE

CHAPTER LXI

ANATOMY AND MALFORMATIONS—INJURIES AND WOUNDS—TORSION

Surgical anatomy.—The testicles are contained in the scrotum, separated by a median septum. The left hangs lower than the right. The organs are suspended in a vertical position by the spermatic cords, with the body turned a little outwards and the upper end tilted slightly forwards.

The gland consists of the testicle and the epididymis.

The testicle is covered by the visceral layer of the tunica vaginalis, which is adherent to it. This serous membrane covers the globus major and the outer part of the body of the epididymis, and dips in between the epididymis and the testicle on the outer side to form the digital fossa. The surfaces are lubricated by a small amount of serous fluid.

The testicle is covered by a dense fibrous capsule, the *tunica albuginea*. At the back of the testicle this forms a mass, the mediastinum testis, from which septa radiate through the gland to the inner surface of the tunica albuginea. In this connective-tissue framework are small collections of polyhedral cells like the cortical cells of the suprarenal capsules, and containing yellow granules. These surround capillary blood-vessels and are named the "interstitial cells" of the testicle. Between 150 and 200 compartments are formed by the fibrous septa, and contain the convoluted *tubuli seminiferi*, 300 to 400 in number. By the union of these tubules larger tubes (*tubuli recti*) are formed, and these form a plexus (rete testis) in the mediastinum. From the larger tubes *vasa efferentia*, 12 to 20 in number, emerge and enter the head of the epididymis.

The *epididymis* consists of a head (globus major), a body, and a tail (globus minor). It is attached to the back of the testis by the vasa efferentia, which enter the globus major, the body being attached only by areolar tissue. After entering the globus

2 w 753

major each vas efferens becomes coiled into a cone (conus vasculosus), and they all terminate in a single collecting tube (tube of the epididymis), which is coiled and twisted (15 to 20 feet long) to form the epididymis, and ends in the vas deferens.

Certain vestigial remains are found in relation to the testis and epididymis. The *vas aberrans* is a narrow coiled diverticulum 2–12 in. long, arising from the lower end of the canal of the epididymis. It originates in the Wolffian duct. The organ of Giraldès, or *paradidymis*, is part of the Wolffian body, and consists of several small, irregular masses of convoluted tubules situated on the front of the cord immediately above the head of the epididymis.

The *hydatids of Morgagni* are one or more small pedunculated bodies attached to the front of the globus major and testicle. They consist of blood-vessels and connective tissue, and may contain a canal lined by ciliated epithelium. They are remains of part of Müller's duct.

The spermatic cord contains the *vas deferens*, which lies behind the other structures and has the deferential vessels in close relation to it, the spermatic artery and plexus of veins (pampiniform plexus), lymphatics, sympathetic nerves, the remains of the connection between the tunica vaginalis and peritoneum (processus vaginalis), areolar tissue, fat, and smooth muscle fibres (internal cremaster).

The *veins* are arranged in two groups. The spermatic veins, surrounding the spermatic artery, arise from the upper part of the testicle and run in front of the deferential veins, which form the second group and surround the vas deferens.

According to Jamieson and Dobson,[1] the collecting *lymphatic vessels*, four to eight in number, ascend with the veins in the cord and in the subperitoneal tissues over the psoas as far as the point where the spermatic vessels cross the ureter ; here they part from the blood-vessels and extend fan-wise into the lumbar glands. The *lymphatic glands* are those glands of the lumbar group in front of and by the sides of the aorta and vena cava below the level of the renal veins, and are members of the external group. The glands of each testicle communicate with each other.

Descent of the testicle.—The testicle is developed in close relation to the kidney, and is invested by a layer of peritoneum, the mesorchium. Strands of non-striped muscle fibres (gubernaculum testis) connect the testicle with the pillars of the external abdominal ring, the front of the pubes, and with the skin of the scrotum, Scarpa's triangle, and perineum.

The testicle, before it commences to descend, is already low

[1] *Lancet*, 1910, i. 493.

down in the abdomen, and the distance from the external abdominal ring is very small.

By a gradual process of development, especially the development of the pelvis and the growth of the lumbar spine, the testicle comes to lie at the brim of the pelvis and reaches the internal abdominal ring at the sixth month. Preceded by a process of peritoneum (processus vaginalis), and accompanied by some fat and extraperitoneal tissue, the testicle now passes obliquely through the abdominal wall, reaching the external abdominal ring during the seventh or eighth month. At the end of the eighth or during the ninth month it has arrived at the bottom of the scrotum.

ATROPHY OF THE TESTICLE

"Atrophy" of the testicle may be arrest of development or atrophy after full development. Arrest of development is seen in the imperfectly descended and ectopic testicle, or the testicle may descend into the scrotum but remain infantile in its proportions. A varying degree of atrophy of the testicle is present in almost all cases of varicocele. Should both testicles fail to develop, the secondary sexual characteristics of the male do not appear. The voice remains a high-pitched treble, the face is smooth and hairless, the figure plump and rounded. Mental deficiency becomes evident in some cases.

Atrophy after full development may result from many conditions. In the majority, orchitis precedes the atrophy, which is a process of sclerosis. Epididymo-orchitis due to gonorrhœa, mumps, typhoid fever, bacillus coli or other bacterial infection, is the most common. Traumatic orchitis is a not infrequent cause, atrophy following a crush of or blow upon the testicle. Syphilitic orchitis is less common.

Orchitis is said to complicate mumps in 60 per cent. of cases, and atrophy very frequently results. Heller found that of 10 cases, in adults, of mumps complicated with orchitis, atrophy followed in 5. Torsion of the cord produces atrophy of the testicle. Atrophy has been known to follow injuries to the brain and spinal cord in some manner unexplained.

Senile atrophy occurs in extreme old age, but may commence as early as the fiftieth year in exceptional cases.

In cases in which the testicle has not developed, or the atrophy is due to cutting off of the blood supply, the testicle is soft and inelastic. On section there is widespread fatty degeneration, but no sclerosis. When the testicle has atrophied as the result of inflammatory changes due to syphilis or traumatism it is tough, or even hard, and the gland tissue is sclerosed, the tubules being compressed by the increased interstitial fibrous tissue. Occasionally the atrophied testicle following inflammatory disease is soft and flabby, and here the atrophy probably results from interference with the blood supply rather than from sclerosis of the gland tissue.

In conjunction with testicular atrophy the mammæ in rare cases become enlarged, either from an increased deposit of fat or from a true hypertrophy of the glandular tissue. When both testicles are atrophic, sterility ensues. Not infrequently sterility results from atrophy of one testicle and thickening of the epididymis, with blocking of the tube on the second side, the result of an attack of epididymitis.

Treatment consists in the treatment of the conditions causing atrophy. There is no means of arresting atrophy when it has once commenced.

ANORCHISM, MONORCHISM

Congenital absence of one or both testicles is an uncommon condition. It is not possible to obtain reliable proof of this condition during life, as the testicle may be undescended, or imperfectly descended, and very small. The testicle may be absent and the epididymis developed, but much more frequently the testis, epididymis, and part of the vas deferens are wanting. The portion of the vas deferens nearest the seminal vesicle is usually present, but occasionally this also is absent and the seminal vesicle is rudimentary.

In bilateral anorchism the external genitals are rudimentary, and the secondary sexual characteristics of the male do not develop. Other malformations may be associated with these conditions. The kidney and ureter may be absent, rudimentary, or malformed on the side on which the testicle is absent, and there may also be imperforate anus, urethro-rectal and vesico-rectal fistulæ.

INJURIES OF THE TESTICLE

Severe injuries to the testicles are uncommon. Kicks, falls astride, the blow of a cricket-ball, the impact of a wheel in carriage accidents, are the types of violence by which the injury is produced.

Extensive ecchymosis of the scrotum rapidly follows.

The testicle has been dislocated on to the pubes, the perineum, or even the thigh, but the more frequent form of injury consists in hæmorrhage into the testicle or epididymis. The blood may accumulate under the tunica albuginea, or form small collections in the substance of the testicle. Rupture of the tunica albuginea follows more severe crushes. Epididymitis and orchitis ensue.

Symptoms.—Severe shock results from a blow on the testicle, and Kocher quotes two deaths from shock caused by such an injury. In less severe cases there is a heavy, depressing pain, with nausea and vomiting. The testicle becomes tense and greatly increased in size, and the epididymis rapidly enlarges. The scrotum is swollen with effused blood, and widespread ecchymosis rapidly appears. The scrotum and testicle are intensely tender. Under treatment the pain and swelling subside, but epididymitis frequently follows and the hæmatocele persists. At a later date atrophy of the testicle frequently occurs. Suppuration occasionally follows injury.

Repeated injuries to a partly descended testicle result in fibrosis of an already imperfectly developed organ.

The relation of hydrocele, tuberculosis of the epididymis, and new growths to injury is not clearly defined, although it is common to obtain a history of a blow on the testicle in these diseases. There is danger of attributing to injury diseases of the testicle which were present before the injury was inflicted, and to which the injury merely draws attention.

Treatment.—Dislocation of the testicle is treated by manipulation under an anæsthetic, and, failing that, the displaced organ is exposed by operation and replaced in the scrotum. After severe injury to the testicle the patient should be confined to bed and the scrotum supported on a pillow or slung upon a broad band of strapping which passes between the thighs, and cooling lotions or an ice-bag applied. Where the tension and pain due to extravasation of blood within the tunica albuginea are very great, punctures with a tenotomy knife may give relief. When epididymitis and orchitis develop, hot fomentations should be applied. Very rarely abscess results and necessitates incision.

WOUNDS OF THE TESTICLE

These most frequently occur from the puncture of a trocar in tapping a hydrocele. The puncture in the tunica albuginea may be small and rapidly close, but not infrequently a hæmatocele is the result, and this may recur after tapping.

Incised and stab wounds occur apart from surgical procedures, and the testicle may be prolapsed through a wound in the scrotum and lacerated or incised.

Treatment.—Hæmatocele following puncture of the testicle is treated by rest in bed, support of the testicle, and an ice-bag. The collection should be withdrawn by tapping after some days. An operation may be necessary to remove masses of laminated clot.

An exposed incised testicle should be treated by suture of the tunica albuginea and replacement of the organ.

TORSION OR VOLVULUS OF THE TESTICLE

Torsion of the testicle is comparatively rare. Corner collected 100 cases from the literature and added 9 personal cases. The condition most often arises before or shortly after puberty. About 70 per cent. of cases occur before the age of 20. A case has been described in a child four hours after birth (Taylor). Torsion occurring in adults is uncommon, but a few cases have been described after the age of 40. The right testicle is the more frequently affected (60 per cent.), and the condition is always unilateral.

Etiology.—In the majority of cases the testicle is imperfectly descended, but a few cases are recorded (Edington) in which a fully descended organ was the seat of volvulus.

Abnormality of the cord exists previously to the torsion. According to Lauenstein the cord is broad, and the testicle lies with its long axis horizontal (reversion of the testis). From the lower end of the testicle the vas deferens arises, while the principal group of veins passes to the globus major at the upper end. Rotation of the horizontally placed testicle leads to twisting of these structures. Moreover, the testicle appears to be unduly mobile within the tunica vaginalis. This may be due to the gland hanging loose in the tunica vaginalis by a mesorchium formed of two layers of the serous membrane attached the whole length of the epididymis or only at the upper part. Adhesion to the bottom of the scrotum is said to be deficient in these cases.

The relation of the tunica vaginalis to the testicle and epididymis may be unaltered, but in some cases the epididymis has been found completely within the cavity of the tunica vaginalis.

The exciting cause is sometimes traced to muscular exertion or injury. Crossing the legs has brought on an attack.

Pathology.—Examined from the front the twist is from left to right on the right side, and from right to left on the left side. The pedicle is twisted from half a turn to four or five turns. The twist affects the cord; or, where the epididymis and testicle are separated by a considerable interval, the mesorchium formed by the tunica vaginalis between the structures may be twisted. The testicle and epididymis are engorged with blood from the venous obstruction. The organ is a deep purple colour, and patches of extravasated blood are found in the substance of the testis. Infection of the strangulated organ occurs early, especially if a hernia is present, and gangrene supervenes in 88 per cent. of cases, according to Scudder. The tunica vaginalis is filled with blood-stained fluid.

Symptoms.—There are recurring attacks of torsion after an injury or exertion, or occasionally during sleep there is a sudden attack of severe pain in the testicle, extending to the lower part of the abdomen and even to the loin. Collapse and vomiting follow, and the patient is pale and sweating, with a drawn, anxious expression. The temperature may be subnormal at first, but is not infrequently raised to 100° or 102° F. after a few hours. The pulse is rapid, abdominal distension has been observed, and constipation is often present. There may be a history of an imperfectly descended testicle, and not infrequently of several previous attacks of testicular pain and swelling. The skin over the testicle may be red and œdematous. A hard, very tender, tense swelling occupies the upper part of the scrotum close to the external abdominal ring, and the testicle is absent from the scrotum. The swelling is dull on percussion, irreducible, and shows no impulse on coughing unless a hernia is present above the testicle.

The attacks may last for one or several days and then pass off, leaving the testicle painful and tender, and after a time the organ atrophies.

Less severe attacks occur in some cases, and gradual atrophy of the testicle follows a series of slight attacks of pain and swelling. The cord is felt hard and tender at the area of torsion.

An acute attack frequently results in suppuration or gangrene of the testicle.

The number of attacks varies. In a case under my care a man of 24 had six attacks in three years, only one of which lasted more than twenty-four hours. The right testicle was finally a small, round, hard body, the size of a hazel-nut, lying near the external abdominal ring.

Diagnosis.—The conditions most likely to be mistaken for torsion of the cord are strangulated hernia and inflammation of the lymphatic glands of the groin.

In strangulated hernia the testicle is found unaltered and completely descended, collapse and vomiting are more severe, and constipation absolute. In lymphadenitis a source of infection can be demonstrated, the testicle and cord are normal, and collapse, vomiting, and constipation are absent.

Other sources of difficulty in diagnosis which may only be cleared up by operation are appendicitis in an inguinal hernia, embolism of the spermatic artery, and epididymo-orchitis in an imperfectly descended testicle.

Treatment.—Manipulation without operation has been successful in untwisting the cord in one known case. At an early stage, if the diagnosis is not in doubt and the testicle is sufficiently descended to permit of the necessary manipulations, an attempt may be made to carry out this treatment.

In the great majority of cases, however, immediate operation is necessary, the diagnosis from strangulated hernia being in doubt or the condition of the patient so gravè that radical measures are necessary. The testicle may be exposed, the cord untwisted, and fixed by sutures. In the majority of cases orchidectomy is necessary, and, if a hernia is present also, radical cure should be carried out. In chronic cases the testicle should be removèd, as atrophy is certain.

LITERATURE

Corner, *Male Diseases in General Practice.* 1900.
Cotte, *Lyon Méd.,* 1911, p. 758.
Dowden, *Brit. Med. Journ.,* April 29, 1905.
Edington, *Lancet,* June 25, 1904.
Lexer, *Arch. f. klin. Chir.,* 1894, p. 201.
Low, *Trans. Med. Soc. Lond.,* 1908, 1909.
Perry, *Birmingham Med. Rev.,* 1898, p. 270.
Scudder, *Ann. of Surg.,* 1901, p. 234.
Taylor, *Brit. Med. Journ.,* Feb. 20, 1897.
Van der Poel, *N.Y. Med. Rec.,* June 15, 1895.

CHAPTER LXII

CONGENITAL MALPOSITION — IMPERFECTLY DESCENDED TESTICLE—ECTOPIA TESTIS

THE testicle may fail to descend (Fig. 239), or may partly descend. Its retention in the abdomen or inguinal canal is cryptorchism, which may be unilateral or bilateral. The testicle may occupy some abnormal position not in the track of normal descent—this is ectopia testis.

Etiology.—Imperfect descent may be due to one or to several factors.

The mesorchium or peritoneal fold may be adherent, or it may be too long, so that the organ swings loosely and does not engage in the inguinal canal. The spermatic vessels or vas deferens may be short, or the testicle or epididymis is said in some cases to be too large to pass the inguinal canal. Usually, however, the organ is small and atrophied, and the imperfect descent is probably due, in part, to this. The de-

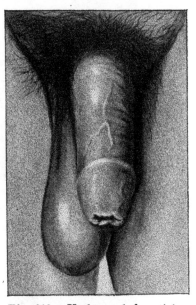

Fig. 239.—Undescended testicle.

velopment and attachments of the gubernaculum testis may be deficient. The inguinal canal, abdominal ring, or scrotum may be poorly developed. In ectopia testis the testis is drawn into an abnormal position by the fibres of the gubernaculum testis attached in that area, or the testicle is pushed into an abnormal position by a hernia.

Pathological anatomy.—The testicles are normally in the scrotum at birth, but the descent may be delayed.

761

A retained or imperfectly descended testis may reach the scrotum during the first year, but after that time it will not do so. In infants the testicles may temporarily disappear and **return** to the scrotum.

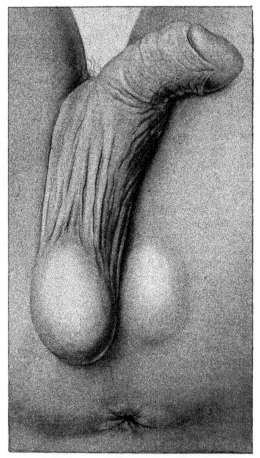

Fig. 240.—Perineal ectopia of left testicle (S. G. MacDonald's case).

Dukes found 9 cases of imperfectly descended testis in 2,000 public-school boys, and Corner states that this condition was present in 6·7 per cent. of 2,500 cases of inguinal hernia (children and adults) treated at St. Thomas's Hospital.

The right side is slightly more often affected than the left.

In imperfect descent the organ may be retained within the abdomen, or it may be in the inguinal canal, or at the external abdominal ring immediately outside the canal.

The ectopic testis may lie in the perineum (Fig. 240), Scarpa's triangle, in front of the pubes, or on the abdominal wall above Poupart's ligament.

Eccles considers it extremely doubtful if the testis is ever spontaneously passed into the upper part of the thigh through the femoral ring.

The communication of the tunica vaginalis with the peritoneal cavity (processus vaginalis) is usually open.

The imperfectly descended testicle is smaller and remains infantile in size (Fig. 241), but it is also said to develop to its proper size and then become atrophic.

The body and globus minor of the epididymis are frequently separated from the body of the testicle by a broad band of tissue, the mesorchium.

In structure the imperfectly descended testicle (Fig. 242) shows an

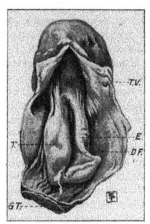

Fig. 241.—Operation specimen of imperfectly descended testicle and hydrocele surrounding it.

T., Poorly developed testicle. E., Epididymis. D.F., Vas deferens. G.T., Gubernaculum testis. T.V., Tunica vaginalis.

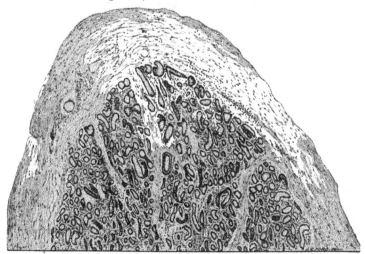

Fig. 242.—Section of undeveloped imperfectly descended testicle.

increase in the fibrous stroma, the tubules are smaller and fewer in number, and spermatoblasts and spermatozoa are absent. The interstitial cells of the testicle are present and fully developed. The scrotum on the side of the undescended testis is frequently undeveloped and smooth, the dartos muscle being absent. Sometimes, however, it is normal in appearance, and only smaller in size from the absence of the testicle.

Value of the imperfectly descended and ectopic testicle. —The testicle is incapable of producing spermatozoa, and if the abnormality is bilateral the individual is sterile. To this there appear to be a few exceptions, spermatozoa being present in the seminal fluid. The appearance of spermatozoa in these cases is delayed to the age of 20 or 22, and usually lasts only one or two years. Spermatozoa have, however, been found in rare cases as late as 35 years of age. Very rarely the subjects of double cryptorchism have been fertile. In these cases it is supposed that the imperfect descent results from obstruction rather than from congenital deformity.

Of 27 cases in which a microscopical examination was made the testicle was ill-developed and atrophic in 15, apparently normal with spermatogenesis in 10, tuberculous in 1, and malignant in 1 (Rawling).

The internal secretion of the testicle, which is believed to be furnished by the interstitial cells, is not abolished, and the development of manly characteristics is not necessarily arrested. The individual may be fully developed and virile.

Symptoms.—The great majority of cases seek advice on account of a swelling in the groin, which, on examination, is found to be the imperfectly descended testis with or without a hernia. The patient (or the parents if the patient is a child) is usually aware that the testicle is not in the scrotum, but this may not have been noticed. Pain is present and is the prominent symptom in about 25 per cent. of cases. It may be moderate and constant, or in recurrent attacks, or it may, less frequently, be very severe.

Complications. 1. Inflammatory.—The misplaced testis is subject to the inflammatory diseases which affect the normally placed organ. Thus, epididymitis may occur in gonorrhœal and other forms of urethritis and orchitis, in mumps, and the organ may become the seat of tuberculous disease. The abnormal position renders it especially liable to traumatism, and recurrent attacks of inflammation from this cause are common. Adhesions form between the testicle and the external abdominal ring and render the testicle less movable. The pain is usually severe, and it may be aecompanied by vomiting and collapse. There is a firm, exquisitely tender swelling in the position of the abnormally placed testis. Fluid may be present in the tunica vaginalis, and fluctuation is detected, but more often the sac is tense and fluctuation cannot be obtained. The skin may be unchanged, or red and œdematous.

Strangulated hernia or acute inflammation of lymphatic glands of the groin may simulate this condition. The history of recurrent attacks of inflammation and the absence of the testicle from the scrotum are important points in diagnosis. The general symptoms are seldom so severe in inflammation of the misplaced testis; the onset is more gradual, and the temperature is more likely to be raised than in strangulated hernia, where the onset is sudden, the collapse more profound, the vomiting more severe, and the constipation more complete. Local pain and tenderness are more pronounced in the inflamed testis. The diagnosis from inflammation of lymphatic glands in the groin depends upon the absence of any cause of lymphadenitis, the empty scrotum, the position of the swelling, and the history.

After the attack of inflammation has subsided the testicle remains tender, and eventually atrophy occurs after one or several attacks. The hydrocele may persist after the inflammation has subsided. Suppuration is a rare complication of the inflamed misplaced testis.

2. **Hernia.**—Incomplete closure of the processus vaginalis, and consequent hernia of the abdominal contents, is frequently associated with imperfect descent of the testis, and this is more likely to occur when the testis is retained in the inguinal canal than if it lies at the external abdominal ring. Corner found the communication open in 80 per cent. of 200 cases. In these cases the hernia usually occurs in infancy and is of the congenital variety. In a few cases no hernia is found. The most frequent form of hernia is a bubonocele; scrotal hernia is less common, and interstitial, crural, and perineal hernias are rare. Irreducible hernia, and very rarely strangulated hernia, have been noted.

3. **New growths.**—Any of the new growths that affect a fully descended testis may be present in the imperfectly descended organ. It is widely believed that malignant growths (Fig. 243) more often affect an imperfectly descended than a normally placed testis. Eccles found that of 40 cases of sarcoma of the testis the testicle was imperfectly descended in only 1, and in that case it was retained within the abdomen. It is significant, however, that of 57 consecutive cases of malignant disease of the testicle treated at the London Hospital, Russell Howard found that 9 were

cases of retained testis (16 per cent.)—an unduly large proportion. Of 54 cases of malignant disease of the testicle admitted
to the Massachusetts General Hospital, 6 (11 per cent.) were in
imperfectly descended testicles; and Schädel found that 5 in 41
cases (12 per cent.) of malignant disease were in partly descended
organs. There appears, therefore, to be some foundation in fact

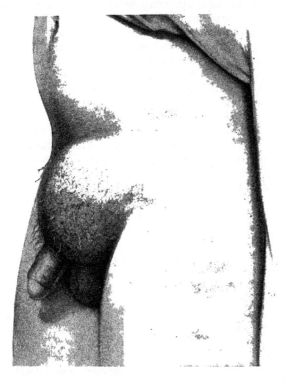

Fig. 243.—Malignant growth of imperfectly descended testicle.

for the view that the imperfectly descended testis is more liable
to the development of malignant disease.

The majority of malignant growths which affect the undescended
testis are sarcomatous in nature, while those found in the normally
placed organ are more frequently epithelial in type. The round-,
spindle-, and mixed-celled, and myxo-sarcoma, are the varieties
observed.

4. **Torsion of the cord.**—This condition, which is considered
elsewhere (p. 758), is especially frequent in association with im-

perfect descent of the testis. Torsion may take place when the testicle is in the inguinal canal or outside the external ring.

5. **Varicocele.**—Occasionally a displaced testicle is associated with varicocele, which may be felt underneath the skin. I have met with a large mass of varicose veins of the cord protruding from the external abdominal ring when an imperfectly developed testis occupied the inguinal canal above it.

6. **General changes and concomitant malformations.**— When both testicles are imperfectly descended and badly developed the general development of the body is likely to be affected. This is dependent upon the absence of the internal secretion of the testis. If the imperfectly descended testes are well developed, or one only is affected, there is no lack of growth. Other congenital deformities may be present, such as cleft palate, hare-lip, spina bifida, talipes, absence of one kidney, ectopia vesicæ, hypospadias, cleft scrotum, etc.

Treatment.—The testicle should not be left undisturbed, even where it is giving rise to no inconvenience at the time of the examination. The tendency of the development of hernia, the certainty of recurrent attacks of inflammation, the imperfect development or atrophy of the organ, the possibility of infection and of torsion, and the predisposition to the development of malignant disease, all render operative interference imperative.

Operation consists in (1) placing the testis in the scrotum, or (2) replacing the organ in the abdomen, or (3) removing the testicle.

If both testicles are retained within the abdomen operation is unnecessary. In such cases single or double inguinal hernia may be present, and operation for the radical cure of hernia becomes necessary. During this operation search should be made for a small testicle in the inguinal canal which may have escaped observation. If such a testicle is found it should be returned to . the abdomen if its fellow is retained, or removed if the second organ is normal and descended.

If both testicles are partly descended an attempt to bring them down into the scrotum by operation should only be made when there appears to be some prospect of success, the structures of the cord allowing a fair degree of downward excursion. Failing this, the testicles should be replaced within the abdomen. It is known that the testicle in these cases does not furnish active spermatozoa, but the internal secretion of the organ is usually active and is preserved. Corner recommends that the testicle be placed in the scrotum on one side and replaced in the abdomen on the other.

Where one testicle is fully descended and the other is only

imperfectly descended an attempt may be made to place the latter in the scrotum and retain it there. In the majority of cases, however, it will be better to remove the partly descended testicle at once and close the inguinal canal. The necessity for this course depends upon the recurrent attacks of inflammation due to trivial causes, the eventual destruction of the testicle by fibrosis, the development of hernia—all of which are certain to occur if the testicle is left untouched.

The age at which operation for partly descended testicle should be undertaken would be after the fourth year and before puberty. The best age for operation is from 8 to 10 years.

1. **Orchidopexy** consists in placing the testicle in the scrotum and fixing it there. An incision is made from a little below the external abdominal ring along the line of the inguinal canal to within an inch of the anterior superior iliac spine. The external ring is defined and the external oblique aponeurosis split as far as the internal ring. The peritoneal sac is now examined. If the communication between the tunica vaginalis and the peritoneal cavity remains open, this must be cut across just above the testicle and the lower end closed to form a tunica vaginalis, while the upper end, or the hernial sac if the communication has already closed, is dissected from the structures of the cord and ligatured at the internal ring. The testicle should now be thoroughly freed from all adhesions and the cord put upon the stretch. Steady, firm traction may considerably lengthen the cord. Bands of adhesions of the cord, strands of cremasteric muscle, and the coverings of the cord should be sacrificed in attempting to elongate the pedicle. In order to permit further elongation, some of the veins of the cord may be ligatured and cut across, the vas deferens, its artery and vein, being preserved. The epididymis may be separated from the testicle as high as the globus major and the testicle turned .upside down. The scrotum is now prepared for the reception of the testicle by introducing the finger or a pair of dissecting forceps into it from the inguinal wound. The testicle is then sutured to the bottom of the scrotum by invaginating the scrotum with the finger and suturing the testicle with silk, or a silk thread may be passed through the scrotum from without, carried through the tunica albuginea, and through the scrotum again from within outwards, and tied over a small pad of lint or gauze, or the ends may be attached to a wire cage fixed to the perineum. Corner recommends that a flap of tunica vaginalis and tunica albuginea be turned down from the lower pole of the testicle and sutured to the scrotum. The inguinal canal is now repaired as in a hernia operation, and the cord sutured to the external abdominal ring.

Mamourian, after opening the parietal layer of the tunica vaginalis, makes an opening at the lower end of the scrotum and draws the loose membrane through, stitching it with a purse-string suture so that a tuft projects.

If the testicle cannot be implanted in the scrotum without tension, the operation should be abandoned and the organ removed.

Results.—The imperfectly descended testicle is small, and it remains small after it has been transplanted into the scrotum. There is a tendency for the testicle to ascend again after this operation. It is doubtful if the spermatogenetic function of a small transplanted testicle becomes active, although there appears to be some evidence in support of this having occurred in a few cases. The internal secretion is preserved.

In 40 cases of attempted scrotal placement Rawling had 4 fair results, 3 promised unfavourably, 8 were not traced, 25 were failures. From these results he regards scrotal placement as doomed to failure from the beginning.

In perineal, pubic, and crural ectopia an attempt may be made to place the testicle in the scrotum. Should these operations fail, orchidectomy should be performed.

2. Replacement of the testicle in the abdomen. — The object of this operation is to save the internal secretion of the testicle. It is indicated, therefore, in bilateral cryptorchism before puberty. It is known that whatever spermatogenetic function the testicle may possess is lost after being retained in the abdomen for some time. Rare cases of paternity in double retained testis (cryptorchid) are known.

After the inguinal canal has been opened the testicle is placed in a bed in the extraperitoneal tissue and retained by a suture. The inguinal canal is then closed. The testicle may be placed within the peritoneal cavity, but cases of torsion of the cord have been known to occur after this operation.

3. Orchidectomy.—This is performed if one testicle is fully descended and the second imperfectly descended and atrophied. The testicle is dissected as before, the cord ligatured, and the inguinal canal closed.

LITERATURE

Bland-Sutton, *Pract.*, 1910, p. 19.
Cautwell, *Amer. Journ. of Surg.*, 1909, p. 322.
Coley, *Ann. of Surg.*, Sept., 1908.
Corner, *Male Diseases of General Practice.* 1910.
Eccles, McAdam, *The Imperfectly Descended Testis.* 1903.
Howard, Russell, *Pract.*, 1907, p. 794.

LITERATURE (continued)

Moschkowitz, Ann. of Surg., Dec., 1910.
Rawling, Pract., Aug., 1908.
Raymond, Amer. Journ. of Urol., Sept., 1909.
Zacharias, Arch. f. Gyn., 1909, p. 506.

INVERSION OF THE TESTICLE

The fully descended testicle may be displaced within the scrotum. In the usual displacement the free border of the organ looks backwards and the epididymis lies in front. Less frequently the free border faces downwards and the long axis is horizontal. Reversion of the testicle has been described, the upper pole being directed downwards and the vas deferens being attached to the tail of the epididymis, which was at the upper part of the organ. These congenital displacements are of importance in tapping a hydrocele and in other operations on the testicle.

CHAPTER LXIII

INFLAMMATION OF THE EPIDIDYMIS AND TESTICLE

INFLAMMATION of the testicle or epididymis may follow injury, but the two chief paths of infection are the urethra and vas deferens and the blood stream. In the two former the epididymis is affected, while in the latter the testicle is usually involved. In the majority of cases the epididymis is first affected (epididymitis). The testicle may be affected by spread of the inflammation (epididymo-orchitis). Less frequently the testicle is affected alone (orchitis).

EPIDIDYMITIS

This, the most common form of inflammation of the testis, may be acute or chronic. It occurs at any age, but is most frequent in early adult life.

Etiology.—Epididymitis may follow an injury, such as a blow or a kick, or may develop from a metastatic deposit in acute specific fevers such as smallpox, but in the great majority of cases it takes origin in a urethral infection. Gonorrhœa is the most frequent cause, the epididymitis appearing in the third or fourth week of the disease in 20 per cent. of cases. Less frequently epididymitis develops as a complication of old-standing chronic inflammation of the prostatic urethra following gonorrhœa. The passage of instruments in stricture of the urethra or enlargement of the prostate, lithotrity, prostatectomy, and the use of strong instillations in posterior urethritis are common causes. Chronic infection of the bladder, prostate, and prostatic urethra of non-gonorrhœal origin, such as bacillus coli infection, may give rise to acute epididymitis without any obvious exciting cause.

Pathology.—The infection reaches the epididymis by spread along the lumen of the vas deferens, or in some cases along the lymphatic vessels of the cord. Rarely, as in acute specific fevers, the blood stream is the path of infection.

In severe acute epididymitis the whole of the epididymis is involved, and forms a large mass in which the testicle is embedded. In less severe cases the tail only of the epididymis is affected. The

enlargement is due to inflammatory exudation around and between
the convolutions of the duct of the epididymis; small cavities
filled with pus are formed in localized dilatations of the ducts.
The walls of the duct are infiltrated, the epithelium is shed, and
the lumen contains a mixture of pus, epithelium, and spermatozoa.
The tunica vaginalis contains a moderate amount of fluid in about
one-third of the cases. The vas deferens is thickened and inflamed
and denuded of epithelium, and contains pus. There may be redness and œdema of the scrotum.

When the acute attack has subsided the swelling and tenderness disappear. Not infrequently, however, a nodular fibrous
thickening at the tail of the epididymis may persist for many
years or remain permanently.

Symptoms.—There is for some hours or one or two days dull,
heavy aching, and the epididymis and cord are tender. In severe
cases this is followed by an initial rigor, the temperature rises to
101° or 102° F., and the pain becomes severe and sickening in
character. Dragging pain along the cord, severe pain along the
inguinal canal and in the lower abdomen, and pain in the loins
are often experienced. Nausea and sickness are not uncommon.
The epididymis rapidly becomes swollen and forms a large, very
tender mass, in the front of which the testicle is embedded. It
attains its full size in from two to three days, and then remains
stationary. Some fluid can usually be detected in the tunica
vaginalis, and the skin of the scrotum is red and œdematous.
There is tenderness of the cord and along the line of the inguinal
canal, and the vas is felt per rectum to be thickened and tender.
The acute symptoms continue for from five to eight days and then
gradually subside, and the temperature returns to normal in ten
or fourteen days from the onset. The enlargement of the epididymis subsides slowly, lasting from fourteen days to four or six
weeks, and it may persist as a nodule at the tail of the organ.
When a urethral discharge has been present before the onset of
the epididymitis it disappears, and only reappears when the epididymitis subsides. Epididymitis may be bilateral, but the inflammation in one epididymis has partly or completely subsided
before the other is affected; double simultaneous epididymitis is
very rare. The extent to which the testicle proper is involved,
so far as it can be estimated clinically, is very small in the majority
of cases. When it is not concealed by an acute hydrocele the
testicle is found to remain unchanged in size and consistence, and
is not tender. In a few cases it shares in the inflammation, and
is tense, tender, and exquisitely painful (epididymo-orchitis).

Complications and sequelæ.—In epididymitis secondary

to urethral disease there is invariably infection of the prostatic urethra. Acute prostatitis not infrequently precedes the onset of epididymitis, but the prostate may escape. Seminal-vesiculitis is often present. Abscess formation is an unusual complication of epididymitis. Very rare in gonorrhœal epididymitis, it is more frequent in the form which results from other infections, such as epididymitis complicating stricture, enlarged prostate, etc. The abscess may form either at the head or at the tail of the epididymis. The scrotum is red and œdematous, and the epididymis quickly becomes adherent. The skin becomes thin and glazed, and the abscess ruptures on the surface. After discharging for a week or more the sinus heals, and when the epididymitis has subsided a fibrous track remains, binding a dimpled scar on the surface of the scrotum to the epididymis.

A fibrous nodule may persist after acute epididymitis, and is usually situated at the tail. Obliteration of the lumen of the epididymal duct at this point is not infrequently the result. When this is bilateral, or when the second testicle is imperfectly developed or atrophied, sterility results. Benzla found that in soldiers of the German army who had suffered from gonorrhœa 10·5 per cent. of those who had not had epididymitis were childless, while of those who had suffered from unilateral and from bilateral epididymitis the percentages were respectively 23·4 and 41·7. Atrophy of the testicle does not follow epididymitis when there has been no orchitis.

Tuberculous disease is stated to be a sequel of acute gonorrhœal epididymitis. This is not, however, my experience. The acute epididymitis which occasionally precedes chronic tuberculosis of the testicle is tuberculous in nature.

Treatment.—In the early stage it will be impossible to foretell the severity of the attack, and the patient should in all cases be confined to bed. Calomel, 4 gr., is given, followed by a smart saline purge, while local treatment of the urethra, if this has preceded the attack, should at once be discontinued. A low diet should be prescribed, with plenty of fluid, and if the pain is severe a hypodermic injection of morphia should be given. The scrotum should be supported ; this may be done by means of a well-fitting suspender or by a sand-bag or cushion of wool or other material placed between the thighs, or by slinging the scrotum in a triangular bandage, the base of which is carried transversely below the scrotum and the ends tied to a waistband, while the apex is brought forwards over the scrotum and penis and folded over the waistband in the middle line, a slit being made through which the penis protrudes. The testicle may also be supported on a piece of adhesive plaster, 4 in. wide, carried across from thigh to thigh, or a well-padded tray of cardboard may be made, with a semicircle cut out of the upper border to embrace the base of the scrotum, and slung round the waist.

During the first twenty-four or thirty-six hours a small bag of finely crushed ice applied to the testicle gives great relief. If this is not obtainable or is unsuccessful in relieving pain, and in any case after the first few hours, hot fomentations of boric lotion, or lead and opium lotion, should be applied, and changed every hour or two hours. Extract of belladonna in glycerine (equal parts) may be painted over the scrotum, and fomentations applied over this.

Guaiacol has been recommended in the acute stage. An ointment containing 6–10 per cent. is applied daily, care being taken not to cause dermatitis. Tucker recommends the local application of a saturated solution of magnesium sulphate on gauze kept constantly wet with the solution. The following ointment is recommended by Maurange : Methyl salicylate 20 parts, guaiacol 2½ parts, lanoline 15 parts, vaseline 25 parts ; this is applied after shaving the scrotum, and is covered with cotton-wool, a double spica woollen bandage being then applied over all. Painting the scrotum with nitrate of silver solution, 10 per cent., has been found useful. If acute hydrocele is present some relief of pain may be obtained by tapping it with a fine trocar.

Puncture of the testicle, at one time much in vogue, is now abandoned.

When the pain and tenderness in a severe attack have subsided the fomentations may be discontinued. In this and the later stages potassium iodide given internally and applied locally as an ointment (half strength of the unguentum potassii iodidi, B.P.) is of considerable value. Iothion (containing 80 per cent. iodine with equal parts of lanoline and vaseline) has been recommended.

The time during which the patient is confined to bed varies with the severity of the attack ; from ten to fourteen days is usual in a moderately severe attack. The application of a Julien suspender, by which pressure may be applied by means of packing, enables the patient to get about sooner when this is imperative. A relapse of the epididymitis is not uncommon if the patient is allowed to leave his bed too soon ; this should be guarded against.

Operative treatment of acute epididymitis has been recommended by various observers. Bazet advised epididymotomy and packing of the wound with ichthyol and glycerine (10 per cent.), and Belfield advocated incision and drainage. Baernamann in 1903 treated 28 cases by puncture.

Hagner makes an incision 2 in. long at the junction of the testicle and epididymis, and opens the tunica vaginalis. The testicle and epididymis are delivered, and the epididymis punctured in many places with a knife. If pus escapes the opening is enlarged and the cavity washed out with antiseptic solution by means of a fine-pointed syringe. The tunica vaginalis is washed and drained. The wound heals in ten days. Hagner operated in 25 cases, and claims that the pain at once disappears and the duration of the disease is shortened.

Puncture of the inflamed epididymis with a hypodermic needle has also been advocated.

In the subacute stage strapping the testicle is sometimes employed. This is carried out by a number of short strips of adhesive plaster applied from behind forwards and from above downwards, and crossing each other along the front of the testicle. The first strip confines the testicle to the lower extremity of the scrotum, the others apply gentle pressure over it.

Recurrent attacks of acute epididymitis may complicate catheter life in cases of enlargement of the prostate or other conditions where sepsis is present in the deep urethra. Where other methods of treatment have failed vasectomy has been practised with success.

In chronic epididymitis the inflammatory nodule is situated at the lower end of the epididymis. This may be bilateral, or the second testicle may be poorly developed and azoöspermia results. In sterile marriages the fault lies with the male partner in over 15 per cent. of cases, and in a large number of these there is azoöspermia due to chronic epididymitis of the globus minor.

For such cases Martin has introduced the operation of epididymo-vasotomy, by which an anastomosis is formed between the vas deferens and the head or upper end of the epididymis. The testicle is exposed and delivered from the scrotum and the head of the epididymis and the adjacent portion of the vas exposed by incising the coverings of the testicle. The most convenient method is to open the tunica vaginalis, when the globus major will be found lying in the cavity at the upper pole of the testicle. The vas is drawn through an opening in the tunica vaginalis at the level of the globus major. A portion of this part of the epididymis is excised, when a milky fluid will ooze from the cut surface ; this contains motile spermatozoa. The vas is incised longitudinally and its lumen opened ; the edges of this incision are stitched to the edges of the wound in the epididymis. Martin used fine silver wire ; I have found fine catgut sufficient for the purpose, but the silver wire is preferable, as it passes readily through the eye of the finest needle. The operation requires delicacy of touch, but presents no great difficulty. The needles must be rounded and very fine, as the wall of the vas cuts very easily. Before undertaking the operation the urethra, prostate and seminal vesicles must be examined, and any disease of these organs—such as stricture, chronic prostatitis, or seminal-vesiculitis—treated. Where there is chronic prostatitis of a severe grade the operation is contraindicated, as it is certain that it would be unsuccessful.

Martin records several cases. I have performed the operation in five cases. Motile spermatozoa have been found in the seminal fluid after the operation where previously azoöspermia existed.

LITERATURE

Baernamann, *Deuts. med. Woch.,* 1903, No. 40.
Bazet, *Amer. Journ. of Urol.,* May, 1906.
Benzla, *Arch. f. Derm. u. Syph.,* 1898, p. 33.
Ernst, *Berl. klin. Woch.,* March 8, 1909.
Hagner, *Ann. of Surg.,* 1908.
Martin, *Univ. of Pennsylvania Med. Bull.,* March, 1902.
    Therap. Gaz., Dec. 15, 1909.
Tucker, *Therap. Gaz.,* April, 1907.

ORCHITIS

In orchitis there is inflammation of the testicle proper. This may be combined with epididymitis, or it may follow an attack of epididymitis (epididymo-orchitis), but more frequently it occurs independently.

Etiology. — A urethral form of epididymo-orchitis following gonorrhœa or complicating stricture, enlarged prostate, etc., is rarely observed. Injury, such as from a blow or a kick, is the most frequent cause. Orchitis occurred in 5·6 per cent. of cases of operation for varicocele recorded by Corner and Nitch. Orchitis is the form of inflammation of the testis which follows metastatic infection, as in mumps, typhoid fever, smallpox, scarlet fever, influenza, malaria, and tonsillitis. The pain is usually severe, but it may be a dull, persistent aching radiating along the cord and into the loin and back. The testicle is enlarged, very tender, and may sometimes reach the size of a goose's egg. It is smooth, firm, and of uniform consistence, and the epididymis can be felt on its posterior aspect. The temperature is raised, and occasionally there is high fever.

There is no difficulty in differentiating orchitis from epididymitis by palpation. Hydrocele is excluded by the absence of translucency.

Symptoms.—In mumps the testicle becomes affected about the sixth or eighth day, when the swelling of the glands is subsiding. It occurs in boys and young adults, and is extremely rare in childhood and old age. I have seen a case of orchitis of this nature in a man of 58 years in whom the general symptoms were very pronounced, and the local symptoms comparatively insignificant. In 23 cases of mumps in an infantry battalion Kocher found 7 complicated with orchitis, and at the same time there were 4 cases of primary orchitis. Orchitis occurred in 9 out of 23 cases of mumps in schoolboys observed by Dukes. The onset of orchitis is preceded by a rise of temperature. The testicle is moderately enlarged and tender. The amount of pain varies; it may be slight or very severe. The epididymis and cord escape. After about four days the swelling subsides and quickly disappears. The second testicle may be attacked when the inflammation in the first is subsiding. In some cases the swelling of the salivary glands is slight; in the case just related it had been overlooked until close questioning elicited a history of slight swelling. In some epidemics of mumps orchitis has occurred when no trace of swelling of the salivary glands could be found. In such cases high fever and marked nervous symptoms may be present.

Atrophy of the testicle follows in a considerable proportion of cases. It is more frequent after the orchitis of mumps than in any other form; Kocher found it in over one-third of such cases.

Typhoid orchitis may occur during the course or convalescence of the disease, the latter being the more frequent. There is a rise of temperature, and occasionally a rigor. The local symptoms may be slight, and the course is usually rapid. Atrophy is a rare sequel.

Orchitis occurring during other specific fevers requires no special description.

Hydrocele is absent in orchitis. Suppuration is not infrequent in orchitis complicating specific fevers. When the temperature remains high and the testicle enlarged and tender, the formation of an abscess may be suspected.

Treatment is similar to that of epididymitis. Puncture of the testicle, at one time largely practised, is now abandoned. When an abscess is suspected an incision into the body of the testicle should be made; protrusion of the testicular gland tissue together with inflammatory material (hernia testis) frequently follows. With antiseptic dressing and pressure applied with adhesive strapping this will heal.

LITERATURE

Corner and Nitch, *Brit. Med. Journ.*, 1906, i. 191.
Dukes, *Lancet*, 1906, i. 861.
Higgens, *Brit. Med. Journ.*, April 18, 1908.
Maidlow, *Brit. Med. Journ.*, April 25, 1908.
Walsh, *Brit. Med. Journ.*, May 30, 1908.

CHAPTER LXIV

SYPHILIS OF THE EPIDIDYMIS AND TESTICLE

SYPHILITIC EPIDIDYMITIS

THE epididymis is rarely affected. Two forms of syphilitic epididymitis have, however, been observed : (a) In the secondary, or sometimes in the tertiary period, a subacute or chronic epididymitis develops in the globus major and may spread over the whole of the organ. The globus minor is rarely affected, nor is the body of the testis involved. The swelling is hard and painless, and usually bilateral, and appears in the third or fourth month, sometimes at a later date. (b) Small gummata are in rare cases found in the epididymis in the tertiary stage. The diagnosis of syphilitic epididymitis is made by the absence of urethral disease, the slow, painless development, the history of syphilis and the effect of antisyphilitic treatment.

SYPHILITIC ORCHITIS

Syphilitic orchitis occurs during the tertiary stage, usually two or three years after the infection, rarely at an earlier period (four to six.months). It either takes a diffuse form or develops as a localized gumma. Active syphilitic lesions may be present when the syphilitic orchitis develops, or the affection of the testicle may be the solitary manifestation of syphilis.

Pathology.—In the diffuse form the tunica albuginea becomes thickened at different spots, and there is effusion of fluid into the tunica vaginalis. The inflammatory thickening spreads to the fibrous framework of the testicle, which is at first densely infiltrated; later fibrous tissue forms. Contraction of the newly formed fibrous tissue causes atrophy of the testicle. Only part of the testicle may be affected, but usually the whole organ is involved.

The testicle on section is firm and may be hard. The thickened fibrous septa can be seen radiating from the rete testis. The tunica albuginea is thickened; the tunica vaginalis contains a small quantity of fluid and is thickened in patches or throughout. Fibrous adhesions form between the walls, and occasionally complete obliteration of the cavity occurs.

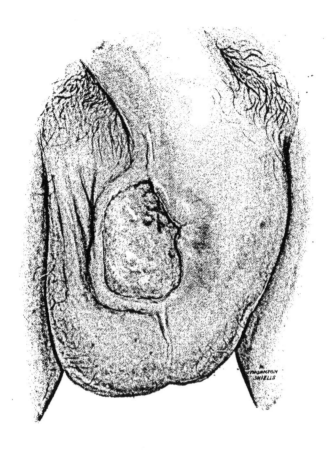

Gumma of testicle ulcerating on surface of scrotum.   (P. 779.)

PLATE 43.

The epididymis and vas deferens are unaffected.

Gummata may exist separately, or they may be found in a testicle the seat of diffuse syphilitic orchitis. There may be a single gumma or several gummata, varying in size from a pea to a chestnut. (Fig. 244.) They are yellowish-white, elastic, and soft in the centre. Around the central caseous portion there is a fibrous capsule of varying thickness, and outside this a greyish cellular ring. The changes in the tunica albuginea and tunica vaginalis are similar to those found in diffuse syphilitic orchitis.

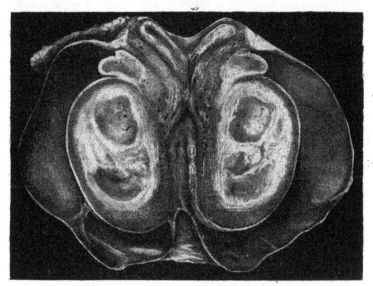

Fig. 244.—Gumma of testicle and hydrocele.

In the early stage the condition may disappear under treatment. Atrophy of the testis frequently follows.

A gumma may soften, form adhesions with the skin of the scrotum, and break through on the surface. A deep, crater-like ulcer with greyish-white base is now formed (Plate 43), or a fungating mass consisting of granulation tissue and necrosing testicular tissue may protrude (hernia testis).

In congenital syphilis diffuse orchitis may occur.

Symptoms.—The testicle becomes slowly and painlessly enlarged. Rarely the onset is sudden and the enlargement rapid, and there are pain and tenderness.

One testicle is affected, and the organ becomes greatly enlarged. A small hydrocele is frequently present. The testicle is oval, and may show one or more nodules, which are firm or hard. Testicular sensation is absent.

Diagnosis.—There is rarely any difficulty in distinguishing tuberculosis. This affects the epididymis and not the body of the testicle until a very late stage; it is rarely accompanied by hydrocele, and there are tenderness and testicular sensation. The formation of sinuses which heal and reopen is characteristic of tuberculosis. Tuberculous nodules may be found along the vas deferens or elsewhere in the genital organs. From new growth of the testicle the diagnosis is made by the history of syphilis and the effect of antisyphilitic treatment. A new growth is more nodular and less uniform in consistence, being soft in some parts and hard in others. The cord is frequently thickened.

Treatment.—Rapid improvement usually takes place under antisyphilitic treatment. Iodides are given alone or combined with mercury, and the testicle may be covered with Scott's dressing. Should any doubt remain in regard to the diagnosis between syphilitic and malignant disease, the testicle, which is already functionless, should be removed.

CHAPTER LXV

TUBERCULOSIS OF THE EPIDIDYMIS AND TESTICLE

THE epididymis is first attacked, the body of the testicle becoming involved later. This forms the primary focus in the genital organs in a large proportion of cases of genital tuberculosis (*see* p. 685). In children the body of the testicle is more frequently affected.

Etiology.—The disease occurs between the ages of 13 and 30, but may develop in adult life, and even in old age. Of 100 cases of genital tuberculosis under my care the genital system was affected alone in 50, the genital and urinary systems in 37, the genital system with tuberculosis elsewhere (lymph-glands, joints, vertebræ, lungs) in 13. Of the 100 cases the epididymis was affected in 72, and in 26 it was the only organ affected; in 16 it was affected with the prostate, in 14 with the seminal vesicle, and in 16 with the prostate and seminal vesicle. The tuberculous epididymitis where this organ only was affected was unilateral in 17 and bilateral in 9; where other parts of the genital system (seminal vesicle, prostate) were affected the disease was bilateral in 15 and unilateral in 31.

There is usually a history of tuberculosis in the family; and frequently there are obsolete and occasionally active tuberculous foci in other parts of the body.

A history of injury is commonly obtained, and experimental work on animals has shown that injury is an important factor in the etiology of tuberculosis of the testicle.

Previous infection with the gonococcus is believed to predispose to the development of tuberculous epididymitis. In the majority of cases there has been no gonorrhœal epididymitis, and in many no gonorrhœal infection of the urethra. Many cases, where the onset is very acute and the diagnosis of preceding gonorrhœal epididymitis is made, are probably instances of acute tuberculous epididymitis, the disease becoming chronic after some weeks.

Pathology.—The bacilli may be conveyed by the blood stream and deposited in the capillaries of the epididymis, or invasion of

the epididymis by way of the vas deferens may occur where the
disease is secondary to tuberculous prostatitis.

Macfarlane Walker has adduced evidence in support of the
view that the tuberculous infection commences in the prostate
and spreads along the lymphatics of the cord to the lower end of
the epididymis. The distribution of the tuberculous tissues, he
holds, suggests two opposing waves of infection—a primary one,
travelling from the prostate along the lymphatics to the epididymis ; and a secondary one, in the lumen of the vas and passing from
the epididymis towards the prostate, due to the flow of infected
secretions from the diseased epididymis.

The tuberculous process does not differ from that found elsewhere. Giant-cell systems are abundant, and bacilli may be
found. At first there is usually a single nodule, which spreads
until the whole epididymis is involved, the organ containing a
number of caseous nodules or a single irregular caseous mass.
Either the head or the tail of the epididymis may be affected, the
latter rather more frequently than the former. The tuberculous
nodule may soften and break down ; the skin becomes adherent
and thinned, and the abscess ruptures on the surface, forming
a fistulous tract, or more rarely a deep, crater-like ulcer. In
the late stage the testicle becomes involved and is the seat of
caseous masses, especially near the rete testis, and there are scattered tubercles throughout the substance of the gland (Plate 44).
If suppuration occurs and the abscess ruptures on the surface a
mass of granulation tissue and degenerating testicular substance
may protrude and form a hernia testis.

Symptoms.—There are two clinical varieties of tuberculous
epididymitis—(1) an acute, (2) a chronic.

1. **Acute tuberculous epididymitis** occurs comparatively
frequently. It is not uncommonly mistaken for gonorrhœal epididymitis, in spite of the patient's protests that no risk of infection has been incurred. There is sudden acute pain in the testicle,
the epididymis is tender and rapidly swells, and in two or at most
three days has reached a large size. There is often a purulent
urethral discharge, due in most cases to tuberculous prostatitis.
Tubercle bacilli may be found in this discharge. After some weeks
softening appears at one part of the epididymis and an abscess
forms and bursts. After this the epididymitis assumes a more
chronic form.

The points which distinguish acute tuberculous epididymitis
from gonorrhœal epididymitis where there is a possibility of recent
or old gonococcal infection are : (1) The pain and tenderness are
usually less acute ; (2) there is abscess formation ; (3) tuberculous

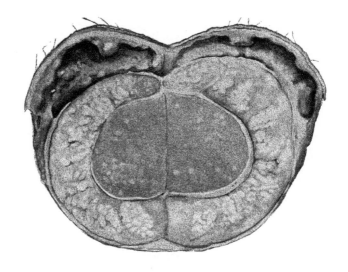

Tuberculosis of epididymis with tuberculous abscess under
skin of scrotum and miliary tubercle of testicle. (P. 782.)

PLATE 44.

lesions are present in the prostate, seminal vesicles, the second epididymis, or urinary organs; (4) the discharge is more watery and the urethral symptoms are slight or absent; (5) tubercle bacilli may be found in the discharge, and gonococci are absent.

2. **Chronic tuberculous epididymitis.**—A nodule develops insidiously in the tail or in the head of the epididymis. The attention of the patient may be attracted to it by some slight injury, when a nodule the size of a pea or bean is discovered; this is tender, hard, and either irregular in shape or smooth. Later the whole of the epididymis becomes involved, and forms a hard, irregular, craggy mass lying vertically on the back of the testicle.

Hydrocele is usually absent, but a small quantity of clear or flocculent fluid is present in the tunica vaginalis in about one-third of the cases. Adhesions between the walls frequently form. The tubercle bacillus is rarely found in the fluid. The vas deferens is frequently invaded, and may show a series of small nodular thickenings or a uniform thickening; or there may be nothing clinically to show that the duct is invaded, but microscopic sections reveal that it is tuberculous. There are tuberculous nodules in the seminal vesicles in 19·4 per cent. of cases, and in the prostate in 22·2 per cent.

Urinary tuberculosis is a frequent complication; it occurred in 37 per cent. of my cases. It is not unusual to find tuberculous epididymitis with tuberculosis of one kidney, usually on the same side.

The genital function of the testicle is destroyed early in the disease by blocking of the vas deferens. When the disease is bilateral the patient is sterile.

Diagnosis.—The diagnosis of chronic tuberculous epididymitis is made on the following points: (1) The insidious onset; (2) the absence of acute inflammation; (3) the hard, irregular, well-defined nodules; (4) breaking down and formation of sinuses which heal and again break down; (5) the presence of tuberculous nodules in the vas deferens and elsewhere in the genital organs; (6) tuberculosis of the urinary organs or elsewhere in the body; (7) a tuberculous family history. A fibrous nodule remaining after acute epididymitis of urethral origin is smooth, tough, and ill defined, and there are no nodules elsewhere. In syphilitic affections the body of the testis is affected and the epididymis remains free.

Course and prognosis.—The tuberculous nodule frequently breaks down and the abscess ruptures, forming a sinus on the skin of the scrotum. After discharging for some months or years this may heal. Later there is reaccumulation of fluid and the fistula again opens, and this may be repeated many times.

The progress is usually very slow, and spontaneous healing of the lesion may be observed, the craggy mass softening and shrinking, and only a tough thickening of the epididymis remaining. At some future date the disease may again become active, or fresh tubercle may develop in the second epididymis or other genital organs.

Acute tuberculous epididymitis subsides after a few weeks to a chronic form, not infrequently after the rupture of an abscess.

The course of chronic tuberculous epididymitis is slow and usually extends over many years. The disease does not, however, remain localized to one epididymis. In a few months, or after a year or more, a tuberculous nodule appears in the second epididymis. At this time nodules will very frequently be detected in the prostate, and in one or both seminal vesicles.

Tuberculous disease of the kidney, either on the same side as the affected epididymis or on the opposite side, may supervene, or the bladder may become infected from the prostate or seminal vesicles. In some cases the genital tuberculosis becomes quiescent, and occasionally it completely disappears, so that no trace of it can be discovered in the epididymis, a healed fibrous track leading to a depressed scar being the only evidence of bygone disease.

In other cases, after remaining quiescent for many years the tuberculous process awakens to renewed activity in the epididymis, or fresh tuberculous deposits appear in the genital organs or elsewhere.

Genital tuberculosis is a comparatively mild form of tuberculosis, and is not in itself dangerous to life : the chief danger is the involvement of the urinary organs. Tuberculous meningitis is a rare sequel.

Treatment. Non-operative treatment includes providing a liberal and nutritious diet and giving cod-liver oil, iodides (syrup of the iodide of iron, 1 teaspoonful thrice daily in milk), iron, and arsenic.

The testicle should be supported in a well-fitting suspensory padded with cotton-wool, and all possible causes of injury such as bicycle- and horse-riding should be interdicted. Local applications such as Scott's dressing are worthless. Residence in a warm climate is beneficial.

Tuberculin treatment can claim many successes. In a large number of cases the tuberculous nodule diminishes in size, becomes less hard and irregular, and eventually soft, and difficult or impossible to detect. This improvement takes place rapidly in some cases, but more usually slowly, and the treatment lasts a year or longer. In some cases, especially the more acute, an abscess forms, and after this is opened healing takes place. The dosage commences at $\frac{1}{10000}$ mg. (T.R.) and rises slowly to $\frac{1}{1000}$ or even $\frac{1}{800}$ mg.

Operative treatment consists in—

1. Conservative measures.
2. Epididymectomy.
3. Castration.

1. *Conservative measures* consist in opening and scraping abscesses as they appear, but no attempt is made completely to eradicate the disease. The wall of the cavity is rubbed with iodine solution or dusted with iodoform and lightly packed with gauze. These measures are used coincidentally with treatment by tuberculin and other general treatment.

2. *Epididymectomy* consists in removal of the epididymis and preserving the testicle. An incision $2\frac{1}{2}$ in. long is made from the external abdominal ring downwards over the testicle. If the organ is adherent to the skin of the scrotum, or if a sinus exists, this part of the scrotum is excised. The testicle is delivered from the wound and turned inwards, and the epididymis exposed by incision of the coverings. Care is taken to interfere as little as possible with the blood-vessels, and the arterial supply of the testis which enters the organ at the upper end of the epididymis is carefully preserved. The epididymis is freed by blunt dissection and detached from the testis, commencing at the lower end. The attachment of the globus major to the testis is cut across, the blood-vessels being avoided, and the epididymis is detached. The vas deferens is now isolated as far as the internal abdominal ring, the inguinal canal being opened up, if necessary, and ligatured. After all bleeding-points have been tied and the inguinal canal repaired, the wound is closed. The advantage of this operation is that the body of the testicle is not removed and its internal secretion is preserved. When one testicle only is affected this is not of such great importance as when the disease is bilateral, but the possibility of future infection of the second epididymis when the disease is unilateral must be considered. The operation of epididymectomy will allow of castration of the second testicle should this be necessary, and the patient will still retain the internal secretion of the first testicle. The objection to the operation is that tuberculosis may already have spread to the body of the. testicle and the operation is not radical.

In the common form of chronic tuberculous epididymitis the disease is confined to the epididymis, and the body of the testicle is only affected at a late stage. In subacute and acute cases the body of the testicle is more likely to be affected.

2 Y

When an isolated tuberculous nodule exists, or when the whole epididymis is converted into a very hard, well-defined mass and the testicle is soft, it is unlikely that the body of the testicle is invaded; but when the limitation of the disease is indefinite and its attachment to the testicle broad, spread to that organ may be surmised. It is frequently impossible, however, to make an accurate diagnosis as to the involvement of the testis. Scraping of the tuberculous testis after epididymectomy, or excision of portions of the body of the organ, is unsatisfactory, and orchidectomy is the only radical form of treatment when the disease has spread into the testis.

Permission for this operation, should it become necessary, must be obtained before commencing the epididymectomy. Necrosis of the testis from interference with its blood supply has been recorded.

The operation of epididymectomy is suitable for early tuberculous disease limited to the epididymis. It is contra-indicated in cases in which the body of the testicle is involved, or where there is advanced disease of the prostate and seminal vesicles or of the urinary organs.

3. *Castration.*—Removal of the testicle may be commenced by isolating and tying the cord, or by dissecting out the testicle and then tying and severing the cord. Of the two methods the former is the better. The penis is fixed to the opposite groin with a stitch; an incision is made about 2 in. long with its centre a little below the external abdominal ring, and the ring defined. The external oblique aponeurosis is slit up as far as the internal ring, and the cord isolated and transfixed with strong catgut. The two halves are carefully tied, one of the ligatures being finally passed round the whole cord and tied. The cord is cut across ¼ in. below the ligature; the lower end of it is stripped downwards and the testicle dislocated from the scrotum and removed, together with any portion of the scrotum which is adherent. The inguinal canal is now closed as in the radical operation for hernia, all bleeding-points· being carefully secured and a small drain placed in the lowest part of the scrotum for two days in case of oozing. Should the vas deferens be diseased at the internal ring it may be dissected up for some distance to the side of the bladder before tying the cord, and then tied and cut.

Von Büngner has introduced a method of forcible avulsion of the vas deferens by which the duct is pulled upon until it gives way at some point in the pelvis. Four-fifths of the length of the vas can thus be removed, and the deeper part is frequently found diseased, although no evidence of this could previously be obtained by the finger. Serious hæmorrhage in the depth of the pelvis has followed this operation in a number of cases, and it is not recommended.

More extensive operations have been practised by Villeneuve, Young, Pauchet, Marion, and others with the object of removing the whole tuberculous genital system.

Pauchet first lays open the inguinal canal and isolates the vas deferens as far as the neighbourhood of the seminal vesicle, cutting it with the cautery between two ligatures. The inguinal canal is now closed and the skin wound prolonged into the scrotum. If the epididymis alone is tuberculous the testicle is preserved, otherwise castration is performed. A transverse prerectal perineal incision is made, the prostate and seminal vesicles are exposed, and both removed if they are tuberculous. Young removes the vesicles and a portion of the prostate by a suprapubic T-shaped incision and separation of the peritoneum from the bladder. Such operations are only called for in exceptional cases of advanced genital tuberculosis.

Bilateral castration has a very deleterious effect, especially on older patients. They lose interest in their affairs, become indolent, irritable, and morose, and in some cases demented and maniacal, and some have committed suicide. It is possible also, judging from experiments on dogs, that the loss of the internal secretion may render the patients less resistant to the tubercle bacillus.

Choice of treatment and results.—If tuberculous disease is apparently limited to one epididymis, and epididymectomy or castration is performed, no further development of the disease may take place. In a considerable number of cases, however, the second epididymis becomes tuberculous, or nodules develop in the prostate or seminal vesicles, either soon after the operation or after a period of some years.

When one epididymis is affected together with the prostate and seminal vesicles, removal of the epididymis or castration is followed by marked improvement, and frequently by disappearance of the prostatic or vesicular disease.

Removal of both testicles in bilateral disease does not prevent the development at a later date of renal tuberculosis, or necessarily cause arrest in the progress of prostatic or vesicular disease, although it has an undoubted influence in causing the arrest of disease which is present, and preventing the appearance of fresh infection.

Of 45 cases of castration collected by König the prostate or vesicles were involved in 31, one testicle being affected in 17 and both in 14. Of the 17 cases in which one testicle was involved

14 were followed for over two years, and there were 10 complete cures, 1 case of improvement, and 1 death. Of the 14 bilateral cases 9 were cured, 2 improved, and 2 died.

Of 26 cases of epididymectomy recorded by Dimitresco 13 were traced for from one to nine years. There were 11 complete cures —7 unilateral, 4 bilateral.

Tuberculin treatment gives good results in chronic tuberculous epididymitis, and may be used either alone or for the treatment of prostatic or vesicular disease after removal of the tuberculous epididymis.

My practice is to treat chronic tuberculous epididymitis with tuberculin and to limit operative procedures to opening and scraping abscesses when they arise. If the disease appears to be spreading is spite of the tuberculin treatment epididymectomy is performed, and if it is already very extensive or has involved the testicle this organ is removed. I have not found it necessary to perform extensive operations for the removal of the pelvic portion of the vas deferens.

LITERATURE

Baudet, *Rev. de Chir.*, 1909, p. 952.
Bolton, *Journ. of Cutan. and Gen.-Urin. Dis.*, Dec., 1899.
von Büngner, *Centralbl. f. Chir.*, Nov. 18, 1893.
Carless, *Pract.*, July, 1901.
Cheyne, Watson, *Brit. Med. Journ.*, Dec. 30, 1899.
Dimitresco, Thèse de Paris, 1897.
Keyes, *Ann. of Surg.*, June, 1907.
König, *Deuts. Zeits. f. Chir.*, 1898, vol. xlvii.
Longuet, *Rev. de Chir.*, Jan., 1900.
Marion, *Arch. Gén. de Chir.*, 1910, p. 151.
Moullin, *Brit. Med. Journ.*, Jan. 13, 1900.
Pauchet, *Rev. de Chir.*, 1909, p. 195.
Poissonnier, *Gaz. des Hôp.*, March 16, 1907.
Southam, *Brit. Med. Journ.*, April 21, 1900.
Tylinski, *Deuts. Zeits. f. Chir.*, 1911, Hefte 4-6.
Walker, Macfarlane, *Lancet*, 1913, i. 435.
Young, *Ann. of Surg.*, 1901, ii. 601.

CHAPTER LXVI

NEW GROWTHS OF THE TESTICLE

New growths of the testicle are comparatively rare. Howard collected 65 cases in 110,000 male patients (0·06 per cent.) admitted to the London Hospital in twenty years.

Etiology.—The etiology of testicular new growths is unknown, but certain facts related to their development are recognized. There is a definite history of recent injury in about one-quarter of cases. Venereal disease has no relation to the occurrence of new growth.

The average age is a little over 30 years. The testicle has been the seat of new growth in an infant and in patients over 80 years. The "fibrocystic" growth occurs between the ages of 25 and 35. Each testicle is about equally affected, and with the exception of a single case of lymphadenoma (Monod and Terillon) the condition is invariably unilateral.

It is generally held that malignant disease occurs frequently in an imperfectly descended testicle. The London Hospital statistics support this view. Of 57 cases 9 occurred in retained testis (15·7 per cent.). The retained testis may lie within the abdomen, in the inguinal canal, or just outside the external ring.

Pathology.—All new growths of the testicle must be regarded as malignant. Tumours described as fibroma, adenoma, chondroma, myxoma, lipoma, and myoma are either the predominating constituents of a mixed growth or are so rare as to be of no clinical interest. An embryonal tumour may remain stationary for many years, but eventually takes on rapid growth.

The following arrangement of new growths is based upon the classification suggested by Nicholson :—

Embryoma ..
{ Fibro-cystic.
  Cystic (dermoid).
  Chorion-epithelioma. }

Carcinoma ..
{ Encephaloid { Alveolar.
                Non-alveolar. }
  Scirrhus. }

Sarcoma .... { Round-celled (lymphadenoma).
               { Myxo-sarcoma.

Endothelioma { Lymphendothelioma.
             { Hæmendothelioma.

An *embryoma* contains elements derived from the three primary
layers, epiblast, mesoblast, and hypoblast. When two or all of
these layers develop a mixed tumour results. (Fig. 245.) When one
element greatly predominates a tumour of corresponding struc-

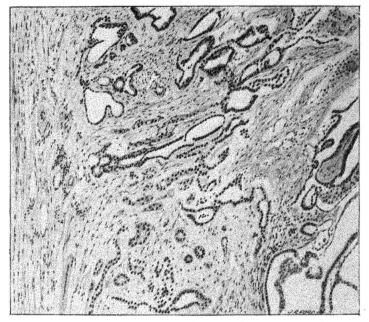

Fig. 245.—Section of portion of a mixed tumour of testicle.

ture results : a columnar-celled carcinoma develops from the
hypoblastic layer, a sarcoma from the mesoblast; and when the
epiblast alone develops, a growth formed of the epiblastic structures mentioned below is produced, or a chorion-epithelioma representing an earlier stage of development of epiblast may be formed.
When one layer is not found, usually the epiblast, it has either
been suppressed or overlooked.

The epiblastic structures found are stratified epithelium lining
cysts, or solid epithelial rods, or the epithelium may be of the
transitional type. Teeth, grey matter, rudimentary retina, and ·
portions of a spinal cord have also been found.

The mesoblastic elements may be connective tissue, embryonic or fibrous, myxomatous areas, hyaline cartilage, bone, unstriped muscle, lymphoid follicles.

Hypoblastic structures comprise columnar epithelium containing goblet cells, ciliated epithelium, alveoli resembling tubular glands.

The solid embryoma may show cystic spaces on section, but the whole tumour may consist of cysts of varying size separated by fibrous tissue, the variety known as " fibro-cystic growth " of the testicle.

Cystic embryomas or dermoids are very rare. They show a thick wall lined partly or completely with epithelium, and containing hair, sebaceous glands, teeth, nervous elements, etc. A process composed of elements from the three germinal layers with a large proportion of nervous tissue, and said to correspond to the anterior end of an embryo, projects into the interior. Barrington has described what appears to be a unique case in which a dermoid was combined with an alveolar carcinoma.

The embryomas all originate within the testicle. The tunica albuginea can be seen, and frequently a thin layer of testicular substance is spread over the tumour (Plate 45).

Of the *carcinomas*, Nicholson looks upon the columnar-celled variety as representing the preponderance in development of the hypoblastic layer in a teratoma. He recognizes, however, an alveolar carcinoma formed of groups of epithelial cells surrounded by a small amount of fibrous tissue carrying blood-vessels, and a non-alveolar which consists of cells embedded in an open meshwork of fibrous trabeculæ.

Sarcoma may be lympho-sarcoma or myxo-sarcoma. These tumours grow very rapidly, and are stated to affect both testicles and quickly form metastases, especially in the skin.

The *endotheliomas* resemble those met with elsewhere.

The comparative frequency of the different varieties is disputed, and until a more uniform view of the pathology is held no reliable information will be obtained in regard to this point.

The origin of the different varieties also is much disputed. Carcinoma is said to develop from the epithelium of the seminal tubules, and sarcoma from the stroma.

The embryomas have been said to arise in the following ways :—
    Cell metaplasia.
    Fœtal inclusion.
    Partial hermaphroditism.
    Fertilization of a polar body.
    An isolated blastoma.
    Remnants of the Wolffian body or Müller's duct.

Shattock has advanced the following theory for the origin of both ovarian and testicular embryomas. The ovarian (or testicnlar) embryoma results from the fertilization of one of the germ cells of the genital ridge by a stray spermatozoon. It is well known that several spermatozoa may penetrate the investing membrane of the ovum, and Shattock suggests that a spermatozoon other than that which fertilizes the ovum may remain alive and become buried in the cells of the segmenting fertilized ovum (morula) and eventually fertilize one of the primordial ova or germ cells of the fœtus, which are developed very early. The longevity of spermatozoa under favourable conditions is not known, but there is reason to suppose that it may be six weeks in fowls.

New growths taking origin in the epididymis are very rare. Rowlands and Nicholson describe a case of squamous-celled carcinoma of the epididymis.

Spread to lymph-glands takes place early. Those first affected are the lumbar glands, which lie along the inferior vena cava and aorta and extend from the bifurcation of the aorta as high as the renal arteries. The inguinal glands are sometimes affected without any involvement of the scrotal tissues. Bland-Sutton mentions a case in which a fibro-cystic growth formed a metastasis by way of the thoracic duct in a gland in the neck.

Symptoms.—In the early stage there is neither pain nor discomfort, but as the growth increases in size the patient complains of the weight of the testicle, and there is dragging pain along the cord, passing up to the groin; there is also pain in the loins. Where secondary deposits form in glands there may be shooting pain from nerve pressure, and œdema of the legs and ascites develop from pressure upon the vena cava.

In the later stage malignant cachexia becomes pronounced.

Enlargement of the testicle is confined to the body of the organ and does not affect the epididymis. The testicle is uniformly enlarged, forms a smooth oval tumour, and retains its normal shape; it may eventually reach the size of a cocoa-nut. As the tumour increases in size one or more rounded nodular swellings appear at the surface. These bosses are softer than the rest of the tumour, and are due to necrosis of the growth, or to a hæmorrhage into its substance. The testicle is heavy when supported by the hand. It is usually very hard, and is insensitive. In rapidly growing neoplasms with extensive degeneration the tumour may be soft, and even give an impression of fluctuation, which has led to puncture of the supposed fluid swelling. Testicular sensation is lost when the growth has destroyed the testicular tissue, but it is present at some part of the swelling in the early

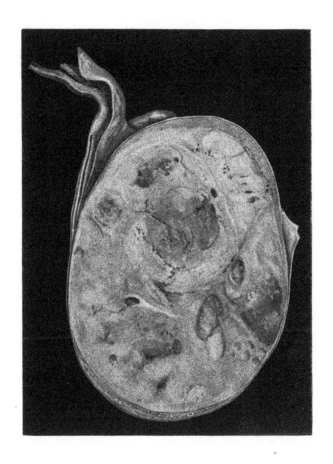

Solid embryoma of testicle; operation specimen. A thin
layer of testicular tissue can be seen surrounding the
growth. (P. 791.)

PLATE 45.

stage of development. The epididymis can be felt unaltered in the early stage; as the growth enlarges, it becomes flattened and stretched over the surface, and cannot be detected on palpation. The globus major may be felt at the upper part of the swelling.

Fluid is not infrequently present in the tunica vaginalis, but is moderate in quantity. It may occupy the whole sac or be confined to the upper or lower pole, the rest of the sac being obliterated.

The cord is usually unchanged, but there may be thickening due to hypertrophy of the cremaster muscle and engorgement of the veins. The veins of the scrotum may be engorged, and in the late stage the growth becomes adherent to the skin of the scrotum and eventually fungates. Enlargement of the lumbar glands forms a deep-seated mass lying alongside the spine at the level of the umbilicus. The inguinal glands may also be enlarged.

When the growth develops in a retained testicle that side of the scrotum is empty, and there is a large, hard, adherent swelling of irregular consistence in the inguinal region. (Fig. 243, p. 766.) There is frequently œdema of the leg from venous stasis, and the surface veins are dilated. In the intra-abdominal retained testis a deeply placed swelling is present, and ascites frequently develops.

The average duration of the disease when first seen was from six to twelve months, and the longest time was eight years in Howard's cases.

Diagnosis.—Difficulties in diagnosis occur in hæmatocele, hydrocele, gumma of the testicle, and tuberculous disease.

In hæmatocele there is usually a history of recent injury and of very rapid development, often with acute pain, or a hydrocele may have been tapped and rapidly filled again.

In cases of longer duration, with an indefinite history and no evidence of injury, the diagnosis may be difficult or impossible. An exploratory operation is the only certain method of diagnosis; puncture with the trocar is unsatisfactory and frequently inconclusive.

In a hydrocele with a thick, hard, sometimes calcareous wall the diagnosis may be difficult. There is usually, however, a history of repeated tappings, and there is no continuous increase in size. Exploratory operation will decide the diagnosis.

In advanced tuberculous disease which has spread from the epididymis to the testicle a large mass is formed and considerable difficulty may exist. Davies points out that in some growths a large part of the tumour is broken down, so that the whole anterior part is soft, while the posterior part retains its firm, irregular outline, giving rise to a condition resembling a tuberculous epididymitis with a soft testicle in front.

The pain and tenderness of the tuberculous testicle, the history and presence of tuberculous nodules in other parts of the genitourinary system or elsewhere in the body, help the diagnosis. Exploratory operation may occasionally be necessary before a diagnosis is finally made.

Syphilitic disease of the testicle produces a hard nodular testicle; the size of the testicle is never so great, the surface is more. nodular, the epididymis is distinct from the testicle, and there.is a history of syphilis and a positive Wassermann reaction. Treatment with mercury and iodides shows rapid improvement in syphilitic orchitis.

Treatment.—Removal of the testicle by operation at the earliest possible date is the only treatment that holds any promise' of cure. Castration by the usual method has been the operation practised until a recent date. The results have, however, been very bad, recurrence taking place in the abdominal lymphatic glands in the great majority of cases soon after the operation.

Recently, Grégoire, Bland-Sutton, Roberts, Davies, and others have advocated a more extensive operation, foreshadowed by Chevassu in his Thesis of 1906, by which the testicle and its lymphatic field as far as the first lymph-glands are removed.

The lymphatic system of the testicle has been investigated by Jamieson and Dobson. The collecting lymphatic vessels, numbering four to eight, leave the mediastinum testis and accompany the veins of the cord lying in the subperitoneal tissues on the psoas to the point where the spermatic vessels cross the ureter. At this point they spread out like a fan and, communicating laterally, empty into the lumbar lymph-glands. (Fig. 246.) The primary lymph-glands lie in front and at the side of the aorta and vena cava below the level of the renal veins. Each testicle has its own set of glands which communicate with each other. The actual distribution of the glands varies much in individual cases. They are contained in an area bounded above by the renal veins and laterally by vertical lines a fingerbreadth outside the aorta and vena cava, and extending below to the level of the bifurcation of the aorta. A gland may be found at the bifurcation of the common iliac artery.

The operation for removal of this lymphatic area may be extraperitoneal or intraperitoneal, the former being the preferable route. An incision is made over the spermatic cord, and extends upwards over the external abdominal ring and inguinal canal to a point

½ in. above and internal to the anterior superior iliac spine. It is then carried upwards to the costal margin at the tip of the 10th rib cartilage. The testicle and cord are dissected out and the abdominal muscles incised until the peritoneum is exposed. The cord is traced into the abdomen, the vas followed into the pelvis, tied, and cut across. The fascia covering part of the iliacus and psoas with its lymphatics and glands is dissected up. This stripping is carried along the psoas, being limited at the outer border of this muscle and by the line of the common iliac artery to the bifurcation of the aorta, the upper limit being at the level of the renal veins. The spermatic vessels are traced to the main vessels and ligatured. In doing this the ureter is separated from the peritoneum. The inferior mesenteric artery is carefully avoided.

This operation has been performed or attempted in 13 cases without as yet giving very encouraging results.

Results.—Chevassu collected statistics of 100 cases in which castration had been performed, and found 19 cures and 81 deaths.

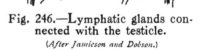

Fig. 246.—Lymphatic glands connected with the testicle.
(*After Jamieson and Dobson.*)

Death took place within the first year in 47 per cent. of the fatal cases. Of the cured cases, 13 were alive and well from four to seven years, and 6 from seven to ten years after the operation.

In the more extensive operation the growths were incompletely removed in 3 cases, 2 are known to have recurred, 1 was well after ten months, and 1 after two years. The remaining cases are too recent to possess significance. In a case of my own, inoperable glands were found under the diaphragm.

Of the London Hospital cases recorded by Russell Howard, only 36 could be traced after the operation. Of these 27 were known to have recurrence of the growth, and only 2 of the remaining 8 were known to be alive three years after operation.

LITERATURE

Barrington, *Lancet,* Aug. 12, 1910, p. 460.
Bland-Sutton, *Lancet,* Nov. 13, 1909, p. 1406.
Calin, *Du Traitement Chirurgical du Cancer du Testicule.*
Chevassu, *Rev. de Chir.,* 1910, p. 628 ; *Tumeurs du Testicule,* 1900.
Davies, Morriston, *Lancet,* Feb. 17, 1912, p. 418.
Ewing, *Surg., Gyn., and Obst.,* March, 1911.
Foulerton, *Lancet,* Dec. 23, 1905, p. 1827.
Grégoire, *Arch. Gén. de Chir.,* 1908, p. 1.
Howard, Russell, *Lancet,* Nov. 18, 1910 ; *Pract.,* 1907, p. 794.
Nicholson, *Guy's Hosp. Repts.,* 1907, xi. 249.
Roberts, *Ann. of Surg.,* 1902, p. 539.
Rowlands and **Nicholson,** *Lancet,* Jan. 30, 1909.
Shattock, *Lancet,* 1908, i. 479.

CHAPTER LXVII

IMPOTENCE AND STERILITY

IN impotence there is inability to perform the sexual act. Sterility implies a loss of procreative power and consists in the absence of living spermatozoa. The two conditions do not necessarily coexist in the same individual.

IMPOTENCE

Impotence may be (1) organic, (2) psychical, (3) atonic.

1. Organic impotence.—Here an organic lesion interferes with some part of the mechanism. The nervous apparatus may be the seat of disease, which affects the lumbar centres of the spinal cord or the nervi erigentes which convey the impulses. Thus, loss of erection is an early symptom in a large number of cases of tabes dorsalis, and may be observed in other syphilitic affections of the spinal cord. Malformations of the genital organs are frequently the cause of impotence. Absence or rudimentary condition of the penis and extreme deformities are incurable causes of impotence. Hypospadias is a frequent cause, and the impotence is due to the fixed downward curve of the penis, which becomes increased on erection, or to the orifice of the urethra being situated at the peno-scrotal junction or in the perineum.

Scarring of the erectile tissue from injury or other cause, and fibrous induration of the corpus cavernosum (p. 848), lead to lateral or vertical deviation of the penis in erection, and prevent coitus.

Phimosis, tumours, and œdema of the penis interfere mechanically with connection, also such conditions as large scrotal hernias, hydroceles, elephantiasis.

Anorchism and complete destruction of the testicular tissue from whatever cause are followed by impotence.

The treatment, where treatment is possible, will be found in the sections in which the different conditions are considered.

2. Psychical impotence.—This is a comparatively frequent form of impotence, and is due to nervousness, fear, or other emotions. It is initiated or increased by a failure, which is frequently attributed to the result of past indiscretion or excess.

In treating these cases it is necessary to gain the confidence of the patient and impress upon him the fact that the impotence is a common condition, that it is temporary, and is due to easily explained and quite easily treated causes, and not to past excess.

It is sometimes wise to forbid connection for a time. The general health, diet, and exercise should receive attention. The bowels should be regulated, the diet full and nourishing, and open-air exercise taken. Small doses of bromides may be given for a few weeks, and later, before marital relations are resumed, such stimulants as strychnine sulphate (gr. $\frac{1}{50}$ to $\frac{1}{20}$) and Johimbin hydrochlorate (gr. $\frac{1}{12}$) should be prescribed.

Other drugs and gland extracts that may be used are: Aphrodine chloride (tablets, $\frac{1}{12}$ gr.), sperminum (essence, 20 to 30 min.), orchitin ($7\frac{1}{2}$ gr.), "lymphoid compound capsules" (one capsule thrice daily), "lymph serum" (10 min. hypodermically).

3. Atonic impotence. — Here there is weakness of the lumbar centres, which leads to absence or weakness of erection or premature ejaculation. This may result from wasting disease such as phthisis, from uræmia, diabetes, anæmia, etc., or from poisons such as lead, antimony, alcohol, tobacco, opium, bromides, cocaine.

In the irritative form, where there is premature ejaculation, there is almost invariably some inflammatory condition of the prostatic urethra, due to gonorrhœa, stricture, sexual excess, irritating hyperacid or phosphatic urine. These conditions are amenable to treatment, and are discussed elsewhere.

STERILITY

The patient is usually potent, but living spermatozoa are absent from the semen. The number of sterile husbands in childless marriages has been calculated at from 10 to 20 per cent.

There may be—(1) aspermia, absence of ejaculation; (2) oligospermia, diminished quantity of semen; or (3) azoöspermia, absence of spermatozoa from the semen.

1. Aspermia.—There may be a want of co-ordination of the ejaculatory muscles, but in the great majority of cases there is obstruction in the urethra, which does not allow the semen to pass. Such conditions are congenital or acquired stricture of the urethra, or disease of the prostate, such as tuberculous disease, malignant growth, stone.

Aspermia follows the operation of suprapubic prostatectomy in 32·5 per cent. of cases.

2. Oligospermia. — The quantity of semen is deficient in fibrous induration of the prostate gland following suppurative or chronic prostatitis.

3. **Azoöspermia** may be due to failure of the testicles to produce spermatozoa, or to obstruction to the passage of spermatozoa from the testicle to the urethra—such conditions as bilateral atrophy, congenital or acquired, bilateral tuberculous disease, syphilitic disease, or malignant growth in a solitary testicle. Bilateral gonorrhœal epididymitis is the most common cause. The globus minor is the seat of a chronic fibrous nodule which surrounds and compresses the duct of the epididymis.

Azoöspermia follows prolonged exposure to the X-rays. It is not known whether this may become permanent or what length of exposure to the rays is necessary. Temporary azoöspermia follows sexual excess.

Diagnosis.—The treatment depends upon a careful diagnosis of the cause. The existence of azoöspermia is established by the microscopical examination of the freshly obtained semen. It is then necessary to find the cause, and the testicles, epididymis, vasa deferentia, prostate, and seminal vesicles are carefully examined for disease. Further, the urethra must be examined with the urethroscope, and the prostatic urethra, verumontanum, and orifices of the ejaculatory ducts inspected by the prostatoscope. The secretion of the seminal vesicles and prostate should be obtained by massage and examined microscopically.

Treatment.—Stricture of the urethra, prostatitis, seminal vesiculitis, and other conditions must be treated. Where both testicles are atrophied the prognosis is bad and treatment useless. Nodules in the globus minor which result from old-standing epididymitis should be treated by short-circuiting the vas deferens and globus major (Martin's operation). This should only be done after treating stricture of the urethra or other cause of obstruction (*see* p. 775). Chronic prostatitis with extensive induration of the gland is a contra-indication of the operation.

PART VIII.—THE TUNICA VAGINALIS

CHAPTER LXVIII

HYDROCELE AND HÆMATOCELE—NEW GROWTHS

HYDROCELE

By hydrocele is understood an accumulation of fluid in the sac of the tunica vaginalis, or in a sac in the cord or epididymis, or on the surface of the testicle apart from the vaginal sac. The common form, and that which is usually denoted by the unqualified name of hydrocele, is a chronic distension of the sac of the tunica vaginalis with fluid, unconnected with disease of the testicle or epididymis. There are, however, numerous other varieties (Fig. 247), some of which are frequently observed, while others are rare. The following varieties will be described either in this or in the next chapter, which deals with the diseases of the cord :—

Acute hydrocele.
Chronic hydrocele.
   1. *Hydrocele of the tunica vaginalis.*
      (*a*) Ordinary hydrocele.
      (*b*) Congenital hydrocele.
      (*c*) Infantile hydrocele.
   2. *Encysted hydrocele* —of the cord ; of the epididymis ; of the testis.
   3. *Diffuse hydrocele of the cord.*

ACUTE HYDROCELE

Acute hydrocele occurs as a complication of acute epididymitis, of gonorrhœal or other origin ; less frequently it complicates orchitis. Rarely, it occurs as the result of punctured wounds or blows or as a complication of specific fevers, such as smallpox or mumps, with or without involvement of the testicle. Acute hydrocele, the fluid of which contained the pneumococcus, has been known to complicate pneumonia.

The fluid, which does not usually exceed 3 oz., is rapidly poured out, and the swelling reaches its full size in two or three days. It is turbid, and contains flakes of lymph and leucocytes. An extensive deposit of fibrin may take place in the wall of the hydrocele (fibrinous or plastic hydrocele), and lead to the formation of

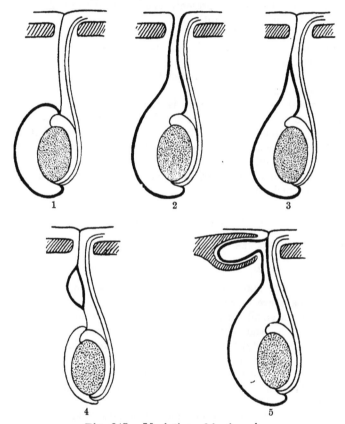

Fig. 247.—Varieties of hydrocele.

1, Vaginal hydrocele. 2, Congenital hydrocele. 3, Infantile hydrocele. 4, Encysted hydrocele of cord. 5, Interstitial hydrocele.

adhesions between the walls of the sac, and occasionally to partial or to complete obliteration of the cavity. Suppuration may follow, and form an empyema of the vaginal sac.

Symptoms.—The local signs consist in the sudden onset and rapid development of a tense, very tender swelling in the scrotum. The swelling is oval or pear-shaped, and the scrotum red and

2 z

sometimes œdematous. The hydrocele is translucent, but if there is extensive deposit of fibrin, or if suppuration has taken place, this character may be lost. In addition to the pain in the swelling there is dragging pain along the cord and in the groin. The symptoms of a specific fever or of acute inflammation of the epididymis or testicle are frequently present, and may obscure the fever caused by the acute vaginalitis.

Acute hydrocele in infants or young children may cause vomiting and prostration, and this, together with a tense, irreducible swelling at the external abdominal ring, gives rise to difficulty in diagnosis from strangulated hernia, which is only cleared up on operation.

Treatment.—The treatment is that of the underlying disease. If the quantity of fluid is small and the tension moderate, no special treatment need be directed to the hydrocele, but the pain of a large, tense, acute hydrocele is relieved by tapping with a trocar and cannula (p. 808).

Should suppuration occur, incision and drainage should be promptly carried out.

CHRONIC HYDROCELE

Hydrocele of the Tunica Vaginalis

(a) Hydrocele: Ordinary Hydrocele

In the normal state the visceral and parietal surfaces of the tunica vaginalis are in contact and glide upon each other, being lubricated by a small quantity of fluid. In hydrocele the sac is distended by a large accumulation of this serous fluid. The average age in this type of hydrocele is 67 years. The right and left sides are about equally affected in unilateral hydrocele. In about one-third of cases the hydrocele is bilateral.

Etiology.—In a small number of cases the commencement can be traced to an attack of epididymitis of urethral origin, or there may be underlying syphilitic or tuberculous disease of the testicle or epididymis. In other cases there is a history of initial or of repeated injury to the testicle. One patient under my care was employed in inspecting and repairing underground electric wires, and blamed the repeated minor injuries received in descending through manholes for the development of a very large vaginal hydrocele. It frequently happens, however, that the injuries are noticed only after the scrotal swelling has attained a considerable size, and is thus more exposed to blows. The wearing of a truss for inguinal hernia, and the occasional appearance of a hydrocele after the operation for varicocele, lend colour to the view that the accumulation of fluid is in some cases due to venous stasis.

In the majority of cases no cause, either local or general, can be found.

The two chief theories are that hydrocele is due (1) to inflammation, (2) to passive congestion. Both of these theories receive some support from the facts stated above, but they do not sufficiently explain the development of the great majority of chronic hydroceles.

Pathology.—In recently formed hydroceles the wall of the tunica vaginalis is usually thin and supple, but where the hydro-

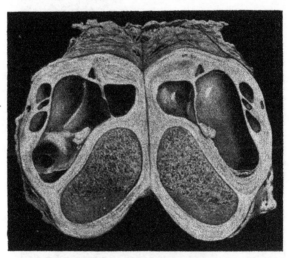

Fig. 248.—Multilocular thick-walled hydrocele.

cele is of long standing, and especially where it has been exposed to recurring injuries and repeated tapping, the serous membrane becomes thick and opaque, and a thick, firm layer of fibrous tissue forms from thickening of the subserous layer. (Fig. 248.) The wall of the hydrocele in such cases may measure ⅛ in. or more in thickness, and is as hard as cartilage. Calcareous deposit may take place, and plates are formed in the wall. Warty pedunculated tags may be found on the inner surface. Partial obliteration of the sac may result from adhesions of the walls. Layers or irregular flakes of buff-coloured fibrin may be found adhering to the wall in cases in which there has been injury, or attempted cure by injection of irritating fluids. There is usually a single cavity, pyriform in shape, which partly surrounds the testicle and epididymis, and

extends upwards for a varying distance along the cord in large
hydroceles, but is oval in the earlier state. An hour-glass shape
is occasionally observed, where a constriction which is due to a
thickening of the tunica vaginalis partly divides the cavity into
two parts (*hydrocèle en bissac*). Multilocular hydrocele is rare, and
the partitions between the separate cysts are formed by adhesions.
(Fig. 248.)

In large hydroceles a hernia of the hydrocele sac through the
coverings of the testicle may be found. (Fig. 249.) A round open-

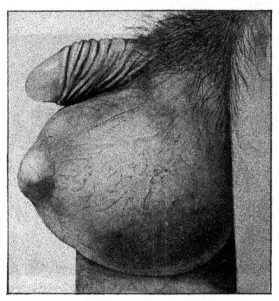

Fig. 249.—Hernia of a large hydrocele.

ing the size of a halfpenny, or larger, bounded by a hard ring of
fibrous tissue, can be felt, and through this the serous membrane
prolapses and forms a soft, secondary, reducible swelling beneath
the skin of the scrotum. In a case under my care the testicle
became prolapsed through this ring into the hernial sac. It could
be replaced in the main sac and again extruded by manipulation.

The testicle usually lies below and behind the sac, but rarely
it occupies a position in front of the hydrocele and is in danger
of being punctured in tapping the sac. In recently formed hydroceles the testicle is unchanged, but in an old-standing hydrocele
it is flattened, fibrous, and atrophied. The epididymis is fre-

quently widely separated from the testicle, and is elongated and flattened.

Hydrocele fluid.—The average quantity of fluid found in a hydrocele is about 6–8 oz. Hydroceles of record size are those of Gibbon the historian, from whose hydrocele, of thirty-two years' duration, first 4 quarts, then a fortnight later 3 quarts, then six weeks later 6 quarts were withdrawn. In another case, recorded by Maisonneuve, the hydrocele contained 21 litres (about 19 quarts).

The fluid is limpid, pale yellow to deep amber colour, has a specific gravity of 1022 or 1024, and contains albumin (6 per cent.), sodium chloride, and carbonate in large quantity. Microscopically, there are a few endothelial cells, occasionally some blood corpuscles, and a very few leucocytes.

The fluid does not coagulate spontaneously, as the fibrin ferment is lacking, but on the addition of blood the ferment is supplied and coagulation takes place.

The fluid may be dark brown, from the presence of altered blood. In some old-standing cases it is charged with innumerable glittering cholesterin crystals, which settle to the bottom of the glass on standing. The presence of these crystals is unexplained: They are more common in old-standing hydroceles than in those of recent origin.

Symptoms.—A small hydrocele forms a smooth oval swelling in the scrotum, replacing the testicle. As it increases in size it frequently becomes pear-shaped by extension of a narrower portion along the cord. The small hydrocele hangs free in the scrotum, but a large hydrocele mounts upwards to the base of the scrotum and is more fixed. (Fig. 250.)

The surface is smooth and regular, and the skin, although it may be stretched, moves freely over the swelling. There is no redness or œdema of the skin, and pain and tenderness are absent.

The consistence varies, but usually the swelling is tense and elastic, and a faint fluid thrill may be obtained. The testicle cannot be felt, but on palpation of the swelling the patient may be able to indicate its position by the testicular sensation. Occasionally the sac is lax and the testicle can be easily palpated. The cord is unaffected. The skin at the base of the scrotum may be dragged down by the large size of the swelling, and the penis may become buried, and the urine issue from a depression at the base of the enormously enlarged scrotum.

The hydrocele is translucent. The examination for translucency is carried out in a darkened room. The upper part of the hydrocele is grasped with the hand nearest the base of the scrotum and squeezed downwards so as to stretch the skin of the scrotum over it and make the sac tense. A strong electric light is placed close to the scrotum behind the swelling, and the surgeon's eye, brought to the level of the hydrocele, searches for translucency and examines the position of the testicle. The latter throws a slightly convex shadow, which appears at the margin of some part of the translucent oval.

The hydrocele is not translucent if the wall is thick or calcareous,

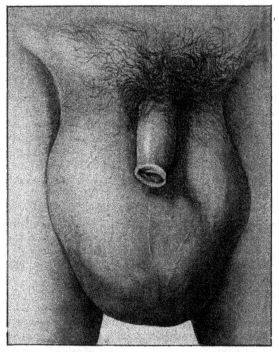

Fig. 250.—Hydrocele of tunica vaginalis.

nor if the contents are purulent or contain blood. In children a scrotal hernia may be translucent.

Diagnosis.—The diagnosis is usually easily made from the characters already given, but difficulty may be met with in the following conditions :—

i. *Scrotal hernia.*—A history can usually be obtained of hernia commencing at the upper part of the scrotum or of hydrocele commencing at the testicle. The hernia may diminish or disappear on lying down, or there is a history that it has done so ;

it has an impulse on coughing; it is resonant, or if dull has the irregular nodular feel of omentum; it is reducible with gurgling, and the testicle can be felt below the swelling. In a hydrocele, on the other hand, there is no variation in size, no impulse on coughing; it is dull on percussion, elastic or tense or fluctuant, irreducible, and the testicle cannot be detected apart from the swelling. The diagnosis may be difficult in an irreducible hernia and in children. The history of previous reducibility is important. The hydrocele may extend along the cord into the inguinal canal and receive a modified impulse on coughing. Difficulty may also occur in old-standing cases where the wall of the hydrocele is thick and opaque and is not translucent.

When a correct diagnosis cannot be made, operation should be recommended and puncture avoided.

ii.. *Hæmatocele.*—The history of an injury, of rapid development of the swelling, of tenderness, and sometimes of the swelling following the puncture of a hydrocele, assists diagnosis. There is frequently ecchymosis of the skin of the scrotum, and there may be creaking or crepitation from subcutaneous effusion of blood.

A hæmatocele is not translucent, and is heavier and less elastic to the touch.

In a difficult case, puncture or an incision into the swelling will give the diagnosis.

iii. *Malignant growth of the testicle.*—There may be difficulty when the wall of a hydrocele is thick and opaque. Irregularity of outline and consistence and steady increase in size are important characteristics of new growth.

Complications. i. **Hernia.**—Inguinal (Fig. 251) or scrotal hernia may coexist with hydrocele, especially where the latter is large and of long standing. At first the two swellings are distinct, but at a later stage they become fused, and diagnosis is rendered difficult, especially when the hydrocele sac is thick and opaque and the hernia irreducible. The hernia may have the following relations to the hydrocele sac: (*a*) It may lie above it, either separated from it or closely united to it. (*b*) It may pass behind it. (*c*) It may invaginate the sac, or may actually rupture into it. The latter condition may give rise to difficulty of diagnosis in a hernia operation. The chief points in diagnosis of a combined hernia and hydrocele are the history, the impulse, reducibility, and tympanitic note of the hernia, and the elastic fluctuant feel and the translucency of the hydrocele.

ii. **Rupture.**—In some cases rupture takes place spontaneously without any apparent cause, or more frequently as the result of traumatism, such as a kick, a blow, or violent muscular effort. I have seen two cases of rupture resulting from coitus. Hastings has recorded three cases and reviewed the literature of the subject. The hydrocele is large, and the wall is usually the seat of irregular fibrous thickening, calcification, or fatty changes. The rupture is slit-like or irregular, and may affect any part of the sac, being slightly more frequent on the anterior aspect. The serous layer of the tunica vaginalis is usually affected alone, but the fibrous layer may also be torn. There is a tearing sensation in most cases, not amounting to pain. Occasionally the rupture has taken place during sleep. The swelling grows large, less defined, and softer, and the scrotum rapidly becomes œdematous on the affected · side; the œdema then extends to the whole scrotum, and affects the penis, and may spread to the abdominal wall and perineum. Discoloration of the scrotum appears in twenty-four hours. The œdema subsides · and disappears, and the hydrocele sac is found to be empty. Cure may follow, but usually the sac refills.

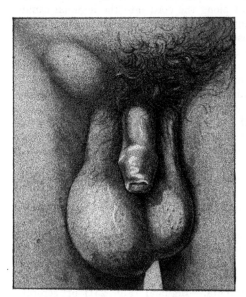

Fig. 251.—Hydrocele and inguinal hernia.

iii. **Suppuration.**—This is rare, and usually follows injury or tapping, but may be spontaneous.

iv. **Hæmatocele.**—A hydrocele may become filled with blood after tapping or injury, or from some unknown cause.

Treatment.—The treatment is (a) palliative, which consists in tapping, or (b) radical, which includes tapping combined with injection of irritating fluids or various operative procedures.

Tapping a hydrocele.—A small-size trocar and cannula should be selected, as the larger sizes cause more pain and are more likely to injure a vein. The trocar and cannula are boiled and the scrotum is washed with antiseptic solution, or a small area is painted with

tincture of iodine. The position of the testicle is defined by examining with a strong light. The surgeon grasps the neck of the scrotum above the hydrocele with the left hand, and squeezes the
hydrocele into the lowest portion of the scrotum, making the skin
over it tense and smooth. (Fig. 252.) The trocar and cannula is
held in the right hand, steadied below the shield with the forefinger 1 in. from the point of the needle. A point on the anterior
surface near the lower pole of the swelling is selected, and care is
taken to avoid the testicle and any large vein. The puncture is
made by a stabbing movement and with confidence, so that the
needle is plunged into the sac for an inch or more.

The trocar is detached by pushing the shield with the forefinger and is then withdrawn, and the cannula pushed in up to
the shield. With the forefinger on the shield the cannula is retained
in position while the pressure is kept up by gradually tightening
the grasp of the left hand.

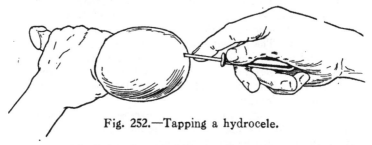

Fig. 252.—Tapping a hydrocele.

The position of the hands is maintained throughout until the
last drops of fluid are squeezed out, when the cannula is withdrawn and the puncture sealed with collodion.

The following accidents may occur :—

i. *Puncture of the testicle.*—This is due to want of care in localizing the testicle.

ii. *Incomplete emptying of the sac* from the cannula slipping out
of the vaginal sac between this and the scrotum, the result of
neglect to hold the cannula in place with the forefinger. The
fluid infiltrates the scrotum. It is useless to attempt retapping
then, as the hydrocele becomes so soft that the needle will not
enter. Retapping will probably be required in a week or ten days.

iii. *Hæmatocele* is due to puncture of a large vein from want
of care or the use of too large an instrument, or to puncture of
the testicle (*see* p. 815).

iv. *Septic complications*, such as cellulitis, should not occur.
In infants a hydrocele may be tapped by making a number of

punctures with a sterilized surgical needle. The fluid oozes away from the surface, and also infiltrates the tissues of the scrotum.

Results of tapping.—In rare cases a cure results from tapping a hydrocele. These cases are probably of the inflammatory type, and not the ordinary chronic hydrocele. Recurrence takes place at a variable period, usually about six months, but sometimes less.

Tapping and Injection.—By this method an attempt is made, by the introduction of irritating fluids after tapping, to cause adhesions of the serous surfaces and thus prevent recurrence by obliteration of the sac. The hydrocele is tapped in the manner already described, and when the last drops of fluid are expressed a syringe containing the irritating fluid is applied to the cannula, the fluid injected and the sac manipulated. Part or all of the fluid is allowed to drain off, and the cannula withdrawn.

The following solutions have been used, viz. tincture of iodine (Edin. tincture), 2–4 drachms ; carbolic acid (1 drachm of crystalline carbolic acid kept liquid with the addition of 10 per cent. of glycerine). Of these the carbolic-acid injection is preferred, as it gives less pain. The patient should be kept in bed for twenty-four hours and on the couch for several days, after which he may get about with the scrotum well slung. Swelling of the hydrocele appears in twenty-four hours and begins to decrease in fourteen days, disappearing in three or four weeks.

The *complications* of injection are (1) excessive inflammation, (2) suppuration, (3) slow absorption of the fluid, (4) recurrence of the hydrocele, (5) carbolic-acid poisoning.

The cases suitable for this operation are thin-walled hydroceles of moderate size. Large hydroceles and those with thick fibrous walls are unsuitable.

Results.—Recurrence takes place in from 8 to 10 per cent. of cases. Multilocular hydrocele may follow. The results are somewhat uncertain, and complications, such as excessive inflammation, may ensue and necessitate a longer convalescence than an aseptic operation. The method has therefore been abandoned by most surgeons.

Operation.—(1) *Excision of the sac.*—The scrotum is shaved and carefully prepared. The hydrocele is made tense with the left hand, and a longitudinal incision 2½ in. long is made on it through the scrotum and covering of the testicle. The coverings are carefully stripped from the hydrocele sac, which is then opened and the fluid allowed to escape. The serous sac is now stripped as far as the epididymis and the attachment to the testicle, and clipped away. All bleeding-points are very carefully ligatured.

Stitch sutures may be necessary, and occasionally a continuous suture may be run round part of the edge of a thick sac. The testicle is returned to the scrotum, a drain inserted for twenty-four hours, and the scrotal wound stitched.

The patient remains in bed for a week, and then gets up with the scrotum slung in a suspensory bandage.

(2) *Jaboulay's operation.*—After exposure of the hydrocele sac it is opened in its whole length along its anterior surface, and each lateral half turned backwards so as to meet behind the testicle. The redundant sac is cut away and the edges of the reduced layers are stitched together behind the testicle, or the sac is turned inside out and drawn up along the cord and stitched in position.

(3) *Wyllys Andrews' " bottle " operation.*—After exposure of the sac and careful dissection of the upper pole or the funicular process, a small opening (2 cm. long) is made at its extreme upper limit, the testicle displaced through this so as to lie outside the sac, the inverted sac drawn up the cord, and the scrotal wound closed.

Jaboulay's and Andrews' operations have the advantage of rapidity, and there are no bleeding-points which might cause a hæmatoma. Only a comparatively small number of cases have been treated by these methods, and the results recorded have, on the whole, been good, but recurrence has taken place in some instances. Cases where the sac is thick, fibrous, or calcified are unsuitable for these operations.

Autoserotherapy.—Gilbert introduced the therapeutic use of the patient's own serous exudations in 1894; the method has been extensively used in cases of pleural and peritoneal effusion, and articles have been published by Lemann and by Marcon. Bertholou employed this method in a case of hydrocele. He punctured the sac with a hypodermic needle and withdrew 2 c.c. of the fluid and injected it subcutaneously in the thigh. After a second injection the hydrocele diminished and disappeared. It had not recurred in a month. I gave the method a trial in 25 consecutive cases of hydrocele, and found that after puncture and hypodermic injection of hydrocele fluid (30–40 minims or more) the hydrocele diminished, and in some cases appeared to be cured. Recurrence took place, however, in all cases after a comparatively short period, varying from weeks to months. In order to determine whether the disappearance of the fluid might be due to leakage from the puncture or reduction of tension, I treated a case of bilateral hydrocele by puncture and injection of fluid from one hydrocele. The punctured hydrocele diminished in size and the fluid almost disappeared, but the unpunctured hydrocele remained unchanged. I concluded that the improvement was due to the puncture, and corresponded to acupuncture used in infants.

Following the idea thus suggested, threads of silk and catgut were introduced through the hydrocele sac, leaving an inch at each end, and by manipulation this was drawn under the skin, so that there was drainage from the hydrocele into the subcutaneous tissues. An immediate diminution in size of the hydrocele followed, but the improvement was not maintained.

LITERATURE

Bertholou, *Journ. de Méd. et de Chir. Pratiques*, June 25, 1910.
Hastings, *Lancet,* 1910, i. 916.
Lemann, *Interstate Med. Journ.,* March, 1911.
Marcon, *Presse Méd.,* Sept. 4, 1909.

(b) Congenital Hydrocele

Here there is a communication between the tunica vaginalis and the peritoneal cavity, due to the normal obliteration of this process not taking place. (Fig. 247,'2.) The testicle may be in the scrotum or it may be imperfectly descended.

The hydrocele is noticed soon after birth. It forms a pear-shaped, translucent elastic or fluctuating swelling, which narrows as it passes up the cord to the abdominal ring.

The swelling increases when the child cries, strains, or coughs. Continuous pressure on the sac empties it, the fluid returning to the abdomen, but it slowly swells again when the pressure is removed. Sometimes the communication with the peritoneal cavity is so small that the fluid is only returned with great difficulty. Congenital hydrocele is most likely to be mistaken for congenital hernia. The features by which they may be distinguished are the dullness in percussion of the hydrocele, the slow disappearance of the swelling on pressure and the absence of the characteristic gurgle and slip of a hernia, the elastic uniform feel, the translucency, and the difficulty of controlling the swelling by pressure on the ring after reduction, whereas a hernia is easily controlled.

Treatment consists in the application of a well-fitting truss and multiple puncture of the hydrocele with a surgical needle. Should this method fail the sac should be excised and the neck ligatured.

(c) Infantile Hydrocele and Bilocular Hydrocele

In this form the tunica vaginalis and the funicular process are distended with fluid, but the communication with the peritoneal cavity is obliterated in the region of the external abdominal ring. (Fig. 247, 3.) It differs from congenital hydrocele clinically in the impossibility of returning the fluid into the abdominal cavity. Multiple puncture will usually cure the condition.

A variant of infantile hydrocele is bilocular hydrocele, in which the funicular process is obliterated at the internal abdominal ring. As the fluid accumulates the sac assumes a bilocular form from the constriction of the external abdominal ring or by a narrow part of the sac itself. The upper loculus develops between the abdominal wall and the peritoneum. The sac should, if possible, be dissected out.

ENCYSTED HYDRO-
CELE OF THE
TESTIS AND EPI-
DIDYMIS (SPER-
MATOCELE)

There are several varieties of these cysts —:

(1) **Multiple small cysts of the epididymis.** —These are usually situated in the head of the epididymis, and less frequently in the body or tail. They form small pea-sized bodies, projecting on the surface of the head of the epididymis;

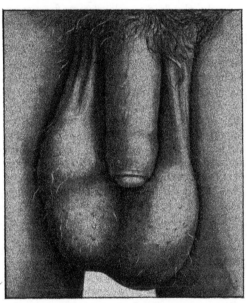

Fig. 253.—Spermatocele.

occasionally they may become pedunculated. The cysts are tense and firm, and contain a transparent or turbid fluid in which spermatozoa may be found. These cysts appear after puberty, and are more common after the age of 40. They are said to arise either in remains of the Müllerian duct or from dilatation of the ducts of the epididymis.

(2) **Single large cysts (spermatocele).**—These arise in connection with the epididymis, either between the globus major and the testicle or above the epididymis. (Fig. 253.) They are situated outside the tunica vaginalis, but may project into the cavity. They are usually single and unilocular, less often multiple, and they may be multilocular. As the cyst increases in

size it separates the testicle and epididymis, and the vasa efferentia may be stretched over it.

The wall consists of fibrous tissue lined with columnar or sometimes flattened epithelium. The fluid is alkaline, opalescent, and milky, and when the glass containing it is swung round the circulating fluid gives a remarkable drift-cloud or shimmering appearance, similar to that seen in the urine in bacilluria. The milkiness is due to spermatozoa, which are actively motile under the microscope. The spermatozoa are present at each tapping.

Rarely, the fluid is colourless and no spermatozoa are present.

Pathology.—There are two views in regard to the pathology of these cysts :

(1) *Retention cyst.*—Communication between the cyst and a seminal tubule has been proved by the injection of mercury into the vas deferens and the discovery of globules in the cyst. The opening into the duct will usually admit a fine bristle.

According to some authorities, these cysts are due to rupture of one of the vasa efferentia.

(2) The second view is that the cysts take origin in *fœtal relics :* (a) The organ of Giraldés (Wolffian body), so that they are analogous to the parovarian cysts in the female. (b) The hydatid of Morgagni ; this is the remains of the duct of Müller, and is the analogue of the Fallopian tube in the female : it normally forms a small pedunculated cyst between the upper pole of the testis and the globus major. (c) The vas aberrans ; this has origin in the tubules of the Wolffian body, and forms a diverticulum of the commencement of the vas deferens. The position of this body is against the view that it gives origin to the cysts.

Encysted hydrocele of the testis is very rare, and forms a single cyst situated beneath the tunica albuginea.

Symptoms.—Small cysts are usually found accidentally as rounded, firm, elastic swellings of the globus major, or connected with the epididymis above and with the outer side of the testicle. In a patient who consulted me there was sudden moderately severe pain in the testicle, followed by the appearance of a small, tense, tender cyst of the globus major. Usually, however, small cysts give rise to no pain or inconvenience. Larger cysts approximate the testicle in size. There is an oval elastic swelling situated immediately above the testicle and inseparably connected with it, but marked off from it by a groove which can be seen on inspecting the scrotum. The upper pole may be larger than the lower, and the cyst resembles an inverted pear. The cyst grows slowly, and never reaches the size of a large vaginal hydrocele. It is usually unilateral, and on the right side, but may be bilateral. When a strong light is used it is always translucent. The patient is often credited by his friends with the possession of a third testicle. The cyst is distinguished from ordinary hydrocele by the slow growth, shape, position, and relation to the testicle and the characters of the fluid.

Treatment.—The cyst rapidly refills after tapping, and the only method of cure is excision of the sac.

HÆMATOCELE

Etiology.—Hæmatocele, an effusion of blood into the vaginal sac, may occur in combination with hydrocele, or independently of it.

(*a*) **Hæmatocele with hydrocele.**—After tapping a hydrocele blood may be rapidly poured into the tunica vaginalis from puncture of a vessel in the wall of the sac, or from puncture of the testicle; or it may apparently follow the rapid removal of fluid from a large hydrocele, and result from rupture of vessels due to lack of support, injury to a hydrocele, such as a blow, or collision with the pommel of the saddle in riding. Bruising of the scrotum is present in the last-named cases. Occasionally the fluid of a hydrocele is found deeply stained with altered blood without any history of injury or of previous tapping.

(*b*) **Traumatic hæmatocele** may rarely develop without a hydrocele having been present, as the result of kicks, blows, or squeezes. In some cases hæmatocele has developed after violent straining, such as lifting heavy weights; here the blood-vessels are probably diseased. Hæmatocele may be associated with growths of the testicle. It occurs in middle and advanced life.

(*c*) **Spontaneous hæmatocele** is occasionally observed in old men. No cause can be ascertained, and there is much difficulty in making a diagnosis from growth of the testicle.

Pathology.—In old-standing hæmatocele the wall of the tunica vaginalis is thickened, and may be hard and even cartilaginous in consistence. The interior is lined with layers of greyish or brown fibrinous false membranes, lying especially on the parietal layer, and the surface may be very irregular. The fluid content varies from red to dark brown, and its consistence from that of hydrocele fluid to syrup. Crystals of hæmatoidin and cholesterin may be found in old-standing cases. Free clots are present in the fluid. The testicle occupies a position similar to that in hydrocele, but it cannot be detected by translucency, and, as the swelling is tender, testicular sensation is no guide. In old-standing cases the testicle is fibrous and atrophied.

Symptoms.—The swelling appears rapidly after a blow or

other injury, or the sac refills in a few hours after tapping of a hydrocele. There is pain, sometimes severe, and the swelling is tender. Discoloration of the scrotum is present in traumatic cases. The swelling is not translucent. On tapping, fluid blood is removed. In chronic cases there is a heavy, smooth, hard, painless, oval swelling, which does not increase in size and is not translucent, and on tapping altered blood is withdrawn. The cord is greatly thickened.

Inflammation and suppuration are the chief complications. The infection may be spontaneous, but it usually follows puncture. The swelling is tender, heavy, and painful, the scrotum reddened and œdematous, and the temperature high.

Diagnosis.—(1) *Hydrocele* is translucent except in very old-standing cases. In hæmatocele the swelling is opaque, heavier, and harder, with less elasticity. Diagnosis is also aided by the rapid onset and history of an injury or by recurrence after tapping.

(2) *New growths.*—In some cases diagnosis may be impossible without an exploratory incision. The steady increase in size of the new growth, the irregularity of contour and consistence, the appearance at some parts of bosses, the detection of hard and soft areas, and the complete loss of testicular sensation, are important points.

Treatment.—In the early acute stage the patient should be confined to bed, the scrotum supported, and an ice-bag applied. After some days or a week the fluid should be drawn off with a trocar and cannula under the strictest aseptic precautions, and moderate pressure applied. This can be obtained by the use of a Jullien suspensory packed with cotton-wool.

In old-standing cases operation is necessary. The sac is freely opened and the contents are turned out. If the sac is supple and the testicle apparently healthy the wall should be clipped away as in hydrocele. If, however, the wall is thick and cartilaginous and the testicle fibrous and atrophied, castration should be performed.

CHYLOUS HYDROCELE (GALACTOCELE, LYMPHOCELE, CHYLOCELE, FATTY HYDROCELE)

The tunica vaginalis is distended with a fluid resembling chyle. A small number of cases have been recorded, the majority of which have occurred in tropical countries. The condition is due to obstruction of the lymphatics by the Filaria sanguinis hominis, and rupture of lymphatic vessels in the wall of the vaginal sac. In 62 cases of filariasis Manson found 6 cases of chylous hydrocele.

The fluid is like milk, and, on standing, a layer of cream-hke fat forms on the surface. When shaken with ether the fluid becomes clear. The appearance of the chylocele may be preceded by attacks of fever and pain. Other evidence of filariasis, such as elephantiasis of the scrotum and legs, is sometimes present.

The cyst resembles an ordinary hydrocele, but is not translucent. Tapping is followed by rapid recurrence. Excision of the sac with the dilated lymphatics of the cord should be carried out.

NEW GROWTHS OF THE TUNICA VAGINALIS

New growths of the tunica vaginalis are very rare, and the few examples recorded belong to the mesoblastic group of tumours.

A few cases of **fibroma** have been observed. Makins has recently described a case, and refers to the literature.

The fibromas spring from the subserous layer of the tunica vaginalis, are usually single, and may reach a large size. The tumour envelops the testicle and is moulded upon it, the organ itself being normal.

Makins's case was a multiple fibroma, and the tumours were attached to the testicle, epididymis, and cord. A similar case is described by Tikhonovich. The tumours are either soft fibromas or composed of hard, pale-white, fibrillar fibrous tissue in bundles.

Myomatous and fatty degeneration are common, and necrosis is frequently present.

Soft fibromas are pyriform, very slowly growing tumours which may reach a very large size, and the origin of which may be ascribed to à blow.

Multiple hard fibromas form a group of nodules not unlike a bunch of grapes. Fibromas are frequently found in the cord in these cases.

The tumours should be removed, the testicle being, if possible, preserved.

A single instance of **lipoma** has been described by Park.

Sarcoma is very rare. In the few recorded cases there was a rapidly forming tumour occurring in a child or an adult, which was usually diagnosed as hæmatocele. These growths are said to belong to the group of endotheliomas.

Pedunculated bodies are sometimes found in the cavity of the tunica vaginalis in adults and old men. These are either an enlarged hydatid of Morgagni attached at the upper pole of the testicle, between it and the globus major, or are composed of fibrous tissue which is sometimes calcified and forms wart-like or leaf-like bodies ; they are attached at the junction of the testicle

3 A

and epididymis, or scattered over the serous surface. The latter have an inflammatory origin. These bodies are found in hydroceles, and give rise to no symptoms. I have felt such a body attached to the outer surface of the testicle near the upper pole, giving rise to no symptoms, and without fluid in the vaginal sac.

LITERATURE

Ballock, *Ann. of Surg.*, 1904, p. 396.
Jacobson, *Diseases of the Male Organs of Generation*, p. 433. 1893.
Makins, *Proc. Roy. Soc. Med.*, Surgical Section, 1912.
Park, *Ann. of Surg.*, 1886, p. 365.
Tikhonovich, *Khirurgia Mosk.*, x. 360.

PART IX.—THE SPERMATIC CORD

CHAPTER LXIX

VOLVULUS—HYDROCELE AND HÆMATOCELE NEW GROWTHS—VARICOCELE

INFLAMMATORY affections of the cord are discussed with those of the testicle and epididymis.

Torsion of the cord is described under Torsion of the Testicle.

VOLVULUS OF THE CORD

McConnell describes a singular case under this title. A boy of 15 was seized with severe pain in the right groin when sitting tailor-fashion with his feet under him. There were nausea, vomiting, and collapse. In the position of the inner half of the right inguinal canal there was a tense, tender, fixed swelling, without impulse on coughing. The right testicle was slightly larger and the cord thicker than the left, but there was no pain or tenderness. On operation the distended sac of an infantile hydrocele was found in the inguinal canal, and projecting into this was a loop of the spermatic cord, twisted on itself for two turns, and purple in colour from greatly distended veins. All the constituents of the cord were included in the twisted loop.[1]

HYDROCELE OF THE CORD

1. DIFFUSE HYDROCELE OF THE CORD

The constituents of the spermatic cord are held together by loose connective tissue rich in lymphatics, and the whole cord is enveloped in a sheath to which each constituent of the abdominal wall contributes a layer, and which is continued down to cover the testicle.

The connective tissue within this sheath is occasionally the seat of diffuse serous infiltration, a form of œdema which has been termed "diffuse hydrocele of the cord." The cause is unknown. There is a smooth, cylindrical swelling of the cord, which is large

[1] *Lancet*, 1912, i. 1056.

at the testicular end. There is dragging weight, but no pain. The testis and epididymis are normal. Posture has no effect, and the swelling is irreducible.

From an omental hernia the swelling is distinguished by the absence or indefiniteness of impulse on coughing, the irreducibility, the uniform "feel," and the difficulty in defining the external abdominal ring. The diagnosis is difficult, and in a stout patient may be impossible without operation.

Treatment consists in incision and drainage combined with elastic pressure.

2. Encysted Hydrocele of the Cord

There is a circumscribed collection of fluid in relation with the cord.

The cyst originates in an unobliterated portion of the funicular process which has closed above and below. (Fig. 247, 4.) It is usually single, but there may be several. The right side is the more often affected, and the condition is found in children and boys, less frequently in adults. Other forms of cyst of the cord result from a blood cyst following trauma, dilatation of the organ of Giraldès, and a partly obliterated hernial sac (hydrocele of a hernial sac).

The cyst contains fluid similar to that of a hydrocele of the tunica vaginalis; it may be mixed with blood after an injury. It forms an oval, well-defined, smooth, elastic, painless, translucent swelling, varying in size from a hazel-nut to a pigeon's egg; it is freely movable, and connected with the spermatic cord.

The cyst usually lies just below the external abdominal ring. When it lies in or immediately outside the canal it may be mistaken for an inguinal hernia. If it lies outside the ring there is no impulse on coughing; but when it lies in the canal there is such an impulse. The swelling can be replaced in the inguinal canal, but cannot be completely reduced. There is no sudden slip, and no gurgling. Pulling on the testicle will sometimes draw a cyst out of the external ring and allow the fingers to slip above it.

The cyst should be dissected and removed.

Hydrocele of a Hernial Sac

This is a rare condition, in which the neck of an empty hernial sac is obliterated by a plug of omentum or by adhesions caused by the prolonged use of a truss. There is a history of a swelling having the characters of a hernia, and this is apparently cured. Later there is the slow development of an irreducible swelling which does not show variations in size. The swelling is transparent, and fluctuation can be obtained. There is no impulse on coughing.

Treatment consists in excision of the sac.

HÆMATOCELE OF THE CORD

1. *Diffuse* hæmatocele of the cord is the more common form, and is due to a blow, kick, or strain. A swelling of the cord rapidly forms, and on palpation may resemble an omental hernia. The diagnosis is usually easy from the history and the absence of impulse, and from the fact that the swelling is irreducible while other signs of strangulation are absent. There may be extensive discoloration of the skin.

In the early stage, when the diagnosis is clear, an ice-bag may be applied. Later, elastic pressure and iodides given internally are recommended. A very extensive and increasing hæmatocele should be incised, the clots cleared out, and a drain inserted.

2. *Encysted* hæmatocele originates either in hæmorrhage into an encysted hydrocele of the cord or in a circumscribed hæmatoma. There is a swelling the size of a pigeon's egg or larger, which is closely incorporated with the cord. The swelling may have appeared rapidly, and may extend downwards and come into relation with the testicle. A history of an injury can usually be obtained.

Treatment consists in incision, removal of clots, and drainage. If a cyst is present it should be removed.

NEW GROWTHS OF THE CORD

Various new growths of the cord have been described, all of which are rare. They include lipoma, fibroma, myoma, myxoma, myxo-lipoma, myxo-fibroma, sarcoma, and carcinoma. Stoerk has described a rhabdo-myo-sarcoma which he believed took origin in the vas deferens. There were metastatic deposits in the inguinal, retroperitoneal, mediastinal, and cervical lymph-glands.

Lipoma is the most common form. It originates in the fatty tissue which is found among the constituents of the cord, or in the extraperitoneal fat. Whether such lipomas drag upon the peritoneum and lead to the formation of a hernial sac, is a disputed point. There is an elongated, smooth, soft, rounded tumour, closely related to the cord and situated near the testicle, just outside the external abdominal ring or in the inguinal canal. (Fig. 254.) In the last-named situation it may possibly be dislodged by traction on the cord and pressure from above so that it lies outside the ring, and it returns to the canal again when pressure and traction are relieved. The tumour has a soft, doughy, or even fluctuating "feel," and, when it is contained in the inguinal canal or lies just outside it, closely resembles an omental hernia. It is not, however, reducible, and does not show rapid variations in size. The tumour may also resemble an encysted hydrocele of the cord, but is not so elastic and well defined, nor is it translucent.

Treatment consists in dissection and removal of the growth and radical cure of the hernia, should this be present as a complication.

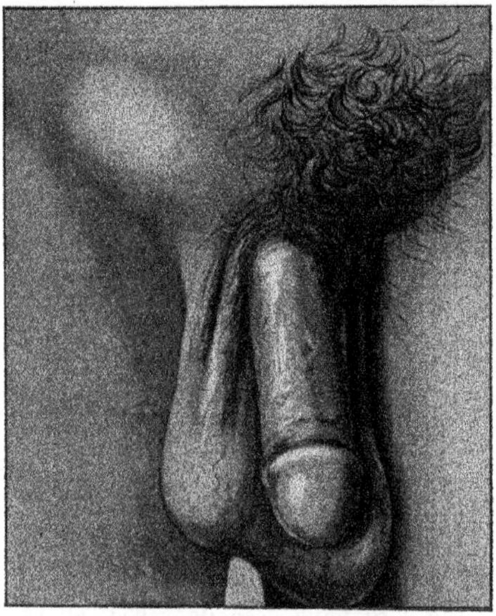

The remaining tumours of the cord are extremely rare.

VARICOCELE

This consists in enlargement of the veins of the spermatic plexus. A moderate degree of varicocele is said to exist in 10 per cent. of male subjects; a marked degree of varicocele is much less frequent. The left side is affected in the great majority of cases (97 per cent.), the right side very rarely (4 per cent.), and both sides still more rarely (2 per cent.) (Corner). Vari-

Fig. 254.—Lipoma of spermatic cord at external abdominal ring.

cocele occurs most frequently between the ages of 15 and 26, less often in the next decade, and rarely after that. Curling found that 23 per cent. of recruits for the English army had varicocele, Senn noted its presence in 25 per cent. of recruits for the American volunteer army, and French statistics state that its frequency in recruits in France is 10 per cent.

The spermatic veins leave the testicle at its upper end and pass upwards in front of the vas deferens and of the deferential veins. The veins are large, intercommunicate freely by lateral branches surrounding the spermatic artery, and form a plexus of convoluted vessels, the pampiniform or spermatic plexus. The veins pass through the inguinal canal into the abdomen, and unite to form two or three large veins which eventually combine into a single vein, the spermatic vein, which opens obliquely into the inferior vena cava on the right side and at right angles into the renal vein on the left. The left spermatic vein is longer and larger than the right. It is crossed by the sigmoid flexure of the colon, and receives one or two colico-spermatic veins.

There is usually a valve at the upper end of each spermatic vein. This may be absent on the left side, and in this case there is a valve in the renal vein near the opening. Valves exist also in the veins of the pampiniform plexus.

In varicocele there is dilatation of the veins of the cord, especially the anterior group, the pampiniform plexus. The veins appear to be greatly increased in number; they are elongated and tortuous, and their walls thickened and rigid. Thrombosis is frequently present. I have dissected from a varicocele of moderate size a rigid, tortuous, thrombosed vein which felt like a very hard vas deferens and measured 5 in. in length. Phleboliths are said to occur. The dilated veins are massed immediately above and behind the testicle, and diminish in size and numbers at the upper part of the cord. Veins covering the testicle beneath the tunica vaginalis may also be dilated and tortuous.

Bennett recognizes four anatomical varieties: (1) Varicocele involving the pampiniform plexus and its efferent veins and extending as far as the abdomen. (2) Varicocele limited to the lower part of the pampiniform plexus. (3) Varicocele involving especially the upper part of the plexus as far as the formation of the spermatic vein. (4) Varicocele affecting the pampiniform plexus, efferent veins, and spermatic veins.

The testicle is very frequently small and soft when compared with its neighbour. This condition may have resulted from a want of development, or from retrograde changes due to the varicocele.

Etiology.—Numerous theories are advanced to explain the occurrence of varicocele, but nothing definite is known in regard to its origin. Anatomically the veins have a very long course, are tortuous and poorly supported, and are liable to pressure by the abdominal muscles in their passage through the abdominal wall. But these anatomical features are common to all subjects, and what has to be explained is the occurrence of varicocele in a few.

In explanation of the frequency with which the left side is affected, it is urged that the left spermatic vein is longer than the right, enters the renal vein at a right angle, and is liable to pressure from a loaded sigmoid flexure.

The condition is reasonably held to be congenital and to result either from persistence of fœtal veins that are usually obliterated, or from congenital malformation of the venous plexus. The following reasons are given for upholding the congenital origin of varicocele : (1) A fully developed varicocele may be found at an early age. (2) The majority of varicoceles are only discovered when fully developed. (3) The testicle is frequently found undeveloped, arrest of development having occurred at an early period. (4) There is an heredity of varicocele or varix of the lower extremity in half the cases. (5) Other vascular abnormalities frequently coexist, such as varices and nævi.

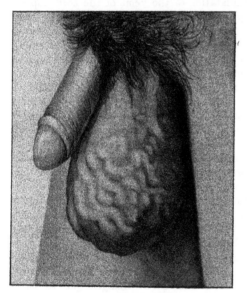

Fig. 255.—Varicocele.

Symptoms.—The scrotum is thin, lax, and lower than normal on the left side, and either there is a fullness immediately above the testicle or the veins can be seen standing out promiuently. (Figs. 255 and 256.) There may be varicose veins on the surface of the scrotum. The swelling increases on standing, especially if this is prolonged, and diminishes when the patient lies down.

On palpation the scrotum is softer than normal, and the enlarged veins are felt like a bag of earthworms. The testicle is usually soft, and often smaller than its neighbour, and the long axis is infrequently horizontal or nearly horizontal. The vas is easily distinguished. Occasionally a thrombosed thickened vein may resemble it, but is more rigid and tortuous.

A slight non-expansile impulse can be detected on coughing. When the patient lies down the veins are emptied, and they refill on resumption of the erect posture, the reflux being uncontrolled by pressure of the finger at the external abdominal ring.

The patient complains of a heavy, dragging sensation, and sometimes of aching pain.

These symptoms vary very greatly in different individuals. Sharp pain is rarely felt. In examining large numbers of recruits for the Territorial forces I found that there were two well-defined groups. In one the subject was well developed and robust, and the varicocele had frequently escaped his notice and caused him no inconvenience. In the second class the subject was ill-grown and pallid, and his tissues were lax; varicose veins and flat-foot were frequent concomitants. Between these extremes were many gradations.

Varicocele occurs in growths of the kidney, and a rapidly developing varicocele, especially on the right side, in an adult or elderly patient should always raise the suspicion of renal growth (*see* p. 198).

Prognosis.—In most cases varicocele tends to improve and eventually disappear spontaneously, and it is very rare in old men. In a subject of brooding habit, and in men of the ill-developed, loosely built type to which I have referred, aching pain is frequent and gradually assumes an exaggerated importance, and hypochondriasis may develop.

Treatment. 1. Palliative. — This consists in reassuring the patient that atrophy of the testicle and impotence will not occur, in advising cold baths, regulated exercise, tonics, and the use of a well-fitting suspensory bandage.

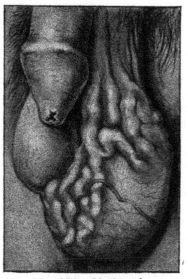

Fig. 256.—Varicocele.

2. **Operation.**—This should be performed when the varicocele is increasing, and when it is causing pain and discomfort. It is necessary when admission to the public services is desired. The hard-and-fast rule by which candidates for the British Army who suffer from varicocele are refused has been condemned by Colonel Howard and others.

General, spinal, or local anæsthesia may be used. The varicocele is grasped in the left hand just below the external abdominal ring, and an incision 1½ in. long is made into its upper extremity, just above the level of the ring.

An incision 1 in. long over the external abdominal ring, transverse to the long axis of the cord, has been used. It has no advantage over the incision here described.

The cord is exposed and the incision carried through its coverings so as to expose the veins. The vas deferens is identified and separated, together with the spermatic artery and a few veins lying behind it. These are returned to the wound, and the varicocele raised up on an aneurysm needle. A strong catgut ligature is now passed and tied round the veins near the external abdominal ring. The testicle is pulled up, and a second ligature is placed about 2 in. below the first. The intervening bunch of veins is cut away, leaving a sufficient projection beyond the ligatures to prevent slipping.

The ends of the upper and lower ligatures are tied together so as to approximate the two stumps, and the cut surfaces are accurately held together by one or two catgut stitches. This shortens the cord and raises the pendulous testicle. If the scrotum is unduly lax an elliptical portion of it may now be removed, or the most pendulous part may be removed in the following manner : An intestinal clamp is placed transversely on the scrotum below the testicles, or in an antero-posterior direction, and mattress stitches are inserted at intervals above it. The redundant portion of the scrotum is cut away below the clamp, which is then removed, the skin being brought together by interrupted silkworm-gut sutures. This procedure is rarely necessary.

The wound is closed without a drain. The patient is confined to bed for two days, and a suspender should be worn for some months after the operation. In this operation the spermatic artery is ligatured, and the blood supply of the testicle depends upon branches of this vessel which pass off high up, and upon the deferential artery.

Hæmorrhage may occur as a postoperative accident due to slipping of the ligature. It may take place in the scrotum or within the abdomen, and in the latter position may be serious and even fatal. If imperfectly tied, the spermatic artery retracts into the abdomen. The hæmorrhage is at first extraperitoneal, but later rupture into the peritoneal cavity takes place. The symptoms are abdominal pain following the operation, and signs of internal hæmorrhage, viz. rapid pulse, pallor, sighing respiration, fainting, thirst, restlessness, etc. Orchitis and hydrocele may follow the operation.

Results.—Corner states that fibrosis of the testicle is present in 90 per .cent. of cases after operation. It may have preceded the operation, but this observer. believes that it is produced more rapidly and in greater degree by the operation. In 55 per cent. of cases there was increase in the size of the testicle due to this fibrosis. In some cases (21 per cent.) atrophy of the testicle has been said to follow radical operation for varicocele. It is well before operating to draw the patient's attention to any lack of development of the testicle that may exist, since he is apt to attribute to the operative measures maldevelopment discovered after the operation. I have frequently seen hydrocele of the tunica vaginalis follow the operation even in the hands of competent surgeons. Corner found that it occurred in 23 per cent. of cases, and appeared soon after the operation. It is the practice of some surgeons to incise the tunica vaginalis and turn it inside out at the time of the varicocele operation in order to prevent the development of hydrocele. Rarely neuralgic pain, present before the operation, persists or even increases. In the majority of cases no further trouble is experienced after the operation. Corner found that 70 per cent. of these patients were definitely improved and well satisfied.

LITERATURE

Bennett, *Brit. Med. Journ.*, 1901, i. 501.
Corner and Nitch, *Brit. Med. Journ.*, Jan. 27, 1906, p. 191.
Hochenegg, *Zeits. f. klin. Med.*, July, 1907.
Howard and others, *Lancet*, Dec. 16, 1905, p. 1786.
Josseraud, Nove, *Lyon Méd.*, 1897, p. 237.
Riccioli, *Il Policlinico*, Dec. 9, 1906.
Stoerk, *Zeits. f. Heilk.*, 1901, S. 1.
Thornburgh, *Med. Rec.*, Aug. 29, 1903.

PART X.—THE SCROTUM

CHAPTER LXX

ELEPHANTIASIS—NEW GROWTHS

INFLAMMATORY diseases and fistulæ of the scrotum are described with those of the urethra and the testicle.

ELEPHANTIASIS AND LYMPH SCROTUM

Etiology.—Elephantiasis of the scrotum and lymph scrotum are diseases of tropical climates due to lymphatic obstruction by the Filaria sanguinis hominis. The distribution extends from 35° N. to 25° S. in the eastern, and from 25° N. to 30° S. in the western hemisphere. It is more common along sea-coasts and the banks of large rivers, and is especially associated with high air temperature and considerable atmospheric humidity, which favour the development of the filaria in mosquitoes and its penetration of the skin of the human subject. In addition to the filaria, secondary bacterial infection by a diplococcus (lymphococcus of Dufongeré) may perhaps assist in producing the disease. Obstruction is not caused by the normal embryo, which measures 130 to 300 μ in length and 7 to 11 μ in breadth, but by miniature ova 50 μ long and 34 μ in breadth. These, according to Manson, are liberated by some damage, such as a blow, to the pregnant adult female worm, and obstruct a sufficient number of lymph-channels and glands to cause lymph stasis.

Obstruction may also be caused by a coiled mass of adult worms blocking an important lymph-channel.

Symptoms and pathology.—Lymph scrotum commences with an attack of fever. associated with redness, swelling, and pain in the scrotum. When the acute symptoms have subsided the scrotum remains swollen and elastic. The surface is soft and smooth, or covered with rugæ, and numbers of clear vesicles appear. If these are punctured they discharge continuously a clear lymph or chyle containing filaria embryos, and this eventually causes exhaustion.

Elephantiasis may begin as lymph scrotum, or there may be recurrent attacks of inflammation with redness and fever, and after each attack the scrotum is larger. After a time the enlargement proceeds slowly and continuously until an enormous size is reached, the largest recorded size weighing 224 lb. (Chevers). The mass is somewhat triangular in shape, with the base upwards. On the anterior and upper aspect is a depression leading into a

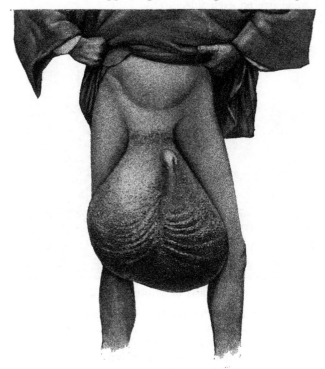

Fig. 257.—Elephantiasis of scrotum.

canal formed by the inverted prepuce, and at the bottom of this is the glans penis. The skin becomes coarse and leathery. Thick rugæ and hypertrophied papillæ stand out (Fig. 257), and the mouths of the follicles are unusually distinct. Inflammation and ulceration and sometimes sloughing of the skin occur.

On section the skin is greatly hypertrophied, and the deeper layer dense, thick, and fibrous. The subcutaneous tissue is greatly increased in bulk, and has a yellowish œdematous appearance, containing a large quantity of fluid.

The thickening of the skin and subcutaneous tissues is greatest at the most dependent part, and they get thinner as they pass up towards the base of attachment. At the sides and posteriorly the skin is softer, supple, and less changed. The testicles he towards the back, and nearer the lower than the upper end of the mass. Each testicle is firmly bound down to the skin by a greatly hypertrophied gubernaculum testis, and there is usually a hydrocele of some size on each side.

The weight of the scrotum drags down the skin of the pubes

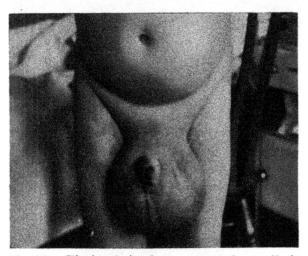

Fig. 258.—Elephantiasis of scrotum not due to filaria.

and perineum. A section of the base is triangular with the apex backwards. Elephantiasis of the legs is frequently present.

In rare cases a non-filarial form of elephantiasis of the scrotum is met with. It is due to blocking of lymphatics from chronic inflammation (chronic ulcers, chronic erysipelas) or cicatrices, or is secondary to chronic ulcers and recurrent erysipelas. Jonathan Hutchinson describes a case due to tertiary syphilitic inflammation. I have operated on a case in which no cause could be discovered for the lymphatic obstruction. The patient, a man of 45, had never left England. Four years before there was a swelling of the scrotum for fourteen days, which subsided, and for two years there had been gradual enlargement. The mass weighed 52 oz. after removal. (Fig. 258.)

Treatment.—In the early stages pressure by elastic bandages is said to cause improvement, but when the disease is fully established nothing short of operation will give relief. Operation is contra-indicated in old or enfeebled patients. The mortality is under 5 per cent. (Manson).

Hernia and abscess formation should be treated.

For two days the patient is confined to bed and the mass suspended so as to empty it, and before operation it should be emptied as far as possible by elastic pressure.

A tourniquet is placed round the base of the mass and carried round the pelvis in a figure of eight. The testicles are exposed by vertical incision and dissected out, the hydroceles opened and inverted, and the penis exposed and isolated by slitting up the tunnel in which it is buried. The incisions are carried round the base, marking out flaps if feasible, and deepened, vessels being clamped as they are cut. The great mass consisting of thick skin and œdematous areolar tissue is removed. The flaps are brought together and sutured over the testicles.

LITERATURE

Castellani and Chalmers, *Manual of Tropical Medicine*. 1910.
Daniels and Wilkinson, *Tropical Medicine and Hygiene*.
Manson, *Tropical Diseases*, 4th ed. 1907.

NEW GROWTHS OF THE SCROTUM

Non-malignant new growths of the scrotum are uncommon. Cutaneous nævi may be met with, and soft and hard fibroma, lipoma, chondroma, and osteoma have been recorded. Sebaceous cysts may occur singly or as multiple tumours (Fig. 259). I have seen a case in which the whole scrotum was closely set with round, hard nodules the size of a pea and larger, and which proved to be sebaceous cysts. The tumours caused no inconvenience, and no treatment was desired. Similar cases are recorded by Hutchinson, Kocher, and others.

A case of intrascrotal hydatid cyst has been recorded.

Masses of varicose veins closely set and with small telangiectatic spots are met with in the scrotum. On cursory examination the condition somewhat resembles a varicocele. (Fig. 260.)

EPITHELIOMA OF THE SCROTUM (CHIMNEY-SWEEP'S CANCER)

Epithelioma of the scrotum is more frequent in chimney-sweeps than in other males, and has thus received the name " chimney-sweep's cancer." In the Report of the Departmental Committee on Compensation for Industrial Diseases (1907) it is stated that the mortality from cancer among chimney-sweeps is twice that among occupied males generally. For the three years 1900–2 the comparative mortality figure for cancer among chimney-sweeps between the ages of 26 and 65 was **133**, as compared with **63** among occupied males at the same ages. The disease commences in a wart (soot wart), most often at the lower and front part of the

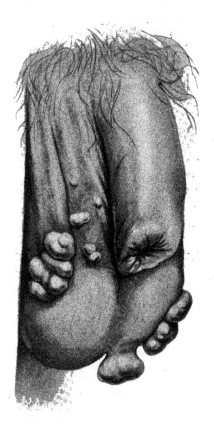

Fig. 259.—Sebaceous cysts of scrotum.

scrotum, and the whole scrotum may be covered with these warts. The warts may remain for long simple, and then one of them begins to grow rapidly, becomes softer, more vascular, bleeds easily, and ulcerates. The ulcer spreads slowly along the skin, the base is indurated, the edges are hard and everted. Other forms in which the growth may commence are a nodule, a cauliflower excrescence, or a horn-like outgrowth on a papilloma. The ulcer spreads over the scrotum, the testicles are exposed and sometimes invaded, and the crura of the penis become involved. The inguinal glands are enlarged at first from inflammatory products, but later from metastatic deposit from the growth. Large masses may form and break down, and ulceration into the femora' or iliac arteries may occur. There is little tendency to the production of distant metastases.

Extension to the inguinal glands is usually long delayed, and has been known to make its appearance some years after successful removal of the primary disease.

Spencer has shown that soot granules are found in the cells of the growth, and also in healthy skin beyond the growth.

The presence of soot granules in the cells of the epididymis gives rise to dark patches which cannot be washed away, and may explain the development of " chimney-sweep's cancer "

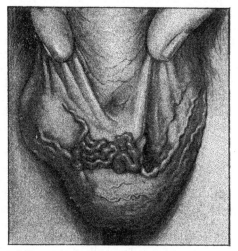

Fig. 260.—Varicose veins of scrotum.

years after the patient has ceased to follow his occupation.

The disease is much more common in England than in any other country, and this was attributed by Butlin (*Brit. Med. Journ.*, 1892, p. 1343) to the burning of hard coal and to deficient protection of the skin from contact with soot, and to insufficient washing.

According to Jacobson the disease is diminishing in frequency. Labourers engaged in work among tar and paraffin are also liable to develop epithelioma of the scrotum.

Treatment.—This consists in preventing the prolonged contact of soot with the skin. The clothes should be protective, and thorough washing should be regularly carried out.

Operation should remove the growth with a wide margin, and the inguinal glands on both sides should be carefully removed with the fat in which they are embedded.

3 B

PART XI.—THE PENIS

CHAPTER LXXI

ANATOMY—CONGENITAL MALFORMATIONS
INJURIES—PREPUTIAL CALCULI

Surgical anatomy.—The penis consists of three masses of erectile tissue—the two corpora cavernosa and the corpus spongiosum.

The corpora cavernosa lie side by side, and form the bulk of the body of the penis. At the root of the penis they separate from each other to form the crura, which are attached to the rami of the pubes and ischium, and are covered by the erectores penis muscles. In the body of the penis they are closely united, and at the anterior part of the organ become partly blended, the septum between the two bodies being vertically perforated to join a comb-like partition (septum pectiniforme). In front they are united in a conical extremity which is capped by the glans penis. The corpora cavernosa are surrounded by a dense white sheath consisting of fibrous and elastic tissue, which forms a common investment, and internally to which each has a separate capsule of similar structure. The blood supply of each corpus cavernosum is derived from the artery to the crus, a branch of the internal pudic artery, and some twigs from the dorsal artery of the penis, and the veins pass to the prostatic plexus and pudendal veins and to the dorsal vein of the penis.

The corpus spongiosum lies in the middle line on the under surface of the penis in a groove between the two corpora cavernosa. Posteriorly it expands into a rounded mass, the bulb, and anteriorly it forms a cap, the glans penis, which envelops the end of the corpora cavernosa. The bulb shows a superficial median division at its posterior extremity. It is attached to the under surface of the triangular ligament and covered by the bulbo-cavernosus muscle. The corpus spongiosum is invested by a sheath which contains more elastic and less fibrous tissue than the corpora cavernosa. The urethra enters the upper surface of the bulbous portion about ½ in. from its posterior extremity and passes for-

834

wards in its substance, piercing it at the conical extremity of the glans penis.

The arterial supply enters the corpus spongiosum at each end, the posterior supply being derived from the artery to the bulb, a branch of the internal pudic; the anterior is the dorsal artery of the penis. The veins pass to the dorsal veins of the penis and to the veins of the bulb.

The skin of the penis is thin, elastic, free from fat or hairs. Anteriorly it forms the foreskin, and on the glans is firmly adherent to the spongy tissue and has no glands. Around the cervix of the penis behind the glans are the glands of Tyson, which secrete smegma.

The superficial fascia is thick, is continuous with that of the abdominal wall and scrotum, and contains smooth muscle fibre. A strong fibrous sheath invests the entire organ and covers the dorsal vessels. The suspensory ligament is a strong fibrous band passing from the pubic symphysis to the base of the penis, and blending with the fascial sheath and passing into the septum scroti. This ligament slings the base of the penis to the pubic symphysis. The lymphatics pass along the dorsum to the inguinal glands, while a few pass from the corpora cavernosa and corpus spongiosum to the pelvic lymph-glands.

The development of the penis and urethra is described at p. 392.

CONGENITAL MALFORMATIONS

Rudimentary development of the penis is not uncommon, and the penis may be so small as to be entirely hidden in the redundant tissues of the pubes and scrotum. Such cases have erroneously been described as absence of the penis. A penis of infantile type may develop after puberty into an organ capable of procreation. The subject may in other respects be normally developed. When rudimentary development of the penis is combined with a bifid scrotum and undescended testes the sex is difficult to distinguish. These, and also cases of hypertrophic clitoris, are frequently regarded as cases of *hermaphroditism,* or the sex of the child may be erroneously diagnosed. Neugebauer collected 58 cases in which the mistake was first discovered after marriage.

In many cases it is impossible to be certain of the sex at birth, and French authors recognize a class of "sexe indéterminé." In the male pseudo-hermaphrodite the descent of one or both testicles into the folds which might represent a bifid scrotum or labia majora may take place, and in one case a hydrocele was demonstrated by its translucency. The folds are also more wrinkled from the development of dartos in the scrotum than in the labia.

Per rectum nothing will be felt to aid the diagnosis. At puberty characters develop in most cases which make the diagnosis certain—the characteristic development of pubic hair extending to the umbilicus in the male, the development of the prostate felt per rectum, and the appearance of secondary sexual characters, such as changes in the voice, the breadth of the shoulders as compared with the pelvis, the appearance of hair on the face; and in the female the commencement of menstruation and the development of the mammæ.

True hermaphroditism is very rare. Corner quotes two cases : one of a woman, aged 21, who had a testicle removed from an inguinal hernia (Bernard Pitts), and another of a man, aged 25, who had a uterus, discovered also at operation (Kellock).

Several cases of *absence of the penis* have been described, and the malformation is usually combined with congenital urethrorectal fistula. The scrotum and testes in these cases have usually been normal in development.

Torsion of the penis is a rare abnormality, and is not seen apart from epispadias or hypospadias. The penis, which is usually poorly developed, but may be large, is rotated to the right one-quarter of or a complete circle.

Adhesion of the skin of the penis to the scrotum may occur alone, when the whole under surface may be webbed, or in combination with hypospadias. The penis is easily separated and the edges of the wound united. A hypospadias operation should then be performed if necessary.

Double penis is very rare, and is usually combined with other deformities, such as extrophy of the bladder, malformation of the kidneys, additional limbs, or atrophy of a limb. The penes may be quite separate and perfectly developed, and functional, or they may be webbed. The testicles may be normal or rudimentary and displaced.

Phimosis

Narrowing of the opening in the prepuce is the commonest of all congenital malformations of the urinary tract. The prepuce may be adherent and the orifice of the foreskin narrower ; it may also be long and project well beyond the glans penis as a loose process.

Phimosis may be acquired in adult life from chronic or recurrent balanitis, and in chronic inflammation in diabetes mellitus in cases of long foreskin. The orifice becomes scarred and contracted. Acquired narrowing of the outlet may also result from the scar following a chancre, from epithelioma, or from an incomplete operation for phimosis.

Complications.—In children frequent micturition and nocturnal enuresis are frequent complications. Irritation leading to masturbation, difficult micturition with ballooning of the foreskin and retention, may result; and hypertrophy of the bladder, with dilatation of the kidneys, umbilical and inguinal hernia, prolapse of the anus, and even extravasation of urine, are ascribed to this cause. Balanitis is a frequent complication both in children and in adults, and gives rise to irritation and discomfort and a purulent discharge. Gangrene of the foreskin has been known to result. Preputial calculi may form. The urethra is infected from this source, and recurrent attacks of urethritis ensue. Stricture has been stated to result (Ortmann).

Paraphimosis is a common complication, and in adult life is a cause of impeded coitus. In cases of long-standing balanitis epithelioma may develop.

Treatment.—Operation is necessary on account of any of these complications. Gradual dilatation of the orifice by means of forceps is tedious and unsatisfactory.

Two methods of **circumcision** are in use: 1. A pair of forceps is placed in the orifice of the foreskin and gentle traction exerted so that the foreskin is pulled forwards. A circumcision clamp (of which there are many varieties) is put obliquely on the foreskin parallel to the corona glandis, if this can be felt, and just beyond the edge of the glans penis. The clamp is held in the left hand and the forceps and clamp are cut off with a scalpel, the edge of which is kept close to the clamp. The skin retracts and the mucous membrane still covers the glans. The edge of this is picked up with forceps, and is cut along the dorsum to the corona and stripped off the glans until the coronal sulcus with yellow smegma is exposed. The redundant mucous membrane is then clipped away. Four bleeding-points will usually be found—a dorsal, two lateral, and a frænal. If the bleeding from these does not quickly cease, they are clamped and tied with fine catgut, and catgut stitches are then inserted through the mucous membrane and skin, bringing them into accurate apposition.

In children the wound should be thickly dusted with boric powder; no dressing is necessary. In adults a dressing of moist antiseptic gauze is kept in position with a bandage. After twenty-four hours the most comfortable dressing is boric or hazeline ointment spread on lint.

2. A preferable method is the following: The foreskin is retracted until the orifice is tense, and on the edge of this three pairs of fine-toothed forceps are placed—two close together on each side of the median line dorsally, and one at the middle line

ventrally. These are raiséd and the foreskin is separated .from the glans with a director. With a sharp-pointed pair of scissors the fores'in is slit up the middle line on the dorsum as far as the postcoronal sulcus, the edge of each flap thus formed being held by one of the pairs of forceps (Fig. 261). The flaps are well stripped off the glans and corona, and from the end of the dorsal incision a

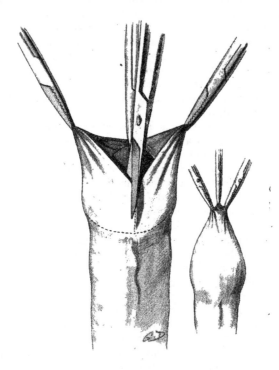

Fig. 261.—Circumcision.

On the right, a dorsal view of the penis with forceps in position, two pairs close together at the dorsal and one pair at the frænal margin of orifice of foreskin. On the left, the foreskin is being cut along the dorsum and the further incisions are marked by dotted lines.

second is carried round one flap of foreskin, leaving just a narrow ledge of mucous membrane below the corona (Fig. 262). This flap is cut away, leaving the lower pair of forceps attached. The same incision is carried round the second side, this time cutting away the two remaining pairs of forceps (Fig. 263).

Complications of circumcision.—1. Insufficient removal of the foreskin, with recontraction.

2. Injury to the glans.

3. Removal of too much skin or of a collar of skin while that at the orifice is left. These complications occur in the clamp method, and are avoided in the second method. The desire to "save something of the foreskin" is a fruitful source of trouble and recontraction. Hæmorrhage may occur in the subjects of hæmophilia, and may be fatal. Jacobson quotes the case of four

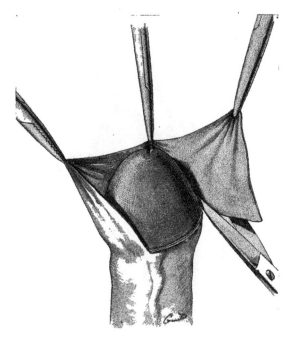

Fig. 262.—Circumcision, dorsal view.

The incision is being carried round the right side, close to the corona glandis.

Jewish infants, each of them descended from a different grandchild of a common ancestress through the female line, four generations back, who died from hæmorrhage consequent on circumcision. Pressure, hot lotion, and suprarenal extract should be used in oozing due to hæmophilia.

PARAPHIMOSIS

This is a complication of phimosis. The foreskin is retracted and the narrow opening is drawn over the corona glandis and cannot be returned. Balanitis is frequently present as a complication.

The orifice of the foreskin is usually rigid, and may either be pulled directly. back until it slips over the corona or may be rolled back and the foreskin reversed as in normal retraction. When paraphimosis has developed there is seen a thick œdematous collar of mucous membrane behind the corona, which may become deepred or even purple. Behind this is a deep sulcus, and there may be another collar, less prominent, above this, and sometimes a

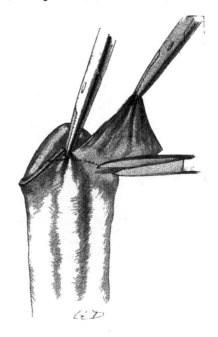

Fig. 263.—Circumcision, ventral view.

The right wing of the foreskin has been removed, and the removal of the left wing is nearly complete. The remaining part of the incision passes below the forceps, as indicated by the dotted line. ꞌ

second sulcus. The glans is congested, deep-red or purple. The site of strangulation may be immediately behind the glans or farther back. Rarely a chronic form is observed following the acute, and the thickening takes the form of a solid œdema.

If left untreated the acute form goes on to ulceration, and relief may be obtained by ulceration of the constriction; very rarely the glans becomes gangrenous.

Treatment.—Immediate reduction should be carried out

whenever possible. The patient may require a general anæsthetic. The penis is grasped between the first and second fingers of one hand on each side, and with both thumbs pressing upon the glans. The œdematous collar is pulled forwards, while at the same time the glans is pressed back. The traction is more important than the pressure. The œdematous folds may be punctured with a needle. The application of a layer of lint soaked in adrenalin (1 in 1,000) and cocaine (10 per cent.) may reduce the congestion of the parts and aid reduction.

If these measures fail a longitudinal incision should be made on the dorsum of the penis through the œdematous folds and the constricting rings. Secondary incisions may be made to relieve œdema.

LITERATURE

Beck, *Med. News,* 1901, p. 451.
Collier, *Brit. Med. Journ.,* 1889, i. 409.
Corner, *Male Diseases in General Practice.* 1910.
Goschler, *Vierteljahrsch. f. pract. Heilk.,* 1857, S. 89.
Hart, *Lancet,* 1866, i. 71.
Jacobson, *Diseases of the Male Organs of Generation,* p. 633. 1893.
Lorthior, *Centralbl. f. d. Krankh. d. Harn- u. Sex.-Org.,* 1901, p. 381.
Murphy, *Brit. Med. Journ.,* 1885, ii. 62.
Neugebauer, *Wien. klin. Runds.,* 1902, p. 631.
Sangalli, *Ann. d. Mal. d. Org. Gén.-Urin.,* 1895, p. 478.

INJURIES OF THE PENIS

Wounds of the penis are usually incised, rarely punctured, and are produced intentionally in certain sects, maliciously from jealousy, or by barbarians in war, or accidentally.

In deep wounds the hæmorrhage is abundant if the penis is erect at the time of the injury, but may be comparatively trifling if it is flaccid.

When the organ is incompletely severed the urethra may escape. If the urethra is cut across, the end will retract and retention of urine occurs. In complete amputation the hæmorrhage should be arrested by ligature of the arteries and by stitching the edges of the sheath of the corpora cavernosa together. The urethra must be identified and drawn up and stitched to the skin, and a catheter tied in.

In partial section the hæmorrhage should be controlled by accurate suture of the fibrous sheath of the corpora cavernosa. When the penis remains attached by a small segment a catheter should be tied in and an attempt made by accurate suture to obtain adhesion. The functional result, though not at first good, may, after some months, be satisfactory. During convalescence the patient should be kept under the influence of morphia, belladonna, and bromides in order to prevent erections, which seriously interfere with healing.   .

The skin of the penis and scrotum may be torn away by the bite of an animal. Immediate Thiersch grafting should be done to prevent cicatricial contraction, or a transverse flap of skin may be raised on the pubes and the penis, with a catheter in the urethra inserted under this. When the flap is adherent to the under surface of the penis it is cut from the abdominal wall, leaving sufficient to wrap around the penis. The two wings meet on the dorsum.

Wounds from firearms are rare, and the indications for treatment are the same as those from cutting instruments. Contusion is seldom met with, and, apart from the injury to the urethra which may result, recovery is usually rapid. Gentle pressure and the use of an ice-bag are indicated.

Fracture of the erect penis may occur during connection. In some cases periurethral induration around a stricture has been a predisposing cause. When the accident has occurred pain was felt so severe as to cause fainting. The pain radiates to the pubis and groin. Several patients have stated that there was a sound like the breaking of a glass rod. The organ suddenly becomes flaccid, and this is followed by enormous swelling from infiltration with blood. If rupture of the urethra takes place there are hæmorrhage from the meatus, pain on micturition, and infiltration of urine or complete retention.

The sequelæ of this injury are traumatic stricture and impairment of erection. The proximal segment becomes erect, but the distal segment beyond the site of fracture remains flaccid or may become erect later. In order to avoid these results, Reclus advises that the fracture be treated by incision, clearing out of the clots, and suture.

Dislocation of the penis has been recorded in a few cases. The skin of the penis remains in position, the attachment of the skin behind the glans is torn, and the glans and body are displaced into the subcutaneous tissue of the pubes, scrotum, or groin.

Rupture of the urethra and subsequent infiltration of urine may complicate the diagnosis. The penis should be replaced in its cutaneous sheath and retained by stitches, and the urethra repaired.

Strangulation of the penis may occur by accident, as from the use of a jugum penis for the treatment of incontinence, or in erotic individuals from instruments such as a ring. Congestion and œdema of the peripheral segment results, the penis becomes enormously swollen, and retention of urine follows. If relief is not obtained sloughing takes place, and urinary fistulæ may form. The treatment consists in removing the strangulating body by the use of vaseline and massage in the earlier stages, or by cutting it across with a chisel or pliers if this is possible.

LITERATURE

Bagaraze, *Ann. d. Mal. d. Org. Gén.-Urin.,* 1908, p. 1028.
Duplay et **Reclus,** *Traité.de Chir.,* 1899, vii. 1250.
Hagen, Bessel, *Arch. f. klin. Chir.,* 1902, p. 75.
Powers, *Ann. of Surg.,* 1909, p. 238.

PREPUTIAL CALCULI

A high degree of phimosis is present, and almost all the cases occur in adults, children being rarely affected. The number of calculi varies. Lewin found from 1 to 10 calculi in six cases, 15 in one case, and between 38 and 70 in eight cases; Lloyd found 11, weighing 70 gr.; Jacobson 11, Corney 22, and Vincent 200 small calculi. The size varies from that of a pea to that of a man's fist.·

The composition varies according to the origin. Kaufmann divides the calculi into three classes :

1. Preputial calculi composed of smegma impregnated with lime salts. These are soft, friable masses consisting of epithelium, cholesterin, fatty acids, and lime, with numerous bacteria.

2. Preputial calculi arising in stagnant urine in the prepuce. These are harder, and may show some lamination. The chief constituents are uric acid, calcium phosphate, ammonio-magnesium sulphate, with traces of carbonic, oxalic, and sulphuric acids.

3. Migrating vesical calculi, which are arrested in the dilated foreskin. A calculus may ulcerate through the floor of the fossa navicularis and lodge in the preputial sac.

The constant symptom is a copious purulent discharge, and pain and difficult micturition are frequently present. The calculi can be felt as a hard mass in the foreskin, and grating can in many cases be elicited.

LITERATURE

Bland-Sutton, *Brit. Med. Journ.,* 1907, i. 1412.
Blodgett, *Boston Med. and Surg. Journ.,* June 21, 1900.
Croft, *Trans. Clin. Soc.,* xviii. 8.
Kaufmann, *Verletzungen und Krankheiten der männlichen Harnröhre und Penis.* 1886.
Lloyd, *Brit. Med. Journ.,* 1882, ii. 580.
Louis, *La Grèce Médicale,* 1899, No. 7.
Sutton, Walton, *Lancet,* Aug. 18, 1900.

CHAPTER LXXII

BALANITIS—HERPES PRÆPUTIALIS — ŒDEMA OF PENIS—PRIAPISM—FIBROUS CAVERNOSITIS— TUMOURS

BALANITIS—BALANO-POSTHITIS

BALANITIS means inflammation of the glans, and posthitis inflammation of the foreskin.

Apart from venereal balano-posthitis, which is the most common variety, inflammation under the foreskin may arise from a number of causes. Non-venereal balanitis is subacute. It occurs in the subjects of phimosis, and may result from intercourse with a woman affected with leucorrhœa, or from want of cleanliness, leading to accumulation and decomposition of smegma. It is frequently met with in patients who are looked upon as gouty.

Balanitis also occurs in diabetes, and the inflammation may spread to the penis and scrotum, causing a very painful form of eczema.

The inflammation usually commences in the sulcus behind the corona glandis, and leads to constant burning and itching. A purulent discharge appears from under the foreskin, and if neglected this may become fetid. Superficial ulceration may be found on the glans and inner surface of the foreskin.

A rare form occurs with intensely red shining patches on the surface of the glans. The margin is sharply defined, and there is no irritation or uneasiness. Long-continued balanitis is a predisposing cause of epithelioma. Diphtheritic and croupous forms have been described.

Treatment.—Occasional attacks of balanitis are treated by washing with a solution of bicarbonate of soda or lead lotion, or, after washing the parts thoroughly with soap and water and carefully drying, tannin and glycerine (glycerinum acidi tannici, B.P.) should be applied with a cotton-wool dab; and this is repeated night and morning. The general health and diet should receive attention, and the urine should be tested for sugar. Diabetic balanitis may be treated on the same lines, or a dusting powder may be prescribed containing boric acid, starch, and zinc oxide, or protection to the skin given by smearing with zinc oxide ointment. The effect of general and dietetic treatment is very marked in these cases. In persistent balanitis circumcision should be recommended, and the danger of the development of epithelioma pointed out.

In diabetic balanitis operation should, if possible, be avoided. In persistent and severe cases circumcision should be done under local anæsthesia and with the strictest antiseptic precautions.

HERPES PRÆPUTIALIS

True herpes zoster of the penis is a rare condition, and differs in no way from that seen elsewhere.

The common variety has been called catarrhal herpes, and is an erythema (Jacobson).

The disease occurs in young or middle-aged men. The onset may be preceded by digestive disturbance, such as dyspepsia and flatulence, and in recurrent attacks these prodromata may be recognized by the patient as a certain warning of the onset. Nervous depression may also be noted. There is intense itching and burning, and a red blush appears on the inner surface of the foreskin near the sulcus, and less frequently on the glans or on the cutaneous surface of the foreskin or the skin of the penis. A group of tiny papules appear, and these become vesicles and then pustules. If protected, they shrivel in a few days and a dark scab forms, which is thrown off, and healing has taken place. Usually friction of the clothes rubs off the pustules, and tiny round punched-out superficial ulcers remain in groups. The "attack" lasts five to six days, but, if care is not taken to protect the ulcers and observe strict cleanliness, secondary infections may prolong the disease. In such cases there are enlargement and tenderness of the groin glands. There is a tendency for herpes to recur at definite intervals, usually of a few weeks or months, and it may persist in this intermittent form for some years, gradually diminishing in frequency and severity, and eventually disappearing. The immediate cause of these attacks may occasionally be ascribed to dietetic errors or sexual excesses.

The relation of herpes to venereal diseases has been much discussed. Syphilitic patients and those who have suffered from soft sore are more liable to develop this condition, but it frequently occurs when there has never been venereal disease, and occasionally when there has been no sexual intercourse.

Diagnosis.—In the ulcerative stage herpes is distinguished from soft chancre by the sequence of papule, vesicle, and pustule, the grouping of the ulcers, and the slight reaction of the surrounding tissues, and frequently by the history of previous attacks; from syphilitic chancre by the absence of induration and of adenitis, the history of the local conditions, and occurrence within a few days after connection. Scrapings of the surface may be examined for the Spirochæta pallida.

Treatment.—Careful washing, followed by the use of an ointment or dusting powder as in balanitis, to act as a protective layer, prevents infection and spread. Lead lotion may be used, and forms a deposit on the ulcer. The most efficacious treatment is to apply nitrate of silver solution (2–4 per cent.) on a pledget of cotton-wool so that a white layer forms over each ulcer. One application may suffice. Arsenic is recommended as a preventive medicine, and should be tried in recurring cases.

Circumcision has not given good results, the vesicles appearing elsewhere.

ŒDEMA OF THE PENIS

Acute œdema of the skin of the penis, usually confined to the foreskin but occasionally involving the whole penis, is observed in venereal diseases, and occurs as a result of paraphimosis, compression of the penis by rings, extravasation of urine, and as an insignificant part of œdema due to systemic diseases.

In rare instances acute œdema develops as an isolated phenomenon without apparent cause. I have met with three cases in which sudden acute œdema occurred in young and middle-aged men. There had been no venereal disease for ten or more years. The onset was sudden and without any warning. The skin was shiny and translucent in appearance, and the œdema ceased at the base of the penis. After lasting from three days to a week the swelling rapidly or gradually disappeared. No evidence of phlebitis of the dorsal vein or any cause for lymphatic obstruction could be found. In one case there had been several attacks at intervals of a year or more.

Chronic œdema of the penis may occur as a part of elephantiasis. Where extensive scarring is present in both groins from bygone suppuration or (in one case) extensive dissection of tuberculous glands, chronic œdema of the penis may be present (Fig. 264); or the lymphatic drain may suffice under ordinary conditions, but is inadequate when some slight attack of balanitis occurs and the penile skin swells up from time to time.

Treatment.—No local treatment is usually necessary in idiopathic œdema; but multiple punctures may afford relief. In more chronic conditions all causes of local irritation should be removed and massage applied to the groins. Lymphatic drainage by buried strands of catgut, after Handley's method for œdema of the arm in breast tumours, may be tried.

PRIAPISM

This term denotes continuous erection, which is usually extremely painful, and is unaccompanied by desire or emission.

Some local cause may be present, such as injury, acute or chronic inflammation, or new growth. Or priapism may be due

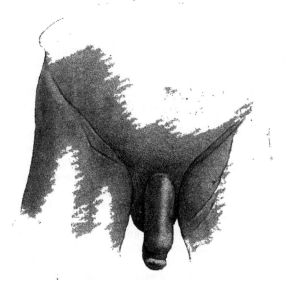

Fig. 264.—Chronic œdema of penis due to extensive scarring following operations on both groins.

to disease of or injury to the cervical or upper dorsal spinal cord. In some cases it is reflex : Hobbs describes a case having a nasal origin. It occurs occasionally in leukæmia. The cause is at present obscure. Priapism has been ascribed to thrombosis, to nervous influences, to the pressure of a hæmatoma on the veins, and to vaso-motor influences. The onset is often sudden. The corpora cavernosa only are rigid. There is constant severe pain; and micturition is difficult. The condition may last several weeks— three or six—or even months, but recovery usually takes place.

Treatment.—Sedatives (bromides, camphor, morphia, chloral) may be tried and ice-bags applied, but these measures have proved ineffectual. Incision of the corpora cavernosa and evacuation of the contents has been immediately successful, but the ultimate result has been a complete loss of erection.

FIBROUS CAVERNOSITIS—INDURATION OF THE CORPORA CAVERNOSA

In this condition there is a fibrous induration of the sheath or in the substance of the corpora cavernosa.

Etiology.—The average age in 20 cases of primary indurative cavernositis under my care was 56½ years; one patient was aged 30, and one 48; the others were all over 50. There are two distinct classes of cavernositis—that which follows a recognized local cause, and that which appears spontaneously.

1. *Secondary indurative cavernositis.*—Gonorrhœal urethritis is the most frequent cause, and the induration succeeds an old-standing periurethritis. Gummatous infiltration is a less common cause (cavernositis syphilitica). Induration of the cavernous tissue may follow injury such as contusions or fracture of the penis or wounds.

2. *Primary indurative cavernositis* was first described by Kirby, of Dublin, and is comparatively uncommon. I have notes of 20 cases that have passed through my hands in eight years.

Gout, diabetes, or rheumatism is sometimes present, and the sclerosis may be ascribed to one of these diseases. Tuffier in 26 collected cases found gout in 15 and diabetes in 11. Dupuytren's contraction may be present.

Smallpox, typhoid fever, pyæmia, and exanthemata have been noted as causes, but in many cases no cause, either local or general, can be found to explain the sclerosis. Sacher gives the frequency of different causes in 187 collected cases as follows: Diabetes and gout 23·5 per cent., syphilis 11 per cent., gonorrhœa 9 per cent., traumatism 8·2 per cent., rheumatism 2·1 per cent.

Pathological anatomy.—The induration may be in the form of a nodule, a plaque, or a cord. The nodule is rounded, regular, and solitary or multiple, and several may coalesce. Plaques vary in thickness, and cords are frequently nodular and situated in the middle line on the dorsum. They are hard, sometimes cartilaginous in consistence. When due to fracture, stricture, or other local cause, the induration may involve the tunica albuginea of the corpus cavernosum and extend into the cavernous tissue. In primary indurative cavernositis the sclerosis is confined to the tunica albuginea and the septum. In the primary form the induration consists of tissue similar to a cheloid. There is hard, fibrous tissue with embryonic cells and very few blood-vessels.

Symptoms.—The patient complains of curvature of the penis during erection (*le strabisme pénien*). The curve may be to the right or the left, or towards the pubes, or very rarely downwards, according to the position of the induration, which occupies the concavity of the curve.

There may be pain on erection, and connection is frequently impossible. Delayed ejaculation is often present. In severe cases

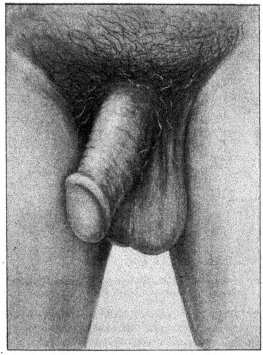

Fig. 265.—Indurative cavernositis of sheath of left corpus cavernosum ; penis displaced to right.

there is distortion of the penis in the flaccid condition, the penis being turned towards the sound side (Fig. 265). In some cases the portion of the penis beyond the indurated mass remains flaccid when erection occurs.

The onset is insidious in primary sclerosis, but may be sudden in traumatic cases. There is a hard nodule or a plaque in the sheath of the corpus cavernosum or along the septum.

The most frequent situation is at the base of the penis on the

3 c

dorsum, and there is usually a saddle-shaped plaque, which spreads laterally, involving part of the circumference. (Fig. 266.) With or without this plaque a hard cord may be felt along the middle line on the dorsum. Plaques or nodules may be found at other parts of the corpora.. The anterior ends of these bodies may be affected so that the mass feels buried in the base of the glans penis. The skin is freely movable over the mass.

The sclerosis may extend to the under surface of the corpora cavernosa, and the urethra and corpus spongiosum are felt like a gutter between the lateral masses.

Diagnosis.—The diagnosis is not difficult. The cartilaginous

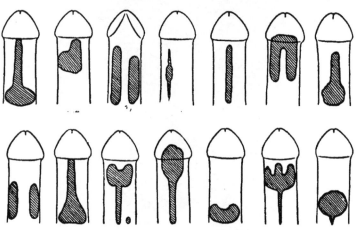

Fig. 266.—Diagrams of distribution of fibrous induration in 14 consecutive cases of indurative cavernositis.

hardness, the absence of signs of syphilis, and the effect of anti-syphilitic treatment distinguish the indurations from gummata. Malignant infiltration of the corpus cavernosum is always secondary to epithelioma of the glans or prepuce; it is more deeply seated in the cavernous tissue, and has a rapid course.

Course and prognosis.—Primary indurative cavernositis slowly extends, but after a time becomes stationary. There is no tendency to resolution. Cartilaginous transformation appears to have occurred in one instance. Ossification has not been authenticated. Sachs found calcification in three cases on X-ray examination.

Treatment.—The effect of treatment is disappointing. Iodide of potash and arsenic have been recommended, and local applica-tions of iodide of potash, mercury, iodoform, and salicylates are used. Applications of the faradic current have been unsuccessful. Electrolysis has in rare cases been followed by improvement. Subcutaneous injections of thiosinamin ethyl iodide, 3 gr., or iodolysin, 15 minims, may be tried. In one case I used local injections into the fibrous mass of fibrolysin (thiosinamin and sodium salicylate, 15 per cent.), 2–3 c.c., and the induration disappeared. Excision has not been successful in relieving the deformity.

LITERATURE

Hopezansky, *Wien. klin. Woch.,* **xxi.** 318.
Kirby, *Dublin Med. Journ.,* 1850.
Trillat, *Gaz. des Hôp.,* 1902, 1045.
Whitacre, *N.Y. Med. Journ.,* March 19, 1910.
Wolbarst, *Therap. Gaz.,* June 15, 1900.

TUMOURS OF THE PENIS

Dermoid cysts are very rare. They occur as small pea-sized bodies in or close to the median raphe on the under surface of the penis. In a young man aged 31, under my care, there was a raised, round swelling the size of a small pea in the skin immediately to the left of the median raphe, 1 in. behind the glans on the ventral surface of the penis. (Fig. 267.) He had noticed it since it began to discharge a little clear fluid eight years previously. There was a tiny granular bud on its surface, and a little clear fluid could be expressed. On section the cyst wall consisted of squamous epithelium.

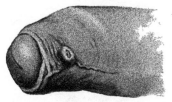

Fig. 267.—Dermoid cyst of penis; displaced raphe.

Mucous cysts have also been described, and sebaceous cysts are sometimes seen.

A horn composed of epithelium growing from the glans penis has been described. Such cases are pathological curiosities.

Examples of lipoma, fibroma, angioma, and chondroma have been recorded.

PAPILLOMA

Soft warts are usually venereal in origin, but occasionally are non-venereal. They are usually collected in the sulcus behind the corona glandis or on the foreskin. (Fig. 268.) The skin of the glans may also be affected. They are soft and friable, and bleed easily. It has been shown that these papillomas may become malignant and infiltrate the penis.

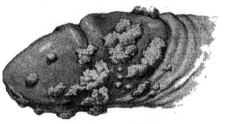

Fig. 268.—Venereal warts on glans penis and foreskin.

Treatment. — The warts should be removed with curved scissors, and solid nitrate of silver applied to the base. Pressure should be used to control bleeding, and adrenalin may be applied to stop any troublesome oozing.

EPITHELIOMA

Malignant growths of the penis are of comparatively frequent occurrence. They form 2½–3 per cent. of all malignant growths.

Etiology. — The disease is chiefly met with between the ages of 50 and 70, is rare before 45, and is most common at the age of 55. Cases occurring at the ages of 21 and 30 have, however, been described.

Phimosis is an important predisposing cause. Epithelioma frequently develops where phimosis is present. Demarquay found that 42 out of 59 cases of epithelioma of the penis had phimosis. Epithelioma in this situation is very rare among the Jews (Travers).

The long foreskin encourages the development of chronic balanitis, and

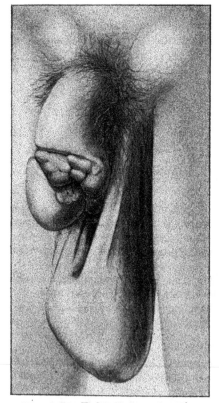

Fig. 269.—Epithelioma of penis.

long-continued balanitis attributable to this cause, or of the type ascribed to gout, is a predisposing cause of epithelioma.

Epithelioma may develop in venereal warts, scars from old

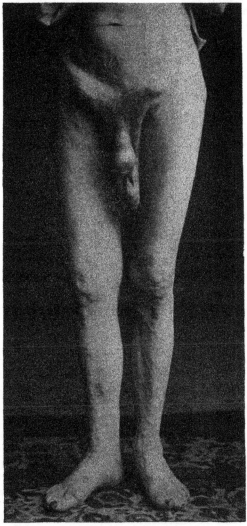

Fig. 270.—Epithelioma of penis, enlargement of groin glands, œdema of right leg.

chancres, or in gummatous induration. Leucoplakia is a rare precancerous condition.

Injuries such as tearing of the frænum have been the starting-point of malignant disease. Infection of the glans penis from carcinoma of the cervix has been recorded in isolated cases.

Pathology.—The epithelioma commences more frequently on the foreskin than on the glans penis, but when the patient comes under observation both are usually affected. Kaufmann states

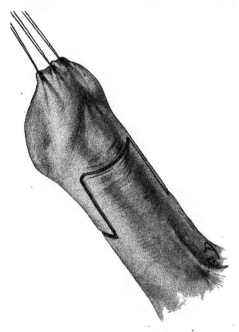

Fig. 271.—Partial amputation of penis for epithelioma of glans. The orifice of the foreskin has been closed over the growth with stitches, which are used for traction. Incision for amputation with ventral flap.

that out of 33 cases the foreskin was first affected in 20 and the glans in 13. The growth usually begins as a wart (87 per cent.), as a deeply seated nodule, or in an ulcer. In the majority of cases it forms a papillomatous or cauliflower-like growth, or it may be composed of nodules. (Fig. 269.) A phimosis is usually present and covers the growth. The end of the penis becomes greatly increased in circumference and club-like, and it is frequently impossible to draw back the foreskin in order to inspect the growth.

A less common form is an epitheliomatous ulcer with irregular depressed base and indurated rolled-over margin. A rare form infiltrates the glans penis.

Extension takes place along the lymphatic channels or into the corpora cavernosa. The lymphatics pass along the dorsum and sides of the penis to the innermost group of the horizontal groin glands, which lie in close relation to the internal saphena

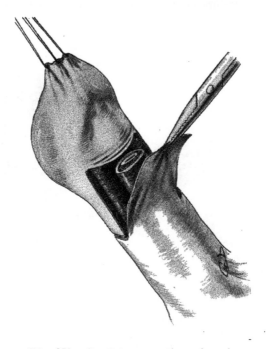

Fig. 272.—Partial amputation of penis.

Ventral flap formed; corpus spongiosum with urethra cut across and dissected up.

vein and the femoral vein. Lymphatic spread takes place comparatively early. Kaufmann found that the glands were normal in only 8 out of 48 cases. The fibrous sheath of the corpora cavernosa resists the invasion of the growth for a long time, but eventually it is destroyed, and in a few cases the cavernous tissue is invaded. Narrowing of the urethra may be observed, but the wall is rarely destroyed. Metastases to viscera such as the lungs and liver are rare.

Histologically the growth is a squamous epithelioma.

Symptoms.—When phimosis is present the patient complains of a purulent and sometimes fetid discharge, which is frequently blood-stained. As already mentioned, there is enlargement of the end of the penis, which may assume very considerable proportions. (Fig. 270.) Only partial retraction of the foreskin is possible, and an irregular warty bleeding mass is seen. In the ulcerative form an epitheliomatous ulcer with irregular base and heaped-up, sometimes irregular and warty edges, is seen. The meatus of the urethra is in some cases invaded. There may be

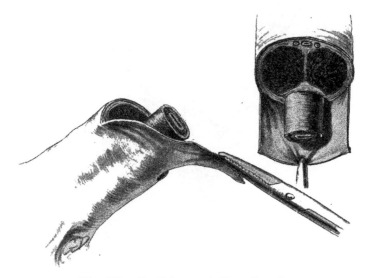

Fig. 273.—Partial amputation of penis.

Two views of stump. The severed corpora cavernosa and the longer corpus spongiosum containing the urethra are seen.

difficulty in micturition. Pain is usually absent until a late stage, and when it appears is of a neuralgic character, radiating to the groins and down the thighs. Hæmorrhage, beyond staining the purulent discharge, is exceptional. Painful erections may occur. The lymphatic glands of the groin are enlarged at a comparatively early period. Cachexia occurs late. The duration extends over two, three, or four years.

Diagnosis.—When phimosis is present the fetid sanious discharge and enlargement of the glans penis may lead to a diagnosis, but it may be necessary to slit up the foreskin before the nature of the disease is evident.

If any doubt remains a portion of the growth should be removed and examined microscopically.

Treatment.—Radical treatment is indicated in all but advanced cases. It is contra-indicated by cachexia, visceral metastases, and any considerable metastasis to the lymph-glands.

Amputation of the penis.—This may be performed by means of a flap or circular or elliptical incision. A tourniquet (a rubber catheter) is placed around the base of the penis and a flap marked out on the dorsum of the organ extending on each side to half the circumference. (Fig. 271.) This is raised from the tunica albuginea, and the skin of the ventral surface, the corpus spongiosum, and the urethra are cut across at the level of the base of the flap, and the urethra is dissected out. (Fig. 272.) Ligatures are placed on the dorsal vessels and the principal arteries of the corpora cavernosa. The tunica albuginea of the corpora cavernosa is united across the face of the cut cavernous tissue. (Fig. 273.) The dorsal flap is punctured near its lower extremity, and the urethra brought through this opening, split, and stitched down. The skin wound is then closed. (Fig. 274.) In the elliptical incision the urethra is cut obliquely and the skin united to the edge of the urethra all round. This operation should be performed when the disease is confined to the glans penis or extends less than an inch beyond it. The inguinal lymph-glands should be removed.

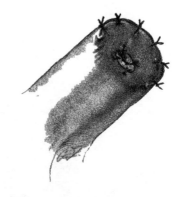

Fig. 274.—Partial amputation of penis.

Flap covering end of stump and urethra appearing through opening near base of flap.

Complete amputation of the penis: Thiersch-Gould operation. (Figs. 275-9.) The patient is placed in the lithotomy position and an elliptical incision made around the base of the penis and carried down along the middle line to the mid-point of the perineum. A sound is placed in the urethra, the scrotum is split, and the bulb exposed. The urethra is cut across with about 2 in. of the bulb, and left hanging. The suspensory ligament is cut across and the penis dissected downwards, the crura being detached from the rami of the pubes and ischium by means of a raspatory. The scrotum is brought together, and the urethra brought down to the perineal part of the wound, trimmed, and stitched to the skin. The groin glands are then removed by a curved incision with the convexity downwards. The dissection

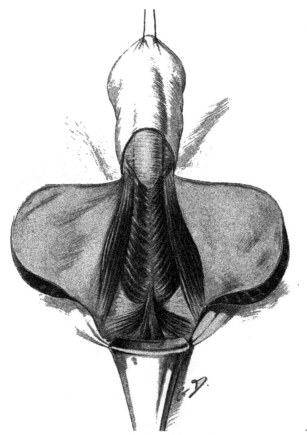

Fig. 275.—Complete amputation of penis (Thiersch-Gould operation).

Scrotum split and retracted ; incision carried round base of penis.

of the fat and glands proceeds from without inwards, and it may be necessary to ligature the internal saphenous vein.

Total emasculation is sometimes performed, and consists in removal of the testicles and the penis.

Results.—Good results are obtained in suitable cases by partial or by total amputation of the penis combined with removal of the groin glands. Of 100 cases Dellinger-Barney found recurrence in 39 per cent. in the first year and 16 per cent. in the second and third years. Only 12 per cent. of cases showed recurrence

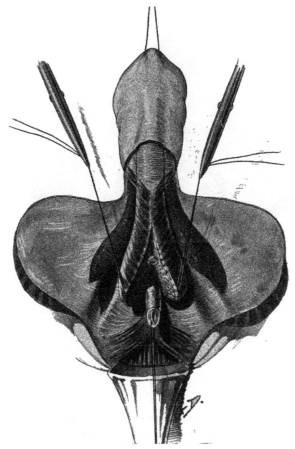

Fig. 276.—Complete amputation of penis.

Crura dissected up, bulb split, and urethra cut across.

after five years. Survivals of three to ten years are not uncommon, and survivals of twelve and twenty-nine years are also recorded.

A patient who came under my care is well without recurrence six years after partial amputation of the penis with removal of epitheliomatous groin glands. In total emasculation for very extensive growths survivals without recurrence for one year, fifteen and sixteen months, and three years have been recorded.

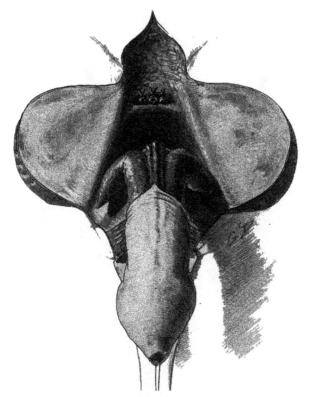

Fig. 277.—Complete amputation of penis.

Penis turned down and dissected off pubic symphysis and triangular ligament; dorsal Vessels ligatured.

Sarcoma and Endothelioma

These growths are very rare. Legueu found only 18 recorded cases of sarcoma. The growth is round-celled, mixed-celled, or spindle-celled, and melanotic sarcoma has been observed. Lymph-glands, lungs, and liver are early involved. Sarcoma is much more rapid in its development and course than epithelioma.

The enlarged glands may reach an enormous size. A few cases of endothelioma have been recorded. The results of operation for sarcoma have been very unsatisfactory, the majority of the patients dying within a few months.

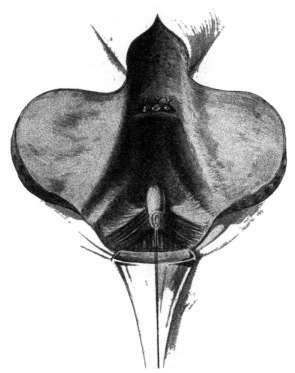

Fig. 278.—Complete amputation of penis.

Penis has been removed ; stump of urethra is seen.

LITERATURE

Bland-Sutton, *Tumours, Innocent and Malignant,* 5th ed. 1911.
Cholzoff, *Zeits. f. Urol.,* 1910, p. 649.
Colmers, *Zieglers Beitr.,* 1903, p. 285.
Dellinger-Barney, *Ann. of Surg.,* 1907, p. 890.
Demarquay, *Maladies Chirurgicales de Pénis.* 1877.
Englisch, *Centralbl. f. d. Krankh. d. Harn- u. Sex.-Org.,* 1902, p. 36.

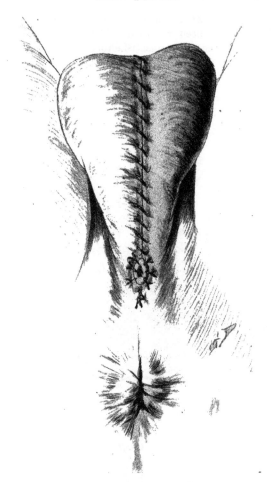

Fig. 279.—Complete amputation of penis.

Operation completed ; urethra implanted in perineum.

LITERATURE (*continued*)

Jacobson, *Diseases of the Male Organs of Generation.* 1893.
Kaufmann, *Verletzungen und Krankheiten der männlichen Harnröhre und Penis.*
    1886.
Kuttner, *Beitr. z. klin. Chir.,* 1900.
Legueu, II*e* Congrès de la Soc. Internat. de Chir., 1908, ii. 63.
Mermet, *Rev. de Chir.,* 1895, p. 382.
Shield, *Lancet,* 1900, i. 75.
Steiner, *Deuts. Zeits. f. Chir.,* 1906, p. 363.

INDEX

PRINTED BY
CASSELL & COMPANY, LIMITED, LA BELLE SAUVAGE
LONDON, E.C.

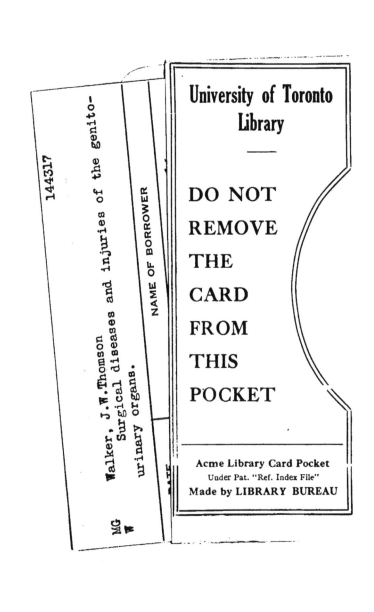